Coronary Heart Disease & Risk Factor Management

A NURSING PERSPE

Coronary Heart Disease & Risk Factor Management

A NURSING PERSPECTIVE

Nalini Jairath, M.Sc.N., Ph.D.
Associate Professor and Senior Research Faculty
School of Nursing
University of Maryland
Baltimore, Maryland

W.B. SAUNDERS COMPANY
A Division of Harcourt Brace & Company
Philadelphia   London   Toronto   Montreal   Sydney   Tokyo

W.B. SAUNDERS COMPANY
A Division of Harcourt Brace & Company

The Curtis Center
Independence Square West
Philadelphia, Pennsylvania 19106

Library of Congress Cataloging-in-Publication Data

Jairath, Nalini.
Coronary heart disease & risk factor management: a nursing perspective / Nalini Jairath.

p.   cm.

ISBN 0-7216-6855-0

1. Coronary heart disease—Risk factors.   2. Coronary heart
   disease—Prevention.   3. Coronary heart disease—Nursing.

I. Title.
[DNLM: 1. Coronary Disease—prevention & control nurses' instruction.   2. Risk
Factors nurses' instruction.   WG300J25c 1999]

RC685.C6J35 1999   616.1′23—dc21

DNLM/DLC   98–36804

CORONARY HEART DISEASE & RISK FACTOR MANAGEMENT:
A Nursing Perspective   ISBN 0-7216-6855-0

Printed in the United States of America.

Last digit is the print number: 9   8   7   6   5   4   3   2   1

My husband, Pankaj Topiwala, my children Jay and Raj, and my mother Juanita Jairath all hold a special place in my heart. In addition, I must thank Dr. Jacqueline Chapman, who has been a mentor and a role model since we first met when I enrolled in the Master's Program at the University of Toronto so many years ago.

CONTRIBUTORS

Howard Brunt, R.N., Ph.D.
Acting Associate Vice President, Research, Office of Research Administration;
Professor of Nursing, University of Victoria, Victoria, British Columbia, Canada
Risk and Coronary Heart Disease

Aggie Casey, R.N., M.S.
Associate Professor of Medicine, Harvard Medical School; Director, Cardiac Wellness
Program, Beth Isreal–Deaconess Medical Center, Boston, Massachusetts
Stress Management

Judy Costello, M.Sc.N.
Clinical Associate, School of Nursing, University of Toronto; Director of Nursing,
Surgical Directorate, The Toronto Hospital, Toronto, Ontario, Canada
Cardioprotective Agents: Antioxidants and Alcohol

Donna D'Agostino, R.N., M.S.N.
Department of Medicine, University of Massachusetts Medical Center, Worcester,
Massachusetts
Cardioprotective Agents: Antioxidants and Alcohol

Catherine Daly-Nee R.N.-C., M.S., N.P.
Acute Care Nurse Practitioner, Cardiac Access Unit, Massachusetts General Hospital,
Boston, Massachusetts
Risk and Coronary Heart Disease

Pam Doyle, N.P., M.S.
Acute Care Nurse Practitioner, Bone Marrow Transplant, University of Massachusetts
Memorial Health Care, Worcester, Massachusetts
Women and Coronary Heart Disease

Michelle Fey, M.S., R.N.

Acute Care Nurse Practitioner, Cardiothoracic/Surgical Intensive Care Unit, Hartford Hospital, Hartford, Connecticut

Communicating Risk to Patients

Margaret I. Fitch, R.N., Ph.D.

Assistant Professor, Faculty of Nursing, University of Toronto; Head, Oncology Nursing and Supportive Care, Toronto-Sunnybrook Regional Cancer Centre, Toronto, Ontario, Canada

Radiation-Induced Coronary Artery Disease

Glenys A. Hamilton, R.N., D.N.Sc., H.L.D. (hon.)

Nurse Researcher, Department of Nursing; Consultant, International Nursing, Center for Clinical & Professional Development, Massachusetts General Hospital, Boston, Massachusetts

Women and Coronary Heart Disease

James A. Fain, Ph.D., R.N., F.A.A.N.

Associate Professor/Director, Collaborative Ph.D. Nursing Program, University of Massachusetts Medical Center, Graduate School of Nursing, Worcester, Massachusetts

Diabetes

Nalini Jairath, M.Sc.N., Ph.D.

Associate Professor and Senior Research Faculty, School of Nursing, University of Maryland, Baltimore, Maryland

Risk and Coronary Heart Disease; Communicating Risk to Patients; Physical Activity

Satya S. Jonnalagadda, Ph.D.

Assistant Professor, Department of Nutrition, Georgia State University, Atlanta, Georgia

Dietary Factors

Elizabeth A. Keating, R.N., M.S.

Oncology Nurse Practitioner, University of Massachusetts Memorial Health Care, Worcester, Massachusetts

Radiation-Induced Coronary Artery Disease

Colleen Keller, R.N., Ph.D.

School of Nursing, The University of Texas Health Science Center at San Antonio, San Antonio, Texas

Ethnicity and Coronary Heart Disease

Susan L. Kozicz, R.N., M.S.

Acute Care Nurse Practitioner, Department of Cardiology, University of Massachusetts Memorial Health Care, Worcester, Massachusetts

Stress Management

Penny Kris-Etherton, Ph.D., R.D.

Distinguished Professor of Nutrition, Department of Nutrition, Pennsylvania State University, University Park, Pennsylvania
Dietary Factors

Lori Anne Lyne, M.S., R.N.

Nurse Practitioner, Baystate Medical Center, Springfield, Massachusetts
Physical Activity

Catherine Pianka, R.N., M.S.N.

University of Massachusetts at Worcester Graduate School of Nursing; Staff Nurse, Cardiothoracic Intensive Care Unit, University of Massachusetts Medical Center, Worcester, Massachusetts
Ethnicity and Coronary Heart Disease

Joseph S. Rossi, Ph.D.

Professor, University of Rhode Island; Director of Research, Cancer Prevention Research Center, University of Rhode Island, Kingston, Rhode Island
Concepts and Theoretical Models

Susan R. Rossi, Ph.D., R.N.

Adjunct Assistant Professor of Nursing, University of Rhode Island College of Nursing; Coordinator, Adherence and Education Programs, Rhode Island Public Health Partnership, University of Rhode Island, Kingston, Rhode Island
Concepts and Theoretical Models; Dietary Factors

Ellen Rukholm, M.Sc.N.

Associate Professor, School of Nursing, Laurentian University, Sudbury, Ontario, Canada
Children and Coronary Heart Disease

Annmarie Donahue Samar, R.N., M.S.

Instructor, Department of Nursing, Worcester State College; Staff Nurse, Critical Care Unit, University of Massachusetts Medical Center, Worcester, Massachusetts
The Pathogenesis of Atherosclerosis

Debra Lee Servello, R.N., M.S.

Cardiac Nurse Practitioner, The Miriam Hospital, Providence, Rhode Island
Blood Pressure Regulation

Kathleen H. Sims, M.S., N.P.

Associate Faculty, University of Massachusetts Graduate School of Nursing; Nurse Practitioner, Department of Cardiology, University of Massachusetts Memorial Health Care, Worcester, Massachusetts
Smoking Cessation

Donna Williams, M.S., R.N.

Regis College Instructor, Regis College, Weston; Cardiac Clinical Specialist, Caritas Norwood Hospital, Norwood, Massachusetts

Nursing Assessment

Donna M. Zucker, R.N., M.S.

Clinical Assistant Professor, University of Massachusetts School of Nursing; Program Coordinator, RN/BS Program, University of Massachusetts School of Nursing, Amherst, Massachusetts

Smoking Cessation

PREFACE

Coronary heart disease (CHD) transcends time and racial, cultural, economic, and geographic boundaries. In the United States, clinicians increasingly refer to CHD as an epidemic. Although this claim initially may seem hyperbolic, between one in four and one in five Americans dies of CHD or related cardiovascular diseases. As such, the need to reduce CHD becomes a national imperative.

Nurses have a long and impressive commitment to CHD risk reduction. In collaboration with other health professionals, we have been involved in early public health initiatives, have directed cardiac rehabilitation programs, and are now in the forefront of cardiac wellness programs. For patients suffering from acute CHD-related events or conditions, nurses at the bedside have often been the primary source of teaching and counseling regarding CHD risk-reduction strategies. We have much to be proud of but also much to learn.

Innovations in our understanding of CHD and CHD risk-reduction interventions continue to develop. Particularly promising is the research regarding vulnerable plaque and mechanisms and interventions for atherosclerotic plaque regression/stabilization. New contenders for official recognition as major CHD risk factors arise continually, along with current contenders, such as homocysteine and some of the apolipoproteins.

This book was created to meet the needs of nurses for a comprehensive scholarly yet practical source of information regarding CHD risk and risk-reduction strategies. To be an effective and equal member of an interdisciplinary health-care team, nurses must share a core knowledge base with physicians, dietitians, exercise physiologists, and other professional colleagues. As such, this book makes a concerted effort to help nurses understand in detail the research and theoretical basis of CHD risk-reduction approaches.

The audience for this book is diverse. Bedside nurses may find concrete information, such as that included in the chapter on ethnicity, particularly helpful. Advanced-practice nurses may find sections addressing their unique role, such as that in the chapter on hypertension, invaluable. Nurse scientists may find that the integrated reviews of the research literature provide support and direction for subsequent studies. Nursing students may find the book helpful in shifting their focus from the treatment to the prevention of disease.

Given this diverse audience, the chapters are designed to be largely independent of previous and subsequent chapters. In general, an overview of the research and theoretical literature is presented, followed by issues related to intervention. It is my sincere hope that you will enjoy this book and find it a valuable guide in practice.

NALINI JAIRATH

ACKNOWLEDGMENTS

The chapter authors and I thank all the colleagues, friends, administrative staff, and computer geniuses who helped with reviewing and preparing the chapters and formatting the illustrations. Linelle M. Blais, Ph.D., of the American Cancer Society, National Office, Atlanta, Georgia, is thanked for her review and helpful comments on the models described in Chapter 3. Kim Gans, Ph.D., M.P.H., L.D.N., Memorial Hospital Division of Health Education, and Stephanie Ounpuu, Ph.D., R.D., University of Guelph, are thanked for their reviews and helpful comments on previous versions of Chapter 6.

The Graduate School of Nursing, University of Massachusetts, Worcester, where I served for many years, and the School of Nursing, University of Maryland, Baltimore, are thanked for their consistent support.

CONTENTS

Fundamentals of
Risk Reduction

CHAPTER 1

Risk and Coronary Heart Disease

Catherine Daly-Nee
Howard Brunt
Nalini Jairath

Heart disease is a major health problem in the industrialized world and a growing one in developing nations. In the United States alone, heart disease is the number one killer, claiming a life every 34 seconds and resulting in 925,000 deaths annually. In addition, approximately 59 million out of 255 million Americans have some form of heart disease, with an estimated 19% of all disabilities attributed to cardiovascular conditions. The economic impact of heart disease continues to increase, from an estimated $128 billion in 1994 to a projected $137.7 billion in 1995. Furthermore, as the population continues to age, the economic, social, and psychological burden will increase.

Given its magnitude, understanding the epidemiology of coronary heart disease (CHD) is a major concern for clinicians and researchers alike. Simply stated, *epidemiology* is the science of health events in human populations. Epidemiologists study the distribution of states of health and determine deviations from health in human populations. Frequently the focus is on the natural history of disease and the factors that affect the original development of disease. Such knowledge can be used in developing strategies for disease prevention. Since the 1940s, epidemiologic studies have also made a major contribution to our understanding of risk factors and risk-reduction strategies.

This chapter is designed to give nurses and other clinicians an understanding of the basic epidemiologic concepts, approaches, and studies that have shaped current knowledge regarding CHD risk factors and risk reduction. Therefore, using a primarily epidemiologic perspective, we will discuss issues related to disease causation, the concept of risk, risk-factor identification in regard to decision making, and CHD risk-reduction strategies. The epidemiology of CHD risk factors and major epidemiologic studies will then be briefly addressed.

EPIDEMIOLOGIC MODELS OF DISEASE CAUSATION

Traditionally, epidemiologists conceptualized disease as having a single cause or etiology; the idea was that a causative agent infected a "host" to produce a disease. The environment and its composite factors served as a reservoir

3

for the agent to reside in or reproduce in. From this perspective, risk for disease was minimized when the host, agent, and environment were in equilibrium; and risk was increased when the host, agent, and environment were in disequilibrium.

The recognition of chronic diseases of noninfectious origin as major causes of morbidity and mortality has revolutionized modern epidemiology. Conceptualizations of disease causation have expanded to acknowledge the many factors that contribute to the development of diseases such as CHD. These many factors of disease causation are understood in terms of a "web of causation" composed of interconnected risk factors and protective factors. The multiple intersections in the web reflect specific risk factors or outcomes, and the strands of the web symbolize diverse causal pathways. From this perspective, in the prepathogenesis state, the host, agent, and environment may begin to interact and thus form the web of causation ultimately associated with the specific disease (MacMachon, Pugh, & Ipsen, 1960). Consequently, modern epidemiologic interventions focus on the identification and prediction of the results of breaking the strands of this causal web (Krieger, 1994).

Epidemiologists have viewed CHD in two ways: (1) as a syndrome reflecting a constellation of diseases such as angina, myocardial infarction, and so forth; and (2) as a discrete disease entity. Despite controversy about the correct view (Stehbens, 1992), the web-of-causation model presented in this chapter has several implications for intervention with individual clients and with populations.

First, the presence of one or more CHD risk factors does not guarantee that disease is an inevitable consequence, although it increases the probability of disease occurrence. Second, complex host-agent-environment interactions yet to be identified may contribute to disease occurrence in individuals with no known risk factors, as illustrated by the occurrence of myocardial infarction in clients with no known risk factors. Third, the web-of-causation model raises the possibility of effective CHD risk reduction through indirect strategies not specifically targeting an identified CHD risk factor. For example, although smoking is a CHD risk

factor, a smoker's CHD risk may be reduced by addressing other factors as well.

In conclusion, the current epidemiologic conceptualization of CHD disease causation is inherently probabalistic and multifactorial. A probabalistic relationship exists between the number and severity of CHD risk factors and the likelihood of CHD occurrence.

EPIDEMIOLOGIC PERSPECTIVES ON THE MEANING OF RISK

As already noted, the concepts of CHD risk and CHD risk factors underlie current approaches to CHD prevention and treatment. *Risk* is defined as the probability of an unfavorable event, whereas *risk factor* is defined as a specific factor associated with an acquired disease. Risk for CHD may be understood in terms of absolute, relative, and attributable risk.

Absolute risk, or *incidence,* is the rate of occurrence of a disease as in the rate of CHD in a particular population. *Relative risk* compares the incidence of a disease in a population exposed and not exposed to an occurrence. For example, the rate of CHD in postmenopausal as compared to premenopausal women might be compared for relative risk. *Attributable risk* addresses the difference between the incidence in the exposed versus the unexposed population. When based on per 1,000 members of the population, the term *population attributable risk* is employed (Kaplan & Stamler, 1983). Thus, attributable risk provides information about the impact of a particular occurrence or factor upon the rate of disease occurrence, as in the increased risk for CHD directly attributable to smoking.

Although the term *risk factor* first appeared in the Framingham Heart Study reports in the mid-1960s, epidemiologists actually use the term more generically to denote a risk marker, risk determinant, or modifiable risk factor. A *risk marker* is an attribute or exposure associated with an increased probability of a specific outcome. A *risk determinant* is an attribute or exposure that has been proved to increase the probability of occurrence of an outcome. A *modifiable risk factor* is a risk determinant that may be modified by intervention, thus reducing the probability of a specific outcome.

Modifiability of a risk factor is based on epidemiologic data that establishes the existence of a relationship between the risk factor and incidence of disease (i.e., absolute risk). Reduction in the modifiable risk factor is associated with a reduction in the incidence or outcomes related to the disease.

Within the context of CHD, such factors as earlobe creases would be identified as risk markers, familial hyperlipidemia as a risk determinant, and cigarette smoking as a modifiable risk factor. From the CHD risk-reduction perspective, modifiable risk factors are of special interest because of the potential of reduced CHD-related morbidity and mortality.

EPIDEMIOLOGIC APPROACHES TO RISK-FACTOR IDENTIFICATION AND DECISION MAKING

Epidemiologic data provides information regarding the distribution of a risk factor across a population and its relationship to CHD risk. Data may be obtained through population-based surveys, health questionnaires, and direct measurement. The resultant information is used to identify the subset of the population that warrants focused treatment. This subset is usually identified by establishing a *threshold,* or cutoff value, for the risk factor based on such considerations as (1) the relative risk versus benefits of treatment, (2) the percentage of the population with values below or above a particular threshold, and (3) the sensitivity and specificity associated with using a specified screening approach and screening threshold.

The threshold may be used to screen people into two categories: the *positives,* those likely to be at a higher risk for the disease, and the *negatives,* those likely to be at a lower risk for the disease (Mausner & Bahn, 1974). A highly *sensitive* approach and screening threshold increases the likelihood of correctly identifying these at-risk people. Likewise, a highly *specific* approach and screening threshold increases the likelihood of accurately identifying the people who are at less risk. An ideal screening approach and threshold is both highly specific and sensitive.

For example, the desirable cutoff point (threshold) for initiating treatment for hypercholesterolemia is 200 mg/dl. If this cutoff point is increased to 250 mg/dl, specificity is increased, and nearly everyone whose cholesterol values are truly negative for predicting CHD will be identified. Unfortunately, increased specificity is very frequently associated with decreased sensitivity, resulting in a larger proportion of false negative results. That is, the screening approach with reduced sensitivity fails to identify many people whose cholesterol levels place them at increased risk for CHD.

On the other hand, if the cutoff point is decreased to 180 mg/dl, the sensitivity of the approach is increased at the expense of specificity. Nearly everyone who could be at risk for developing CHD is identified. But many people not at risk would be included in the larger percentage of the population with cholesterol levels above this cutoff point. These people would require further testing, with resultant anxiety and added expense and inconvenience. The benefits of this additional testing for individuals actually at low risk for CHD would be questionable.

Therefore, as with other CHD risk factors, such as blood pressure, the selected thresholds for screening and intervention represent a compromise between the need for high sensitivity and high specificity.

CHD RISK-REDUCTION STRATEGIES

Intervention is possible once risk factors are identified and host-agent-environment interactions delineated. Epidemiologists conceptualize intervention in terms of disease prevention. Prevention can occur at various stages in disease progression and is characterized as primary, secondary, or tertiary in nature. Regardless of the stage of disease development or progression, the effectiveness of epidemiologic interventions is predicated on an understanding of factors influencing the risk-taking behavior of the host individual. The degree of risk acceptable to the individual client depends upon several factors, but for most, the initial factor is recognition, or identification, of a specific event, condition, or other cue as being potentially threatening. Nevertheless, individuals may live with diseases and afflictions without recognizing the eventual outcome in terms of morbidity or mortality. Whether or not such potential outcomes are recognized may be influenced by past personal experiences, organized education, or even false information.

Once a potential threat is recognized, the individual must learn to live with the uncertainty of its outcome. Mishel (1990) postulates that clients learn to integrate these uncertainties into their lifestyles and use *probabalistic thinking* when dealing with health issues. Probabalistic thinking forces the individual to confront the absence of guarantees in life. Because of the probabalistic nature of chronic diseases such as CHD, the clinician cannot guarantee that risk-reduction efforts will translate into health benefits or a survival advantage. Therefore, individuals must use probabilistic thinking to appraise their chances for success and then make choices based on that appraisal.

Whereas an individual may know that a particular behavior or failure to modify a risk is potentially damaging, individual tolerances for acceptable risk vary. Risk-tolerant people will maintain a risky behavior that risk-averse people will avoid. With these considerations in mind, epidemiologically based interventions will now be briefly addressed.

Primary Prevention

The goal of primary prevention is to limit the incidence of disease by controlling causes and risk factors during the prepathogenesis stage of the disease process. Whereas clinicians focus on encounters with individual clients, epidemiologists focus on health-promotion activities for populations, with the goal of *social immunization*. Epidemiologists and clinicians alike postulate that with education and support, individuals are less likely to adopt and maintain habits injurious to their health.

Within the context of CHD risk reduction, epidemiologists favor early intervention before potentially damaging behavior patterns are established. In general, primary prevention interventions for CHD risk reduction focus on heightening awareness of risk and risk factors, improving knowledge of CHD risk-reduction

strategies, providing models or guidelines for desired behavior, and modifying environmental exposure to factors that can cumulatively increase the risk of CHD development and progression. As described in Chapter 7, education of teenagers regarding the health risks of smoking provides a clear example of primary prevention strategies for smoking.

Secondary Prevention

The goals of secondary prevention are to "cure" patients and reduce the more serious consequences of disease through early diagnosis and treatment. Interventions occur during the window of time between disease onset and presentation of clinical symptoms requiring treatment. The basis of secondary prevention is (1) effective screening to identify individuals at higher risk for CHD relative to the population, followed by (2) early intervention to reduce modifiable risk factors. As with primary prevention, interventions focus on education and environmental modification. Blood pressure reduction strategies, as described in Chapter 9, illustrate one approach to secondary prevention. Another example of population-focused secondary prevention is the annual Great American Smokeout. With resources for smoking cessation readily available, smokers are challenged to stop smoking on Smokeout Day and donate the proceeds to charity.

Tertiary Prevention

The goal of tertiary prevention is to reduce the progression of clinically manifest disease before it causes additional disability, acute illness, and finally death. Traditionally, tertiary prevention and intervention are typified by comprehensive cardiac rehabilitation programs. By virtue of the inclusion and exclusion criteria, costs, and hospital-based focus, these programs focus primarily upon the individual client. In contrast, epidemiologists favor population-based, public health initiatives.

THE EPIDEMIOLOGY OF CHD

CHD risk-reduction approaches are partially predicated upon epidemiologic research. This research complements basic and applied research regarding the pathophysiology of CHD and the effectiveness of specific risk-reduction strategies. It is beyond the scope of this chapter to discuss all epidemiologic studies regarding CHD risk, so we will briefly describe only the major epidemiologic studies and the pertinent conclusions regarding CHD risk factors.

Landmark prospective population studies that provided the initial insights into CHD risk factors were pioneered by epidemiologists such as Ancel Keys, who hypothesized that atherosclerotic disease was not the inevitable result of aging as previously believed but was related to environmental factors such as dietary fat consumption. One of the earliest and still most influential studies is the ongoing Framingham Heart Study, initiated in 1949. The initial focus of the Framingham Heart Study included the identification of modifiable and nonmodifiable risk factors and the acquisition of information about CHD disease progression over time. The original study sample included 5,209 individuals between the ages of 30 and 60 years, 2,336 men and 2,873 women. Among the original sample, 5,127 people, men and women, were free of CHD at the start of the study (Dawber, 1980). Each subject was assessed for coronary and cardiovascular risk factors.

Currently, a cohort of adult members of the Framingham, Massachusetts, community continues to be evaluated biannually for CHD and associated risk factors. Over a 20-year period, an additional 80% of the original cohort has continued to participate in the study. The Framingham Heart Study has clearly established that high cholesterol, hypertension, and cigarette smoking are the three CHD risk factors with the largest population attributable risk. In addition to this classic triad of factors (which will be discussed in detail in the next section of this chapter), gender, family history, and age have also been identified as nonmodifiable risk factors.

The Framingham Heart Study has provided the impetus for additional studies investigating specific risk factors such as high cholesterol, hypertension, smoking, gender, and sedentary lifestyle. Secondary analysis of Framingham Heart Study data also continues to provide insights into CHD development.

The American Heart Association has recently categorized putative CHD risk factors in terms of the strength of supportive research and the amenability of the factor to modification for CHD risk reduction (Pearson & Fuster, 1996). Figure 1–1 presents an overview of CHD risk factors according to category and ranking of the quality of evidence supporting an association with cardiovascular disease. As the legend indicates, Category I risk factors are those for which interventions have been "proved" to lower risk; Category IV risk factors are those for which no intervention can lower risk (i.e., these are nonmodifiable risk factors). In between are Categories II and III. Within each category, the quality of supportive evidence can range from poor or nonexistent to very strong or very consistent.

Pertinent findings and seminal studies for specific risk factors will now be addressed, starting with Category I factors.

The Classic Triad

Elevated cholesterol, smoking, and hypertension are Category I risk factors. They are frequently termed the *classic triad* in recognition of their magnitude and prevalence as CHD risk factors.

ELEVATED CHOLESTEROL

A large body of research (Caggiula & Mustad, 1997) indicates a strong and consistent relationship between elevated cholesterol levels and increasing risk of coronary heart disease. Hypercholesterolemia is estimated to account for 40% of all myocardial infarctions (Riegel, 1991). Although the thresholds for diagnosis and the magnitude of hypercholesterolemia and dyslipidemia vary internationally, hypercholesterolemia remains a concern, especially in industrialized Western European nations. Based on the current National Cholesterol Education Program (NCEP) definition of elevated serum cholesterol as ≥200 mg/dl, an estimated 52% of American adults have elevated serum cholesterol, and 20%, or about 37.2 million, of American adults have levels of 240 mg/dl or above (American Heart Association, 1994). Furthermore, an estimated 36.5% of American youth age 19 and under (26.7 million young people)

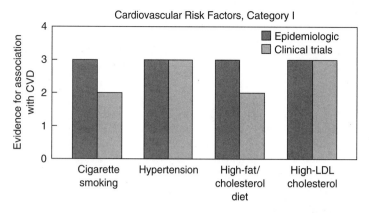

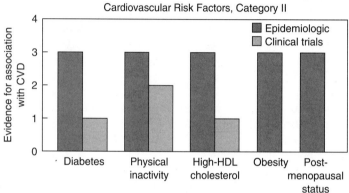

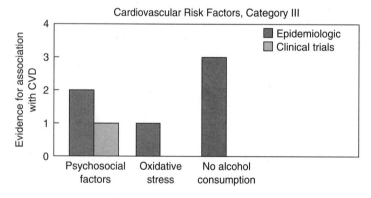

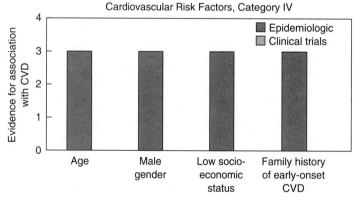

FIGURE 1–1 Cardiovascular risk factors and the evidence supporting their association with disease: Category I risk factors, if modified, have been "proved" to lower CVD risk. Category II risk factors, if modified, are likely to lower CVD risk. Category III risk factors, if modified, might lower CVD risk. Category IV risk factors cannot be modified. From Pearson, T., & Fuster, V. (1996). Twentieth Bethesda Conference—Matching the intensity of risk factor management with the hazard for coronary disease events. *Journal of the American College of Cardiology, 27*(5), 962. Reprinted with permission from the American College of Cardiology.

CVD = Cardiovascular Disease; HDL = High Density Lipoprotein; LDL = Low Density Lipoprotein; 0 = Evidence poor or nonexistent; 1 = weak, somewhat consistent evidence; 2 = Moderately strong, rather consistent evidence; 3 = Very strong, consistent evidence have serum cholesterol levels of 170 mg/dl or higher, which is the level comparable to the 200 mg/dl cutoff point in adults (American Heart Association, 1994). Because, in general, serum cholesterol levels increase from young adulthood until middle age in both men and women, these findings raise the possibility that elevated cholesterol levels will escalate in American adults over time.

Among the major epidemiologic studies that have contributed to our knowledge of hypercholesterolemia as a major CHD risk factor are the three that provided most of the initial evidence: the Framingham Heart Study, the Seven Countries Study, and the Japanese Migrants' Study. The previously described Framingham study examined the association between elevated cholesterol levels and CHD mortality and morbidity based on a history of angina, stroke, transient ischemic attacks, intermittent claudication, and congestive heart failure. Data analysis indicated that cholesterol level was directly related to the 30-year overall morbidity and mortality rates for individuals under 50 years of age. For each 10 mg/dl increase in serum cholesterol, the overall death rate increased by 5% and the cardiovascular-related death rate by 9% (Anderson, Castelli, & Levy, 1987). However, for people older than 50, overall mortality was not correlated with serum cholesterol levels. This finding suggests an age-related uncoupling between cholesterol levels and CHD risk.

The relationship between diet, serum cholesterol levels, and CHD risk was examined in two other studies: the Seven Countries Study and the Japanese Migrants' Study. These studies provided critical new insights into the relationships between cultural conditions and the existence of certain risk factors. In the Seven Countries Study, baseline data on diet and other potential risk factors were collected from men aged 40–59 years ($N = 12,763$) in Yugoslavia, Finland, Italy, the Netherlands, Greece, the United States, and Japan. Data analysis indicated that dietary saturated-fat consumption was associated with total serum cholesterol levels within and between populations. Risk varied widely according to other risk factors, such as elevated cholesterol, hypertension, left ventricular hypertrophy, and cigarette smoking.

Later follow-up of the cohorts also indicated that increased intake of dietary fat was consistently and strongly associated with higher rates of CHD and total mortality (Reign, 1991). Similarly, the incidence of coronary death paralleled the distribution of dietary fat, with Americans and eastern Finns having the highest incidence of coronary-related deaths, and the Japanese and Greeks having the lowest incidence.

The Japanese Migrant's Study, described in detail in Chapter 14, followed Japanese men who had migrated to the United States and had adopted the Western high-fat diet. Data analysis indicated that the incidence of coronary heart disease increased in the Japanese migrants to the United States relative to Japanese men who did not migrate. Furthermore, the greater the acculturation to the American diet was, the greater the cholesterol elevation and subsequent CHD risk.

These population-based prospective studies provided the basis for numerous primary and secondary prevention studies involving diet and drug treatment to reduce serum cholesterol levels. For example, two large placebo-controlled trials, the Lipid Research Clinics Coronary Primary Prevention Trial (LRC-CPPT) and the Helsinki Heart Study, addressed primary prevention of hyperlipidemia in middle-aged men. In the LRC-CPPT, cholestyramine and dietary modifications were used to reduce serum cholesterol. The regimen was associated with an amazing 19% decrease in the incidence of CHD relative to the placebo group but a minimal 2% decrease in mean LDL cholesterol (Lipid Research Clinics Program, 1984).

In the Helsinki Heart Study, gemfibrozil was used for cholesterol reduction in a sample of 4,081 men between 40 and 55 years of age with no clinical evidence of CHD. LDL cholesterol was reduced by 11%, and HDL cholesterol was increased by 11%. In addition, triglyceride counts were 35% lower than those of the placebo group. The group receiving gemfibrozil attained the greatest benefit and exhibited the highest LDL/HDL ratio (>5). Furthermore, data analysis indicated that the 71% decline in the incidence of CHD events within this group was attributable to aggressive reduction of total serum cholesterol (Manninen, Tankanen, Koskinen, et al. 1992).

Several studies have also established the benefits of cholesterol reduction for secondary prevention (see Table 1–1). Lowering serum cholesterol levels is postulated to stabilize plaques, decrease vasospasm, and permit endothelial healing. The angiographic documentation of coronary atherosclerosis coupled with rigorous design and sampling criteria make three studies especially noteworthy: Cholesterol Lowering Atherosclerosis Study (CLAS), Familial Atherosclerosis Trial (FATS), and Monitored Atherosclerosis Regression Study (MARS). Although sample sizes and baseline cholesterol values varied, all three studies were placebo-controlled, with the experimental group receiving diet therapy with or without pharmacologic agents. On average, treated patients were half as likely to experience overall progression of their coronary lesions. Furthermore, the experimental subjects were three times as likely as the control group to experience a regression of selected lesions (Jones & Gotton, 1994). Further clinical trials supported these findings, with a 25% decrease in recurrent coronary events and a 10% reduction in overall mortality (Grundy, 1994, 1997).

As a result of these and other studies, considerable controversy exists nationally and internationally regarding both screening and treatment approaches for cholesterol reduction. In the United States the NCEP has determined that a 5% reduction in CHD incidence may translate to 75,000 fewer heart attacks and 25,000 fewer deaths per year. This analysis favors wide-spread screening of the population despite cost-benefit considerations. Prospective studies offer no compelling support for the screening or treatment of elevated cholesterol in populations other than that of the white male of <60 years who has a cholesterol level above the 90th percentile (Hulley, Walsh, & Newman, 1992; Brett, 1989). The NCEP contends that the expense of coronary artery bypass graft surgery and treatment of myocardial infarction does not outweigh the cost of widespread screening. Other national groups and western nations, including Canada and Great Britain, have reviewed the research data and choose not to spend scarce health care resources on a universal cholesterol-lowering campaign (Forrester and Shah, 1997; Dunnigan, 1993; Hulley, Walsh, & Newman, 1992).

The Canadian experience clearly indicates the dilemma faced by health planners and policymakers. Screening of all adults 18 years and older would result in half of the adult Canadian population having to "enter the health care system as patients," and half of these having to be treated with drugs (Little & Horlick, 1989). Therefore, the Canadian Task Force on Periodic Health Care Examination suggests targeting men 35–59 years of age for screening (Morgan & Lindsay, 1994). Moreover, the Toronto Working Group on Cholesterol Policy emphasizes that an individual's cholesterol level is integrated within a highly complex matrix of

TABLE 1–1 Major Cholesterol Studies

Name of Study	Duration in Years	Intervention	No. of Patients	Percent Change in Cholesterol
LRC-CPPT	5	Diet	1,900	
		Diet/cholestyramine	1,906	−9
Helsinki Heart Study	5	Diet	2,030	
		Diet/gemfibrozil	2,051	−10
CLAS-1	2	Placebo	94	
		Colestipol/niacin	94	−26
FATS	2.5	Placebo/colestipol	46	−4
		Lovostatin/colestipol	38	−23
		Niacin/colestipol	36	−34
MARS	2.2	Placebo	124	−1.8
		Lovostatin	123	

Based on Forrester, J., Merz, N., Bush, T., et al. (1996). Twenty-Seventh Bethesda Conference—Task Force 4. Efficacy of risk factor management. *Journal of the American College of Cardiology, 27*(5), 992–993. Used with permission from the American College of Cardiology.

interrelated CHD risk factors and may prove to be a less important risk factor to control than smoking or hypertension. Similar arguments are made by other industrialized nations.

In conclusion, as patient-care advocates and health-care promotion advisors, nurses and other clinicians must be aware of the effect of elevated serum cholesterol on CHD morbidity and mortality. In addition, the ever changing guidelines and interventions must be reviewed and evaluated, based upon epidemiologic data and analytic approaches. These interventions and guidelines will be further discussed in Chapter 6.

HYPERTENSION

Hypertension, typically defined as systolic blood pressure ≥ 140 mm Hg or diastolic blood pressure ≥ 90 mm Hg, has been called the "silent killer." An estimated one in four adult Americans are diagnosable as hypertensive given adequate screening (American Heart Association, 1994). This condition predisposes people to various aspects of cardiovascular diseases through a direct pathologic effect on the vasculature and promotion of the atherogenic process. Hypertension is one of the most important risk factors for stroke, which accounts for about one of every 15 deaths (American Heart Association, 1994).

Many factors determine whether or not a person develops hypertension. Age, race, socioeconomic status, education, and gender affect the progression of hypertension and response to treatment. Also, other coronary risk factors may have a cumulative effect on this condition. The risk of morbidity and mortality with coronary heart disease is related to increased levels of blood pressure in a direct and continuous manner.

Based on the Framingham Heart Study, national health surveys, population studies, and resultant meta-analyses, the evidence for hypertension as a major CHD risk factor is overwhelming. Meta-analysis of data from nine large prospective observational studies suggests a direct continuous relationship between blood pressure values and CHD risk. In this meta-analysis, the combined sample of 420,000 participants was divided into five groups based on diastolic blood pressure (<79, 80–89, 90–99,

100–109, ≥ 110 mm Hg). People with a diastolic blood pressure in the highest range (≥ 110 mm Hg) had a 10 to 12 times greater risk for coronary heart disease than those people in the lowest range (<79 mm Hg) (MacMahon, Peto, & Cutler, 1990). Furthermore, the Framingham Heart Study data indicates an incidence of sudden death up to two times higher in the hypertensive individuals than in a nonhypertensive cohort (Dawber, 1980).

This study also established that both systolic and diastolic pressures should be considered when evaluating hypertension. Data projections indicate that approximately 14% of males and 23% of females will develop isolated systolic hypertension over a 30-year period, significantly affecting hypertension-related mortality and morbidity.

Several factors influence the development of hypertension, most notably age. Framingham Heart Study data indicated that after age 65, isolated systolic hypertension accounted for 57.4% of any type of hypertension in men and 65.1% in women. Furthermore, 1988–1991 data from the National Health and Nutrition Surveys indicates that hypertension is increasing by 25% in the 35–44 age group, by 50% in the 55–64 age group, and 66% in the 65–74 age group.

In addition to age, some ethnic and racial characteristics influence blood pressure distributions and the rate of hypertension. For instance, African Americans have a rate of hypertension that is among the highest in the world. Studies have shown that 30% of all deaths in males and 20% of all deaths in females of African-American heritage may be attributed to hypertension (National Blood Pressure Education Program, 1993). In addition, African Americans often develop hypertension at an early age and may experience greater disease severity during each decade than other subsets of the general population.

Identifying the reasons for ethnic or racial differences in the incidence of hypertension is complicated because of the presence of multiple interrelated contributory factors. As discussed in Chapter 15, salt intake, obesity, and cigarette smoking, as well as the prevalence of non-insulin-dependent diabetes, vary by ethnicity or racial background.

Education and socioeconomic resources may

also play a role in the genesis or progression of hypertension. In general, residents of the southeastern United States are 1.32 times more likely to die from stroke-related diseases than those who are from other parts of the country. These findings may reflect differences in access to adequate medical care as well as variations in educational and socioeconomic status. Currently in the United States the incidence of unrecognized hypertension is approximately 15%, down from 50% in 1971–1972 (Furberg, Berglund, & Manolio, 1994). In comparison, the incidence of unrecognized hypertension is lower in European countries, where universal health care is provided through government efforts.

Three major epidemiologic studies indicate that hypertension can be successfully treated such that cardiovascular damage is reduced. The United Kingdom–Medical Research Council (UK-MRC) trial studied 4,396 patients aged 65–74 years. With intervention, a 19% reduction in stroke and cardiovascular events occurred (MRC Working Party, 1992) The STOP-Hypertension trial (Swedish Trial of Old Patients with Hypertension) studied 1,627 patients aged 70–84 years. Their results corroborated the findings of the UK-MRC trials, with a 13% reduction in cardiovascular events (Dahlof, Lindholm, Hannson, et al., 1991).

Most significantly, the SHEP (Systolic Hypertension in the Elderly Program) showed a 36% reduction in stroke, 25% reduction in coronary heart disease, and an overall 27% reduction in cardiovascular mortality. Published in 1991, this report was based on a sample of 4,736 people aged 60–80 years. The combined results of the SHEP, the UK-MRC, and STOP-Hypertension reports demonstrate that it is clearly beneficial to treat persons up to age 84 for hypertension.

Intervention research has also focused on several additional issues related to the potential decrease in mortality and morbidity with treatment. As discussed in Chapter 9, these include the (1) threshold for intervention, (2) selection of first-line treatment agents, (3) relative benefits of pharmacologic versus nonpharmacologic intervention or combination therapy, and (4) compliance with treatment regimens. Although pertinent studies are too numerous to review, a promising area of research is evaluating the benefits of nonpharmacologic intervention. For example, Langford and colleagues compared outcomes of 496 former drug trial participants randomly assigned to a salt-restricted diet or a weight-reduction plan with a control group. Those with hypertension who required a return to use of pharmacologic agents were identified. Data indicated that those following a sodium-restricted regimen were two times as likely not to need medication.

Of even more significance was the discovery that people on a weight-reduction diet were 3.5 times as likely to remain off medications (Langford, Blaufox, & Oberman, 1985). Furthermore, an additional Australian study established that weight reduction was as effective as metopropanol in blood pressure reduction for a selected hypertensive population. Despite the initial promise of these studies, we must emphasize that additional research is warranted, and that the most recent treatment guidelines continue to recommend the use of drugs earlier when other CHD risk factors are present.

In conclusion, hypertension is a major risk factor for CHD. Substantial progress has been made in identification of at-risk populations. Debate continues regarding the optimal treatment regimen for various groups of hypertensive patients. Compliance with pharmacologic and nonpharmacologic treatment regimens is poor, and clinicians and researchers alike are increasingly recognizing that instead of examining compliance, it may be more profitable to match treatment regimens to patient characteristics.

SMOKING

Smoking is a contributory factor in one out of five deaths each year in the United States (Manley, 1997). Smoking-related illnesses cost the United States about $50 billion annually in medical care and are the number one preventable cause of CHD (American Heart Association, 1994). The increased cost of care and the morbidity and mortality associated with smoking have been extensively chronicled nationally and internationally. Particularly noteworthy is landmark American research by Hammond and Horn (1958) and British research by Doll and Peto (1976), addressing the increased mortality rate from CHD in smokers. Furthermore, as early as 1964, based on extensive research, the U.S. Surgeon General's Advisory Committee Reports identified a direct association between cigarette smoking and long-term health consequences. These reports unequivocally concluded that cigarette smoking was a health hazard of sufficient importance to warrant remedial action. Lamentably, in spite of the magnitude of these numbers and the population attributable risk, in 1993 there were still 40 million smokers in the United States alone (Wynder, 1993).

In addition to its effects upon the respiratory system and overall health, cigarette smoking has many adverse effects on the cardiovascular system. These effects include increased platelet adhesiveness; increased heart rate, with resulting increases in myocardial demand; elevated catecholamine levels; and decreased serum oxygen-carrying capacity. The impact of cigarette smoking and smoking cessation upon cardiovascular mortality and morbidity has been extensively studied. The Framingham Heart Study findings supported the direct relationship between cigarette smoking and the increased risk of myocardial infarction, sudden cardiac death, and CHD mortality in both sexes (Wilhelmsen, 1988). In addition, government data tracking the health of the American populace indicate that smokers have a risk of death secondary to coronary artery disease that is two to three times higher than that of nonsmokers. The sudden cardiac death rate is ten times higher in male smokers and five times higher in female smokers (MMWR, 1992).

Survivors of sudden cardiac attacks who quit smoking have a 19% recurrence of these attacks; however, if they continue to smoke, the rate increases to 27% (Hallstrom, Cobb, & Ray, 1986). In addition, major CHD risk factors such as hypercholesteremia and obesity can have a cumulative effect when combined with cigarette smoking. For example, a male smoker with a total serum cholesterol of >240 mg/dl and a diastolic blood pressure of >90 mm Hg has a risk of dying of CHD that is 14 times greater than a male smoker with lower total cholesterol and diastolic blood pressure.

The research indicates that education, social environment, and social attitudes play a key role in whether a person continues to smoke or stops. An estimated 90% of smokers begin before the age of 20 (Ernster, 1993). Annually, 3 million additional young people, or 3,000 each day, become regular smokers (Guba & MacDonald, 1993). Years of aggressive marketing by tobacco companies popularizing and glamorizing cigarette smoking have encouraged younger and younger people to begin smoking. For example, in one study, over 90% of 6-year-olds surveyed recognized a cigarette company cartoon figure named Joe Camel and his association with cigarettes as readily as they recognized Mickey Mouse. In contrast, only 10% matched the Surgeon General's health warnings that appear on all American cigarette packages with the picture of a cigarette (Fischer, Meyher, & Schwartz, 1991). News organizations subsequently reported the "demise" of Joe Camel following a 1997 decision by the tobacco company to stop using that advertising. Nevertheless, use of strategies to promote cigarette consumption by young people with the potential for addiction continues to be a clinical concern because of children's vulnerability to sophisticated marketing approaches and their susceptibility to lifelong cigarette addiction. Research indicates that if the temptation to begin smoking is resisted during the teen years, the likelihood of starting smoking later in life is reduced.

As with hypertension, cultural and racial differences also exist in smoking patterns and the impact of smoking (Willems, Hunt, & Schorling, 1997). The reasons for these differences have not been clearly delineated but may partly reflect social norms. Social norms have influenced the terminology and criteria used to define cultural and racial groups in pertinent studies. For example, studies examining "blacks" may or may not have been restricted to African Americans. The actual research study designations may be opposed to the currently accepted terminology.

As discussed in detail in Chapter 15, Native Americans have an alarmingly high rate of smoking, 77% for males and 67% for females (Gillum, Gillum, & Smith, 1984). The research also indicates that the rate of smoking in "blacks" is higher than the general population. Some studies have found a 32% rate of smoking for black males, 28% for white males, 24.5% for white females, and 23.9% for black females (American Heart Association, 1994). In contrast, Hispanics have shown a consistently lower rate of smoking than blacks or whites (25.6% for men and 13.4% for women). Yet, studies by Escobedo and Remington (1989) suggest that the magnitude of these differences is narrowing.

Gender also appears to influence smoking patterns. The American Heart Association (AHA) reported in 1994 that 30.1% of men and 29.6% of women smoked. The National Health Interview Survey in 1991 found that one in four American women (23.5%) smoked, (MMWR, 1993), whereas one in three smoked in 1965. Still, 22.2 million U.S. women continue to smoke, including a high percentage of pregnant women.

Fear of weight gain makes some women continue smoking (Wydner, 1993) An additional factor affecting women smokers is the cumulative effect of smoking and the use of the birth control pill. Studies show that women smokers who use oral contraceptives are up to 39 times more likely to have a heart attack and 22 times more likely to have a stroke than women who neither smoke nor use the birth control pill (American Heart Association, 1994). However, educational level is quickly replacing gender as the sociodemographic variable most highly predictive of differences in smoking prevalence. Among high school dropouts, the incidence of smoking is 40% versus 15.7% in those with some college education (Guba et al., 1993).

In addition to the direct effects of smoking upon CHD risk, research on the hazards of smoking has turned to the association between exposure to *environmental tobacco smoke* (ETS) and adverse health effects. The subject of "passive smoking," or exposure to ETS, was first raised in the 1972 report of the U.S. Surgeon General based on epidemiologic studies reported by the Environmental Protection Agency. The lethality of smoking is also underscored by a spate of new studies linking passive smoking to CHD risk in spouses/partners of smokers, to asthma in children, and to low birth weight in infants.

In conclusion, epidemiology has made a major contribution to our understanding of smoking as a CHD risk factor. However, the new frontier for epidemiologists may be wide-scale interventions not only for primary prevention but also for secondary and tertiary prevention.

Additional CHD Risk Factors

The AHA has recently categorized putative CHD risk factors in terms of the strength of supportive research and the amenability of the factor to modification for CHD risk reduction (Pearson & Fuster, 1996). The classic triad of hypertension, elevated cholesterol, and smoking are Category I factors. Other risk factors distributed across Categories II through IV are being investigated from the dual perspectives of CHD risk factors and cardioprotection. Although several of these factors are discussed in detail in subsequent chapters, a brief synopsis of current knowledge is presented here.

PHYSICAL ACTIVITY

An estimated 60% of U.S. adults live a "sedentary lifestyle" (Jones & Gotton, 1994). Several epidemiologic studies indicate that increased or higher levels of physical activity reduce CHD risk whereas decreased or lower levels are associated with increased CHD risk. The Harvard Alumni Study (Paffenbarger, Hyde, Wing, et al., 1990) is especially noteworthy because of its large sample size (16,936 males) and longitudinal tracking of subjects over a long timeframe. In this study, Harvard University alumni who reported a sedentary lifestyle had a 31% greater risk of cardiovascular-related mortality than those who reported a greater degree of physical activity. As discussed in detail in Chapter 8, physical activity influences CHD risk through diverse mechanisms, including indirect effects on blood pressure, cholesterol, weight, and diabetes control. To illustrate, research indicates that less fit persons have a 30–50% greater risk of developing high blood pressure, a major independent CHD risk factor (American Heart Association, 1994).

Despite controversies regarding quantification of a possible dose-response relationship between physical activity and CHD risk, it is generally agreed that exercise of low to moderate intensity for 20 minutes, three times per week, benefits the cardiovascular system and contributes to overall good health. Additional research is needed to determine the effectiveness of population-based interventions to increase physical activity. Such interventions must consider economic, educational, social, and cultural factors. For example, people with lower incomes and a less than twelfth-grade education are more likely to be sedentary (American Heart Association, 1994).

In conclusion, manipulation of the level of physical activity is particularly attractive to clinicians. The risks of increased physical activity are relatively low compared with risks associated with other CHD risk-reduction approaches, such as use of antihypertensive and antilipidemic medications. Decreasing sedentary behavior and increasing physical activity in at-risk populations is an exciting and necessary intervention for CHD risk reduction. Preliminary evidence suggests that the benefits of increased physical activity pertain to women as well as men (Folsom, Arnett, Hutchinson, et al., 1997).

PSYCHOSOCIAL FACTORS

As discussed in Chapter 10, the relationship between CHD risk and several psychosocial factors continues to be investigated. Promising models explaining the interrelationships between various psychosocial factors are also being developed (Holahan, Moos, Holahan, et al., 1997). Based on Framingham Heart Study data, the *Type A personality,* characterized as aggressive, ambitious, and having a competitive drive and a chronic sense of urgency, was associated with increased CHD risk. More recently, however, data from the Western Collaborative Group Study of Type A Behavior and CHD indicates that subcomponents of Type A behavior, not Type A behavior per se, are associated with increased CHD risk (Ragland & Brand, 1988). These subcomponents pertain to cynicism, anger, and hostility and may exert their effects through altered cardiovascular reactivity. Additional research is needed to determine the generalizability of findings to women.

Depression and lack of social support, which have been variously defined, are also associated with increased CHD risk. But, unlike the research on personality traits, research regarding the role of psychosocial factors in CHD risk reduction or cardioprotection is limited.

In conclusion, despite the importance of psychosocial factors, interventions are relatively crude and warrant additional investigation regarding their effectiveness. As a result, many clinicians prefer to use general stress-reduction approaches and support groups to address diverse psychosocial factors linked to CHD development.

GENDER

Research examining the CHD risk and risk patterns in women is severely limited (Drown, 1997). An emphasis on age-gender interaction is replacing the classic view that male gender is a CHD risk factor. In fact, cardiovascular diseases are a leading cause of death and disability in women. By the year 2000, a projected 38% of all women in the United States will be 45 years of age or older. Although males are at higher risk for CHD in the early to middle adult years, postmenopausal females have an increasing risk of CHD that ultimately surpasses that of males in the sixth or seventh decade of life. After menopause, whether occurring naturally or surgically, women face a two to three times greater risk of developing CHD than prior to menopause (Colditz, Willet, & Stampfer, 1987). Framingham Heart Study data indicates that after age 55, women's risk of CHD increases tenfold (Castelli, 1983). Cardiovascular disease will more than likely continue to be a major problem for women in the next decades.

Given the age-gender interaction, current intervention studies focus on the use of estrogen replacement therapy in postmenopausal women. Estrogen lowers LDL cholesterol and increases HDL cholesterol. Furthermore, decreased estrogen levels are accompanied by decreased cardioprotective effects, based on Nurses' Health Study data (Matthews, Meilahn, & Keller, 1989). Case control studies have linked estrogen use with reduced coronary stenosis. Based on these and many other epidemiologic studies, the 1993 National Cholesterol Education Program (NCEP) has recommended the use of estrogen replacement therapy as an adjunct to other therapy for the reduction of coronary heart disease. In addition, the program emphasizes that the risk-benefit ratio must be weighed in regard to the increased incidence of breast and uterine cancer with hormone replacement therapy. Age-gender interactions and their relation to CHD risk require further investigation.

DIABETES

CHD is two to four times more common in diabetics (Levetan & Ratner, 1995). Furthermore, CHD mortality and morbidity contributed to 75–85% of all deaths in diabetic individuals (Vinicor, 1996). Diabetics frequently have multiple CHD risk factors, such as hypertension, dyslipidemias, obesity, and smoking. In addition, hyperglycemia and hyperinsulinemia have been postulated to affect CHD risk because of their effect on lipid metabolism and renal function. Type II, or non-insulin-dependent diabetes, carries a greater CHD risk than Type I, or insulin-dependent diabetes. Particularly dangerous from the CHD risk perspective is Syndrome X in Type II diabetics. This syndrome is characterized by hypertension, hypertriglyceridemia, low HDL cholesterol levels, and abdominal obesity (Kaplan, 1989).

Given the adverse effect of diabetes upon CHD risk, effective assessment and management of diabetes is imperative. As discussed in detail in Chapter 11, assessment of CHD risk may be based on guidelines from the Centers for Disease Control, Division of Diabetes Translation (1991). Intervention focuses on maintaining better diabetes control and addressing coexistent CHD risk factors. Despite its overall benefit, pharmacologic treatment should be cautiously initiated and closely administered. As discussed in Chapter 11, lipid modifiers such as niacin may increase blood glucose levels and the risk for liver disease; fibric acid derivatives used to treat hypertriglyceridemia may increase LDL cholesterol.

Because diabetes increases CHD risk, diabetics should be routinely and systematically assessed for CHD. Tight diabetic control coupled with modification of other CHD risk factors may help decrease CHD risk in these people. Given the potential strictness of the resultant treatment regimen, issues related to regimen adoptions and adherence should receive additional consideration from clinicians and researchers alike.

CARDIOPROTECTIVE AGENTS: ANTIOXIDANTS AND ALCOHOL

Both clinicians and clients are interested in identifying agents that could reduce CHD risk by their direct effect on the atherosclerotic process. Of particular interest is the role of antioxidants and alcohol. As discussed in Chapter 11, the Nurses' Health Study of women (Gaziano & Hennekens, 1992), the Health Professionals Follow-Up Study of men (Rimm, Stampfer, Ascherio, et al., 1993), and observational epidemiologic studies have all linked antioxidant consumption with a reduced risk for CHD.

Some evidence exists that antioxidants delay or prevent progression of atherosclerosis. In the Physicians' Health Study, male physicians randomly assigned to therapy with beta-carotene showed a 50% reduction in CHD events (Gaziano, Manson, Ridder, et al., 1990). Evidence is still insufficient to warrant the widespread use of antioxidants in primary and secondary prevention of coronary heart disease.

Evidence to support a cardioprotective role of alcohol is stronger. The Nurses' Health Study, with a large cohort of over 87,000 female nurses, showed a 50% lower risk of nonfatal myocardial infarction and of death from coronary artery disease in women who consumed approximately one alcoholic drink per day (Stampfer, Colditz, & Willett, 1988). The benefit of increased HDL, cholesterol, fibrinolysis, and vasodilatation caused by the intake of alcohol may account for these findings.

Pending additional data, clients may elect to use cardioprotective agents such as alcohol and antioxidants on a case-by-case basis, but given the potential for alcohol abuse, extreme caution should be exercised in prescribing alcohol for CHD risk reduction.

CONCLUSION

CHD has a major impact socially, economically, psychologically, and physiologically. It continues to be the leading cause of death in the United States. Over the past 40 years, many epidemiologic studies have been conducted on the subject. The concept of cardiac risk factors was initially presented in the Framingham Heart Study reports, derived from observation of cohorts in the Framingham study. Further epidemiologic theory led to the concept of the web of causation. As a result, CHD is viewed as having multiple causal pathways with various outcomes. This relatively new emphasis has directed CHD risk-reduction interventions and provides the basis for many epidemiologic studies today.

The great strides that have been made in identification and reduction of cardiac risk factors must be acknowledged. In 1950 the annual death rate from CHD in the United States was 424.2 per 100,000; by 1991, the rate had dropped to 186.0 per 100,000 (American Heart Association, 1994). From 1982 to 1992 the death rate from high blood pressure declined 8.6%. In addition, studies show that smoking has declined by more than 37% since 1965 in the United States. Dyslipidemia, hypertension, and tobacco consumption all increase risk for CHD powerfully and are common in the U.S. population. Although these risk factors carry the largest population attributable risk, their amenability to treatment in the vast number of cases provides a window of opportunity. Through education, identification of high-risk persons and groups, and rehabilitation, nurses and other clinicians play a large role at all levels in the continued work to prevent CHD. Our goal should be to break even one small thread in the causal web for CHD.

This chapter has presented the reader with a brief introduction to essential concepts in understanding CHD risk, risk reduction, and the evolution of knowledge regarding risk intervention. In the next chapter, a completely different, though complementary, perspective is presented: CHD risk and risk reduction are addressed in terms of the underlying anatomic and pathologic processes and the proposed mechanisms linking risk-factor modification to disease progression.

References

Anderson, K.M., Castelli, W.P., & Levy, D. (1987). Cholesterol and mortality: 30 years of follow up from the Framingham study. *Journal of the American Medical Association, 257*(16), 2176–2180.

Blankenhorn, D.H., Azen, S.P., Kramsch, D.M., Mack, W.J., Cashin-Hemphill, L., Hodis, H.N., De Boer, L.W.V., Mahrer, P.R., Mastelli, M.J., Vailas, L.I., et al. (1994). Coronary angiographic changes with lovastatin therapy. The Monitored Atherosclerosis Regression Study (MARS). *Annals of Internal Medicine, 119,* 969–976.

Blankenhorn, D.H., Nessim, S.A., Johnson, R.L., Sanmarco, M.E., Azen, S.P., & Cashin-Hemphill, L. (1987). Beneficial effects of combined colestipol-niacin therapy on coronary atherosclerosis and coronary venous bypass grafts. *Journal of the American Medical Association, 257*(23), 3233–3240.

Boyle, P. (1993). The hazards of passive and active smoking. *New England Journal of Medicine, 328*(23), 1708–1709.

Brett, A. (1989). Treating hypercholesterolemia: How should practicing physicians interpret the published data for patients? *New England Journal of Medicine, 321*(10), 676–680.

Brown, G., Albers, J.J., Fisher, L.D., Schaefer, S.M., Lin, J.-T., Kaplan, C., Zhao, X.-Q., Bisson, B.D., Fitzpatrick, V.F., & Dodge, H.T. (1990). Regression of coronary heart disease as a result of intensive lipid-lowering therapy in men with high levels of apolipoprotein B. *New England Journal of Medicine, 323*(19), 1289–1298.

Brunner, D., Manelis, G., Madan, M., & Levin, S. (1974). Physical activity at work and the incidence of myocardial infarction, angina pectoris and death due to ischemic heart disease: An epidemiologic study in Israeli collective settlements (kibbutzim). *Journal of Chronic Disease, 27*(4), 217.

Caggiula, A.W., & Mustad, V.A. (1997). Effects of dietary fat and fatty acids on coronary artery disease risk and total and lipoprotein cholesterol concentrations: Epidemiologic studies. *American Journal of Clinical Nutrition, 65*(5 Suppl.), 1597S–1610S.

Calabrese, G., Mazzotta, A., & Pratesi, G. (1994). Hypertension in the elderly. *Lancet, 344*(8920), 447–449.

Castelli, W.P. (1983). Cardiovascular disease and multifactorial risk: Challenge of the 1980s. *American Heart Journal, 106* (5, part 2), 1191.

Centers for Disease Control (1991). Smoking attributable mortality and years of potential lost life—U.S. 1988. *Morbidity and Mortality World Reports, 40,* 62–71.

Centers for Disease Control (1992). The National Health Interview Survey: Health promotion and disease prevention (NHIS-HPDP). *Morbidity and Mortality World Reports, 41,* 354–355, 361–362.

Centers for Disease Control (1993). Cigarette smoking among adults. U.S. 1991. *Morbidity and Mortality World Reports, 42,* 230–233.

Colditz, G.A., Willett, W.C., Stampfler, M.J., et al. (1987). Menopause and the risk of coronary heart disease in women. *New England Journal of Medicine, 316*(18), 1105–1110.

Cunningham, S. (1992). The epidemiologic basis of coronary disease prevention. *Nursing Clinics of North America, 27*(1), 153–170.

Dahlöf, B., Lindholm, L.H., Hannson, L., Schersten, B., Ekbom, T., & Wester, P.-O. (1991). Morbidity and mortality in the Swedish trial in old patients with hypertension (STOP-Hypertension). *Lancet, 338*(8778), 1281–1285.

Dawber, T.R. (1980). *The Framingham Study: The Epidemiology of Atherosclerotic Disease.* Cambridge, MA: Harvard University Press.

Doll, R., & Peto, R. (1976). Mortality in relation to smoking: 20 years' observations on male British doctors. *British Medical Journal, 2*(6051), 1525–1536.

Drown, D.J. (1997). Where women stand today in prevention of coronary heart disease. *Progress in Cardiovascular Nursing. 12*(2), 34–36.

Dunnigan, M.G. (1993). The problem of cholesterol: No

light at the end of this tunnel? *British Medical Journal,* *306*(6889), 1355–1356.

Ernster, V.L. (1993). Women and smoking [Editorial]. *American Journal of Public Health 83*(9), 1202–1204.

Escobedo, L.G., & Remington, P.L. (1989). Birth cohort analysis of prevalence of cigarette smoking among Hispanics in the United States. *Journal of the American Medical Association, 26*(1), 66–69.

Fischer, P.M., Schwartz, M.P., Richards, J.W., Jr., Goldstein, A.O., Rojas, T.H., et al. (1991). Brand logo recognition by children age 3 to 6 years: Mickey Mouse and Old Joe the Camel. *Journal of the American Medical Association, 266*(22), 3145–3148.

Folsom, A.R., Arnett, D.K., Hutchinson, R.G., Liao, F., Clegg, L.X., & Cooper, L.S. (1997). Physical activity and incidence of coronary heart disease in middle-aged women and men. *Medicine & Science in Sports & Exercise, 29*(7), 901–901.

Foreman, M. (1986). Cardiovascular disease: A men's health hazard. *Nursing Clinics of North America, 21*(1), 65–73.

Forrester, J.S., & Shah, P.K. (1997). Using serum cholesterol as a screening test for preventing coronary heart disease: The five fundamental flaws of the American College of Physicians' Guidelines. *American Journal of Cardiology, 79*(6), 790–792.

Forrester, J., Merz, N., Bush, T., et al. (1996) Twenty-Seventh Bethesda Conference—Task Force 4. Efficacy of risk factor management. *Journal of the American College of Cardiology, 27*(5), 992–993.

Fulwood, R., Kalsbeek, W., Rifkund, B., et al. (1986). Total serum cholesterol levels of adults 20–74 years of age: United States 1976–80. *Vital and Health Statistics (Series II), 236,* U.S. Public Health Service.

Furberg, C.D., Berglund, G., Manolio, T.A., & Psaty, B.M. (1994). Overtreatment and undertreatment of hypertension. *Journal of Internal Medicine, 235*(5), 387–397.

Gaziano, J.M., & Hennekens, C.H. (1992). Vitamin antioxidants and cardiovascular disease. *Current Opinion Lipidology, 3,* 291–294.

Gaziano, J.M., Manson, J.E., Ridker, P.M., Buring, J.E., & Hennekens, C.H. (1990). Beta carotene therapy for chronic stable angina. *Circulation (Suppl. III), 82,* Abstract III-201.

Gillum, R.F., Gillum, B.S., & Smith, N. (1984). Cardiovascular risk factors among urban American Indians: Blood pressure serum lipids, smoking, diabetes, health knowledge and behavior. *American Heart Journal, 107*(4), 765–776.

Grundy, S.M. (1997). Management of high serum cholesterol and related disorders in patients at risk for coronary heart disease. *American Journal of Medicine, 102*(2A), 15–22.

Grundy, S.M. (1994). Heart disease and stroke guidelines for cholesterol management: Recommendations of the National Cholesterol Education Program's Adult Treatment Panel II, (May/June), 123–127.

Grundy, S.M. (1986). Cholesterol and coronary heart disease: A new era. *Journal of the American Medical Association, 256*(20), 2849–2858.

Guba, C., & McDonald, J. (1993) Epidemiology of smoking. *Health Values, 17*(2), 4–11.

Hallstrom, A.P., Cobb, L.A., & Ray, R. (1986). Smoking as a risk factor for recurrence of sudden cardiac arrest. *New England Journal of Medicine, 314*(5), 271–275.

Hammond, E.C., & Horn, D. (1958). Smoking and death rates: Report on 44 months of follow-up of 187,783 men. II. Death rates by cause. *Journal of the American Medical Association, 166,* 1294.

Holahan, C.J., Moos, R.S., Holahan, C.K., & Brennan, P.L. (1997). Social context, coping strategies, and depressive symptoms: An expanded model with cardiac patients. *Journal of Personality and Social Psychology. 72*(4), 918–928.

Hulley, S., Walsh, J., & Newman, T. (1992). Health policy on blood cholesterol: Time to change directions. *Circulation, 86*(3), 1026–1029.

Jones, P.H., & Gotton, A.M., Jr. (1994). Prevention of coronary heart disease in 1994. Evidence for intervention. *Heart Disease and Stroke, 3*(6), 290–296.

Joseph, D. (1993). Risk: A concept worthy of attention. *Nursing Forum, 28*(1), 13–16.

Kannel, W.B. (1990). Coronary heart disease risk factors: A Framingham study update. *Hospital Practice, 25*(7), 119–127, 130.

Kaplan, N. (1989). The deadly quartet: Upper body obesity, glucose intolerance, hypertriglycerides, and hypertension. *Archives of Internal Medicine, 149,* 14.

Kaplan, N., & Stamler, J. (1983). *Prevention of Coronary Heart Disease.* Philadelphia: W.B. Saunders.

Keys, A. (1980). *Seven Countries: A Multivariate Analysis of Death and Coronary Heart Disease.* Cambridge, MA: Harvard University Press.

Keys, A., Menotti, A., Karvonen, M.J., et al. (1986) The diet and 15-year death rate in the seven countries study. *American Journal of Epidemiology, 124*(6), 903–915.

Krieger, N. (1994). Epidemiology and the web of causation: Has anyone seen the spider? *Social Science and Medicine, 39*(7), 887–903.

Langford, H.G., Blaufox, M.D., Oberman, A., et al. (1985). Dietary therapy slows the return of hypertension after stopping prolonged medication. *Journal of the American Medical Association, 253*(5), 657–664.

Lipid Research Clinics Program. (1984). The lipid research clinics coronary primary prevention trials. I. Reduction in incidence of coronary heart disease. *Journal of the American Medical Association, 251*(3), 351–364.

Little, J.A., & Horlick, L. (1989). Consensus reports: Implications for the management of hypercholesterolemia and for future research. *Canadian Medical Association Journal, 140*(4), 369–370.

MacMahon, S., Peto, R., Cutler, J., et al. (1990). Blood pressure, stroke, and coronary heart disease. I. Prolonged differences in blood pressure: Prospective observational studies corrected for the regression dilution bias. *Lancet, 335*(8692), 765–774.

MacMahon, S.W., MacDonald, G.J., Bernstein, L., et al. (1985). Comparison of weight reduction with metoprolol in treatment of hypertension in young overweight patients. *Lancet, 1*(8440), 1233–1236.

MacMahon, B., Pugh, T.F., & Ipsen, J. (1960). *Epidemiologic Methods.* Boston: Little, Brown.

Manley, A.F. (1997). Cardiovascular implications of smoking: The Surgeon General's point of view. *Journal of Health Care for the Poor & Underserved. 8*(3), 303–310.

Manninen, V., Tenkanen, L., Koskinen, P., Huttuinen, J.K., Manttari, M., Heinonen, O.P., & Frick, M.H. (1992). Joint effects of serum triglyceride and LDL cholesterol and HDL cholesterol concentrations on coronary heart disease risk in Helsinki Heart Study: Implications for treatment. *Circulation, 85*(1), 37–45.

Marmot, M., & Elliott, P. (1992). *Coronary heart disease: Epidemiology from aetiology to public health.* New York: Oxford University Press.

Matthews, K.A., Meilahn, E., Kuller, L.H., Kelsey, S.F., Caggiula, A.N., Wing, R.R. (1989). Menopause and risk factors for coronary heart disease. *New England Journal of Medicine, 321*(10), 641–646.

Mausner, J., & Bahn, A. (1974). *Epidemiology: An introductory text.* Philadelphia: W.B. Saunders.

Morgan, P., & Lindsay, E. (1994). Screening in the office for elevated cholesterol levels: Still a dilemma. *Canadian Medical Association Journal, 151*(1), 25–27.

MRC Working Party. (1992). Medical Research Council trial of treatment of hypertension in older adults: Principal results. *British Medical Journal, 304*(6824), 405–412.

Murdaugh, C.L. (1992). The person with coronary heart disease risk factors. In C. Guzzetta & B. Dossey (Eds.), *Cardiovascular Nursing Holistic Practice.* St. Louis: Mosby–Year Book.

National High Blood Pressure Education Program (1993). The fifth report of the Joint National Committee on Detection, Evaluation and Treatment of Hypertension. *Archives of Internal Medicine, 153*(2), 154–183.

Naylor, C.D., Basinski, A., Frank, J., & Rachlis, M. (The Toronto Working Group on Cholesterol Policy) (1990). Asymptomatic hypercholesterol: A clinical policy review. *Journal of Clinical Epidemiology, 43*(10), 1028–1121.

Ockene, I., & Ockene, J.K. (1992). *Prevention of Coronary Heart Disease.* Boston: Little Brown & Co.

Oderkirk, W. (1994). Enthusiasm misplaced? Revisiting cholesterol screening. *Journal of Holistic Nursing, 12*(4), 414–424.

Paffenbarger, R.S., Jr., Hyde, R.T., Wing, A.L., et al. (1993). The association of changes in physical activity level and other lifestyle characteristics with mortality among men. *New England Journal of Medicine, 328*(8), 538–545.

Paffenbarger, R.S., Hyde, R.T., Wing, A.L., et al. (1990). Physical activity, all-cause mortality, and longevity of college alumni. *New England Journal of Medicine, 322,* 1770.

Pearson, T., & Fuster, V. (1996). Twenty-Seventh Bethesda Conference. Matching the intensity of risk factor management with the hazard for coronary disease events. *Journal of the American College of Cardiology, 27*(5), 957–1047.

Pekkanen, J., Nissinen, A., & Vartiainen, E., et al. (1994). Changes in serum cholesterol level and mortality: A 30-year followup. The Finnish cohorts of the Seven Countries Study. *American Journal of Epidemiology, 139*(2), 155–165.

Peto, R., Lopez, A.D., Boreham, J., Thun, M., & Heath, C. (1992). Mortality from tobacco in developed countries: Indirect estimation from national vital statistics. *Lancet, 339*(8804), 1268–1278.

Pierce, J.P., Fiore, M.C., Novotny, T.E., et al., (1989). Trends in cigarette smoking in the United States: Projections to the year 2000. *Journal of the American Medical Association, 261*(1), 61–65.

Pirie, P.L., Murray, D.M., & Luepker, R.V. (1988). Smoking prevalence in a cohort of adolescents including absentees, dropouts and transfers. *American Journal of Public Health 78*(2), 176–178.

Ragland, D.R., & Brand, R.J. (1988). Type A behavior and mortality from coronary heart disease. *New England Journal of Medicine, 318*(2), 65–69.

Rimm, E.B., Stampfer, M.J., Ascherio, A., Giovannucci, E., Colditz, G.A., & Wailed, W.C. (1993). Vitamin E consumption and the risk of coronary heart disease in men. *New England Journal of Medicine, 328*(20), 1450–1456.

Sempos, C.T., Cleeman, J., Carroll, M.D., Johnson, C.L., Bachorik, P.S., Gordon, D.T., Burt, V.L., Briefel, R.R., Brown, C.D., Lippel, K., & Rifkind, B. (1993). Prevalence of high blood cholesterol among U.S. adults: An update on guidelines from the second report of the National Cholesterol Education Program's Adult Treatment Panel. *Journal of the American Medical Association, 269*(2), 3009–3014.

Sempos, C., Fulwood, R., Haines, C., Carroll, M., Anda, R., Williamson, D., Remington, P., & Cleerman, J. (1989). The prevalence of high blood cholesterol among adults in the United States. *Journal of the American Medical Association, 262*(1), 45–52.

Shoplan, D.R. (1993). Smoking control in the 1990s: A National Cancer Institute model for change. *American Journal of Public Health, 83*(9), 1208–1210.

Stampfer, M.J., Wailed, W.C., Colditz, G.A., et al. (1991). A prospective study of postmenopausal estrogen therapy and coronary heart disease. *New England Journal of Medicine, 325*(11), 756–762.

Stampfer, M.J., Colditz, G.A., Wailed, W.C., et al. (1988). A prospective study of moderate alcohol consumption and the risk of coronary heart disease and stroke in women. *New England Journal of Medicine, 319*(5), 267–273.

Stehbens, W.E. (1992). Causality in medical science with particular reference to heart disease and atherosclerosis. *Perspectives in Biology and Medicine, 36*(1), 97–119.

Stokes, J. Dyslipidemia as a risk factor for cardiovascular disease and untimely death: The Framingham study. *Atherosclerosis Reviews, 18,* 49–57.

The Systolic Hypertension in the Elderly Program (SHEP) Cooperative Research Group. (1991). Prevention of stroke by antihypertensive drug treatment in older persons with isolated systolic hypertension: Final results of the Systolic Hypertension in the Elderly Program (SHEP). *Journal of the American Medical Association, 265*(24), 3255–3264.

Valanis, B. (1992). *Epidemiology in Nursing and Health Care* (2nd ed.). East Norwalk, CT, Appleton & Lange.

Vinicor, F. (1996). Features of microvascular disease of diabetes. In D. Haire-Ishu (Ed). *Management of Diabetes Mellitus: Perspectives of Care across the Lifespan.* St. Louis: Mosby–Year Book, 190–214.

Wilhelmsen, L. (1988). Coronary heart disease: Epidemiology of smoking and interventional studies of smoking. *American Heart Journal, 115*(1, part 2), 242–249.

Willems, J.P., Hunt, D.E., & Schorling, J.B. (1997). Coronary heart disease risk factors and cigarette smoking among rural African Americans. *Journal of the National Medical Association, 89*(1), 37–47.

Willson, P.W.F., Garrison, R.J., & Castelli, W.P. (1985). Postmenopausal estrogen use, cigarette smoking, and cardiovascular morbidity in women over fifty: The Framingham study. *New England Journal of Medicine, 313*(17), 1038–1043.

Windsor, R.A., Li, C.Q., Lowe, J.B., Perkins, L.L., Ershoff, D., & Glynn, T. (1993). The dissemination of smoking cessation methods for pregnant women: Achieving the year 2000 objectives. *American Journal of Public Health, 83*(2), 173–178.

Wynder, E.L. (1993). Toward a smoke-free society: Opportunities and obstacles. *American Journal of Public Health, 83*(9), 1204–1205.

CHAPTER 2

The Pathogenesis of Atherosclerosis

Annmarie Donahue Samar

Coronary artery disease is the end-product of a pathogenic process associated with development of atherosclerotic plaque in the coronary vasculature. To appropriately intervene with clients and to integrate theoretical and research perspectives into clinical practice, a knowledge of cellular pathophysiology is essential. Following an overview of atherosclerosis, this chapter will address normal arterial anatomy, the major cellular components involved in atherogenesis, lesion classification, and the six established hypotheses of atherosclerosis. The goal of this chapter is to break down complex physiology into manageable pieces, allowing the clinician to understand and interpret the intricate process of atherogenesis and risk factors in concrete physiologic terms.

OVERVIEW OF ATHEROSCLEROSIS

Atherosclerosis consists of the formation of fibrofatty and fibrous lesions, preceded and accompanied by inflammation (Ross, 1993). Atherosclerosis is essentially an intimal disease, with changes beginning many years before they become clinically apparent. Accumulations of lipid in the intima and associated changes begin in children and may lead to symptom-producing lesions starting at middle age. The mechanisms of atherogenesis are not completely clear. Once symptoms are present, causation is difficult to attribute. However, atherosclerosis can be treated most efficiently prior to lesions becoming clinically obvious (Stary, 1995).

Atherosclerosis is often incorrectly thought of as a twentieth-century disease. Calcified, ulcerated thrombotic plaques similar to those currently described have been identified in Egyptian mummies from 1500 BC to AD 520. Similar evidence of generalized atherosclerosis and significant involvement of the coronary arteries has been found in China, carbon-dated to 2,100 years ago. Extensive coronary atherosclerosis was found in a frozen mummy from Alaska dated approximately AD 400 (Velican, 1989).

Atherosclerosis is a disease in its own right and a contributor to the development of multiple disease states, such as myocardial and cerebral infarction, other cardiac sequelae, and loss of function and gangrene in limbs. Despite considerable research and speculation, the pathogenesis and complex mechanisms of development remain only partially understood. Even with extensive investigation, the true initiating factor or mechanism(s) of atherosclerosis remain unknown. However, atherosclerosis is known to be a multifactorial process associated with genetic, environmental, and lifestyle factors (Teplitz & Siwik, 1994). Lesions result from the many complex interactions between noxious stimuli and healing responses of the arterial wall. This intricate, normally protective process results from an extreme inflammatory, fibroproliferative response to insult occurring in a hyperlipidemic or dyslipoproteinemic environment.

Dyslipoproteinemias are disorders of plasma lipid transport (Schwartz et al., 1993). Atherosclerosis is categorized clinically as a systemic disorder with multi-organ involvement. Single cases demonstrate notable variations in the occurrence and magnitude of lesions (Hort, 1994). Lesions do not occur indiscriminately but at specific lesion-prone sites distinguished by increased permeability of the endothelium to plasma proteins. In animal studies these particular sites demonstrate a significant increase in intimal cholesterol accumulation and a thinner boundary layer (glycocalyx) at the endothelial surface when a high-fat and high-cholesterol diet is consumed (Schwartz, Valente, & Sprague, 1993).

With improved knowledge of the earliest stages of atherosclerosis, researchers are now beginning to relate morphologic changes to disorders of function. Advances in pathology techniques and equipment now allow components of the vessel wall to be studied in reference to clinically apparent dysfunction (Hort, 1994).

NORMAL ARTERIAL WALL ANATOMY AND PHYSIOLOGY

To understand the pathophysiology of atherosclerosis, the clinician must understand the normal structure of the arterial wall and related physiologic processes, especially normal arterial thickening. As a prelude to a discussion of the complex pathologic changes that may occur, much of the information in this section is descriptive.

The normal arterial wall is musculoelastic and made up of three discrete layers (tunicas): intima, media, and adventitia (Fig. 2–1).

INTIMA. The innermost tunica, the intima, is defined as "the region of the arterial wall from and including the endothelial surface at the lumen to the luminal margin of the media" (Stary

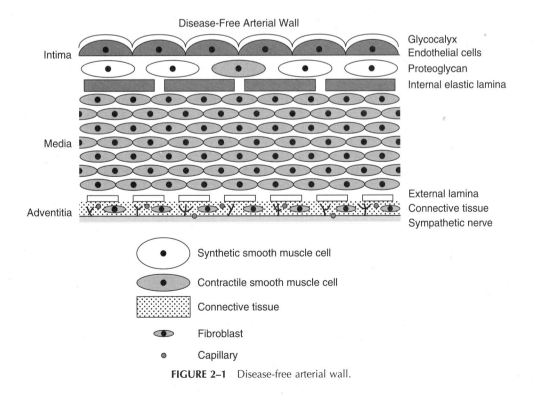

FIGURE 2–1 Disease-free arterial wall.

et al., p. 393, 1992). The intima is made of two layers and is not of consistent thickness. A single thickness of endothelial cells is joined to a basement membrane of proteins, called the *proteoglycan*. This transparent monolayer of endothelial cells is coated with a glycocalyx, or boundary layer, at the luminal surface. The normally slick glycocalyx is made up principally of free polysaccharides, glycosaminoglycans, and glycoprotein and glycolipid side chains proceeding from the plasma membrane. The glycocalyx is in direct contact with the blood coursing through the vessel and constitutes a crucial link between the blood and the tissues (Teplitz & Siwik, 1994). The endothelial cells provide a nonthrombogenic surface to (1) prohibit platelet aggregation and clot formation and (2) regulate the passage of substances in and out of the arterial wall. The endothelium is normally selectively permeable to all proteins in the blood and does not support the adherence of liberal numbers of leukocytes (Stary, Blankenhorn, et al., 1992).

When viewed by traditional light microscopy, the intimal layers may be absent or barely visible. When viewed by electron microscopy, though, the intimal proteoglycan has sparse elastic fibers and broadly spaced, single smooth muscle cells (SMCs) of the synthetic (rough endoplasmic reticulum-rich or immature) type with occasional cells of contractile (myofilament-rich, or adult) type. Isolated macrophages may be found in the proteoglycan layer in disease-free intima near the endothelium (Stary, Blankenhorn, et al., 1992).

MEDIA. The media is the second discrete tunica (layer) of the normal arterial wall, made up almost entirely of SMCs surrounded by a basement membrane similar to that of the intima. The proteins of the basement membrane interact directly with the SMCs via specific receptors. These receptors regulate transport of substances and link extracellular matrix proteins to the SMCs. The layers of smooth muscle are concentric and embedded within a meshwork of the extracellular matrix proteins. This meshwork provides a framework that sustains the integrity of vascular structures (Teplitz, 1994). The margin between the intima and media is called the *internal elastic lamina* and is usually treated as a component of the media (Stary, Blankenhorn, et al., 1992).

ADVENTITIA. The adventitia, the third tunica, is chiefly made up of fibroblasts, with sparse SMCs in loose connective tissues. The media and adventitia are separated by a boundary of elastic fibers called the *external lamina*. A major portion of the strength of the arterial wall is provided by the adventitia (Zierler & Cowan, 1995). Atherosclerotic changes occur primarily in the intimal layer. Secondary alterations can be found in the media, with ensuing arterial dilatation and aneurysm formation. As the incidence of atherosclerotic lesions is increased in areas of physiologic, adaptive intimal thickening, associated processes will now be discussed.

PHYSIOLOGIC ADAPTIVE THICKENING

Atherosclerotic lesions of all types are increased in locations with adaptive intimal thickening. Although these areas are the first to develop advanced lesions, adaptive thickening per se does not imply or foretell an atherosclerotic lesion. It simply identifies locations where, with risk factors present, atherosclerotic lesions develop earlier and more swiftly. When adaptive intimal thickening coincides with sites of early occurrence of advanced atherosclerotic lesions, areas are identified as atherosclerosis-prone (Stary, 1994; Stary, Blankenhorn, et al., 1992).

"Intima, as living, reactive tissue, adapts in thickness to changes in pulse rate, blood pressure, arterial geometry, flow rate, and resistance to flow in distal vascular segments and in supplied organs" (Stary, Blankenhorn, et al., 1992). Normal human arterial intima is of uneven thickness. Areas of thick intima may develop in utero and exist in healthy humans of all ages. These areas are self-limited, do not obstruct blood flow, and are not characteristic of disease.

Thickening, a physiologic adaptation to specific mechanical forces, is related to changes in wall stress or blood flow or both; it may be considered the result of an endeavor by the tissue to sustain pressures and flow. Physiologic adaptive thickening differs from atherosclerosis in that the thickened structure is composed of normal arterial wall elements. Two patterns of adaptive intimal thickening exist: eccentric (focal or abrupt) and diffuse (extensive) intimal thickening (Table 2–1). *Eccentric thickening* is characterized by a focal pattern occurring in areas of arterial branching and orifices. *Diffuse thickening* is characterized by a widespread encircling pattern of thickening. From a morphologic perspective, these two patterns may occur concurrently or contiguously such that differentiation may be difficult (Stary, 1994; Stary, Blankenhorn, et al., 1992).

As discussed, eccentric thickening is associated with areas of turbulent and disturbed flow such as branching and orifices. Shear and tensile stresses are not consistently distributed in eccentric thickening. Histologically, eccentric intimal thickening has three times as many macrophages as the opposing wall without thickening. Eccentric thickening may occur in the aorta and the coronary, renal, cerebral, and carotid arteries (Stary, 1994; Stary, Blankenhorn, et al., 1992). In contrast, diffuse intimal thickening is widespread, frequently has an encircling pattern, and is not obviously related to branching, orifices, and bifurcations of the vessels. The degree of diffuse thickening is less than that of eccentric in coronary arteries (Stary, 1994; Stary, Blankenhorn, et al., 1992).

Areas with adaptive thickening perform differently than other regions. The rates of turnover of endothelial cells, SMCs, and concentrations of *low-density lipoprotein* (LDL) and other plasma components are increased. These changes are not considered aberrant unless they reach a level allied with tissue injury (Stary, 1994; Stary, Blankenhorn, et al., 1992).

TYPES OF ATHEROGENIC LESIONS

A detailed discussion of the progression and classification of atherosclerotic lesions is important to provide a foundation for understanding the hypotheses of atherogenesis. Insight into lesion classification—in particular, of early lesions—and how they progress is essential to understanding the physiologic basis of risk factors and risk-reduction strategies.

Atherogenesis is the sequential process associated with formation of an *atheroma* (lesion that is potentially symptom-producing). Based on autopsy data, the American Heart Associa-

tion's Committee on Vascular Lesions has categorized atherosclerotic lesions and their progression. A stage approach has been used to classify characteristic lesions in terms of sequential pathologic stages I through VI, which range from minimal intimal change to changes associated with clinical manifestations. The roman numerals indicate the usual sequence of lesion progression. This classification system is termed the *Stary system* after its primary originator. The Stary classification system correlates the appearance of both advanced lesions and their precursors as noted in clinical imaging studies, with clinical syndromes and histologic lesion types (Stary, 1989; Stary, Blankenhorn, et al., 1992; Stary, Chandler, et al., 1995).

In early stages, the progression of atherosclerosis is predictable, characteristic, and uniform. In more advanced lesions, progression is less predictable. Advanced lesions may progress in diverse morphologic stages, resulting in different lesion types and clinical presentation's (Stary, Chandler, et al., 1995). Each of six types of lesions identified with its components will now be discussed. Table 2–2 lists the six types with their components and their corresponding Bethesda classification (discussed later under "Bethesda Classification"). Figure 2–2 illustrates the six types. Table 2–3 gives their characteristic locations, in areas of eccentric versus diffuse thickening.

Type I—Isolated Macrophage Foam Cells

Type I (isolated macrophage foam cell) lesions contain enough atherogenic lipoprotein to elicit an increase in monocytes/macrophages and the formation of macrophages containing lipid droplets. These droplets, referred to as *macrophage foam cells* (MFCs), are commonly believed to be the earliest cellular markers of pathologic changes associated with atheroma development. MFCs provide the first evidence that lipid is retained and reacted to in the intima. MFCs occur as small clumps or separate cells that balloon out because of the lipid within them. They develop a foamy appearance, hence the name "foam cells."

When MFCs are present, macrophages without lipid droplets are also seen more frequently

TABLE 2–1 Physiologic Adaptive Thickening: Variants in Normal Intimal Histology

Type of Thickening	Descriptive Terms	Characteristic Composition	Characteristic Location	Characteristic Age of Onset
Eccentric (intimal) thickening (ET)	Intimal cushion Intimal pad Spindle cell pad Intimal bolster Fibromuscular plaque Smooth muscle mass Focal intimal hyperplasia	Distinct upper layer Layer with voluminous proteoglycan Isolated macrophage foam cells Lower musculoelastic layer several times the thickness of the upper layer with compact rows of contractile SMCs and elastic fibers	At bifurcations; tapers into diffuse thickening at its periphery	From birth
Diffuse (intimal) thickening (DT)	Musculoelastic intimal thickening Intimal hyperplasia	Proteoglycan and musculoelastic layers are present but less thick than in ET The same elements as ET	Comparable involvement of all portions of the main coronary arteries, not involved with ET	From birth

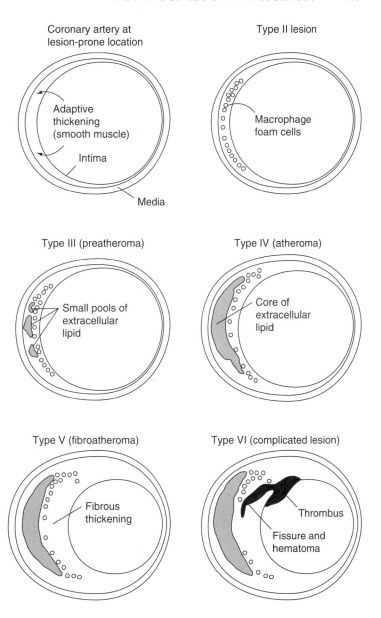

FIGURE 2–2 Cross sections of identical, most proximal part of six left anterior descending coronary arteries. The morphology of the intima ranges from adaptive intimal thickening always present in this lesion-prone location to a type VI lesion in advanced atherosclerotic disease. Other cross sections show sequence of atherosclerotic lesion types that may lead to type VI. Identical morphologies may be found in other lesion-prone parts of the coronary and many other arteries. From Stary, H.C., Chandler, A.B., Dinsmore, R.E., Fuster, V., Glagov, S., Insull, W., Rosenfeld, M.E., Schwartz, C., Wagner, W.D., & Wissler, R.B. (1995). A definition of advanced types of atherosclerotic lesions and a histological classification of atherosclerosis: A report from the Committee on Vascular Lesions of the Council on Arteriosclerosis, American Heart Association. *Circulation, 92*, 1362. Reprinted with permission of the American Heart Association.

than in normal intima. Stary reports that macrophages occur six times more frequently and MFCs five times more frequently in areas of eccentric thickening than in areas of diffuse thickening. Macrophages are found in only the immediate subendothelial area, whereas foam cells are found deep in the proteoglycan layer. With Type I lesions, lipid accumulates intracellularly only. Research supports the role of Type I lesions as a cellular marker of pathologic atherosclerotic changes, especially in areas of

adaptive thickening (Stary, 1989; Stary, Chandler, et al., 1994).

Type II—Fatty Streak, Superficial or Submerged

Type II (fatty streak) lesions are composed of layers of MFCs and lipid-laden smooth muscle cells under an intact endothelium (see Fig. 2–2). Thinly scattered particles of extracellular lipid

TABLE 2-2 Six Types of Lesions Identified with Components

Lesion Type	Lesion Subtype	Chief Histology	Chief Growth Mechanism	Earliest Onset	Clinical Correlation	Clinical Classification: Bethesda Phase
Type I *Initial first evidence of lipid accumulation*		Isolated macrophage foam cells with only intracellular accumulation; no tissue injury	Lipid accumulation	From first decade	Clinically silent	Early lesion: Bethesda Phase 1
Type II *Fatty streak*		Layers of SMCs with intracellular and extracellular lipid and increased MFCs; no tissue injury	Lipid accumulation	From first decade	Superficial-visible or submerged-concealed; clinically silent	Early lesion: Bethesda Phase 1
Type III *Preatheroma*		Type II changes with greatly increased extracellular lipid and small lipid pools; microscopic evidence of tissue injury	Lipid accumulation	From third decade	Small white elevations; clinically silent	Intermediate lesion: Bethesda Phase 1
Type IV *Atheroma with lipid core* *Atheroma with necrotic core*		Type III changes without small lipid pools Pools join to form an extensive lipid core that dissolves intimal architecture and significantly thickens intima; massive structural injury	Lipid accumulation	From third decade	Clinically silent or detectable	Advanced/raised lesion: Bethesda Phase 2
Type V *Fibroatheroma*		Type IV changes with the earliest fibrotic changes to the proteoglycan layer; increased synthetic SMCs; new fibrous connective tissue above lipid core	Accelerated smooth muscle and collagen increase	From fourth decade	Clinically silent or detectable	Advanced/raised lesion: Bethesda Phase 2

Classification	Description		Age	Clinical	Bethesda
	Type Va Multilayered multiple lipid cores				Bethesda Phase 5
	Type Vb Calcific				Bethesda Phase 5
	Type Vc Fibrotic; no lipid cores; minimal amount of lipid				
Type VI *Complicated surface defects*	Type IV or V lesions with disruptions to the surface; thrombotic deposits or hematoma	Thrombosis; hematoma	From fourth decade	Clinically silent or detectable	Advanced/raised/complicated lesion: Bethesda Phase 3 or 4
	Type VIa Disruption of surface fissure ulceration				
	Type VIb Hematoma; hemorrhage				Bethesda Phase 3 or 4
	Type VIc Thrombosis				Bethesda Phase 3 or 4

TABLE 2–3 Lesion Occurrence
in Adaptive Thickening

Lesion Type	Characteristic Location
Initial type	In eccentric and diffuse thickening (more in eccentric)
Type II: fatty streak	Submerged in eccentric periphery of both eccentric and diffuse thickening (more in and at the periphery of eccentric thickening)
Type III: preatheroma	Only in eccentric thickening
Type IV: atheroma with lipid core	Only in eccentric thickening
Type IV: atheroma with necrotic core	
Type V: fibroatheroma	Only in eccentric thickening but frequent extensions beyond eccentric thickening
Type VI: complicated lesion with surface defect	Only in eccentric thickening but frequent extensions beyond eccentric thickening

are present in the intracellular matrix. Although the number of intimal smooth muscle cells is no greater in atherosclerotic tissue than in non-atherosclerotic tissue, the number of macrophages or MFCs is increased relative to Type I lesions.

The location of MFCs depends on the depth of the proteoglycan layer. MFCs tend to build up in the lower part of the proteoglycan layer in one or more layers. Lipid deposits occur near the endothelium and are grossly visible in areas of diffuse thickening or at the periphery of eccentric thickening. These visible lipid deposits are known as *superficial fatty streaks*. They may appear as yellowish smooth streaks, patches, or spots. In areas of eccentric thickening with associated wider proteoglycan layers, the foam cells are chiefly invisible from the endothelial surface. The terms "submerged" and "concealed" have been applied to this morphologic representation of fatty streaks (Falk, 1994; Stary, 1989; Stary, Chandler, et al., 1994). Although fatty streaks may be identifiable within the first decade of life, their significance is questionable. Advanced lesions do be-

gin with fatty streaks, but it is unclear whether or not the presence of fatty streaks indicates a greater chance of advanced lesions developing.

Type III—Preatheroma

Type III (preatheroma) lesions are transient lesions between the Type II, fatty streak, and the Type IV, atheroma, categories. Stary's autopsy study (1989) found Type III lesions in coronary artery areas with eccentric thickening. Type III lesions contain all the characteristics of Type II lesions in addition to a greatly increased number of extracellular lipid particles. These particles form multiple, individual pool-like aggregates in the musculoelastic layer of eccentric thickening. They occur beneath the layers of MFCs in the bordering proteoglycan layer (see Fig. 2–2). Aggregates replace intracellular matrix, increase intracellular space, and disrupt the coherence of structural SMCs. Type III lesions increase arterial wall thickness, but Stary and colleagues noted no loss of lumen and noted that preatheromas appear as small white elevations (Stary, 1989).

Type IV—Atheroma, Lipid or Necrotic Core

Type IV (atheroma) and higher lesions are considered to be advanced lesions, characterized by disintegration and derangement of the intima of the artery. Even these advanced lesions may not be clinically apparent or angiographically discernible (Stary, 1994). Type IV lesions have all the components of Type III lesions except for the individual pools of extracellular lipid particles. In Type IV lesions, the Type III pools in the musculoelastic layer of eccentric thickening are joined to a dense, extensive lipid core (see Fig. 2–2). Fused lipid particles are grossly visible beneath the proteoglycan layer and are identical to lipid droplets found within the cytoplasm of lipid-laden cells (Stary, Chandler, et al., 1995).

The term *necrotic core* is commonly used to describe these lesions, although Stary and colleagues use *lipid core* because lipid is the actual chief component. Type IV lesions are the first of the advanced lesions in that the lipid core, or mass of extracellular lipid, causes intimal disorganization by dissolving the intimal architecture, separating the musculoelastic layer, and thus disrupting and displacing cells into inner and outer sections.

The core significantly thickens the intima, and resultant changes are generally detectable by the human eye. The increase in lipid is hypothesized to develop from continued insudation from the plasma. Stary (1989) reported a few scattered, occasionally dead, widely separated SMCs in the core, at times only a few dead ones. MFCs border, but are not found within, the core on the lumen aspect. Type IV lesions slow the flow mildly or not at all and therefore are not detectable clinically (Stary, 1989, 1994).

Type IV lesions may have great clinical significance. The abundant concentrations of macrophages, MFCs, and lymphocytes in the periphery make these lesions vulnerable to rupture and fissure (Stary, Chandler, et al., 1995).

Type V—Fibroatheroma

Type V (fibroatheroma) lesions are identical to Type IV (atheroma) lesions except for changes in the makeup of the proteoglycan layer. Type V lesions are characterized by a slow, progressive conversion of the proteoglycan layer into a fibrous cap, increased numbers of synthetic rather than contractile SMCs, and prominent new fibrous connective tissue (see Fig. 2–2). The cells are enmeshed in a thick network of collagen and capillaries (Stary, 1989, 1994; Stary, Chandler, et al., 1995).

Type V lesions are the earliest lesions to demonstrate significant changes to the proteoglycan layer. The collagenous cap is generally formed gradually over a period of years (Ferrel, 1994). When platelets and fibrin deposited on the endothelial surface are incorporated into the cap, its development and thickening are accelerated. The cap's SMCs are of varied structure and are stratified in compact, parallel layers around the circumference of the vessel.

Lipid droplets in caps are rare or nonexistent. Type V lesions are seen in areas of eccentric thickening, with some extensions beyond, especially when thrombotic deposits are incorpo-

rated. These lesions may be clinically detectable or quiescent depending on the degree of narrowing they cause, but they are clinically significant, as they can develop fissures, hematoma, or thrombus (Stary, 1989, 1994; Stary, Chandler, et al., 1995).

Three subtypes of Type V lesions (Types Va, Vb, and Vc) exist. When a lipid core is part of this lesion, it is referred to as Type Va. When a lesion's lipid core and other parts are calcified, Type Vb is the term used. When the lipid core is not present, and widespread lipid is minimal, the lesion is referred to Type Vc. The regions surrounding the core, particularly the region above, are thickened and remodeled by layers of collagen in Type Vc (Stary, 1994).

Type Va lesions may be called *multilayered fibroatheroma,* as they are often multilayered and irregularly stacked with several lipid cores divided by substantial layers of reparative fibrous tissue, chiefly collagenous. An explanation for the multilayered architecture may be found in repetitive disruptions of lesion surface, hematomas, and thrombotic deposits. Mechanical forces may play a role in the development of Type Va lesions. Type Vb (calcific) lesions are made up largely of calcium and increased fibrotic connective tissue. Accumulated remnants of dead cells and lipid may be replaced by mineral deposits. Mineralization is the dominant Type Vb feature. Type Vc (fibrotic) lesions have absent lipid cores, and lipid, in general, is minimal (Stary, Chandler, et al., 1995).

Type VI—Complicated Lesions

Type VI (complicated) lesions have the underlying morphology of Type IV or V lesions, with disruptions of the surface and with thrombotic deposits or hematoma (see Fig. 2–2). Morbidity and mortality from atherosclerosis, as well as aneurysms, are often associated with Type VI lesions. Type VI lesions may be grouped by their complicating features, which may be superimposed on any type of lesion or, less often, on intima. The nature of the complicating features depends on individual tissue reactions and personal risk factors.

Type VIa lesions have a disruption of the surface, which may be fissures or ulcerations. Type VIb lesions have a hematoma or hemorrhage. Type VIc lesions have thrombosis. A lesion with all three subtypes is termed a Type VIabc lesion (Stary, Chandler, et al., 1995).

Bethesda Classification

The Twenty-Seventh Bethesda Conference endorsed Stary's classification system and delineated a five-phase model to link plaque morphology and progression to clinical disease. The model implies diverse morphologic progression of advanced lesions, resulting in different lesion types and clinical presentations (Fig. 2–3). Phase 1 includes Types I, II, and III, which develop over a period of years. In Phase 2 plaque may not necessarily be stenotic but is prone to rupture because of a high lipid content, as occurs in Types IV and Va lesions. Phase 2 can evolve into Phase 3 complicated lesions or Phase 4 acute syndromes. Phases 3 and 4 can further progress to Phase 5, the more stenotic and fibrotic Type Vb or Vc le-

sions. Phase 5 lesions are usually clinically apparent, with evidence of occlusion and angina. Some Phase 5 lesions, however, may remain clinically silent owing to collateral vessel development (Fuster et al., 1996)

THE CAST OF CELLULAR CHARACTERS

To date, we have looked at morphologic presentation in our discussion of lesion classification and only alluded to the prevalence and function of certain cell types and cellular factors. In this section these cellular "players" will be discussed in detail to assist the reader in understanding cutting-edge research and clinical practice implications.

A variety of regulatory molecules are involved in the atherosclerotic process, including growth factors, cytokines, and chemicals such as lipids and nitric oxide. The roles of regulatory molecules in atherogenesis include cell migration

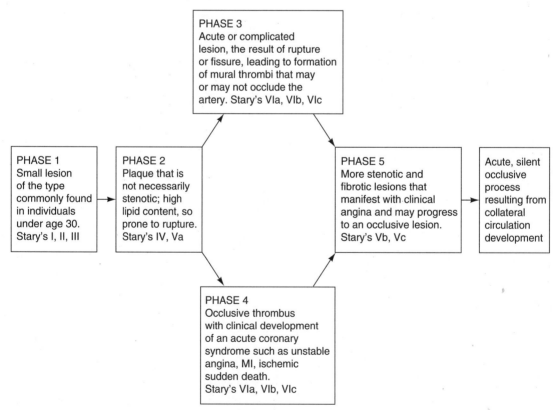

FIGURE 2–3 Bethesda classification for the process of plaque progression, based on the five phases of Stary's classification system.

and recruitment, cell proliferation, and control of lipid and protein synthesis. The same modifiers may have a part in vascular functioning, as in vasodilatation, vasoconstriction, and coagulation. The terms *growth factor* and *cytokine* are frequently used interchangeably. Originally cytokines were identified as mediators of inflammation and immunity, and growth factors as mediators of cell proliferation and chemotaxis. But both cytokines and growth factors can function as regulators of inflammation and growth in atherogenesis. *Chemotaxis* is the movement of white blood cells to an area of inflammation in response to chemical mediators released by neutrophils, monocytes, and injured tissue (Ross, 1993).

The four major cell types involved in the atherosclerotic process (endothelial cells, SMCs, platelets, and monocyte-macrophages) will now be addressed.

Endothelial Cells

Endothelial cells are the primary site of development of atherosclerosis and are often called collectively the *endothelium*. The endothelium is a highly dynamic, multifunctional organ whose central role is to sense and respond to changes in stress and blood flow. In systemic and coronary arteries, the endothelium has a significant effect on vascular tone, platelet adhesion, and aggregation. "Endothelial cells may be viewed as a mechanotransducer sensing local blood flow and converting signals of increased shear stress into vessel wall relaxation thereby optimizing tissue perfusion according to the metabolic needs" (Zeiher et al., 1995). The transparent endothelium has a significant role in vasodilatation and in modulating or inhibiting vasoconstriction in response to numerous vasoactive stimuli (Harrison, 1995; Zeiher et al., 1995).

Three principal endothelial attributes prevent clotting in disease-free arteries. The first is the smoothness of the endothelium, which prevents contact activation of the intrinsic clotting system. Second is the presence of the glycocalyx, a mucopolysaccharide that adheres to the luminal surface of the endothelium and repels clotting factors and platelets. Third, thrombodulin, a protein bound with the endothelial membrane, binds thrombin. Clotting is thus deterred by inactivating thrombin and by the action of protein C. Protein C is activated by the thrombodulin-thrombin structure and inactivates Factors V and VIII (Guyton & Hall, 1996).

Unlike other cells, endothelial cells invariably develop in a strict single layer (i.e., *monolayer*) in all vascular sites. The monolayer's properties of cell-to-cell attachment and "contact inhibition" are important because they regulate the capacity of endothelial cells to multiply and respond to injury. Alterations in endothelial cells may be the initiating component of atherosclerosis. Endothelial cells augment the lesion by the secretion of growth-stimulating factors (Ross, 1986; Teplitz & Siwik, 1994).

Endothelial cells also govern the type of lipoproteins and plasma contents that enter the subendothelial space. They bind LDL through specific high-affinity receptors and mildly oxidize it so that it is acknowledged and ingested by macrophages. In addition, endothelial cells secrete vasoconstrictors, vasodilators, growth factors, and growth inhibitors in response to numerous stimuli. Endothelial cells may have a significant impact on monocytes and SMCs. Vasoconstrictors secreted include endothelins, *platelet-derived growth factor* (PDGF), and endothelium-derived constricting factor. Vasorelaxors secreted include *endothelium-derived relaxing factor* (EDRF), *nitric oxide* (NO), and prostacyclin. NO or a related compound has been postulated to account for the biologic activity of EDRF. Prostacyclin inhibits platelet activation (Ross, 1986; Teplitz & Siwik, 1994).

Shear forces, which likely increase in the presence of hypertension, the chemical irritants in tobacco smoke, diabetes without glycemic control, and other risk factors, may also contribute to chronic endothelial injury or dysfunction. When endothelial injury occurs, smoothness and glycocalyx-thrombodulin layer are lost. The break in endothelial integrity initiates clotting by Factor XII and platelet stimulation. The activation is even more powerful when contact with subendothelial collagen takes place (Fuster, Gotto, Libby, et al., 1996; Guyton & Hall, 1996).

Endothelial cells may have an early pivotal role in atherogenesis by oxidizing and thus mildly modifying LDL. Modified LDL is hypothesized to stimulate the expression of adhesive glycoproteins on the endothelial glycocalyx, leading to early involvement in monocyte recruitment (Fuster, Gotto, Libby, et al., 1996). It is noteworthy that all major cell types of the vessel wall can modify LDL (Table 2–4).

Smooth Muscle Cells

SMCs ordinarily are the dominant cellular element of the media, and they play a major role in the reparative and proliferative processes of atherosclerosis. They are not normally present in the luminal layer of the intima but may be detected in atherosclerotic intima. SMCs are the primary cell type in fibrous plaques, and SMC proliferation is widely accepted as a basic mechanism in atherogenesis. Furthermore, SMC proliferation determines the extent of the lesion and whether clinical sequelae will evolve (Ross, 1986, 1993; Teplitz & Siwik, 1994).

Vascular SMCs may have the appearance of

TABLE 2–4 Endothelial Cells

Function	Related Properties
Permeability barrier	Presence of glycocalyx; basement membrane; size of vesicles; tight cell junctions
Thromboresistance	Smoothness; "slippery" glycocalyx; thrombodulin bond with endothelial membrane; swift metabolism of platelet-aggregating agents; synthesis and secretion of prostacyclin and plasminogen activator
Modulation of vascular tone	Synthesis and secretion of prostacyclin, endothelial-derived relaxing factor, and endothelin; expression of leukocyte adhesion molecules, leukocyte chemotactic proteins, growth factors, and scavenger receptors
Inflammation and immune response	

Adapted from Stary, H.C., Blankenhorn, D.H., et al. (1992). A definition of the intima of human arteries and of its atherosclerosis-prone regions: A report from the Committee on Vascular Lesions of the Council on Arteriosclerosis, American Heart Association. *Circulation, 1,* 391–405. Adapted with permission of the American Heart Association.

foam cells, leading to some confusion in lesion classification among researchers. They are capable of many functions, including formation of extensive connective tissue matrix and amassment of lipid. SMCs have receptors for LDL and for growth factors, including PDGF, and can synthesize prostacyclin, prostaglandin E, and other prostaglandin derivatives. An important feature of SMCs is their capacity to migrate from the media to the intima in response to specific chemoattractants and then replicate (Ross, 1986).

As part of the healing response, SMCs lose contractile capacities and contain fewer myofibrils. Contractile-type SMCs contain myofibrils that allow vasoconstriction and vasodilatation in response to endogenous and pharmacologic stimuli. Moreover, SMCs gain the synthetic capacity to divide and produce collagen. Synthetic-type cells are also able to express genes for cytokines and growth-regulatory molecules and react to growth factors by expressing appropriate receptors and synthesizing extracellular matrix. In the synthetic state, SMCs express LDL receptors and thus can "ingest" lipid. Synthetic SMCs can also produce their own mitogenic factors leading to autostimulation and proliferation.

Ross suggests that following appropriate stimulation, SMCs in lesions may have changed from contractile to synthetic type (Ross, 1993). The proposed change from contractile to synthetic would have significant impact on the ability of a lesion to react to diverse agonists and on the development of atherosclerosis. Once involved in the atherosclerotic lesion, vascular SMCs may activate their own development and recruitment by secreting growth regulatory factors and laying down matrix. SMCs may return to a contractile state when the endothelial layer is reestablished or upon chronic endothelial activation (Ross, 1986, 1993; Teplitz & Siwik, 1994). Thus, risk reduction may play a role in SMC function (Table 2–5).

Platelets

Platelets are not cells, but disk-shaped cytoplasmic fragments without a nucleus or DNA. Platelets are essential for blood coagulation and control of bleeding. They play a role in athero-

TABLE 2–5 Smooth Muscle Cells

Function	Related Properties
Contractility	Ability to influence the content of contractile proteins; responsiveness to vasoactive substances; synthesis and secretion of collagen, elastin, and proteoglycan
Maintenance of vessel wall structure	Ability to proliferate by expressing growth factor receptors; ability to synthesize and secrete growth factors; ability to migrate
Lipid metabolism	Removal of lipoproteins by the expression of LDL receptors or phagocytosis

genesis through (1) direct adhesion to subendothelium in a hypercholesterolemic environment or after endothelial injury and (2) release of mitogenic (cell-division–stimulating) and chemotaxic (white-blood-cell–attracting) products or factors (Ross, 1993; Teplitz & Siwik, 1994). Table 2–6 details the functions and related properties of activated platelets.

Platelets can be thought of as circulating receptacles of multiple granules containing potent biochemical mediators. Platelets do not adhere to disease-free endothelium or to themselves unless activated. When platelet activation occurs, platelet granule contents are released, with resultant stimulation of adherence and aggregation. Release of granule contents in turn attracts more platelets to the site, and clotting mechanisms ensue. Within 3–5 days after release of platelet granule contents, SMCs migrate, and proliferation begins.

Platelet granule mitogens, or substances stimulating cell division and SMC migration, include *epidermal growth factor* (EGF) and PDGF. Additional significant effects of platelet activation are platelet-mediated SMC proliferation and stimulation of connective tissue formation. PDGF is considered to be the most potent growth factor. It is exceptionally important in atherosclerosis, as it is both chemotactic and mitogenic. PDGF effects include enhanced synthesis of collagen Type I, LDL receptors and

scavenger receptors on the macrophages. As will be discussed in the subsequent section addressing the lipid-insudation-irritation hypothesis, LDL has a significant role in atherogenesis. PDGF promotes increased LDL uptake and accelerated output of *insulin-like growth factor* (IGF), prostaglandins, and monocyte chemoattractants. EGF increases DNA synthesis in SMCs (Ross, 1993; Teplitz & Siwik, 1994).

Additional platelet-derived factors include the potent vasoconstrictors, serotonin, norepinephrine, and histamine. These amines increase proliferation and migration of cultured SMCs in the presence of serum. Further damage to vessel walls can occur by vasoconstriction and increasing shear stress. Activated platelets release factors that are involved in cell adhesion and attract more platelets to the clot. Ross (1993) reports laboratory evidence that if platelets are kept out of a site of endothelial injury, the typical intimal proliferative lesions will not develop (Ross, 1993; Teplitz & Siwik, 1994).

Monocytes/Macrophages

Monocytes/macrophages are the scavenger cells of the body. A part of the mononuclear phagocyte system, they are present in all stages of atherosclerosis. Monocytes/macrophages are the principal inflammatory mediators of cells in an atherogenic environment. Circulating monocytes are recruited to the intima by the expression of adhesive glycoproteins on the glycocalyx. Adhesive glycoprotein production is thought to be induced by mildly oxidized LDL. Endothelium is critical in this process, as it is believed to mildly oxidize the LDL (Fuster, Gotto, Libby, et al., 1996; Ross, 1986, 1993; Teplitz & Siwik, 1994).

One of the first cellular reactions that occurs is the binding of monocytes to endothelium. With monocyte adhesion to the vessel wall, monocyte chemotactic protein-1 and colony-stimulating factor are secreted, and more monocytes are attracted to the site. Once monocytes enter the intima, substances associated with atherogenesis may participate in the activation of monocytes that differentiate to fixed tissue macrophages. Macrophages are the hallmark of the inflammatory response and produce one of the most powerful chemoattrac-

TABLE 2–6 Activated Platelets

Function	Related Properties
Remodeling of the intima	Direct adhesion to subendothelium in a hypercholesterolemic environment or after endothelial injury; release of mitogenic (cell-division–stimulating) and chemotaxic (white blood cell–attracting) products or factors.
Procoagulant	Activation causes adherence, aggregation, and release of platelet granule contents, including factors involved in cell adhesion, attraction of additional platelets, and support of fibrin production.
Maintenance and growth of vessel wall structure	Granule mitogens include epidermal EGF, which increases DNA synthesis in SMCs. Granule mitogens include the most potent growth factor, PDGF. PDGF is exceptionally important in atherosclerosis as it is both chemotaxic and mitogenic. PDGF effects include enhanced synthesis of collagen Type I, LDL receptors and scavenger receptors. PDGF promotes LDL uptake, accelerated output of IGF, prostaglandins, and monocyte chemoattractants.
Modulation of vascular tone	Platelet-derived factors include the potent vasoconstrictors serotonin, norepinephrine, and histamine.
Tissue destruction	Granule contents include substances such as ADP and epinephrine that can cause further vessel damage through the above mentioned vasoconstriction and increased shear force.

tants, leukotriene B4 (Fuster, Gotto, Libby, et al., 1996; Ross, 1986, 1993; Teplitz & Siwik, 1994).

Macrophages possess receptors for native, or natural, LDL and for modified, or oxidized, LDL. By producing reactive oxygen species, macrophages play an important role in atherogenesis. Reactive oxygen species include oxygen radicals in the form of superoxide, hydroxyl radicals, and hydrogen peroxide. They are produced when oxygen is incompletely reduced and is unstable with an unpaired electron. Reactive oxygen species oxidize cells, with resulting direct cell membrane damage.

Oxidized lipids are often unrecognizable by LDL receptors. Oxidized lipids bind with scavenger receptors of macrophages and enter the cells, converting them to foam cells. Unregulated amounts of lipids are taken up and amassed in the cytoplasm. Normal scavenger function is demonstrated by subendothelial localization of the monocyte/macrophage, lipid accumulation, and phagocytosis of extracellular material. Macrophages or MFCs (foam cells) can damage nearby tissue by liberating toxic substances such as cholesterol (esterified and

oxidized). Thus, macrophages can injure endothelium and precipitate events leading to the proliferative lesions of atherosclerosis (Fuster, Gotto, Libby, et al., 1996; Ross, 1986, 1993; Teplitz & Siwik, 1994).

Macrophages play another role in the fibroproliferative process associated with atherogenesis by synthesizing and releasing specific growth factors for three cell types. These growth factors are PDGF for connective tissue cells, including SMCs and fibroblasts, *fibroblast growth factor* (FGF) for vascular endothelial cells, and EGF for epithelial cells. Finally, macrophages release digestive enzymes, such as proteases, which break down extracellular matrix proteins, and heparinases, which break down heparin, thereby damaging neighboring cells (Ross, 1986, 1993; Teplitz & Siwik, 1994). Table 2–7 summarizes the functions and related properties of monocytes/macrophages.

HYPOTHESES OF PATHOGENESIS OF ATHEROSCLEROSIS

As apparent from the previous discussion, the process of atherosclerosis/lesion formation is

TABLE 2-7 Monocytes/Macrophages

Function	Related Properties
Remodeling of the intima	Synthesis and secretion of collagenase and elastase, growth factors for SMCs and endothelial cells, chemotactic factors for SMCs, and angiogenesis factors.
Inflammatory and immune response	Principal inflammatory mediators of cells in atherogenic environment, activation of immune response; binding of monocytes to endothelium with subsequent release of chemotactic protein-1 and colony-stimulating factor; production of one of the most powerful chemoattractants, leukotriene B4.
Scavenger functions	Lipid metabolism; uptake of native and oxidized LDL; phagocytosis and removal of dead cells and immune complexes; fibrinolysis and removal of mural thrombi and other deposited plasma proteins.
Tissue destruction	Release of superoxides, hydrolases, and digestive enxymes, which may damage neighboring cells.

Adapted from Stary, H.C., Blankenhorn, D.H., et al. (1992). A definition of the intima of human arteries and of its atherosclerosis-prone regions: A report from the Committee on Vascular Lesions of the Council on Arteriosclerosis, American Heart Association. *Circulation, 1,* 391–405. Adapted with permission of the American Heart Association.

complex. Scientists and clinicians have understood the process in terms of anatomic stages and involved cellular processes. Both the anatomic and the physiologic information has been integrated by researchers to develop hypotheses of atherogenesis. Some hypotheses build on earlier ones. None explains all the research findings, and none is universally accepted. Each, however, accounts for some part of the findings and, more importantly, explains physiologic consequences in concrete terms.

These hypotheses are an integral component of a discussion of the pathogenesis of atherosclerosis, and they build on previously discussed material to provide a framework for the nurse practicing risk reduction. Six major hypotheses will now be discussed, including the central concepts, proposed mechanisms for atherogenesis, supportive evidence, and relationship to other hypotheses. Pertinent research will be presented to explain the relevance and limitations of the hypotheses for clinicians.

Response-to-Injury Hypothesis

The response-to-injury hypothesis was first proposed by Virchow in 1856, elaborated on by Ross and Glomset (1973, 1976), and has been frequently updated. "Central to the response-to-injury hypothesis is the proposal that the different risk factors somehow lead to endothelial dysfunction, which can elicit a series of cellular interactions that culminate in the lesions of atherosclerosis" (Ross, p. 804, 1993). The process of development of a fibrous lesion in response to injury can be likened to that of wound healing. However, the process differs from wound healing in that the primary origin of connective tissue is the SMC. The second difference is that the causative factors tend to be chronic, so atherosclerotic progression is unlikely to be interrupted (Ross, 1993).

This hypothesis suggests that the precipitating event in the atherosclerotic process is damage to the endothelial cells. Endothelial damage with resultant arterial injury occurs particularly at arterial bifurcations and includes accelerated trapping of lipoprotein and the presence of distinct adhesive glycoproteins on the endothelial cell surface. Monocytes and T lymphocytes attach to glycoproteins and migrate between the endothelial cells.

The injury is attributed to factors that alter the permeability of the intimal membrane. These factors might include cigarette smoke, hypertension, increased hemodynamic forces (shear stress), hyperlipidemia, catecholamines, angiotensin II, or oxidative stress. The growth regulatory factors and chemoattractants that influence the response to endothelial injury are secreted by the altered endothelium, its cleaving leukocytes, and perhaps underlying smooth muscle. As discussed in the previous section on platelets, an immediate platelet response occurs with injury to endothelial cells. The platelet response consists of platelet adherence to the subendothelial layer, then aggregation and release of granule contents (Ross, 1993; Teplitz & Siwik, 1994).

The injury also initiates a regeneration of endothelial cells in an attempt to recover the opening caused by the injury. With an endothelial wound or injury, contact between cells is disturbed. Cells nearest to the site of injury will sustain existing attachments and extend into the wound in an effort to reestablish intercellular contacts. With an injury that is too big to allow this, the cells at the border may replicate or proliferate.

Hypothetically, chronic injury causes cells at the border to undergo enough doubling to approach senescence. The phenomenon of *senescence* will be discussed in detail when the clonal-senescence hypothesis is presented. Cells distant from the injury could replicate, but they would be unable to participate in wound closure owing to the restrictions of the monolayer (Ross, 1993).

Acute or chronic injury will cause endothelial dysfunction. Monocytes will migrate further into the vessel wall, become macrophages, amass lipid, and become foam cells. The foam cells with accompanying lymphocytes become the fatty streak. The lesion in the vessel wall advances by accumulating alternating layers of SMCs, foam cells, and connective tissue. Arteries may contain areas of retracted endothelial cells, exposing foam cells. These provide sites for platelet activation leading to the formation of mural thrombi. "Many of these exposed macrophages seem, as in other inflammatory responses, to be attempts by the macrophages to remove accumulating lipid by circulating back to lung, liver, spleen and lymph nodes" (Ross, p. 803, 1993).

The response-to-injury hypothesis is important for several reasons, most notably because it indicates that atherosclerosis may be reversed. This inference is consistent with animal studies demonstrating that the endothelium regenerates. Repeated balloon-induced local injuries are progressively less able to elicit endothelium-dependent relaxation in response to platelets (Teplitz & Siwik, 1994). The response-to-injury hypothesis has also been extended to describe development of coronary thrombus in an artery with advanced plaque. Endothelial injury may lead to platelet deposition succeeded by SMC proliferation and extracellular matrix synthesis. Chronic endothelial loss over a plaque may augment the chance of arterial thrombosis (Farb, Burke, Tang, et al., 1996).

Clonal-Senescence Hypothesis

The clonal-senescence hypothesis focuses on the relationship of age to atherogenesis and may provide important clues about the unequal distribution of atherosclerosis throughout the arterial tree. "Senescence may be defined as a constellation of deteriorative changes in structure and function of an organism, generally occurring after sexual maturation, which results in a progressive decline in the efficiency of homeostasis and in the success of the reaction to injury" (Martin, p. 484, 1977). This hypothesis arises from the observation that cells from different arteries age at distinct, or different, rates and that some segments of the aorta are more likely to develop atherosclerosis and mature more quickly. *Clonal senescence* is the limited replicative lifespan of individual clones of cells such that replication ceases after a certain point, termed the *Hayflick limit* (Benditt, 1977; Hayflick, 1980; Martin, 1977).

Observations of human fibroblasts over a duration of months illustrate the Hayflick limit. Human fibroblasts divide numerous times, gradually stop dividing, inevitably die, and are replaced by their descendants. The new cells resulting from division do not make the organism younger; aging is exhibited in cell lineages, not individual cells. Aging of cell lineage may be an innate property of cells (Hayflick, 1980; Martin, 1977).

As articulated by Martin and Sprague (1972), the clonal-senescence hypothesis is based on the premise that cell reproduction is significantly affected by negative feedback control of chalones. *Chalones* are substances secreted by SMCs and are thought to be part of the natural cell growth control mechanism. A different chalone exists for each cell type. Chalones possibly inhibit mitosis of stem cells, therefore reducing the number of newly differentiated progenies of SMCs.

The numbers of both stem cells and chalones are hypothesized to decrease with advancing age. Martin and Sprague demonstrated that SMCs from the atherosclerotic-prone abdominal aorta had decreased growth potential as compared to equivalent cells from the relatively atherosclerosis-free thoracic aorta. Because intimal SMCs are closely related to medial SMCs, they are subject to similar regulatory controls. Martin and Sprague's hypothesis indicates that under equilibrium conditions, loss of SMCs is compensated by the liberation of regional stem cells capable of producing a new distinct progeny. This research suggests that there are regions within the vascular tree (abdominal aorta) with relatively rapid rates of clonal senescence of medial cells accompanied by depletion of stem cells. The unproductive, differentiated SMCs are not replaced at appropriate frequencies, leading to a decline in diffusible inhibitory macromolecule and multifocal proliferation of intimal SMCs. As the proliferations could be monoclonal, the clonal-senescence hypothesis and the monoclonal hypothesis (discussed next) do not appear to be mutually exclusive (Hayflick, 1980; Martin, 1977).

Monoclonal Hypothesis

The monoclonal hypothesis, or the single-cell hypothesis, suggests that a proliferation of monoclonal SMCs make up the atherosclerotic plaque. Benditt (1977) and co-researchers propose that plaque is distinguished by an accumulation of cells that are progeny of a solitary, "parent," mutated SMC located adjacent to the plaque. With respect to this hypothesis, plaque formation is thus analogous to a benign tumor of the artery wall resulting from mutation of a single cell (Benditt, 1977).

A research team headed by Benditt (1977) initially studied spontaneous and induced lesions in chickens and observed that cells of early spontaneous lesions were subtly distinct from typical SMCs. Cells appeared smaller, with little or no intracellular junctions, and they produced more collagen than elastin. The spontaneous lesion cells were thought to have originated from either (1) some small cell population

ordinarily not observed and subject to a stimulant of some kind or (2) SMCs altered by mutation. A sharp contrast existed with plaque cells from the induced lesions. These had all the characteristics of normal SMCs, including intercellular junctions and a greater proportion of elastin than collagen. Benditt (1977) and colleagues proposed that genetically altered plaque cells would be expected to be monoclonal, like the cells of a benign tumor. Plaque cells arising in response to injury or other stimulus would be polyclonal. The stimulus would have its effect on multiple normal cells in multiple locations (Benditt, 1977).

Studies dating back to the 1970s involving genetic testing of black females, using an X-linked marker to determine phenotype, support the monoclonal hypothesis. The goal of these studies was to determine if plaque SMCs were monoclonal or polyclonal. Black females were studied because of their tendency to be heterozygous for an X chromosome gene that codes for the marker *glucose-6-phosphate dehydrogenase* (G6PD). The findings were felt to be generalizable to atherogenesis across all ethnic groups in both men and women. Consistent with the monoclonal hypothesis, results indicated 80% of atherosclerotic plaques are monoclonal or consist of one type of cell (Benditt, 1977, 1988; Pearson, Wang, Solez, and Heptinstall, 1975).

Pearson, Wang, Solez, et al. (1975) performed similar research, first, to determine if Benditt's findings could be validated and, second, to examine the use of the same cellular marker to resolve issues in the progression of fatty streak to fibrous plaque. Research data indicated that although most (89.7%) fibrous plaques were monoclonal, most fatty streaks were polyclonal. Only 17.8% were monoclonal. Thus, these findings present evidence that is both supportive and not supportive of the monoclonal hypothesis.

The monoclonal hypothesis remains important because it provides a link between certain risk factors and coronary heart disease. Smoking may be linked to atherogenesis, as cigarette smoke is known to contain mutagens. High-fat diets have been linked with some cancers as well as with atherosclerosis. Benditt has proposed that both disease states may be caused by similar mechanisms. The use of human as opposed to animal models is a strength of the supportive evidence for the monoclonal hypothesis (Benditt, 1977; Kolata, 1976).

Thrombogenic Hypothesis or Encrustation Theory

The thrombogenic hypothesis, or encrustation theory, of atheroma formation is based on the assumption that plaque is (1) initiated with the organization of small mural thrombi and (2) transformed into an aggregation of tissue in the intima. Arterial wall cells migrate to it, reproduce, and secrete typical substances. Thrombus formation is proposed to be the chief mechanism of atherosclerotic development (Velican & Velican, 1989).

As proposed by Duguid (1946), atherosclerosis may develop from mural thrombi and, even more frequently, from minuscule fibrin deposits on areas of damaged intima. Although Duguid found fibrinous deposits in a large number of aortas and microthrombi incorporation in plaque, it is a fact that methods to detect fibrin within the intima are inadequate. Furthermore, microthrombi are not visible on gross examination, so reported prevalence rates may be based on those found incidentally on microscopic examination (Friedman, 1969; Velican & Velican, 1989).

In subsequent research by Friedman and associates, treated wire coils placed in an animal artery resulted in complete dissolution of the coil and the formation of white thrombi with chief components of fibrin, platelets, and metallic salts within 72 hours. Almost no red or white blood cells were found within the thrombi, and thrombi were initially unattached to the vessel wall except at the site of initial puncture with the wire coil. After a week, fibroblastic tissue grew from the adventitia via the initial puncture and began to cover and replace the thrombus. Initially the fibroblastic blood vessels were thin and poorly developed, but after 3 weeks thrombi were completely covered and infiltrated by the fibroblasts. After 12 weeks the thrombi were completely replaced by a flat, dense, fibrous plaque covered with endothelial cells that resembled the typical pearly plaque of atherosclerosis with multiple macrophages in central and basal portions (Friedman, 1969).

As with the response-to-injury hypothesis, the thrombogenic hypothesis postulates that endothelial damage is a prerequisite to atherogenesis. Proponents argue that thrombi or platelet deposits do not occur on intact endothelium. Friedman (1969) voiced his support of the notion that plaque, if not actually beginning as a thrombus, certainly increased in size from thrombus deposition. Fuster and co-investigators (1992) report that when thrombi are small they can contribute to plaque growth, and when they are large they can contribute to acute coronary syndromes (Ferrell & Fuster, 1994; Friedman, 1969).

Ferrell and Fuster (1994) give expanding support to the proposition that expansion of existing lesions occurs swiftly and sequentially in response to endothelial injury. This conclusion agrees with the response-to-injury hypothesis. Steps include cap fissuring, formation of thrombus, and fibrotic construction.

It has long been accepted that plaque disruption leads to thrombus formation. Current use of thrombolytics, platelet inhibitors, and anticoagulation is based on the recognition that platelets are the elements that initiate the process of thrombosis. Multiple researchers have reported that, experimentally, plaque does not develop without platelets. When Friedman and co-investigators treated animals with antibodies to rabbit platelets, lesions did not form. Fuster and colleagues (1992) recount that accumulating evidence suggests recurrent episodes of mural thrombosis, as opposed to one episode, lead gradually to vascular occlusion (Ferrell & Fuster, 1994; Friedman, 1969). As a result, currently, the majority of myocardial ischemic events are believed to be precipitated by thrombosis. This hypothesis has been supported by pathologic, angiographic, and angioscopic evidence (Davies et al., 1994). The heterogeneity of atherosclerotic plaque implies that various mechanisms are potentially involved in thrombus development.

Hemodynamic Hypothesis

The hemodynamic hypothesis suggests all pathogenic mechanisms implicated in atherogenesis are mediated, at least in part, by mechanical forces of hemodynamic stress and turbulent flow. The hemodynamic hypothesis proposes that atheromas occur at sites in the arteries that experience the full stress and impact of the blood. Specific hemodynamic conditions include bending and twisting of coronary vessels during the cardiac cycle, vasomotion/spasm, and increased shear stress. Local mechanical factors, including wall shear stress and mural tensile stress, potentiate atherogenesis (Farb, Burke, Tang, et al., 1996; Glagov, Zarins, Giddens, et al., 1988; Velican & Velican, 1989).

Atherogenesis has been demonstrated to occur with and without the widely identified risk factors. Velican and Velican (1989) conclude that risk factors such as smoking, hypertension, high cholesterol levels, and diabetes aggravate the natural history of atherosclerosis but are not the initiating factor(s). The initiating factor appears to be "a special pattern of hemodynamic stress, present in vessels larger than 1 mm in which a pulsatile pressure of higher than 100 mm Hg exists" (Velican & Velican, p. 181, 1989). The onset of atherosclerosis does not require the specialized architecture of the native arterial wall. It can occur in grafted veins and in the neointima of arterial prostheses.

The supposition that hemodynamic forces are significant in the initiation and localization of plaques was established after extensive observation that lesions do not occur by chance. Coronary arteries may be extensively atherosclerotic while the unidirectional and less intricate renal and mesenteric arteries are disease-free. Particular sites and configurations are much more susceptible. In areas of SMC proliferation, it is assumed that the vessel wall is stressed beyond the limits of its optimal adaptability. Intimal thickening may be predicted by the laws of hydrodynamics, severity of atherosclerosis may be firmly linked to the extension and degree of intimal thickening (Glagov, Zarins, Giddons, et al., 1988; Velican & Velican, 1989).

SMCs respond to hemodynamic and mechanical forces with counteracting mechanisms. Connective tissue components and myofibrils are produced to allow the removal of stressing forces from the cells via a negative-feedback mechanism. The same lipoprotein level exists throughout flowing blood, yet the onset and growth of atherosclerotic lesions differ region-ally, which indicates local hemodynamic factors are key in determining when and if a plaque will develop (Velican & Velican, 1989).

Hemodynamic stress may be viewed as "limited to any of the identifiable mechanical forces which are exerted per unit wall area by the blood pressure and/or flow" (Velican & Velican, p. 12, 1989). Tension created by the blood pressure appears to be related to vessel diameter, with total force or tension being the product of the radius of the vessel and the blood pressure. Shear stress is dependent in part on branching, vessel curvature, and tapering. The torsion, twisting, bending, and rhythmic compression that take place with each systole must be considered (Velican & Velican, 1989).

Turbulent flow has long been investigated as a possible determinant of plaque location. Turbulence is likely to arise in the same areas where atherosclerosis develops. Hemodynamic stresses result in functional and ultrastructural wall changes. The most significant changes are those related to augmented endothelial permeability. Atherogenesis appears to occur when the arterial wall is unable to adapt to hemodynamic stress and thus preserve sufficient trans-intimal passage and clearance of plasma components. The actual mechanism(s) of initiation is not clear. Lowering of the potential energy barrier for diffusion molecules, "fatigue," and "leaky" intercellular junctions have been discussed (Glagov, Zarins, Giddens, et al., 1988; Velican & Velican, 1989).

Hemodynamic forces are not universally considered an initiating factor in atherosclerosis but are universally considered a significant factor in lesion progression. The number of platelets attaching to an endothelial injury is determined by the degree of injury and the transport of the platelets. Thrombus composition changes based on the shear stress. At high shear rates with mild injury, initial platelet deposition rate and maximal extent of deposition are both significantly higher. Maximum platelet deposition or thrombus formation is noted after 20 to 30 minutes, and thrombus is dislodged by flowing blood after longer exposure (Fuster, Badimon, Cohen, et al., 1988). Andre, Arbeille, Drouet, and co-workers (1996) found that, at high shear stress, plaque is made up chiefly of platelets, thus explaining their significant role in vascular disease; these investigators found that raising the shear rate effected a marked augmentation in thrombus growth (Andre, Arbeille, Drouet, et al., 1996).

Computer modeling of simulated vessel walls that contain plaques of different configurations suggests the local concentration of tensile stress contributes to intimal tearing. Plaques with stiffer caps create elevated areas of circumferential stress during systole that affect the point of insertion of the cap into the vessel wall. Models with layers of fibrous tissue or with a plate of very rigid material (such as calcium) lead to very high shear stress, which explains the frequency of intimal tears into fibrous and calcified plaques (Davies, 1990).

Lipid-Insudation-Irritation Hypothesis

The lipid-insudation-irritation hypothesis focuses on the relationship between fatty materials from the circulating blood that infiltrate into the vascular wall and the initiation of atherogenesis. Cholesterol deposits develop and serve as irritants causing inflammation and proliferation of cells. Lipid deposits exceed lipid removal. This hypothesis is supported by the universal observance that individuals with elevated blood cholesterol have a greater incidence of atherosclerosis. The lipid-insudation-irritation hypothesis has fostered a family of theories, the "lipid hypotheses" (Benditt, 1977; Fuster, Badimon, Badimon, et al., 1992; Velican & Velican, 1989).

Anitschkow and Chalatow (1913) observed a disease resembling human atherosclerosis in rabbits fed a high-cholesterol diet. These investigators made the first attempt to correlate blood lipid changes and the onset of fatty streak–like lesions. Studies demonstrating fatty deposits in infants and children facilitated acceptance of this theory and led to acceptance of the questionable assumption that the natural evolution of atherosclerosis is from fatty streaks to fibrous plaques (Benditt, 1977).

Schwartz, Valente, and Sprague (1993) report that the two principal events in atherogenesis are the influx and accumulation of LDL at atherosclerosis-prone sites and the induction of blood monocytes to these same sites. LDL, and possibly additional lipoproteins, cross the endo-

thelium and are oxidized by reactive oxygen species of surrounding cells. Selwyn, Kinlay, Libby, and Ganz (1997) report that native LDL has little effect on arterial wall cells. Research by Rangswamy, Penn, Saidel, and Chisolm (1997) indicates that exogenously introduced native LDL does not produce typical atherosclerotic changes. Movement of LDL from the plasma and into the intima/media is accelerated after oxidation (Bjorkerud & Bjorkerud, 1996; Schwartz, Valente, & Sprague, 1993; Selwyn, Kinlay, Libby, et al., 1997; Rangaswamy, Penn, Saidel, et al., 1997). The binding property of native LDL to components of the extracellular matrix prolongs the intimal residence period of native LDL and increases the likelihood of oxidation. The elastin of atherosclerotic lesions has two to four times the binding capacity for LDL as does normal arterial elastin (Penn & Chisolm, 1994).

These findings indicate how important it is to gain an understanding of oxidized LDL's suggested causal role in atherosclerosis. Oxidation is a very significant part of the atherogenic process. Oxidized or glycated (associated with diabetes) LDL is no longer recognized by the normal LDL receptors. The oxidized or glycated LDL is taken up by non-down-regulating macrophage scavenger receptors, with the subsequent formation of foam cells. The scavenger receptor provides a mechanism for the ongoing uptake of modified lipoproteins and formation of the fatty streak that is a crucial factor in atherogenesis (Bjorkerud & Bjorkerud, 1996; Schwartz, Valente, & Sprague, 1993; Selwyn, Kinlay, Libby, et al., 1997; Rangaswamy et al., 1997). Table 2–8 summarizes the potential role of oxidized LDL in atherosclerosis.

Oxidization is the addition of oxygen atoms. LDL is oxidized by free radicals of SMCs, macrophages, and probably endothelial cells. Oxidized or modified LDL has many biologic consequences; it is cytotoxic and therefore has a role in foam cell necrosis and possible core development. Oxidized LDL has chemotactic properties, inhibits monocyte migration, causes inactivation of EDRF (endothelial-derived relaxing factor) and is antigenic (capable of causing the production of an antibody), so it contributes to autoimmune inflammation and induces an increased expression of colony-stimulating factors. *Colony-stimulating factors* are pro-

TABLE 2–8 Potential Role of Oxidized LDL in Atherosclerosis

- Produces cytotoxic effects causing injury to endothelium, SMCs, and macrophages
- Produces cytotoxic effects on macrophages, causing foam cell necrosis and possibly core development
- Stimulates increased production and release of monocyte chemotactic protein-1 (MCP-1) by endothelial cells
- Is chemoattractant for monocytes (MCP-1)
- Is chemoattractant for SMCs
- Inactivates endothelial derived relaxing factor (EDRF)
- Inhibits migration of endothelial cells (reversible)
- Inhibits migration of macrophages (reversible)
- Stimulates the expression of "sticky" glycoproteins in the glycocalyx, which increase monocyte adhesion
- Stimulates increased expression of granulocyte and monocyte colony-stimulating factors, increasing available monocytes
- Increases growth-factor production
- Increases cytokine production
- Binds avidly to collagen owing to negative charge
- Is taken up by non-down-regulating scavenger receptors leading to foam cell formation; degree of oxidation correlates with diminishing recognition by normal LDL receptors
- Is antigenic (capable of causing the production of antibodies so contributes to autoimmune inflammation)

Note: Dozens of new products are produced when LDL is oxidized.

teins present in human serum that promote monocyte differentiation.

Native LDL promotes growth of SMCs, and collagen synthesis is increased by SMCs leading to the fibrous plaque. As mentioned, oxidized LDL is a cytotoxin. Together, LDL and oxidized LDL produce the typical model of plaque: extreme intimal growth alternating with central extensive cell death (Bjorkerud & Bjorkerud, 1996; Schwartz, Valente, & Sprague, 1993).

Lesion-prone sites demonstrate increased endothelial permeability to plasma proteins, including LDL, albumin, and fibrinogen, and show a significantly increased cholesterol accumulation in animals fed a high-fat, high-cholesterol diet. Atherosclerosis-prone areas have a thinner glycocalyx and greater endothelial turnover. Increased spontaneous monocyte recruitment occurs without microscopically visible plaques. The mechanisms involved in the mi-

gration of monocytes into the subendothelial space are not fully understood. Contact with the endothelial cells is essential, as is monocyte adhesion. Once migration begins, guidance is provided by chemoattractants.

Monocyte chemotactic protein 1 (MCP-1) is one chemoattractant derived from SMCs and endothelial cells. There are many other chemoattractants, including oxidatively modified LDL. MCP-1 is thought to be of particular significance because of its monocyte specificity. Minimally modified or slightly oxidized LDL increases the expression and synthesis of MCP-1 in endothelial cells and SMCs. Oxidatively modified LDL may indirectly increase monocyte recruitment. Once converted to macrophages, some of these cells are affected by migration inhibition factors and thus stay within the intima. As mentioned, one migration inhibition factor is thought to be oxidized LDL (Fogelman, 1994; Schwartz, Valente, & Sprague, 1993).

Oxidized LDL is viewed as responsible for dysfunction leading to lesion formation and general endothelial dysfunction. Rangaswamy, Penn, Saidel, and Chisolm (1997) introduced endogenous native and oxidized LDL into the bloodstream of rats and measured endothelial injury and proliferation. Oxidized LDL infusion was found to increase the number of damaged endothelial cells in the aorta fivefold over native LDL. Rangaswamy and co-researchers concluded that if oxidized LDL is present in high enough concentrations, endothelial injury will occur with increased cell turnover and interference with normal endothelial function, including altered permeability (Rangaswamy, Penn, Saidel, et al., 1997).

Selwyn and co-investigators (1997) report that processes triggered by oxidized LDL are reversible within hours during a single experiment. These findings validate LDL reduction strategies. Born (1994) reports that atherogenic uptake of LDL is accelerated by epinephrine and norepinephrine in rat and rabbit species. Linkage was demonstrated between increased atherosclerosis and conditions associated with elevated catecholamine concentrations, including episodic increases with cigarette smoking and stress and the sustained increases of pheochromocytoma. Born's research indicates primary passage of LDL into the endothelium is accelerated by catecholamines. A potential method of slowing atherosclerosis may be by pharmacologically antagonizing the catecholamines (Born, 1994; Selwyn, Kinlay, Libby, et al., 1997).

In conclusion, all six hypotheses are relevant to risk reduction when considering their potential as a framework for risk-reduction strategies. The response-to-injury and thrombogenic hypothesis support an intervention or strategy that decreases endothelial damage. Risk factors associated with this type of damage include cigarette smoking, hypertension, increased hemodynamic forces (shear stress), hyperlipidemia, catecholamines, angiotensin II, and oxidative stress. The response-to-injury hypothesis indicates atherosclerosis may be reversed, so this hypothesis can also be used as a framework for atherosclerosis-regression approaches.

The clonal-senescence hypothesis is compatible with risk-reduction strategies aimed at reducing the effects of chronic injury, such as blood pressure control, and provides a framework for understanding increasing age as a risk factor. The monoclonal hypothesis provides support to all risk-reduction strategies designed to decrease endothelial injury, specifically those that decrease cell mutation and are linked to prevention of cancer, such as cessation of cigarette smoking and low-fat diets. The thrombogenic hypothesis can be used as a framework for the current use of thrombolytics, platelet inhibitors, and anticoagulation. The hemodynamic hypothesis supports all strategies aimed at lowering blood pressure and decreasing wall stress, which this hypothesis implies initiate atherogenesis. The lipid-insudation-irritation hypothesis clearly supports all strategies that decrease blood cholesterol levels, as well as the use of antioxidants and improved diabetic control as risk-reduction approaches. Table 2–9 summarizes the risk factors and risk-reduction strategies associated with each of the six hypotheses.

EMERGING ISSUES

Our knowledge of the pathogenesis of atherosclerosis is constantly evolving. Emerging issues include (1) the relationship between plaque-formation atherogenesis and clinical outcomes and

(2) the role of specific risk factors in plaque formation.

Researchers are currently seeking to clarify the concept of endothelial dysfunction versus actual injury. Rangaswamy (1997) and co-workers discuss the possibility that insult to endothelium could be sublethal, leading to dysfunction rather than actual injury. Similarly, Fuster and colleagues (1996) discuss the concept of chronic minimal injury. Dysfunction may lead to activation of endothelium, with a production of adhesive glycoproteins. A shortened life span of the cell population may be another impact of a dysfunction level insult. Compromised barrier function and increased endothelial permeability may lead to entry and accumulation of LDL (Fuster, Gotto, Libby, et al., 1996; Rangaswamy, Penn, Saidel, et al., 1997).

Identification of plaques at risk is a focus of current research. Risk of rupture appears to be related to plaque composition, but the exact pathogenic mechanisms are unclear. Biomechanical factors such as shear stress and vasospasm, along with tissue changes of the fibrous cap, appear to be significant. Van der Wal, Becker, Van der Loos, and Das (1993) found the sites of rupture to be associated with a localized accumulation of T cells and macrophages and a decrease in SMCs.

Van der Wal and colleagues postulate that "plaques at risk" should be identified based on lesions with occasional local areas dominated by inflammatory cells, large atheromatous pools, and essentially no fibrous caps. Davies, Woolf, Rowles, and Richardson (1994) validate these conclusions. SMC proliferation, often viewed as harmful after interventions, can be seen as essential for plaque stability. Farb and co-researchers (1996) studied plaque underlying acute coronary thrombosis. Their research indicated that the definition of thrombosis-prone plaque should be expanded to include SMC-rich and proteoglycan-rich plaques with chronic endothelial loss. Therefore, the decision to intervene based on the degree of luminal obstruction may need to be replaced by evaluation of plaque profile and constituent elements. However, coronary angiography is unable to differentiate between plaques at risk and more stable fibrotic or calcified plaque. For this reason, new imaging techniques are under development (Davies, Woolf, Rowles, et al., 1994;

TABLE 2–9 Atherosclerosis Hypotheses with Associated
Risk Factors and Risk-Reduction Strategies

Hypotheses	Risk Factors and Risk-Reduction Strategies
Response-to-injury	• Strategies are to decrease endothelial damage. • Risk factors include smoking, hypertension, increased hemodynamic forces, hyperlipidema, catecholamine excess, angiotensin II, and oxidative stress. • Hypothesis provides framework for atherosclerosis regression techniques.
Clonal-senescence	• Strategies are to reduce effects of chronic injury, such as blood pressure control. • Hypothesis provides framework for understanding age as a risk factor.
Monoclonal	• Strategies are to decrease endothelial injuries, specifically those that decrease cell mutation and are linked to prevention of cancer, such as cessation of smoking and low-fat diets.
Thrombogenic/encrustation	• Strategies are to decrease endothelial damage. • Risk factors include smoking, hypertension, increased hemodynamic forces, hyperlipidema, catecholamine excess, angiotensin II, and oxidative stress. • Hypothesis provides framework for use of thrombolytics, platelet inhibitors, and anticoagulation.
Hemodynamic	• Strategies are to lower blood pressure and decrease wall stress.
Lipid-insudation-irritation	• Strategies are to decrease blood cholesterol levels. • Hypothesis provides framework for use of antioxidant therapy, strategies that improve diabetic control, and pharmacologic antagonizing catecholamines.

Farb, Burke, Tang, et al., 1996; Fuster, Gotto, Libby, et al., 1996; Van der Wal, Becker, Van der Loos, et al., 1993).

New insights into atherogenesis also include the especially significant finding that the core area of the plaque is detectable earlier in lesion development than commonly thought, before formation of the fibrous plaque. The core has been detected in its earliest stage at the transition of fatty streak to fibrous plaque and is recognized by typical lipid deposits (cholesterol clefts), partial loss of cells, or both. Research by Guyton and Klemp (1996) calls into question the assumption that sources of core lipids are foam cells or tissue lipoproteins. Guyton and Klemp looked at the amount of free cholesterol, cholesterol ester, fatty acyl patterns, and the size of lipid droplets in the early core. Their research suggests the following:

1 Early core lipids reveal a notable amount of free cholesterol—63% of the total cholesterol—whereas foam cells and tissue lipoproteins have abundant esterified cholesterol in contrast to free cholesterol.

2 A discrepancy exists between the cholesterol ester fatty acyl patterns of the core lipids and the foam cell lipids.

3 The lipid processing known to go on in the foam cells is not apparent in early core lipids.

4 A marked size difference exists between extracellular oily droplets and foam cell droplets.

The mechanisms contributing to the vesicular-rich, free-cholesterol early core are unknown. Guyton and Klemp (1996) point to a direct extracellular process, potentially lipoprotein aggregation and fusion (Stary, Chandler, et al., 1994).

If subsequent research supports these findings, current hypotheses of atherosclerosis will need to be reevaluated; furthermore, the staging typology, with its underlying assumptions of progression from macrophage foam cells to fatty streaks, will need to be revisited. It is possible that the roles of the cellular components will also need to be clarified.

Other emerging issues focus on risk factors for atherogenesis. Guyton and Hall (1996) report experimental studies suggesting excess iron levels in the blood can lead to atherosclerosis. Iron may be involved in the formation of free radicals that injure arterial walls (Guyton & Hall, 1996).

A significant amount of attention has also been directed toward increased homocysteine levels being a factor in the pathogenesis of atherosclerosis. Homocysteine is an essential amino acid. Clinical and experimental studies suggest that elevated homocysteine levels can be responsible for atherogenic and thrombotic changes. Pyrodoxine (vitamin B_6) is a necessary cofactor in the process of converting homocysteine into cysteine, an amino acid valuable as a source of sulfur in metabolism. Folate and cobalamin (vitamin B_{12}) are cofactors required to remethylate homocysteine into methionine, another essential amino acid. Deficiencies in these cofactors are seen in two thirds of individuals with elevated homocysteine levels (Futterman & Lemberg, 1997a; Pasternak, Grundy, Levy, et al., 1996).

Homocystinuria is usually an inherited enzyme defect associated with impaired metabolism of homocysteine. Individuals with homocystinuria have increased urine and serum levels of homocysteine and premature atherosclerosis with often extensive and multifocal vascular disease. The precise level of homocysteine associated with increased risk is unknown, although risk of premature vascular disease is 30 times greater in people with elevated homocysteine levels than in control subjects.

The mechanisms are unclear, but homocysteine has been shown to affect several factors in the clotting cascade, with negative effects on the endothelium. The effects may include direct damage to the endothelium, induction and proliferation of SMCs, enhanced oxidation of LDL, and promotion of thrombogenesis. Supplementation of the cofactors—folate, B_6, and B_{12}—has been shown to lower homocysteine levels. Prevention studies are being undertaken (Futterman & Lemberg, 1997a; Pasternak, Grundy, Levy, et al., 1996).

Coffee intake is being studied as a possible causative agent in atherosclerosis. Although yet unpublished at the time of this writing, studies have been discussed in the public media linking the consumption of coffee, especially unfiltered coffee, with increased lipid levels. An unpublished, at the time of this writing, study at the University of Bergen attempted to correlate dietary intake with homocysteine levels. Results indicated a correlation between coffee intake and homocysteine levels: intake of nine or more cups of coffee resulted in a 20% increase in homocysteine.

CONCLUSION

Scientists and clinicians have worked for several hundred years to solve the puzzle of atherosclerosis. Evaluating and caring for clients with coronary artery disease demands both a knowledge of the pathogenesis and progression of atherosclerosis and the integration and application of current scientific discovery. As discussed in Chapter 1, many factors contribute to the disease of atherosclerosis. This chapter has presented normal arterial wall anatomy and physiology, a detailed typology for lesion classification, a description of the major cell types involved, and an explanation of the six accepted hypotheses of atherogenesis. Extensive research on the pathogenesis of atherosclerosis exists, yet no single etiologic event or pathologic mechanism has been identified as the initial causative agent. All information presented here should be considered in an attempt to explain the multifactorial nature of atherosclerosis. The web of causation addresses the diversity of often interconnected pathogenetic mechanisms.

References

Alexander, R.W. (1994). Inflammation and coronary artery disease. *New England Journal of Medicine, 334*(7), 468–469.

Andre, P., Arbeille, B., Drouet V., Hainaud, P., Bal dit Sollier, C., Caen, J.P., & Drouet, L.O. (1996). Optimal antagonism of GPIIb/IIa favors platelet adhesion by inhibiting thrombus growth: An ex vivo capillary perfusion chamber study in the guinea pig. *Arteriosclerosis, Thrombosis and Vascular Biology, 16*(1), 56–63.

Becker, R.C., (1994). Thrombolytic retreatment for coronary arterial reclusion. In R. Becker (Ed.), *The Modern Era of Coronary Thrombolysis* (pp. 175–193). Norwell, MA: Kluwer Academic Publishers.

Benditt, E.P. (1977). The origin of atherosclerosis. *Scientific American, 236* (2), 74–85.

Benditt, E.P. (1988). Origins of human atherosclerotic plaques: The role of gene expression. *Archives of Pathology Laboratory Medicine, 112* (October), 997–1001.

Berne, R.M., & Levy, M.N. (1996). *Principles of Physiology*, 2nd ed. St. Louis: Mosby.

Bjorkerud, B., & Bjorkerud, S. (1996). Coronary effects of lightly and strongly oxidized LDL with potent promotion of growth versus apoptosis on arterial smooth muscle cells, macrophages, and fibroblasts. *Arteriosclerosis, Thrombosis, and Vascular Biology, 16,* 416–424.

Born, G.V.R. (1994). New determinants of the uptake of atherogenic plasma proteins by arteries. *Basic Research in Cardiology, 89* (Suppl. I), 103–106.

Davies, M.J., (1990). A macro and micro view of coronary vascular insult in ischemic heart disease. *Circulation, 82*(3) (Suppl. II), 3846.

Davies, M.J., Woolf, N., Rowles, P., & Richardson, P.D., (1994). Lipid and cellular constituents of unstable human aortic plaques. In H. Just, W. Hort, & A.M. Zeiher (Eds.), Arteriosclerosis: New insights into pathogenetic mechanisms and prevention. *Basic Research in Cardiology, 89* (Suppl. I), 33–39.

Duguid, J.B. (1946). Thrombosis as a factor in the pathogenesis of coronary atherosclerosis. *Journal of Pathological Bacteriology, 58,* 207.

Falk, E. (1992) Why do plaques rupture? *Circulation, 86* (Suppl.), 30–42.

Farb, A., Burke, A.P., Tang, A.L., Liany, Y., Manran, P., Smialek, J., & Vinnani, R. (1996). Coronary plaque erosion without rupture into a lipid core: A frequent cause of coronary thrombosis in sudden coronary death. *Circulation, 93,* 1354–1363.

Ferrell, M., & Fuster, V. (1994). Mechanism of acute myocardial infarction. In R. Becker (Ed.), *The Modern Era of Coronary Thrombolysis* (pp. 1–13). Norwell, MA: Kluwer Academic Publishers.

Florentin, R.A., Nam, S.C., Janakidevi K., Lee, K.T., Reinter, J.M., & Thom, W.A. (1973). Population dynamics of arterial smooth-muscle cells: In vivo inhibition of entry intro mitosis of swine arterial smooth-muscle cells by aortic tissue extracts. *Archives of Pathology, 95,* 317–320.

Fogelman, A.M. (1994). From fatty streak to myocardial infarction: An inflammatory response to oxidized lipids. *Circulation, 90*(4), I–B.

Friedman, M. (1969). *Pathogenesis of Coronary Artery Disease.* New York: McGraw-Hill.

Fuster, V., Badimon, L., Badimon, J.J., & Chesebro, J.H. (1992). The pathogenesis of coronary artery disease and the acute coronary syndromes. *New England Journal of Medicine, 326,* 242–250.

Fuster, V., Badimon, L., Cohen, M., Ambrose, J.A., Badimom J.J., & Chesebro, J. (1988). Insights into the pathogenesis of acute ischemic syndromes. *Circulation, 77*(6), 1213–1220.

Fuster, V., Gotto, A.M., Libby, P., Loscalzo, J., & McGill, H.C. (1996). Task Force 1. Pathogenesis of coronary disease: The biologic role of risk factors. Twenty-Seventh Bethesda Conference. Matching the intensity of risk factor management with the hazard for coronary disease events. *Journal of the American College of Cardiology, 27*(5), 964–975.

Fuster, V., Stein, B., Ambrose, J.A., Badimon, L., Badimon, J.J., & Chesebro, J.H. (1990). Atherosclerotic plaque rupture and thrombosis: Evolving concepts. *Circulation, 82*(3), (Suppl. II), 47–59.

Futterman, L.G., & Lemberg, L. (1997a). Homocysteine and coronary artery disease. *American Journal of Critical Care, 6*(1), 72–77.

Futterman, L.G., & Lemberg, L. (1997b). Endothelium: The key to medical management of coronary artery disease. *American Journal of Critical Care, 6*(2), 159–167.

Glagov, S., Zarins, C., Giddens, D.P., & Ku, D.N. (1988). Hemodynamics and atherosclerosis. *Archives of Pathology Laboratory Medicine, 112,* 1018–1031.

Guyton, A.C., & Hall, J.E. (1996). *Textbook of Medical Physiology,* 9th ed. Philadelphia: W.B. Saunders.

Guyton, J.R., & Klemp, K.F. (1996). Development of the lipid-rich core in human atherosclerosis. *Arteriosclerosis, Thromboses, and Vascular Biology, 16,* 4–11.

Hayflick, L. (1980). The cell biology of human aging. *Scientific American, 242,* 58–65.

Henry, P.D., (1994). Hyperlipidemic endothelial injury and angiogenesis. *Basic Research in Cardiology, 89,* (Suppl. I), 107–114.

Hort, W., (1994). Arteriosclerosis: Its morphology in the past and today. *Basic Research in Cardiology, 89,* (Suppl. I), 1–15.

Kolata, G.B. (1976). Atherosclerotic plaques: Competing theories guide research. *Science, 194,* 592–594.

Loscalzo, J. (1990). Lipoprotein (a): A unique risk factor for atherothrombotic disease. *Arteriosclerosis, 10,* 672–679.

Martin, G.M. (1977). Cellular aging—clonal senescence. *American Journal of Pathology, 89,* 484–511.

Pasternak, R.C., Grundy, S.M., Levy, D., & Thompson, P.D. (1996). Task force 3: Spectrum of risk for coronary heart disease. Twenty-Seventh Bethesda Conference. Matching the intensity of risk factor management with the hazard for coronary disease events. *Journal of the American College of Cardiology, 27* (5), 978–990.

Pathobiological Determinants of Atherosclerosis in Youth (PDAY) Research Group (1993). Natural history of aortic and coronary atherosclerotic lesions in youth: Findings from the PDAY study. *Arteriosclerosis and Thrombosis, 13* (19), 1291–1298.

Pearson, T.A., Wang, A., Solez, K., & Heptinstall, R.H. (1975). Clonal characteristics of fibrous plaques and fatty streaks from human aortas. *American Journal of Pathology, 81* (2), 379–387.

Penn, M.S., & Chisholm, G.M. (1994). Oxidized lipoproteins, altered cell function and atherosclerosis. *Atherosclerosis, (108),* (Suppl.), S21–S29.

Rangaswamy, S., Penn, M.S., Saidel, G.M., & Chisholm, G.M. (1997). Exogenous oxidized low-density lipoprotein injures and alters the barrier function of endothelium in rats in vivo. *Circulation Research, 80* (1), 37–43.

Ross, R. (1986). The pathogenesis of atherosclerosis—An update. *New England Journal of Medicine, 314* (8), 488–497.

Ross, R. (1993). The pathogenesis of atherosclerosis: A perspective for the 1990's. *Nature, 362* (29), 801–809.

Schwartz, C.J., Valente, A.J., & Sprague, E.A. (1993). A modern view of atherogenesis. *American Journal of Cardiology, 71,* 9B–14B.

Selwyn, A.P., Kinlay, S., Libby, P., & Ganz, P. (1997). Atherogenic lipids, vascular dysfunction, and signs of ischemic heart disease. *Circulation, 95* (1), 5–7.

Stary, H.C. (1994). Changes in components and structure of atherosclerotic lesions developing from childhood to middle age in coronary arteries. *Basic Research in Cardiology, 89* (Suppl. I), 17–32.

Stary, H.C. (1989). Evolution and progression of atherosclerotic lesions in coronary arteries of children and young adults. *Arteriosclerosis, 9* (Suppl. I), 19–32.

Stary, H.C., Blankenhorn, D.H., et al. (1992). A definition of the intima of human arteries and of its atherosclerosis-prone regions: A report from the Committee on Vascular Lesions of the Council on Arteriosclerosis, American Heart Association. *Circulation, 1,* 391–405.

Stary, H.C., Chandler, A.B., et al. (1995). A definition of advanced types of atherosclerotic lesions and a histological classification of atherosclerosis: A report from the Committee on Vascular Lesions of the Council on Arteriosclerosis, American Heart Association. *Circulation, 5,* 1355–1374.

Stary, H.C., Chandler, A.B., et al. (1994). A definition of initial, fatty streak and intermediate lesions of atherosclerosis: A report from the Committee on Vascular Lesions of the Council on Arteriosclerosis, American Heart Association. *Arteriosclerosis and Thrombosis, 5,* 840–856.

Stein, Y., & Stein, O. (1973). Lipid synthesis and degradation and lipoprotein transport in mammalian aorta. *Ciba Foundation Symposium, 12,* 165–183.

Teplitz, L., & Siwik, D.A. (1994). Cellular signals in atherosclerosis. *Journal of Cardiovascular Nursing, 8* (3), 28–52.

Van der Wal, A.C., Becker, A.E., Van der Loos, C., & Das, P.K. (1994). Site of intimal rupture or erosion of thrombosed coronary atherosclerotic plaques is characterized by an inflammatory process irrespective of the dominant plaque morphology. *Circulation, 89* (1), 36–44.

Vane, J.R., Annggard, E.E., & Botting, R.M. (1990). Regulatory functions of the vascular endothelium. *New England Journal of Medicine, 323,* 27–36.

Velican, C., & Velican D. (1989). *Natural History of Coronary Atherosclerosis.* Boca Raton, FL: CRC Press, Inc.

Zeiher, A.M., Schachinger, V., Saurbier, B., & Just, H. (1994). Assessment of endothelial modulation of coronary vasomotor tone: Insights into a fundamental functional disturbance in vascular biology of atherosclerosis. In H. Just, W. Hort, & A.M. Zeiher (Eds.), Arteriosclerosis: New Insights into Pathogenetic Mechanisms and Prevention. *Basic Research in Cardiology, 89,* (Suppl. I), 115–128.

Zierler, B.K. & Cowan, M.J. (1995). Pathogenesis of atherosclerosis. In S.L. Woods, E.S., Froelicher, C.J., Halpenny, & S.V. Motzer (Eds.), *Cardiac Nursing,* 3rd ed. Philadelphia: J.B. Lippincott Co.

CHAPTER 3

Concepts and Theoretical Models

Susan R. Rossi
Joseph S. Rossi

Prevention of coronary heart disease (CHD) often involves changing long established lifestyle behaviors that influence more than one risk factor and involve a number of different problem areas. Risk factors might include smoking, high cholesterol and dietary fat intake, being overweight, engaging in insufficient activity or exercise, and being subjected to high stress. More and more, nurses and other clinicians have come to recognize the value that CHD theory and research have in practice. Ultimately, it is the clinician who translates theory into practice and implements research findings through intervention.

Health behavior change is a complex process that includes multiple antecedents, processes, and consequences. In this chapter, three commonly recognized problem areas (smoking, high dietary fat intake, and inactivity) that can influence CHD development are emphasized. Four theoretical perspectives of health behavior change applicable to CHD risk reduction are discussed: the health-belief model, social learning theory, the theory of reasoned action, and the transtheoretical model of behavior change. Two related concepts, self-efficacy and social support, are also considered.

This chapter complements the previous chapters and provides another perspective of CHD risk and risk reduction. As readers may have varying levels of familiarity with, and interest in, the different concepts and theoretical approaches, most individual sections of the chapter are designed to be understandable without it being necessary to read previous sections. Review of the entire chapter is recommended to obtain the comprehensive knowledge base helpful in understanding subsequent chapters and in structuring CHD risk-reduction interventions.

HEALTH-BELIEF MODEL

The *health-belief model* (HBM) is a cognitively focused behavioral prediction model that represents a public health approach to understanding, predicting, and explaining why health-related behavior occurs (Becker, 1974; Becker & Maiman, 1975; Fishbein, Bandura, Triandis, et al., 1991; Janz & Becker; 1984; Rosenstock, 1990). According to the HBM, the likelihood that an individual will take action to prevent illness depends upon the individual's perception that (1) personal vulnerability to the condition exists; (2) the consequences of developing the condition are potentially serious; (3) the precautionary behavior is likely to be effective against developing the condition; and (4) the benefits from reducing the threat of developing the condition exceed the costs of taking action (Rosenstock, 1990). These four factors, which are themselves influenced by mediating variables, indirectly influence the probability of someone performing protective health behaviors in that they influence that person's perceived threat of the illness and expectations about outcome. Figure 3–1 presents a schematic description to help the reader understand the HBM components and their interrelationships in the ensuing discussion.

The HBM has been used in intervening with health screening, illness, sick-role, and precautionary behaviors (e.g., Rosenstock, 1974; Kirscht, 1974; Becker, 1974; Janz & Becker, 1984). The model has undergone some modifications since its original formulation. In the process of translation from theory to practice, various versions of the HBM have emerged. Unfortunately, the existence of various versions

has led to some difficulty in evaluating some of the variables specified in the model, as well as posed problems in rigorous testing of the HBM's effectiveness in predicting health behavior across studies. Some forms of the HBM include additional variables, such as cues to action, general susceptibility to illness, the value of health, and self-efficacy.

The most commonly described form of the HBM has four key components of perception: (1) susceptibility, (2) severity, (3) effectiveness and (4) cost. *Perceived susceptibility* refers to the probability an individual assigns to personal vulnerability in developing the condition. The concept of perceived susceptibility has been found to be predictive of a number of health-protective behaviors. From the HBM perspective, the likelihood an individual will engage in precautionary behaviors (e.g., quit smoking, eat a diet low in fat and cholesterol, exercise) to prevent CHD depends on how much that individual believes the disease will develop. In general, it has been found that people tend to underestimate susceptibility to disease. The individual who smokes but is adversely affected by the death of a smoking parent from a heart

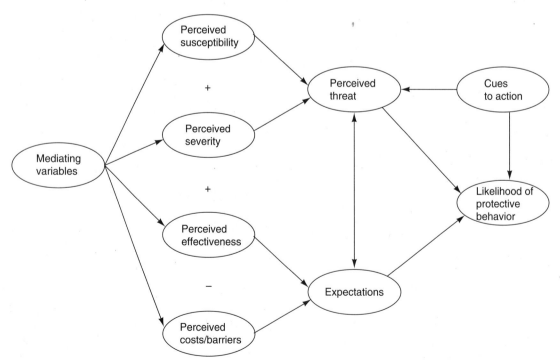

FIGURE 3–1   Heuristic depiction of health-belief model.

attack is more likely to attempt to stop smoking than the individual who feels invulnerable to CHD.

Perceived severity refers to how serious the individual believes the consequences of developing the condition are if current behavior patterns remain unchanged. An individual is more likely to take action to prevent CHD (e.g., change dietary habits to lower cholesterol levels) if he or she believes that possible negative physical, psychological, or social effects resulting from the disease pose serious consequences (e.g., altered significant social relationships, reduced independence, pain, suffering, disability, or even death). Models of health belief frequently refer to health threats perceived by the individual. The combination of perceived susceptibility and perceived severity constitute the notion of a threat. The general consensus is that perception of a threat alone is not enough to motivate an individual to change behavior.

Perceived effectiveness refers to the benefits of engaging in the protective behavior. Motivation to take action to change a behavior requires the belief that the precautionary behavior is likely to be effective against the condition. For example, the individual who is not convinced that there is a causal relationship between smoking and health problems is unlikely to quit smoking to prevent CHD if there is a strong belief that such action will not protect against the disease.

Perceived cost refers to the barriers that impede precautionary behavior adoption. The combination of perceived effectiveness and perceived cost constitutes the notion of outcome expectation. Belief alone is not enough to motivate an individual to act. Action usually follows a cognitive weighing of the personal costs associated with the protective behavior (e.g., not eating bacon, making time in a busy schedule to exercise) against the benefits expected from the protective behavior. In other words, expectations of outcome determine whether action is taken. Benefits have to outweigh the costs involved. For example, an individual is more likely to engage in behaviors to prevent CHD, (e.g., quit smoking) if the perceived positive aspects of smoking cessation (e.g., breathing easier, reduced risk of heart attack) outweigh the perceived negative aspects involved in

changing (e.g., initial weight gain, nicotine withdrawal symptoms).

Cues to action involve stimuli that motivate an individual to engage in the precautionary behavior (Rosenstock, 1990). The stimulus that triggers action may be internal or external. For example, angina, a painful symptom, may act as an internal cue to initiate action. External cues, such as a spouse's sudden hospitalization for a heart attack, or the death of a parent from heart disease, may also trigger behaviors to protect against CHD (quitting smoking, reducing dietary fat, exercising) in an individual who would not have considered making such behavior changes before. The four previously discussed factors central to the HBM may also interact to trigger action. For example, when perceived susceptibility and severity are high, little stimulus may be required to initiate action. More intense stimuli may be needed to initiate action if perceived susceptibility and severity are low.

Some formulations of the HBM have included *self-efficacy* as a key factor. Self-efficacy is influenced by mediating variables and in turn influences expectations. Its use in the model has been criticized on the basis that differentiation between it and the concept of barriers (costs) is unclear (Weinstein, 1993). In addition, some forms of the HBM refer to *general susceptibility to illness* as a key factor in the model. Yet substitution of the general case over specific consequences is appropriate only if the intention of the precautionary behavior is to improve overall health (Weinstein, 1993).

The *value of health,* another variable that is sometimes included, refers to interest in and concerns about general health (Rosenstock, 1990). The extent to which an individual values health has also been recognized as an important factor in influencing the belief in a threat to health (Becker & Maiman, 1975). According to this view of the HBM, individuals concerned about being healthy in general are more likely to exercise regularly to protect against CHD than individuals who place little value on health.

Although both cues to action and the value of health have been included in some forms of HBM, their importance in predicting health behavior is unclear, because neither variable has been systematically studied (Rosenstock, 1990).

Mediating factors (demographic, structural, and social variables) have also been explored in applying the HBM. Mediating variables (e.g., educational level) are believed to indirectly affect behavior by influencing an individual's perceptions of susceptibility, severity, benefits, and barriers (Rosenstock, 1990). Becker and Maiman (1975) added the concept of motivation to the HBM. This concept has also been interpreted as readiness to change behavior (Baranowski, 1992).

SOCIAL LEARNING THEORY

Bandura's (1986) *social learning theory* (SLT), also referred to as *social cognitive theory,* is a behavioral prediction theory that represents a clinical approach to health behavior change (Fishbein, Bandura, Triandis, et al., 1991). This theory has been widely applied to health behavior with respect to prevention of disease, promotion of health, and modification of unhealthy lifestyles for a number of different risk behaviors. The SLT emphasizes what people think and the effect of those thoughts on their behavior (Perry, Baranowski, & Parcel, 1990).

The SLT proposes that behavior can be explained in terms of *triadic reciprocity* among three key concepts that operate as determinants of each other. *Reciprocal determinism* forms the basic organizing principle of SLT. This important concept states that there is a continuous, dynamic interaction between the individual, the environment, and behavior. Thus, a change in one of these factors affects the other two. The SLT involves numerous key concepts, which are pictorially associated with each of the three main constructs in Figure 3–2. This schematic description will help the reader understand SLT components and their interrelationships in the ensuing discussion.

Bandura (1986) conceptualized influences on behavior that involved the concept of *person* in terms of basic human capacities that are cognitive in nature. Key concepts associated with the notion of personhood include personal characteristics, emotional arousal/coping, behavioral capacity, self-efficacy, expectations, expectancies, self-regulation, observational/experiential learning, and reinforcement (Perry, Baranowski, & Parcel, 1990).

Personal characteristics have been operationalized as multiple, interacting determinants such as demographics (e.g., gender, race, ethnicity, education), personality, cognitive factors (e.g., thoughts, attitudes, beliefs, knowledge, ability to symbolize representations of reality and attribute meaning to behavior), motivation, and skills.

Emotional arousal/coping can interfere with learning and thus influence behavior. This influence on behavior involves a response to emotional stimuli with various approaches, strategies, and activities that are appropriate to use in dealing with arousing situations (e.g., fear).

Behavioral capacity refers to an individual's command of the knowledge and skills necessary for performing a behavior. *Self-efficacy* refers to an individual's confidence in his or her ability to perform a behavior in various situations. Self-efficacy has been recognized as an important mediating variable among knowledge, attitudes, skills, and behavior (Baranowski, 1992).

Expectations are beliefs associated with the outcome of a behavior. *Expectancies* are the values an individual attributes to the anticipated outcome of performing a behavior. *Self-regulation* refers to the individual's ability to manage or control behavior. Individuals use goal-setting, self-monitoring, and self-reinforcement to regulate performance of a behavior.

Observational/experiential learning refers to the acquisition of a behavior. Learning can occur through observation of another's performance of a behavior or through personal experience. For example, modeling an observed behavior is a learning strategy that individuals sometimes employ. *Reinforcement* is concerned with consequences that influence the probability that a behavior will be repeated. Individuals are motivated to perform behaviors through rewards and incentives (Perry, Baranowski, & Parcel, 1990).

In the SLT the relationship between behavior, person, and environment is interactive. The stereotypic picture of the relatively young chief executive officer who develops CHD provides an illustration of how variables associated with person (e.g., personal characteristics) interact with the environment and behavior. Consider a person in his or her late 30s to early 40s who is

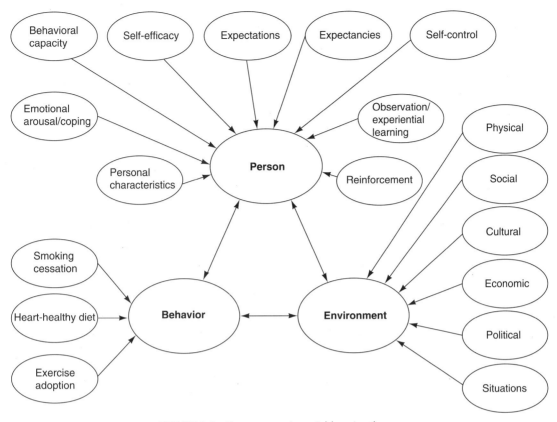

FIGURE 3–2   Key concepts in social learning theory.

obsessed with achievement, advancement, and recognition. This individual is a highly competitive workaholic who is driven to get things done quickly. Such individuals are sometimes described as being hostile and might be found operating in a highly stressful environment. Although simplistic and stereotypic, this picture represents a classic example of a *Type A personality*. From the SLT perspective, the individual's predominant personality type might be expected to negatively influence his behavior. Thus the individual is less likely to take the time to acquire the cognitive and behavioral skills necessary to successfully perform CHD risk-reduction behavior.

Influences on behavior that involve the concept of *environment* can be physical, social, cultural, economic, political (Ockene & Ockene, 1992), or situational (Perry, Baranowski, & Parcel, 1990) in nature. In the SLT the person's perceptions of the environment are referred to as *situations.* This key variable can facilitate or inhibit behavior.

In this reciprocal, interactive scheme in which multiple determinants of behavior are assumed, *behavior* exerts an influence on both the environment and the person. The environment and past experience with a particular behavior can also provide reinforcement for acting in a particular way. For example, as Americans have demanded the availability of healthier, low-fat, higher-fiber food choices in their environment in order to reduce CHD risk, more and more eating establishments have changed their food preparation procedures and menus accordingly. A wider variety of "heart healthy" choices are available now. To reduce their CHD risk, consumers have begun to take advantage of greater environmental choices by engaging in behaviors like the following: purchasing more fruits and vegetables, substituting lower-fat products readily available in supermarkets in place of high-fat ones, changing food preparation methods to broiling and baking instead of frying, and ordering the lower-fat food choices being offered in more restaurants.

Interactions are also assumed to occur between problem behaviors (e.g., eating high-fat foods, lack of exercise, smoking) and physiologic factors (e.g., nicotine, caffeine addiction) (Ockene & Ockene, 1992). An individual's performance of the associated behaviors can have an important impact on CHD prevention. Engaging in exercise can trigger hunger, stimulating the desire for a high-fat dessert. Finishing a meal can trigger the desire for a cigarette. An individual may turn to smoking to relax in a high-stress environment.

To effectively prevent CHD, an individual needs to engage in multiple healthy behaviors, like smoking cessation, exercise adoption, and low-fat/cholesterol eating habits. An individual who is highly motivated to change and decides to reduce CHD risk may make multiple changes in lifestyle: attempt to quit smoking, cut down on dietary fat intake, and increase exercise.

The SLT assumes that most behaviors are learned responses and can be unlearned or modified. Thus, learning through observing the behavior of others (i.e., modeling behavior) is important from the SLT perspective. The SLT also places heavy emphasis on learning both cognitive and behavioral skills for coping with situations and making changes in health behavior. An individual who wants to quit smoking to reduce CHD risk but lacks the cognitive and behavioral skills to effectively cope with stressful situations is less likely to stop smoking despite espoused motivation to do so.

Self-Efficacy

The concept of self-efficacy is recognized as one of Bandura's (1977) most important contributions to the SLT and thus warrants more detailed discussion. Self-efficacy refers to the *confidence* an individual has in his or her own ability to successfully carry out a particular behavior. The importance of the role self-efficacy plays in performing behavior has been widely recognized across multiple problem areas relevant to CHD risk reduction, including smoking cessation and maintaining a low-fat diet and weight control (Table 3–1).

Bandura (1977) proposed that the actual performance of a particular behavior is highly related to an individual's belief in his or her ability

TABLE 3–1 Recognition of Importance of Self-Efficacy across Problem Areas Relevant to CHD Risk Reduction

Problem Area	Source
Smoking cessation	DiClemente, 1986
	Velicer, DiClemente, Rossi, & Prochaska, 1990
Diet	Prochaska, 1992
	Rossi, 1993
Exercise adoption	Marcus, Selby, Niaura, & Rossi, 1992
	Sallis et al., 1986
	Sallis, Pinski, Patterson, & Nader, 1988
Weight control	Bernier & Avard, 1986
	Clark, Abrams, Niaura, Eaton, & Rossi, 1991
	Rossi, Rossi, et al., 1995

to perform that behavior in specific situations. An individual with low self-efficacy is likely to have lower expectations of successfully performing the behavior and hence be more affected by situational temptations that are counterproductive to promoting and maintaining healthy behavior change. In contrast, an individual who has high self-efficacy not only expects to succeed but is actually more likely to do so. For example, the likelihood that an individual will successfully perform a CHD risk-reduction behavior such as exercising depends strongly on how confident the individual is of actually being able to do activities, such as walking, jogging, climbing stairs, riding a bike, using a treadmill, or participating in aerobics on a regular basis.

Several factors influence an individual's self-efficacy, including persuasion by others, observation of others' behavior (modeling), previous experience with performing the behavior, and physiologic feedback (Bandura, 1986). For example, to reduce CHD risk, an individual is more likely to attempt to stop smoking if a physician recommends doing so, the individual is able to observe other people who have been able to quit or are coping well with trying to quit, the individual has had past experience with smoking cessation such as having quit smoking for 24 hours or more, or the individual is able to cope with the physical symptoms of nicotine withdrawal. Self-efficacy exerts such a strong influence on behavior change that the factor of confidence has been found to outperform the factor of past performance in predicting future behavior (DiClemente, 1986).

THEORY OF REASONED ACTION

The *theory of reasoned action* (TRA) is a widely used behavioral prediction theory that represents a social-psychological approach to understanding and predicting the determinants of health behavior (Ajzen & Fishbein, 1980; Fishbein & Ajzen, 1975). Over the years, the TRA has been applied to diverse health-related behaviors, from weight loss, smoking, and alcohol ingestion to breast cancer screening.

The TRA states that the intention to perform a particular behavior is strongly related to the actual act of performing that behavior. Two basic assumptions that underlie the TRA are that (1) most behavior is under volitional control, and (2) people are rational beings. From the perspective of the TRA, we behave in a certain way because we choose to do so, and we use a rational decision-making system in choosing and planning our actions. The TRA was designed to predict behavior from inten-

tion. It proposes quasi-mathematical relationships among beliefs, attitudes, intentions, and behavior. Figure 3–3 illustrates the key components of the TRA and their relationships.

Predicting behavior is the ultimate goal of TRA; therefore, beginning with that component and working backward facilitates an understanding of the relationships between the key variables. According to TRA, behavior is influenced by the intention to perform the behavior. Intention, in turn, is influenced by three major variables: subjective norms, attitudes, and self-efficacy.

Subjective norms involve people's perceptions of what significant others believe about their ability to perform the behavior. For example, their intention to cut down on dietary fat consumption by giving up bacon, red meat, and pastry could be partly determined by what they believe their spouse thinks about their ability to do so.

Attitudes can be conceptualized in terms of values. For example, an individual may believe that cutting down on dietary fat intake is a beneficial behavior to perform for preventing CHD. Thus, that action conforms to a value held by the individual. *Self-efficacy* is the confidence an individual feels that he or she can

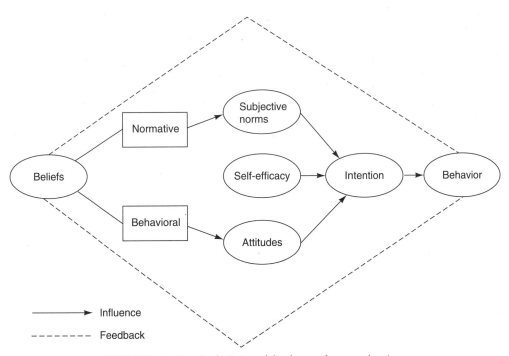

FIGURE 3–3 Generic depiction of the theory of reasoned action.

successfully perform a behavior. A modified version of the TRA includes the addition of *perceived control* over modifying the behavior and has been referred to as the *model of planned behavior* (Fishbein, Bandura, Triandis, et al., 1991).

Two of the variables that influence intention—subjective norms and attitudes—are in turn influenced by beliefs. Two general types of beliefs are considered in the TRA: normative and behavioral beliefs. *Normative beliefs* are situationally based social expectations that are considered the rule. Normative beliefs influence subjective norms, whereas beliefs about the behavior, *behavioral beliefs,* influence attitudes. Attitudes toward a behavior are determined by the expectations an individual has about the outcome of performing the behavior and the extent to which an individual values the outcome. Thus, from a TRA perspective, the likelihood that an individual will engage in CHD risk reduction depends on how much that individual is convinced that healthy alternative behaviors will result in preventing CHD risk and the degree to which the individual perceives the resulting benefits as outweighing the costs of obtaining them.

The majority of the TRA research has focused on the prediction of behavioral intention rather than on behavior itself (Baranowski, 1992). Unfortunately, because the correlation between behavior and intention has not been particularly impressive, research on attitudes and behaviors is often dismissed (Ajzen & Fishbein, 1980). Despite this shortcoming, Sonstroem (1988) has suggested that the TRA can still be a useful perspective as long as (1) situation-specific attitude and intention measures are employed that specify congruent action, target, context, and time and (2) the interactions between personal determinants and situations are emphasized.

SOCIAL SUPPORT

Social support is a relevant concept for CHD prevention and is distinct from the previously discussed theoretical perspectives. Changing multiple health behaviors (e.g., smoking, high dietary fat intake, inactivity) is a difficult task for any individual to accomplish. Assistance from the social environment (i.e., social support) can facilitate behavior change. The social environment includes other human beings people tend to interact with on a regular basis (e.g., family, friends, co-workers, etc.), but there is no universally agreed upon definition of social support. Most definitions of social support are relational in nature and involve one individual meeting another's basic needs through interpersonal interaction. Depending on the investigator, however, the focus of the interaction varies. For example, some focus on actions (Berkman & Syme, 1979; House, 1981). Others focus on information (Cassel, 1974, 1976; Cobb, 1976). Kaplan, Cassel, and Gore (1977) defined social support as the degree to which an individual's social needs are met through interaction. Cohen and Syme (1985) defined it as "resources provided by other persons" (p. 4). Gottlieb (1983) maintained that "social support consists of verbal and non-verbal information or advice, tangible aid, or action that is proffered by social inmates or inferred by their presence and has beneficial emotional or behavioral effects on the recipient" (p. 28).

Although a general consensus exists that social support is a complex, multidimensional concept, considerable variation can be found among researchers, both across and within disciplines, with regard to the components that constitute social support. In general, components of social support can include emotional, informational, tangible, or affirmational support (Table 3–2).

For example, Kaplan, Cassel, and Gore (1977) refer to the concept's components as *basic needs.* Caplan and Killilea (1976) label these components *elements.* Components of social support have also been referred to as *resources* (Gottlieb, 1983). Whether specified explicitly or implicitly, social support generally involves interaction between the individual providing support and the individual receiving it. Specifications of mutual obligation, reciprocity, or component flow (unidirectional versus exchange) of support vary from one investigator to another. Further, an analysis of the literature shows that the various components of social support may themselves take on many different forms (Table 3–3). For example, *emotional support* can involve feeling loved, being liked, being needed; it may

TABLE 3–2 Components of Social Support

Author	Emotional	Informational	Tangible	Interaction	Appraisal	Direction
Berkman & Syme (1979)	E			1		
Brandt & Weinert (1981)	E	Info	T			
Caplan & Killilea (1976)	E	Info	T	1		U
Cassel (1974, 1976)	E	Info		1	A	
Cobb (1976)	E	Info		1		R
Cohen & Syme (1985)	E	Info	T		A	U
Cronenwett (1985)	E	Info	T			
Gore (1978)	E		T		A	U
Gottlieb (1983)	E	Info	T	1	A	U
House & Kahn (1985)	E	Info	T			
Kahn & Antonucci (1980)	E		T	1	A	
Kaplan et al., (1977)	E		T	1		
Norbeck (1981)	E		T		A	
Weiss (1973)					A	

Components of social support specified by authors may be emotional = E, informational = INFO, or tangible = T in nature. Some authors specify or imply the type of relationship that occurs in social support as being between individuals (1 in the table) or affirmational (A). Sometimes the direction in which social support flows is specified as being unidirectional (U), meaning that one individual provides components of social support to another without exchange, or reciprocal (R), meaning an exchange of components occurs.

include esteem, trust, or intimate social relationships. *Informational support* can be verbal or nonverbal in nature and consist of advice, suggestions, guidance, feedback, or directives.

Tangible support, or *instrumental support,* consists of material resources such as goods, supplies, skills, services, money, time, labor, or modification of the environment. Some authors

TABLE 3–3 Forms of Social Support Components

Emotional Support

Feeling Loved	*Being Liked*	*Being Needed*	*Involves Trust*	*Esteem*	*Involves Intimate Relationships*
Cobb, 1976 Gore, 1978 House & Kahn, 1985 Kahn & Antonucci, 1980	Kahn & Antonucci, 1980	Gore, 1978	House & Kahn, 1985	Cohen & Syme, 1985 House, 1981	Berkman & Syme, 1979

Informational Support

Advice	*Suggestions*	*Guidance*	*Feedback/ Directives*
Gottlieb, 1983 House & Kahn, 1985	House & Kahn, 1985	Weise, 1973	House & Kahn, 1985

Tangible Support

Material Resources

Goods	*Supplies*	*Skills*	*Services*	*Money/Time/ Labor*	*Environmental Modification*
Cobb, 1976	Kaplan et al., 1974	Caplan & Killilea, 1976	Cobb, 1976	House & Kahn, 1985	House & Kahn, 1985

use the term *appraisal support,* instead of *affirmational support,* generally referring to feedback, social comparisons, or reassurance.

The impact of social support on health, both physical and emotional well-being, morbidity, and mortality, has been well explored. Several epidemiologic studies suggests that social support may be an important factor in preventing CHD (Berkman & Syme, 1979; Marmot & Syme, 1976; Riegel, 1989; Tilden & Weinert, 1987). It may act as a mediator that buffers the individual from physiologic and psychological stress, although explanations as to exactly how social support buffers stress differ.

Social support can be negative or positive in nature. Removing sources of negative support can be just as important as providing social sources of positive support. Suppose one spouse smokes, and the other does not. One of the reasons the individual smokes is because of the belief that the behavior promotes relaxation. In the mistaken belief that commenting on the negative consequences of smoking constitutes being supportive, the nonsmoking spouse repeatedly reminds the smoker about all the bad things that will happen if the habit is not stopped. Unfortunately, to the individual who is not ready to quit smoking, rather than being supportive, this behavior is perceived as nagging. The tension that is created between the two individuals leads to an increase in stress, and so the smoker continues to smoke. In this case, stress is more likely to be reduced if the negative support (i.e., coercion and nagging) is stopped. Positive support is more likely to create an atmosphere in which the individual becomes more open to considering information about smoking cessation.

The three types of social support identified as important in the SLT context are informational, material, and emotional support (Caplan & Killilea, 1976). *Informational support* is characterized by situations in which one individual provides another with knowledge. In this process, both individuals are helped toward obtaining personal goals. In providing this type of social support to reduce the risk of CHD, the nurse or other health care provider might choose to teach specific strategies for coping that an individual can use in response to stress instead of lighting up or eating foods high in fat.

Material support involves a transaction in which goods or services are provided to help the individual achieve a personal goal. Providing access to equipment like a treadmill or activities such as aerobics programs to individuals who want to reduce CHD risk through exercise are examples of material support.

Emotional support involves the attempts of one individual to increase the other's self-esteem with regard to performing a behavior. One of the values of a support group is that it provides a network of individuals who can motivate and provide emotional support and reinforcement for each other. Providing a forum in which individuals feel comfortable about sharing feelings, hopes, fears, problems, successes, and failures with others who will listen to them and on whom they can depend is important. For the individual who wants to reduce CHD risk, emotional support might come from a spouse, family members, the nurse, a friend, a jogging partner, or a more formal group of people trying to control their weight.

In applying the SLT to facilitate engagement in the CHD risk-reduction behavior of exercise, the nurse and other clinicians might try to motivate an individual by attempting to

1 Increase the perception of health costs of a sedentary lifestyle.
2 Increase the perception of benefits of activity by employing selective reinforcement.
3 Provide opportunities for the individual to learn from observing the practice of healthy behavior.
4 Ensure social support, or focus on skill acquisition, mastery, and competency to enhance self-efficacy.

LIMITATIONS OF THE HBM, SLT, AND TRA PERSPECTIVES

For a number of reasons, the HBM, SLT, and TRA are all limited in their usefulness for CHD prevention. The most important reason concerns the kind of model they represent—a behavioral prediction rather than a behavioral change model. Becker, Bandura, and Fishbein discriminate between behavioral prediction models and behavior change models (Fishbein, Bandura, Triandis, Kanfer, et al., 1991). As the term implies, behavioral prediction models *predict* behavior. In seeking to account for *why* behavior occurs, this type of model is concerned with the factors that influence (i.e., determine) behavior. Behavioral prediction models assume that people continue to behave in a particular way unless some kind of stimulus interrupts their behavioral status quo.

In contrast, behavior change models seek to *explain how* behavior change occurs. This type of model is concerned with change as a process, focusing on (1) the stimuli that disrupt behavior and (2) the activities, strategies, and approaches that people use as they move through different states, steps, or stages in attempting to change behavior. The theory of self-regulation and self-control and the transtheoretical model of behavior change (discussed later in this chapter) are examples of behavior change models.

As behavioral prediction models, all three theoretical perspectives (HBM, SLT, TRA) presented as applicable to CHD risk reduction focus on the determinants of behavior. Becker, Bandura, and Fishbein agree that the HBM, SLT, and TRA share assumptions about eight key variables they and others have identified as the primary determinants of behavior. These eight variables are intention, environmental constraints, skills, attitudes, social norms, self-image, emotions, and self-efficacy (Fishbein, Bandura, Triandis, et al., 1991).

From the behavioral prediction perspective, the likelihood that an individual will perform a particular CHD risk-reduction behavior like reducing dietary fat consumption depends on the assumptions that the individual (1) possesses a strong positive intention to reduce fat or has made a commitment to cut down on fat; (2) has ample opportunity to cut down on fat as well as a lack of environmental restrictions that might prevent the performance of fat-reduction behaviors; (3) has acquired the necessary skills required to reduce dietary fat intake; (4) has a positive attitude toward reducing dietary fat and believes the anticipated CHD risk-reduction advantages of reducing fat will outweigh the negative costs expected in obtaining those benefits; (5) perceives that social pressure (i.e., social norms) to cut down on fat is greater than continuing to maintain high-fat eating habits; (6) perceives the behavior of cutting down

on fat as consistent with self-image or at least, does not consider this behavior to be a violation of personal standards; (7) has feelings toward cutting down on fat that are more positive than negative; and (8) is confident that she or he is capable of cutting down on dietary fat.

These eight common variables represent components of the HBM, SLT, and TRA that are valuable keys to the kind of behavioral change that could reduce CHD risk. Although these models do not explicitly endorse a behavior change perspective, their focus on the determinants of behavior can provide insights as to which factors prompt efforts to change. Examining CHD risk reduction from any of these perspectives could help us identify the variables the contribute most to change behavior. Knowledge of the direction and magnitude of such variables could be useful not only in developing and designing interventions to accelerate behavior change, but as indicators of progress toward that change.

One problem with the HBM, SLT, and TRA is that in focusing on the determinants of behavior, they fail to provide a comprehensive picture of the process of change involved in preventing CHD risk. While they are particularly useful for understanding why change occurs, these perspectives do not provide information about who changes, when change is likely to occur, or more importantly, *how* change occurs. Some of the components of the HBM, TRA, and SLT overlap or complement each other, but none were designed to supply critical information about the strategies, approaches, or activities people use to intentionally and successfully help themselves *throughout* the change process. To facilitate behavior change, it is important to understand how people change.

Perhaps the biggest problem with using the HBM, SLT, or TRA to study CHD risk prevention is that they fail to provide information on the change process once action has been initiated. They do not provide behavioral insights about people who have recently changed, people who make changes but then revert to old, unhealthy behaviors, or people who are able to successfully maintain long-term behavior change.

Current relapse rates indicate that most change is not linear. Prochaska (1992) aptly points out that taking action is *not* equivalent to simply changing behavior. Many people take action only to return to the unhealthy behavior several times before establishing new, healthier lifestyle patterns. The HBM and TRA, in particular, are more concerned with the motivation and intention to perform a particular behavior than with the behavior itself (Baranowski, 1992). Understanding what motivates people and predicting intentions to perform CHD risk behaviors may be useful, but such predictions do little to explain behavior change.

The TRA may be useful for exploring the complex interrelationships between attitudes and behavior. The predictive power associated with the relationships found between intention and behavior can be maximized using the more narrow specification of parameters (Sonstroem, 1988). However, there are difficulties with using the TRA to study behavior change to reduce CHD risk. The mathematical relationships specified in the theory rely on a simple additive model that predicts behavior from intention. The validity of using simplistic additive models to predict behavior is questionable for two reasons. The first reason is based on the need to use mediating variables to explain the relationships between attitude and behavior (Liska, 1984). The second reason concerns the influence of direct previous experience on attitudes, intentions, and behavior (Fazio & Zanna, 1981; Sherman, Presson, Chassin, et al., 1982). Additive models also make the questionable assumption that deficiencies in one component can be compensated by higher scores in other components.

The view of health behavior embodied in the SLT has merit but is not without its share of difficulty in operationalization. Among other things, the SLT has been criticized for ignoring or minimizing the importance of the role of affect by subsuming it within cognitive structures (Turk & Kerns, 1985). The SLT has also been criticized for failing to incorporate developmental and emotional theoretical perspectives (Sinacore-Guinn, 1993). Over the years, clinicians have made practical use of various components of the SLT, most notably reciprocal determinism, modeling, and the concept of self-efficacy. Perceived self-efficacy has been largely recognized as the theory's most valuable contribution to understanding health behavior.

Consequently, rather than being used as a whole, the SLT is often operationalized simply in terms of self-efficacy.

The problem with using self-efficacy alone to study behavior change as it relates to CHD risk reduction is that a single concept can address only the one aspect of behavior it represents and cannot provide a comprehensive picture of the complex process of change likely to underlie multiple problem behaviors.

As a single independent concept, social support has this same limitation with regard to the study of CHD risk reduction. Although the concept of social support is relevant to CHD risk reduction within a larger context of study, the concept suffers from serious definitional, methodologic, and conceptual problems. The main problem is a lack of consensus in the literature regarding the concept's definition, constituent components, operationalization, and measurement. Views differ on the focus, delivery, experience, and interpretation of social support. Greater utility of the concept of social support will depend on its successful integration into more comprehensive models of health behavior.

Over the past 20 years, clinicians have used the HBM, SLT, TRA, and other models or theories to better understand, study, predict, and intervene in high-risk health behavior problems. Despite the considerable strides made in reducing the incidence of heart disease in this country, CHD still ranks as the leading cause of mortality among adults (MMWR, 1993). More than 500,000 Americans die of CHD each year (Public Health Service, 1991). These statistics suggest that a greater impact on behavior change is needed. Furthermore, the literature indicates that in translating from theory to practice, clinicians tend to focus on interventions that are action-oriented (Prochaska, 1992). Unfortunately, most people are not ready to quit smoking, cut down on dietary fat consumption, or increase exercise. Consequently, action-oriented interventions are appropriate for only a minority of individuals and do not meet the needs of the majority of individuals who could benefit from change but are not ready to do so. As changing behavior is tantamount to preventing or reducing CHD risk, use of a behavioral *change* model (versus behavioral prediction model) would seem more appropriate for understanding, explaining, and reducing CHD risk. The challenge posed today is to implement models of health behavior that incorporate a wide range of thoughts, attitudes, feelings, and activities that characterize individuals throughout the entire process of change, including initial motivation, relapse, and success. The notion of *motivational readiness* is an organizing principle that has been particularly successful and useful in this regard.

TRANSTHEORETICAL MODEL

One promising model of behavior change that emphasizes motivational readiness is the *transtheoretical model* (TTM) (Prochaska, DiClemente, & Norcross, 1992). This model is often referred to as the *stages-of-change model,* because its central organizing concept states that people move through a series of stages as they change from unhealthy to healthier behavior. Over the past 15 years, the TTM has received considerable empirical support. Effective CHD risk reduction involves changing multiple risk factors, such as smoking, high-fat/cholesterol diets, and sedentary behavior. The TTM is particularly relevant to primary prevention of CHD because it is rapidly emerging as one of the most promising models applied to multiple risk-factor reduction (Emmons, Marcus, Linnan, et al., 1994; Prochaska, DiClemente, & Norcross,

1992; Prochaska, Velicer, Rossi, et al., 1994; Rossi, 1992b).

The TTM is a general model of behavior change positing that intentionally changing behavior involves making use of different strategies and activities—that is, *processes of change*—to move through different degrees of motivational readiness, or *stages of change.* This model also incorporates a series of intervening or outcome variables, including the pros and cons of changing behavior *(decisional balance),* confidence in the ability to change across problem situations *(self-efficacy),* and the temptation to engage in the problem behavior *(situational temptation).* The model has been found to be generalizable to a wide variety of problem areas. At present, the TTM has been adapted to more than 40 different problem areas. Figure 3–4 represents a heuristic depiction of the model, only portions of which have been empirically tested to determine the direction of the relationships between constructs.

Integrating the successful components of competing models is an inherently strong approach to model building. One of the advantages of using the TTM for preventing CHD is that it represents a "meta-model" that preserves and incorporates some of the best concepts found in the HBM, SLT, and TRA, among many other theories. In addition, the TTM integrates other concepts, including self-efficacy

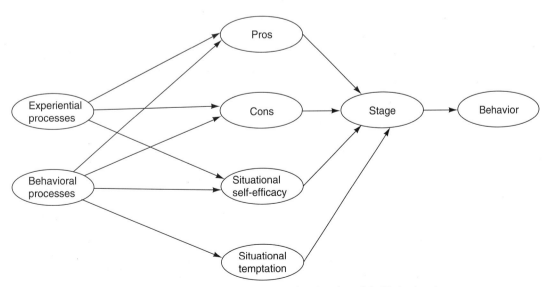

FIGURE 3–4   Heuristic depiction of the transtheoretical model of behavior change.

and social support. Its application to important CHD risk factors (e.g., smoking, dietary fat intake, exercise, and weight control) also make this model particularly useful for primary CHD prevention.

The TTM is currently conceptualized in terms of several major dimensions. The core concept, around which the other dimensions are organized, is stage of change. These stages represent ordered categories along a continuum of motivational readiness to change a problem behavior. A set of independent variables known as the processes of change effect transitions between the stages of change. Intervening or outcome variables also included in the model consist of the pros and cons of change, self-efficacy, and situational temptations. For CHD risk, other intermediate or dependent variables that might be considered are age, gender, cigarette smoking, high dietary fat intake, high cholesterol, high blood pressure, diabetes, being overweight, physical inactivity, family history of CHD, genetic factors, low educational level, and high stress.

Stages of Change

The central organizing concept of the TTM is, as mentioned, the notion of stages of change. Five ordered categories of readiness to change have been defined: precontemplation, contemplation, preparation, action, and maintenance (Prochaska, DiClemente, & Norcross, 1992). For some problem areas, a sixth stage, termination, has also been proposed. Each of these stages provides a temporal or developmental dimension that presents when particular changes occur. The amount of progress people make in changing behavior is a function of their stage of change. Helping individuals advance even one stage of change in a treatment program eventually doubles their chances of taking action in the next 6 months (DiClemente, Prochaska, Fairhurst, et al., 1991; Prochaska, DiClemente, & Norcross, 1992). The idea that there are specific, discrete stages to the change process has now been supported by a great deal of research on how people change, either on their own, in the natural environment, or with professional help, such as in intervention studies, hospitals, or clinics.

Individuals in the *precontemplation stage* of change have no intention of changing their problem behavior in the near future, usually defined as within the next 6 months (Table 3–4). Many precontemplators do not feel that they have a problem and may deny the existence of a problem even when confronted with evidence of it. When precontemplators do acknowledge that they have a problem, they often do not consider it serious enough to require behavior change. Some may be demoralized from repeated unsuccessful attempts to change. In any case, for the precontemplator the costs of changing behavior clearly outweigh the benefits. Precontemplators often feel that they are being pressured into change by family, friends, employer, or society in general. Coerced change is rarely successful; as soon as the pressure is off, precontemplators typically revert to old behavior patterns. Defensiveness and resistance to recognizing or modifying a problem are the most distinctive characteristics of the precontemplation stage.

Individuals in the *contemplation stage* of change acknowledge that they may have a problem and are seriously considering change within the next 6 months (see Table 3–4). Unfortunately, contemplators typically do not act on their intentions and frequently remain stuck in this stage of change for lengthy periods of time ("chronic contemplators"). Contemplators substitute thinking for action, constantly struggling with weighing the costs and benefits of changing behavior. Indecision and lack of commitment are the most distinctive characteristics of the contemplation stage.

Individuals in the *preparation stage* of change intend to act on their problem in the immediate future, for example, within the next 30 days (see Table 3–4). This stage of change is characterized by small steps toward action, such as reducing the number of cigarettes smoked per day or quitting smoking for 24 hours. Preparation is also characterized by recent unsuccessful attempts at behavior change. It is this combination of intention to change with a behavioral pattern of recent attempts to change that distinguishes individuals in the preparation stage from those in contemplation. The preparation stage has now been well defined within the TTM (DiClemente, Prochaska, Fairhurst, et al., 1991). The validity of this stage

TABLE 3–4 Stages of Change for Three Risk Behaviors

Stage of Change	Smoking	Diet	Exercise
Precontemplation	Individual smokes and does not intend to quit in the next 6 months.	Individual does not consistently avoid eating high-fat foods and does not intend to in the next 6 months.	Individual does not exercise and does not intend to in the next 6 months.
Contemplation	Individual smokes but intends to quit in the next 6 months.	Individual does not consistently avoid eating high-fat foods but intends to in the next 6 months.	Individual does not exercise for 20 minutes three times a week but intends to in the next 6 months.
Preparation	Individual smokes but intends to quit in the next 30 days and has made at least one serious 24-hour quit.	Individual does not consistently avoid eating high-fat foods but intends to in the next 30 days.	Individual does not exercise for 20 minutes three times a week but intends to in the next 30 days.
Action	Individual has quit smoking for 6 months or less.	Individual has consistently avoided eating high-fat foods for 6 months or less and has a dietary fat intake of 30%* or less of total daily calories.	Individual has exercised for 20 minutes three times a week for 6 months or less.
Maintenance	Individual has quit smoking for more than 6 months.	Individual has consistently avoided eating high-fat foods for more than 6 months and has a dietary fat intake of 30%* or less of total daily calories.	Individual has exercised for 20 minutes three times a week for more than 6 months.

*Dietary target can be set at any level of fat intake desired (e.g., 30%, 25%, 20%).

has not yet been established across as wide a range of problem behaviors as the other stages of change.

The *action stage* is a period of active engagement in changing the problem behavior and is what most people, including clinicians, think of as behavior change (see Table 3–4). The period of action is usually described as lasting for 6 months, as this typically encompasses the period of greatest risk of relapse for many problem behaviors. To reach the action stage, individuals must meet strict criteria of behavior change, such as quitting smoking, achieving a specified degree of weight loss, reducing dietary fat to 30% or less of total daily calories, or exercising on a regular basis.

The action criterion depends on the problem behavior and should represent the established consensus of experts in the field. For example, the American College of Sports Medicine (1991) has recommended that healthy adults exercise at least three times a week for at least 20 minutes each time. Therefore, this criterion has been adopted as defining action for exercise (Marcus, Rossi, Selby, et al., 1992; Marcus, Selby, Niaura, et al., 1992). A significant problem for the field of weight control is the lack of a clear consensus for action (Rossi, 1995; Rossi, Rossi, Velicer, et al., 1995). Modification of the target behavior to an acceptable criterion and significant overt efforts to change are the most distinctive characteristics of the action stage.

After 6 months of continuous successful action, individuals achieve the *maintenance stage* (see Table 3–4). In this stage, people continue to work on preventing relapse and consolidating the gains made during the action stage. Situational temptations to engage in the problem behavior decline, and efficacy in coping with tempting situations increases. Maintenance is thus a continuation of the change process and not a static period. There is still a risk of relapse, and for some individuals and for some problem behaviors maintenance may be a lifelong struggle. For others, the temptation to engage in the problem behavior may decline eventually to such low levels that the problem may no longer be a salient issue for them. Such individuals may be considered to have reached the *termination stage* of change. For example, people who have been ex-smokers for 5, 10,

20, or more years often think of themselves as nonsmokers. Whether a termination stage for some problems, like weight control or diet, can be attained has not been established and would probably be a controversial subject. In general, stabilizing behavior change and avoiding relapse are the most distinctive characteristics of the maintenance stage.

The stages of change are temporally related. Individuals progress over time from precontemplation to contemplation, preparation, action, and finally to maintenance. The stages are assumed to be invariant, with individuals needing to complete the tasks and consolidate the gains of one stage before they are ready to progress to the next. The 6-month time frame that has been used to characterize most of the stages is somewhat arbitrary but has been well validated (Prochaska, DiClemente, & Norcross, 1992). Early research on the model in the area of smoking cessation examined other time periods, but these did not work as well. However, for some problem behaviors, other time periods might be more appropriate.

As with most behavior problems, the majority of individuals do not progress linearly through the stages for problem behaviors relevant to CHD risk prevention (e.g., smoking, high dietary fat intake, weight control, and inactivity). A cyclical pattern is more common; individuals reaching the action or maintenance stage relapse and then recycle to an earlier stage of change. Relapse is a common phenomenon, especially for addictions like smoking, and on any one attempt the likelihood of successful change is probably small. Fortunately, most relapsers do not regress all the way back to the precontemplation stage. Some of the gains made before the relapse episode are preserved, so that subsequent action attempts are more likely to be successful. From this standpoint, relapse is viewed not as failure but as an opportunity to learn from previous mistakes, to weed out unsuccessful change strategies, and try new ones.

Although relapse was once considered one of the stages in the model, it is now more appropriately viewed as an event that terminates further movement through action or maintenance, initiating the process of recycling. In the case of smoking cessation, individuals who relapse to the contemplation stage are better prepared to make subsequent action attempts than contemplators who have been unable to quit even for 24 hours and who remain in the contemplation stage (DiClemente, Prochaska, Fairhurst, et al., 1991).

These results serve as the basis for incorporating the occurrence of a recent relapse episode into the definition of the preparation stage of change. Unfortunately, some individuals get caught in a recycling loop without making progress toward successfully resolving their problem behavior. Such individuals may be perseverating on strategies that were successful in helping them make progress between earlier stages of change but may not be appropriate for making further progress. For example, seeking information about a problem behavior (consciousness raising) is a recommended strategy for individuals moving from precontemplation to contemplation, but it may become a technique for procrastination, thus delaying further progress, when employed by individuals in the preparation or action stages of change.

Processes of Change

Meta-analyses of models of how people change have identified a common set of processes underlying the modification of problem behaviors (Prochaska, DiClemente, & Norcross, 1992). These processes of change are overt and covert change strategies and techniques that can be employed by nurses and other health-care professionals, or by people changing on their own or with the aid of self-help programs. Ten to twelve processes have been consistently replicated across time, problem behaviors, sex, age, geographic region, and response formats (Prochaska, Velicer, DiClemente, et al., 1988; Prochaska, DiClemente, & Norcross, 1992; Rossi, 1992a). Brief descriptions of the processes of change are given in Table 3–5.

Structural analyses indicate that the processes are organized into two general second-order (hierarchical) constructs, reflecting the tendency of individuals to use more than one process of change at a time (Prochaska, Velicer, DiClemente, et al., 1988). This model has been replicated across nine different problem behaviors, including those relevant to CHD risk prevention (e.g., smoking cessation, exercise adop-

tion, dietary fat reduction, and weight control) (Rossi, 1992a). The two higher-order factors are the experiential and the behavioral processes of change. In general, the *experiential processes* may be characterized as incorporating the cognitive, evaluative, and affective aspects of change, whereas the *behavioral processes* include more specific, observable change strategies. But second-order factors are not independent. Across nine different problem behaviors, the correlation between the experiential and behavioral factors ranged from .51 to .91 (median $r = .77$), indicating a general tendency to use (or not use) all of the processes of change (Rossi, 1992a).

The processes of change and the stages of change are integrally related. Transitions between stages are mediated by the use of distinct subsets of change processes (DiClemente, Prochaska, Fairhurst, et al., 1991; Prochaska, DiClemente, & Norcross, 1992). For example, *consciousness raising* is an experiential process reflecting an individual's attempt to seek out information concerning the problem behavior. Employment of this process predicts successful movement from the precontemplation stage to the contemplation and preparation stages. The process of *self-reevaluation* is characteristic of the change from contemplation to action, whereas *stimulus control* is most frequently employed by individuals progressing from action to maintenance.

Process use by stage varies somewhat depending on the problem being changed. In general, use of the experiential processes of change tends to peak in the contemplation or preparation stages, whereas use of the behavioral processes tends to peak in the action or maintenance stages. Precontemplators use the processes least of all. When individuals (or treatment programs) mismatch processes to stages, action attempts are likely to fail.

These results suggest that stage-specific interventions may accelerate progress through the stages of change. Interventions relevant to primary CHD prevention that have been tailored to a participant's stage of change and have proved successful include smoking cessation and exercise adoption (Marcus, Banspach, Lefebvre, et al., 1992; Prochaska, DiClemente, Velicer, et al., 1993). Stage-matched interventions to reduce dietary fat consumption

TABLE 3–5 Processes of Change

Experiential Processes		Behavioral Processes	
Name	*Description*	*Name*	*Description*
Consciousness raising	Raising awareness about the problem (e.g., smoking, diet, exercise).	Counterconditioning	Substituting other thoughts or behaviors in place of the problem behaviors.
Dramatic relief	Motivation to change based on emotional experience related to the problem behavior.	Helping relationships	Accepting and using social support to change the problem behavior.
Environmental reevaluation	Reappraising the impact the problem behavior has on others.	Interpersonal systems control	Avoiding social cues from other people that trigger the unhealthy behavior.
Self-reevaluation	Reassessing thoughts, feelings, and knowledge about the problem behavior.	Reinforcement management	Rewards for changing behavior.
		Self-liberation	Recognizing choices, using will power, making a commitment to change behavior.
Social liberation	Awareness of changes in the environment that affect the problem behavior.	Stimulus control	Avoiding situations, places, or things that trigger the problem behavior.

have been and are currently being developed and tested. Consideration of the processes of change and their relationship to the stages of change is important from the standpoint of providing guidance for the development of successful intervention programs. Such programs should apply not only to individuals who are ready to change a problem behavior but also to the vast majority of people who are neither prepared nor motivated to change.

Decisional Balance

Part of the decision to move from one stage to the next is based on the relative weight given to the pros and cons of changing behavior such as stopping smoking, reducing dietary fat, and so on (Table 3–6). The pros represent positive aspects of changing behavior, including facilitators of change. The cons represent negative aspects of changing behavior and may be thought of as barriers to change.

The decision-making component of the TTM is based on a model first conceptualized by Janis and Mann (1977). These researchers assumed that sound decision making involves careful assessment of all relevant considerations, which are then evaluated in a decisional "balance sheet" of potential gains and losses. The anticipated gains (or benefits) and losses (or costs) can be categorized into eight major types of consequences: gains for self, losses for self, gains for significant others, losses for significant others, approval from significant others, disapproval from significant others, self-approval, and self-disapproval.

Gains and losses for self and others represent utilitarian considerations that go into making

the decision to change behavior, whereas approval and disapproval for self and others represent instrumental (nonutilitarian) considerations, such as self-esteem, social approval, internalized moral standards, and ego ideals. Thus, both individuals and normative reference groups are taken into account regarding instrumental objectives as well as value-based appraisals.

Although the Janis and Mann (1977) model proposes eight specific categories of decision making, only two general dimensions, the pros and cons of behavior change, have been supported consistently by factor analytic studies (Prochaska, Velicer, Rossi, et al., 1994). Within the context of the TTM, the pros and cons were first examined for the problem of smoking cessation (Velicer, DiClemente, Prochaska, et al., 1985). The existence of a specific functional relationship between decision making and an individual's stage of change was found. Subsequent longitudinal research verified the relationship between the stages of change and decisional balance and established the predictive validity of the construct (Prochaska, Velicer, Guadagnoli, et al., 1991; Prochaska, DiClemente, & Norcross, 1992; Prochaska, Velicer, Rossi, et al., 1994). These studies and others across a wide range of problem behaviors have found that the comparative weighing of the pros and cons varies depending on the individual's stage of change. In general, the pros of healthy behavior increase as a function of stage, whereas the cons decrease.

In the precontemplation stage, the cons of changing a problem behavior will be judged by individuals to outweigh the pros. In the action and maintenance stages, the pros outweigh the cons. The positive aspects of changing a prob-

TABLE 3–6 Decisional Balance

Decisional Balance	Smoking	Diet	Exercise
Pros	Benefits of smoking	Reasons to reduce dietary fat intake	Benefits of exercise
Cons	Costs of quitting	Reasons not to reduce dietary fat intake	Barriers to exercising

Note: For the problem of smoking, the pros refer to the benefits of continuing to smoke, and the cons refer to the barriers to quitting. For diet and exercise, the pros refer to the benefits of adopting the healthy behavior (e.g., reasons for cutting down the dietary fat, reasons to exercise regularly), and the cons refer to the barriers of adopting the healthy behavior change.

lem behavior begin to outweigh the negative aspects of change in the contemplation or preparation stage. That the pros and cons are evaluated approximately equally in the contemplation stage is not surprising. The resulting indecision and lack of commitment is largely responsible for so many individuals becoming stuck in the contemplation stage, substituting thinking for action while continually struggling with weighing the costs and benefits of changing behavior.

The pros and cons of behavior change serve primarily as intermediate outcome variables in the TTM. The shift in decisional balance tends to be especially striking across the early stages of change, especially the increase in the pros from precontemplation to contemplation. Thus, decisional balance tends to be an excellent indicator of an individual's decision to move out of the precontemplation stage.

The relationship between the stages of change and decisional balance has been shown to be remarkably consistent across a diverse set of problem behaviors, including many relevant to CHD prevention (Prochaska, Velicer, Rossi, et al., 1994). Especially noteworthy is the fact that not only is the form of the relationship replicated across problem behaviors, but so is the magnitude of the change in decisional balance across the stages of change. In progressing from precontemplation to action, the pros of change tend to increase by about one standard deviation, whereas the cons of change tend to decrease by about one half of a standard deviation. These results have led to the development of strong and weak principles of behavior change (Prochaska, Velicer, Rossi, et al., 1994).

Self-Efficacy

As with decisional balance, self-efficacy serves primarily as an intermediate outcome variable in the TTM. This component of the model was originally based on the cognitive-social learning theory proposed by Bandura (1977) but has since been elaborated on considerably. Within the context of addictive behaviors like smoking, efficacy has typically been conceptualized psychometrically as unidimensional (DiClemente, 1986). Yet, clinicians who have focused on the situational determinants of relapse have ac-

knowledged the multidimensional nature of the construct (Brownell, Marlatt, Lichtenstein, et al., 1986). The discrepancy between these alternative views was resolved through the use of hierarchical structural modeling. The existence of a single general higher-order construct consisting of several primary, situationally determined factors was demonstrated (Velicer, DiClemente, Rossi, et al., 1990). For smoking cessation, three first-order dimensions were found: positive/social, negative/affective, and habit/addictive. Similar hierarchical models have been found for other problems relevant to CHD prevention such as weight control and dietary fat reduction (Clark, Abrams, Niaura, et al., 1991; Rossi 1993; Rossi, Rossi, Prochaska, et al., 1992; Rossi, Rossi, Velicer et al., 1995). In general, the number of primary efficacy dimensions is expected to be determined by the nature of the problem area, insofar as the situational determinants and temptations for relapse are likely to be problem-specific (Table 3–7).

The hierarchical nature of the model suggests that self-efficacy may be conceptualized either as a single global concept or in terms of separate types of situations. A global self-efficacy score may be useful as a general screening implement—for example, as an aid in determining an individual's readiness to change behavior. In the area of smoking cessation, dramatic differences in efficacy have been demonstrated according to an individual's stage of change, essentially increasing in linear fashion from the precontemplation stage to the maintenance stage (DiClemente, Prochaska, Fairhurst, et al., 1991; Prochaska, Velicer, Guadagnoli, et al., 1991). Once individuals are involved in an intervention program, the separate-scale scores might be used to monitor the effectiveness of the intervention and to help point out potentially troublesome situations that need to be targeted specifically in an effort to prevent relapse. Self-efficacy has been effectively utilized in this way in a computer-based expert system used for interventions aimed at smoking cessation (Velicer, Rossi, Ruggiero, et al., 1995).

Operationalization of the self-efficacy construct within the TTM has typically taken the form of asking respondents how *confident* they are that they would not engage in a problem behavior across a range of problem situations.

TABLE 3–7 Self-Efficacy and Temptation

Problem	Situations		
Smoking	Positive social situations	Negative affective situations	Habit-craving
Diet	Positive social situations	Negative affective situations	Difficult situations
Exercise	All situations	All situations	All situations

Note: A single overall self-efficacy scale covering general confidence in all situations is used for exercise. Smoking and diet use this total-score approach for measuring self-efficacy and temptation as well. However, for diet and exercise, subscale scores for three specific types of situations are also measured.

A companion construct, *temptation,* measured using a parallel instrument, asks respondents how tempted they would be to engage in a problem behavior across the same problem situations. As with self-efficacy, there is a strong relationship between temptation and stage of change, with an essentially linear decrease from precontemplation to maintenance (DiClemente, Prochaska, Fairhurst, et al., 1991; Prochaska, Velicer, Guadagnoli, et al., 1991).

Although the two measures are correlated, they are not completely overlapping (Velicer, DiClemente, Rossi, et al., 1990). For smoking cessation, confidence scores peak after about 18 months of prolonged abstinence (Rossi Redding, Snow, et al., 1989). Temptation scores, on the other hand, continue to decrease for up to 3 to 5 years after cessation. These results suggest that temptation may be a more sensitive measure of relapse potential than confidence and that even individuals who have been in the maintenance stage for several years are not completely free of risk.

CONCLUSION

Prevention of CHD risk involves modifying multiple behaviors that can be influenced by intentional changes in lifestyle. These may include modification of smoking; reduction of dietary cholesterol, fat, or sodium intake; exercise adoption; weight control; stress reduction; and adherence to medication or medical regimens to control problems like blood pressure or diabetes. Four models of health behavior applicable to CHD risk reduction were discussed in this chapter, including the health belief model, social learning theory, the theory of reasoned action, and the transtheoretical model of behavior change. Two concepts, self-efficacy and so-

cial support, were also examined. However, these behavioral prediction models do not identify who changes, when change is likely to occur, or, more importantly, *how* change occurs.

National heart disease and CHD mortality statistics suggest that interventions designed to prevent CHD risk have not been as successful as expected, partly because interventions are not appropriately targeted to an individual's motivational readiness to change risk behaviors. Since changing an individual's behavior is tantamount to preventing or reducing CHD risk, use of a behavioral change model such as the transtheoretical model of behavior change (TTM) is more appropriate for understanding, explaining, and impacting this problem.

This section of the book has provided the reader with a clear overview of existing theoretical and research-based perspectives pertinent to CHD risk reduction. In the next section, concrete information regarding patient assessment and intervention for major CHD risk factors will be discussed. The goal of this section is to provide the reader with a strong, comprehensive overview of the research supporting identification of risk factors and evaluating the effectiveness of pertinent CHD risk-reduction interventions. Depth of knowledge is essential given the ever changing state of our understanding of CHD risk factors and risk reduction. In addition, for effective collaboration and appropriate decision making, all clinicians, including nurses, must be able to address CHD risk reduction using a common knowledge base regarding research and theory.

References

Ajzen, I., & Fishbein, M. (1980). *Understanding Attitudes and Predicting Social Behavior.* Englewood Cliffs, NJ: Prentice-Hall.

American College of Sports Medicine, (1991). *Guidelines*

for Exercise Testing and Prescription, 4th ed. Philadelphia: Lea & Febiger.

Bandura, A. (1977). Self-efficacy: Toward a unifying theory of behavior change. *Psychological Review, 84,* 191–215.

Bandura, A. (1986). *Social Foundations of Thought and Action: A Social Cognitive Theory.* Englewood Cliffs, NJ: Prentice-Hall.

Baranowski, T. (1992). Beliefs as motivational influences at stages in behavior change. *International Quarterly of Community Health Education, 13,* 3–29.

Becker, M.H. (1974). The health belief model and personal health behavior. *Health Education Monographs, 2,* 324–473.

Becker, M.H., Maiman, L.A. (1975). Sociobehavioral determinants of compliance with health and medical care recommendations. *Medical Care, 13,* 10–24.

Berkman, L.F., & Syme, S.L. (1979). Social networks, host resistance, and mortality: A nine-year follow-up study of Alameda County residents. *American Journal of Epidemiology, 109,* 186–204.

Bernier, M., & Avard, J. (1986). Self-efficacy, outcome, and attrition in a weight-reduction program. *Cognitive Therapy and Research, 10,* 319–338.

Brandt, P., & Weinert, C. (1981). The PRQ: A social support measure. *Nursing Research, 30,* 277–280.

Brownell, K.D., Marlatt, G.A., Lichtenstein, E., & Wilson, G.T. (1986). Understanding and preventing relapse. *American Psychologist, 41,* 765–782.

Caplan, G., & Killilea, M. (1976). *Support Systems and Mutual Help: Multidisciplinary Explorations.* New York: Grune & Stratton, Inc.

Cassel, J. (1974). An epidemiological perspective of psychosocial factors in disease etiology. *American Journal of Public Health, 64,* 1040–1043.

Cassel, J. (1976). The contribution of the social environment to host resistance. *American Journal of Epidemiology, 102,* 107–123.

Clark, M.M., Abrams, D.B., Niaura, R.S., Eaton, C.A., & Rossi, J.S. (1991). Self-efficacy in weight management. *Journal of Consulting and Clinical Psychology, 59,* 739–744.

Cobb, S. (1976). Social support as moderator of life stress. *Psychosomatic Medicine, 38,* 300–314.

Condiotte, M.M., & Lichtenstein, E. (1981). Self-efficacy and relapse in smoking cessation programs. *Journal of Consulting and Clinical Psychology, 49,* 648–658.

Cronenwett, L.R. (1985). Network structure, social support, and psychological outcomes of pregnancy. *Nursing Research, 34,* 93–99.

DiClemente, C.C. (1986). Self-efficacy and the addictive behaviors. *Journal of Social and Clinical Psychology, 4,* 302–315.

DiClemente, C.C., Prochaska, J.O., Fairhurst, S.K., Velicer, W.F., Velasquez, M.M., & Rossi, J.S. (1991). The process of smoking cessation: An analysis of precontemplation, contemplation and preparation stages of change. *Journal of Consulting and Clinical Psychology, 59,* 295–304.

Emmons, K.M., Marcus, B.H., Linnan, L., Rossi, J.S., & Abrams, D.B. (1994). Mechanisms in multiple risk factor interventions: Smoking, physical activity, and dietary fat intake among manufacturing workers. *Preventive Medicine, 23,* 481–489.

Fazio, R.H., & Zanna, M.P. (1981). Direct experience and attitude-behavior consistency. *Advances in Experimental Social Psychology, 14,* 161–202.

Fishbein, M., & Ajzen, I. (1975). Belief, attitude, intention, and behavior. In *An Introduction to Theory and Research.* Reading, MA: Addison-Wesley.

Fishbein, M., Bandura, A., Triandis, H.C., Kanfer, F.H., Becker, M.H., & Middlestadt, S.E. (1991). *Factors Influencing Behavior and Behavior Change.* Final Report of the Theorist's Workshop, Washington, DC.

Gore, S. (1978). The effect of social support in moderating the health consequences of unemployment. *Journal of Health and Social Behavior, 19,* 157–165.

Gottlieb, B.H. (1983). *Social Support Strategies: Guidelines for Mental Health Practice.* Beverly Hills, CA.: Sage Publications, Inc.

Greene, G.W., Rossi, S.R., Reed, G.R., Willey, C., & Prochaska, J.O. (1994). Stages of change for reducing dietary fat to 30% of energy or less. *Journal of the American Dietetic Association, 94,* 1105–1110.

House, J.S. (1981). *Work Stress and Social Support.* Reading, MA.: Addison-Wesley Publishing.

House, J.S., & Kahn, R.L. (1985). Measures and concepts of social support. In S. Cohen & S.L. Syme (Eds.), *Social Support and Health* (pp. 83–108). New York: Academic Press.

Janis, I.L., & Mann, L. (1977). *Decision Making: A Psychological Analysis of Conflict Choice, and Commitment.* New York: The Free Press.

Janz, N.K., & Becker, M.H. (1984). The health belief model: A decade later. *Health Education Quarterly, 11,* 1–47.

Kahn, R.L., & Antonucci, T.C. (1980). Conveys over the life course: Attachment, roles, and social support. In P.B. Brim (Eds.), *Lifespan Development and Behavior,* vol. 3 (pp. 253–286). New York: Academic Press.

Kaplan, B. Cassel, I., & Gore, S. (1977). Social support and health. *Medical Care, 15* (Suppl. 51), 47–58.

Kirscht, J.P. (1974). The health belief model and illness behavior. *Health Education Quarterly, 11,* 1–47.

Liska, A.E. (1984). A critical examination of the causal structure of the Fishbein/Ajzen attitude-behavior model. *Social Psychology Quarterly, 47,* 61–74.

Marcus, B.H., Banspach, S.W., Lefebvre, R.C., Rossi, J.S., Carleton, R.A., Abrams, D.B. (1992). Using the stages of change model to increase adoption of physical activity among community participants. *American Journal of Health Promotion, 6,* 424–429.

Marcus, B.H., Rossi, J.S., Selby, V.C., Niaura, R.S., & Abrams, D.B. (1992). The stages and processes of exercise adoption and maintenance in a worksite sample. *Health Psychology, 11,* 386–395.

Marcus, B.H., Selby, V.C., Niaura, R.S., & Rossi, J.S. (1992). Self-efficacy and the stages of exercise behavior change. *Research Quarterly for Exercise and Sport, 63,* 60–66.

Marmot, M.G., & Syme, S.L. (1976). Acculturation and coronary heart disease in Japanese-Americans. *American Journal of Epidemiology, 104,* 225–247.

MMWR (1993). Public health focus: Physical activity and the prevention of coronary heart disease. *Morbidity and Mortality Weekly Report: CDC Surveillance Summary, 42* (35), 669–672.

Norbeck, J.S. (1981). Social support: A model for clinical research and application. *Advances in Nursing Science, 3,* 43–59.

Ockene, I.S., & Ockene, J.K. (1992). Helping patients to reduce their risk of coronary hart disease: An overview. In I.S. Ockene and J.K. Ockene (Eds.), *Prevention of Coronary Heart Disease.* Boston, MA.: Little, Brown and Company.

Perry, C., Baranowski, T., & Parcel, G. (1990). How individuals, environments, and health interact: Social Learning Theory. In K. Glanz, F.M. Lewis, & B.K. Rimer (Eds.), *Health Behavior and Health Education, Theory,*

Research and Practice (pp. 161–186). San Francisco: Jossey-Bass.

Prochaska, J.O. (1992). A transtheoretical model of behavior change: Implications for diet interventions. In M. M. Henderson, D.J. Bowen, and K.K. DeRoss, (Eds.), *Proceedings of the Conference on Promoting Dietary Change in Communities Applying Existing Models of Dietary Change to Population-Based Interventions* (pp. 37–49). Seattle, WA: Fred Hutchinson Cancer Center.

Prochaska, J.O. (1994). Strong and weak principles for progressing from precontemplation to action based on twelve problem behaviors. *Health Psychology, 13,* 47–51.

Prochaska, J.O., DiClemente, C.C., & Norcross, J.C. (1992). In search of how people change: Applications to addictive behaviors. *American Psychologist, 47,* 1102–1114.

Prochaska, J.O., DiClemente, C.C., Velicer, W.F., & Rossi, J.S. (1993). Standardized, individualized, interactive and personalized self-help programs for smoking cessation. *Health Psychology, 12,* 399–405.

Prochaska, J.O., Velicer, W.F., DiClemente, C.C., & Fava, J. (1988). Measuring processes of change: Applications to the cessation of smoking. *Journal of Consulting and Clinical Psychology, 56,* 520–528.

Prochaska, J.O., Velicer, W.F., Guadagnoli, E., Rossi, J.S., & DiClemente, C.C. (1991). Patterns of change: Dynamic typology applied to smoking cessation. *Multivariate Behavioral Research, 26,* 83–107.

Prochaska, J.O., Velicer, W.F., Rossi, J.S., Goldstein, M.G., Marcus, B.H., Rakowski, W., Fiore, C., Harlow, L.L., Redding, C.A., Rosenbloom, D., & Rossi, S.R. (1994). Stages of change and decisional balance for 12 problem behaviors. *Health Psychology, 13,* 1–8.

Public Health Service. (1991). *Healthy People 2000: National objectives: Full report, with commentary.* Washington, DC: U.S. Department of Health and Human Services, Publication PHS 91-50212.

Riegel, B. (1989). Social support and psychological adjustment to chronic coronary heart disease: Operationalization in Johnson's behavioral system model. *Advances in Nursing Science, 11,* 74–84.

Rosenstock, I.M. (1990). The health belief model: Explaining health behavior through expectancies. In K. Glanz, F.M. Lewis, B.K. Rimer (Eds.), *Health behavior and health education: Theory, research, and practice.* San Francisco: Jossey-Bass, 39–62.

Rosenstock, I.M. (1974). The health belief model and preventative health behavior. *Health Education Monographs, 2,* 354–386.

Rossi, J.S. (1992a). Common processes of change across nine problem behaviors. Paper presented at the 100th annual convention of the American Psychological Association, Washington, DC (August).

Rossi, J.S. (1992b). Stages of change for 15 health risk behaviors in an HMO population. Paper presented at the 13th annual meeting of the Society of Behavioral Medicine, New York, NY (March).

Rossi, J.S. (1995). Why do people fail to maintain weight loss? In D.B. Allison & F.X.Pi-Sunyer (Eds.), *Obesity Treatment: Establishing Goals, Improving Outcomes, and Reassessing the Research Agenda* (pp. 97–102). New York: Plenum Press.

Rossi, J.S., Redding, C.A., Snow, M.G., Fava, J., Rossi, S.R., Velicer, W.F., Prochaska, J.O., & DiClemente, C.C.

(1989). Smoking habit strength during maintenance: A termination stage for smoking cessation? Paper presented at the 97th annual convention of the American Psychological Association, New Orleans, LA (August).

Rossi, J.S., Rossi, S.R., Velicer, W.F., & Prochaska, J.O. (1995). Motivational readiness to control weight. In D.B. Allison (Ed.), *Methods for the Assessment of Eating Behaviors and Weight-Related Problems* (pp. 387–430). Newbury Park, CA: Sage.

Rossi, S.R. (1993). Application of the transtheoretical model to dietary fat reduction in a naturalistic environment (doctoral dissertation, University of Rhode Island, 1993). *Dissertation Abstracts International,* DA9421916.

Rossi, S.R., Rossi, J.S., Prochaska, J.O., & Velicer, W.F. (1992). Application of the transtheoretical model of behavior change to dietary fat reduction. *International Journal of Psychology, 27,* 628.

Sallis, J.F., Haskell, W.L., Wood, P.D., Fortmann, S.P., Vranizan, K.M., Taylor, C.B., & Solomon, D.S. (1986). Predictors of adoption and maintenance of physical activity in a community sample. *Preventative Medicine, 15,* 331–341.

Sallis, J.F., Pinski, R.B., Patterson, T.L. & Nader, P.R. (1988). The development of self-efficacy scales for health-related diet and exercise behaviors. *Health Education Research, 3,* 283–292.

Sherman, S.J., Presson, C.C., Chassin, L., Bensenberg, M., Corty, E., & Olshavsky, R.W. (1982). Smoking intentions in adolescents: Direct experience and predictability. *Personality and Social Psychology Bulletin, 8,* 376–383.

Sinacore-Guinn, A.L. (1993). The measurement and construct validity of the theory of systemic-subjective control (doctoral dissertation, Columbia University, 1993). *Dissertation Abstracts International,* AAC 9318281.

Sonstroem, R.J. (1988). Psychological models. In R.K. Dishman (Ed.), *Exercise adherence: Its impact on public health* (pp. 125–153). Champaign, IL: Human Kinetics Books.

Tilden, V.P., & Weinert, C. (1987). Social support and the chronically ill individual. *Nursing Clinics of North America, 22,* 613–620.

Turk, D.C., & Kerns, R.D. (1985). Assessment in health psychology: A cognitive behavioral perspective. In P. Karoly (Ed.), *Measurement Strategies in Health Psychology* (pp. 335–372). New York: John Wiley & Sons.

Velicer, W.F., DiClemente, C.C., Prochaska, J.O., & Brandenburg, N. (1985). Decisional balance measure for assessing and predicting smoking status. *Journal of Personality and Social Psychology, 48,* 1279–1289.

Velicer, W.F., DiClemente, C.C., Rossi, J.S., & Prochaska, J.O. (1990). Relapse situations and self-efficacy: An integrated model. *Addictive Behaviors, 15,* 271–283.

Velicer, W.F., Rossi, J.S., Ruggiero, L., & Prochaska, J.O. (1995). Minimal interventions appropriate for an entire population of smokers. In R. Richmond (Ed.), *Interventions for Smokers: An International Perspective* (pp. 69–92). Baltimore: Williams & Wilkins.

Weinstein, N.D. (1993). Testing four theories of health-protective behavior. *Health Psychology, 12* (4), 324–333.

Weiss, R.S., (1973). Transition states and other stressful situations. Their nature and programs for their management. In G. Caplan and M. Killihea (Eds.), *Support Systems and Mutual Help.* New York: Grune & Stratton.

CHAPTER 4

——
——
——
——
——
——
——
——
——
——
——
——
——

Nursing Assessment

Donna Williams

An estimated 6.2 million Americans have significant coronary heart disease (CHD), resulting in 550,000 deaths per year (American Heart Association, 1993). An additional 12 million Americans have undiagnosed cardiovascular disease (Expert Survey Cardiology II, 1992). The cost of cardiovascular disease in the United States—including CHD, stroke, and hypertension—is estimated to be $151.3 billion per year (American Heart Association, 1995). Nurses, as the largest health-care providers in the United States, have an opportunity to identify individuals, families, or populations that have CHD or the potential for its development.

This chapter introduces the reader to the research and theoretical basis of CHD risk-factor identification and assessment. Subsequent chapters provide more detailed information regarding pertinent clinical trials and other intervention research. This chapter focuses primarily on the assessment of the individual at risk whom the nurse may see in primary care, acute care, or an occupational setting.

Issues related to characterization of risk associated with specific factors, as well as cumulative or combined risk, will be addressed. The principles of assessment for the potential or presence of CHD remain the same across care settings (Rossi & Leary, 1992). This chapter specifically addresses assessment of CHD risk within the context of acute illness and the interplay between assessment of long-term CHD risk and short-term potential for ischemia or infarction. Although assessment is addressed within the paradigm of nursing, the material contained in this chapter is relevant for any clinician involved in CHD risk assessment.

GOALS OF ASSESSMENT

Individuals at risk for the development of CHD can be identified for purposes of preventive management long in advance of symptoms (Kannel, 1990; McCance, 1983). The goals of assessment are to identify those at risk for the development of disease, detect current conditions, reduce morbidity and mortality, and provide a framework for intervention and prevention. Figure 4–1 depicts the way in which the manifestation of CHD risk factors varies with the extent of disease progression.

In *primary prevention*, interventions are designed to lessen or eliminate cardiac risk factors to prevent development of CHD. Reduction of risk factors in youth can have the greatest impact; interventions in adulthood may slow or

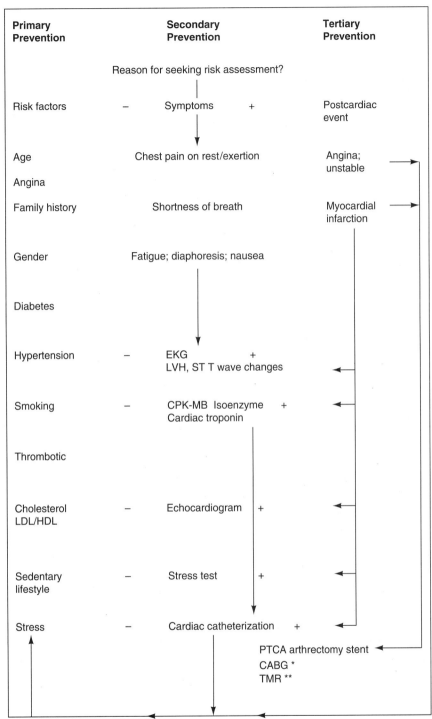

Primary Prevention	Secondary Prevention	Tertiary Prevention

Reason for seeking risk assessment?

Risk factors   −   Symptoms   +   Postcardiac event

Age   Chest pain on rest/exertion   Angina; unstable

Angina

Family history   Shortness of breath   Myocardial infarction

Gender   Fatigue; diaphoresis; nausea

Diabetes

Hypertension   −   EKG   +
                     LVH, ST T wave changes

Smoking   −   CPK-MB Isoenzyme   +
                 Cardiac troponin

Thrombotic

Cholesterol   −   Echocardiogram   +
LDL/HDL

Sedentary   −   Stress test   +
lifestyle

Stress   −   Cardiac catheterization   +

PTCA arthrectomy stent
CABG *
TMR **

* Asymptomatic men over 40 with specific occupations or with two or more risk factors.

** Transmyocardial revascularization with laser currently an experimental procedure; therapy available only in clinical trial sites.

FIGURE 4–1 CHD individual risk assessment.

reverse progression of disease and reduce morbidity and mortality (Cummins, 1994).

In *secondary prevention* the goal is to identify early disease development and halt progression, avoiding complications and cardiovascular events. In *tertiary prevention*, interventions are aimed at reducing dysfunction, minimizing disability, and postponing death. Individuals with known disease are at highest risk for morbidity and mortality (Pearson & Fuster, 1996). Individuals post unstable angina or myocardial infarction are susceptible to rethrombosis of a disrupted atherosclerotic plaque after discharge. Coronary artery bypass graft patients and those who have undergone angioplasty, arthrectomy, or stent placement may experience reocclusion, thrombosis, or restenosis from 1 month to 1 year after the procedure (Califf, Armstrong, Carver, et al., 1996). Despite the increased risk, many individuals treated in the United States for myocardial infarction with percutaneous transluminal coronary angioplasty or coronary artery bypass surgery have cholesterol abnormalities as a result of a high-fat diet, and 50% smoke (Martin, Hulley, Browner, et al., 1986; Cavender, Rogers, Fischer, et al., 1992). The proportion of patients with CHD receiving risk-factor interventions is low (Pearson & Fuster, 1996) even though risk-factor modification is most cost-effective and efficient for individuals with known CHD (Swan, Gersh, Graboys, et al., 1996).

Nurses play a key role in assessing the risk factors that lead to disease expression and in intervening to help individuals modify risk behaviors. Nurse case-managed systems post discharge have been successful in altering risk factors and in supporting sustained behavioral change in a cost-effective manner (DeBusk, Miller, Superko, et al., 1994; Pearson, McBride, Houston, et al., 1996).

Cardiac rehabilitation programs, which are frequently nurse-managed, also attest to the successful and pivotal role of nurses in CHD risk reduction. Patient participation in cardiac rehabilitation is associated with decreased readmission rates, diminished need for cardiac medications, and higher return-to-work rates (Ades, Huang, & Weaver, 1992; Levin, Perk, & Hedlack, 1991). Cardiac rehabilitation programs have also been reported to reduce risk factors, improve functional abilities (Lavie, Milani, &

Littman, 1993), retard the progression of disease (Oldridge, Guyatt, Fischer, et al., 1998). Finally, economic data support cardiac rehabilitation as an efficient use of health-care resources (Pashkow, 1993).

IDENTIFYING RISK FACTORS FOR DEVELOPMENT OF CHD

Epidemiologic observational studies and efficacy clinical trials link specific risk factors with subsequent CHD (Kannel, 1990). An attempt is made to predict the development of disease by evaluating the presence and intensity of risk factors (Millar, 1992). The development of CHD involves multiple modifiable and nonmodifiable factors, each of which must be considered in formulating a cardiac risk profile (Kannel, McGee, & Gordon, 1976; Kannel, 1987).

Major nonmodifiable cardiac risk factors include age, male gender, family history of CHD, and low socioeconomic status. Modifiable risk factors include diabetes, hypertension, hypercholesteremia, obesity, physical inactivity, cigarette smoking, and stress. Postmenopausal risk may be modified by hormone replacement therapy. Elevated serum levels of homocysteine, a circulating amino acid, are now recognized as an independent risk factor for premature atherosclerosis, one that can be modified (Futterman & Lemberg, 1997). Thrombogenic factors, including elevated fibrinogen levels, may be an independent predictor of future CHD (Ernst & Resch, 1993).

As indicated in Table 4–1, CHD risk factors may be grouped into four categories according to their ability to be modified and their responsiveness to interventions (Pearson & Fuster, 1996). The categorization scheme also addresses the clinical usefulness of measuring, or quantifying, the risk factor. Category I includes risk factors for which interventions have been proved to lower the incidence of CHD. Category II includes risk factors for which interventions will likely lower the incidence of CHD. Category III includes risk factors that if modified might lower the incidence of CHD. Category IV includes nonmodifiable risk factors associated with CHD. Specific risk factors, the underlying basis for their designation as risk factors,

TABLE 4–1 Cardiovascular Risk Factors Categories

| Risk Factors | Evidence for Association with CHD | | Clinical Measurement |
	Epidemiologic	Clinical Trials	Usefulness
Category I Risk factors for which interventions have been proved to lower CDH risk			
Cigarette smoking	+ + +	+ +	+ + +
Elevated LDL cholesterol	+ + +	+ + +	+ + +
High-fat/cholesterol diet	+ + +	+ +	+ +
Hypertension	+ + +	+ + +	+ + +
Left ventricular hypertrophy	+ + +	+	+ +
Thrombogenic factors (fibrinogen)	+ + +	+ + +	+
Category II Risk factors for which interventions are likely to lower CHD risk			
Diabetes mellitus	+ + +	+	+ + +
Physical inactivity	+ + +	+ +	+ +
Low HDL cholesterol	+ + +	+	+ + +
Elevated triglycerides	+ +	+ +	+ + +
Obesity	+ + +	−	+ + +
Postmenopausal status	+ + +	−	+ + +
Category III Risk factors associated with increased CHD risk that if modified might lower risk			
Psychosocial factors	+ +	+	+ + +
Lipoprotein (a)	+	−	+
Elevated homocysteine	+ +	−	+ + +
Oxidative stress	+	−	−
No alcohol intake	+ + +	−	+ +
Category IV Risk factors associated with increased CHD risk that cannot be modified			
Age	+ + +	−	+ + +
Male gender	+ + +	−	+ + +
Low socioeconomic status	+ + +	−	+ + +
Family history of CHD	+ + +	−	+ + +

CHD = coronary heart disease.
LDL = low-density lipoprotein.
HDL = high-density lipoprotein.
+ = weak, somewhat consistent evidence.
+ + = moderately strong, rather consistent evidence.
+ + + = very strong, consistent evidence.
− = evidence poor or not existent.
Adapted from Pearson, T., & Fuster, V. (1996). Twenty-Seventh Bethesda Conference—Matching the intensity of risk factor management with the hazard for coronary events. *Journal of the American College of Cardiology, 27*(5), 957–1047. Used with permission from the American College of Cardiology.

and specific assessment issues will now be addressed

Age

Advancing age is correlated with greater risk for coronary heart disease in men and women (Hopkins & Williams, 1986). In the United States, the fastest growing segment of the population is the elderly (Gerber, 1990). Symptoms of CHD may increase in severity with advancing age while interventions become more limited because of concern for side effects (Weaver, Litwin, Martin, et al., 1991). But 85% of all heart disease deaths in the elderly are due to coronary heart disease (Wei & Gersh, 1987). Therefore, although age is not modifiable, it must be factored into the assessment of an individual's overall risk for CHD.

Gender

In the general population, men are considered to be at higher risk for cardiovascular disease than women. Yet the incidence of myocardial infarctions in men and women overall is similar. In addition, myocardial infarction is the leading cause of death in women over the age of 40 (American Heart Association, 1990). Women under the age of 65 develop CHD 10 years later than men do, but their incidence surpasses that of men after the age of 75 (Murdaugh, 1990). Framingham Heart Study data indicate that a higher proportion of unrecognized myocardial infarction occurs in women (Kannel & Abbott, 1984). Moreover, women experience a higher mortality from myocardial infarction than men (Tofler, Stone, Muller, et al., 1987). The mortality rates are highest for black women in the United States, with black women dying at an earlier age (Gillum & Grant, 1982; Kasl, 1984; Haywood, 1984; Murdaugh & O'Rourke, 1988).

Several gender-specific issues are associated with CHD risk. First, a decreased exposure to endogenous estrogen resulting from late menarche, multiparity, or early menopause may be linked to elevated risk of CHD (Valle & Lemberg, 1994; Conti, 1993). Second, menopause is known to increase CHD risk threefold (Kannel, 1990). The increased incidence in postmenopausal women remains unexplained; however, it is known that estrogen loss adversely affects lipid metabolism. Menopause without hormone therapy causes LDL levels to increase and HDL levels to decline (Matthews, Meilahn, Kuller, et al., 1989). In contrast, women who receive oral estrogen and progestin therapy have no increase in risk (Stampfer & Colditz, 1991; PEPI, 1995). Third, oral contraceptives have been associated with increased incidence of myocardial infarction through the promotion of thrombosis (Psaty, Heckbert, Atkins, et al., 1993). The factors of older age, cigarette smoking, and hypertension multiply this risk (Stadel,

1981; Dalen & Hickler, 1981; Stampfer, Willett, Colditz, et al., 1988).

Given these gender differences, the clinician should evaluate a woman's reproductive history with respect to exposure to estrogen. Assessment should focus on age of menarche, parity, onset of menopause and perimenopausal symptoms, and history of exogenous estrogen use, whether through contraceptives or hormone replacement therapy.

Family History

A family history of myocardial infarction is an independent risk factor for CHD. A parental family history of CHD increases risk for development of subsequent disease one and a half to two times over those individuals without a family history. Women may have a higher risk if their mother had CHD; men may be more affected by the paternal history of CHD (Roncaglioni, Santoro, D'Avanzo, et al., 1992; Goldberg, 1992; Scholtz, Rosenman, & Brand, 1975; Barrett-Connor & Khaw, 1984; Colditz, Stampfer, Willett, et al., 1986).

Historically, the Framingham study of siblings, along with twin studies, have supported the role of genetic factors in CHD onset and manifestations (Snowden, McNamara, Garrison, et al., 1982; Kannel, Feinlieb, McNamara, et al., 1979; Feinlieb, Garrison, Fabsitz, et al., 1977). Trends suggest that for both men and women, risk is highest when other siblings have CHD—indeed, three to four times the risk of the individual without a sibling family history (Roncaglioni, Santoro, D'Avanzo, et al., 1992). However, the interplay between genetic influence and other risk factors is not fully understood. Inherited, or genetically based, hyperlipidemias undoubtedly play a role. Elevated serum cholesterol may be familial, with correlations demonstrated among siblings, parents, and offspring (McCance, 1983). Familial hypercholesterolemia, hyperlipidemia, and hypertriglyceridemia may occur in individuals and require more than dietary modification to reduce risk of premature CHD (Chait, Brunzell, Denke, et al., 1993). The majority of individuals with elevated cholesterol may have some genetic tendency that has been affected by a high-fat diet and/or obesity (Nicolosi & Schaefer, 1992). A family history of premature CHD can help the clinician identify an individual at risk, but, as discussed in detail in Chapter 1, disease initiation may require the presence of other CHD risk factors (Kannel, 1990).

A family history should include all first-degree relatives (parents, siblings, children) and second-degree relatives (grandparents, aunts, uncles). In both men and women, relative risk rises as the number of relatives with disease increases. A history of myocardial infarction in two or more first-degree relatives triples the risk for CHD. Risk increases if myocardial infarction occurred at an earlier age, less than 55 years (Roncaglioni, Santoro, D'Avanzo, et al., 1992; McCance, 1983). Therefore, the clinician should note the ages of occurrence of cardiac events in all male and female first-degree relatives. Genograms or familial charts may be used to summarize these relationships.

Diabetes

Multiple studies have demonstrated that the presence of diabetes, defined as a fasting plasma glucose greater than 126 mg/dl, greatly increases the risk of cardiovascular disease (Report of the Expert Committee on the Diagnosis and Classification of Diabetes, 1997). Risk in men doubles and in women increases five to seven times (American Heart Association, 1993; Kannel & McGee, 1979; Heyden, Heiss, Bartel, et al., 1980). In the absence of identifiable diabetes, impaired glucose tolerance, defined as a 2-hour plasma blood glucose of 200 ml/dl (Davidoff, 1997; NDDG, 1979; World Health Organization, 1980), may also increase cardiovascular risk (Orchard, 1992).

As discussed in Chapter 11, the underlying basis of the increased CHD risk is complicated. Diabetics are more likely to have multiple cardiovascular risk factors, including hypercholesteremia, obesity, and hypertension (Sivarajan Froelicher, Berra, Stepp, et al., 1995; Wingard, Barrett-Connor, Criqui, et al., 1983). Diabetes associated with high cholesterol levels increases the risk for CHD development (Chait, Brunzell, Denke, et al., 1993). Diabetes mellitus and obesity have a greater impact on women's risk for CHD than on men's (Goldberg, 1992). In secondary and tertiary prevention, the presence of diabetes increases the risk of death after myocardial infarction and coronary artery bypass graft surgery (Pasternak, Grundy, Levy, et al., 1996).

In 80–90% of cases, diabetes is Type 2, adult-onset, non-insulin-dependent diabetes mellitus (NIDDM) (Keller, Fleury, & Bergstom, 1995). Risk factors for development of NIDDM include family history of diabetes, obesity, age over 40, and a history of gestational diabetes (Ratner, 1992). Individuals often perceive NIDDM as a less serious form of diabetes and minimize its importance in terms of contributing to cardiovascular risk. Symptoms of diabetes may include polydipsia, polyuria, polyphagia, and weight loss.

Other vascular diseases, such as peripheral vascular disease and carotid artery disease, may also be present in the diabetic individual with CHD. Peripheral vascular disease occurs in up to 15% of the population over age 50 and is strongly associated with CHD and the risk factors of smoking and diabetes (Criqui, Froneck, Barrett-Connor, et al., 1985).

Assessment of the diabetic patient for CHD risk focuses upon the degree of diabetic control. Diabetic control and impaired glucose tolerance can be evaluated using glycohemoglobin concentration as a marker of glucose control in the prior 6–8 weeks (Pasternak, Grundy, Levy, et al., 1996).

Blood Pressure

In the United States, systemic hypertension affects 40% of the population and is broadly defined as a blood pressure higher than 140/90 mm Hg (Uber & Uber, 1993). In addition, *cardiovascular reactivity*, displayed by an abrupt increase in blood pressure and heart rate during the daily stress of life, is being identified as a potential risk factor for the development of hypertension and CHD (Thomas & Liehr, 1995). Black Americans have an increased incidence of hypertension, experience it at an earlier age, and are more likely to have severe hypertension than white Americans (Kirn, 1989). Individuals with obesity, a family history of hypertension, and lower socioeconomic status are more at risk for the development of hypertension (Gifford, 1993).

During the assessment process, the severity of hypertension should be determined using a staging system (Table 4–2). Increased systolic and diastolic blood pressures are major risk factors for CHD (Stokes, Kannel, & Wolf, 1989). Several issues pertain to the accuracy and interpretation of blood pressure measurements. Use of the lowest pressure available to determine the need for intervention is not valid; the average of a series of pressures more accurately determines risk (Kannel, 1990). The Joint National Committee on Detection, Evaluation, and Treatment of high blood pressure (Gifford, 1993) recommends that accurate identification of hypertension be based on diastolic and systolic blood pressure measurements on two or more occasions. Diastolic measurements aid in further classifying hypertension.

Finally, the hypertensive reading(s) should be verified using the highest blood pressure reading measured on the contralateral arm (Frohlick, Grim, Labarthe, et al., 1988). In addition to blood pressure levels, assessment of end-organ damage such as left ventricular hypertrophy, decreased renal function, and retinopathy can assist in classifying hypertensive severity and cardiovascular risk (Pasternak, Grundy, Levy, et al., 1996).

TABLE 4–2   Stages of Hypertension

Very severe hypertension	Diastolic pressure ≥120 mm Hg
Severe hypertension	Diastolic pressure: 110–119 mm Hg
Moderate hypertension	Diastolic pressure: 100–109 mm Hg
Mild hypertension	Diastolic pressure: 90–100 mm Hg
Isolated systolic hypertension	Systolic pressure: ≥160 mm Hg Diastolic pressure: <90 mm Hg
Borderline hypertension	Systolic pressure: 140–159 mm Hg Diastolic pressure: <90 mm Hg

Based on data from Gifford, R. (1993). Fifth Report of the Joint National Committee on Detection. Evaluation and treatment of high blood pressure. Bethesda, MD, NIH, NHLBI (NIH publication number 93-1088).

Hypercholesterolemia

Elevated dietary lipid intake promotes the development of atherosclerosis. High serum cholesterol levels are prevalent in people of the United States; more than 52 million Americans could benefit from reduced cholesterol intake (Semjos, Cleeman, Carroll, et al., 1993). Among people in the United States, cholesterol levels greater than 200 mg/dL, LDL cholesterol greater than 130 mg/dL and HDL cholesterol less than 35mg/dL are associated with increased risk of heart disease development (Grundy, 1993). Major epidemiologic studies support a strong correlation between elevated total cholesterol levels and CHD (Stamler, Wentworth, & Neaton, 1986). A strong correlation has also been established between low-density lipoproteins (LDL) and CHD. Elevated levels of high-density lipoproteins (HDL) are inversely related to CHD (Grundy, 1993; Grundy, 1986; Dawber, 1980).

LDL cholesterol is considered the major atherogenic factor, and its level guides dietary and drug intervention strategies. LDL levels increase with age and weight gain, they also may be elevated in the presence of hypothyroidism, nephrotic syndrome, and estrogen deficiency (Pasternak, Grundy, Levy, et al., 1996). A low HDL (<35 mg/dL) is a major risk factor for CHD. A high HDL cholesterol is a negative risk factor. In multiple clinical trials, for every 1 mg/dL increase in HDL cholesterol, a 2–3% reduction of risk for CHD occurred (Gordon, Probstfield, Garrison, et al., 1989).

Controversy exists as to whether fasting triglycerides are an independent risk factor for CHD; however, elevated triglycerides with a low HDL have been associated with increased risk. Elevated levels of triglycerides may also be related to CHD in women (Castelli, 1986, 1988). The combination of elevated triglycerides with a low HDL may be associated with a more atherogenic form of LDL cholesterol (Chait, Brunzell, Denke, et al., 1993). Normal triglyceride levels are below 200 mg/dL, borderline high levels are 200–400 mg/dL, high levels are 400–1,000 mg/dL, with very high levels greater than 1,000 mg/dL. Type 2 diabetes is frequently associated with elevated triglyceride, elevated LDL levels, and low HDL levels

(Grundy, 1993). Clotting-factor abnormalities are also associated with hypertriglyceridemia.

Assessment focuses on determination of the lipid profile and dietary factors contributing to lipid abnormalities. Nonfasting serum measurement of total cholesterol and HDL is recommended as an initial screen for all adults 20 years and older for primary prevention (Grundy, 1993). For individuals with elevated cholesterol levels or a low level of HDL, a fasting lipid profile that includes analysis of LDL, HDL, and triglycerides is needed to determine the appropriate level of intervention. LDL cholesterol analysis is indicated if total cholesterol is more than 240 mg/dL, or if the HDL cholesterol is less than 35mg/dl and total cholesterol levels are between 200 and 239 mg/dl. Individuals with elevated LDL levels (LDL >130mg/dL) with two or more risk factors require consideration for intervention.

In secondary prevention, patients with evidence of CHD, should have LDL cholesterol levels below 100 mg/dL (Grundy, 1993). Angiographic studies have demonstrated lower rates of progression of atherosclerotic plaques and regression of lesions in individuals with LDL cholesterol levels less than 100 mg/dL (Gould, Rossouw, Santanello, et al., 1995). Measurement of lipids done during the immediate recovery from an acute cardiac event may be falsely lowered (Swan, Gersh, Grayboys, et al., 1996). Apolipoprotein B, a major protein of LDL cholesterol, has been linked to CHD in women but is not included in routine evaluation for CHD at this time (Kwiterovitch, Coresh, Smith, et al., 1992).

Dietary assessment tools to evaluate lipid intake can include dietary histories, food diaries, and food-frequency questionnaires. Research tools for dietary assessment such as the Food Record Rating may be too complex and time-consuming to be used in acute clinical practice (Remmell, Gorder, Hall, et al., 1980; Remmell & Benfari, 1980). Many food-frequency questionnaires can be self-administered, are easily scored, and provide direction for intervention (Glanz, 1992). Multiple tools are available from the American Heart Association and the National Institutes of Health to evaluate the amount of saturated fat and cholesterol in foods. Nutritional assessment should not only address current eating patterns and usual sources of dietary fat and cholesterol, but also food preparation practices, including shopping practices and frequency of eating out (Fair & Berra, 1995). Chapter 6 contains additional information regarding dietary management of patients with dyslipidemias.

Obesity

Obesity, defined as a body weight 20% over the desirable level, contributes to cardiac risk (NIHCDP, 1985). A 30% increase in CHD occurs for each 10% gain in weight (Kannel, 1990; Hubert, Feinlab, McNamara, et al., 1983). Obesity contributes to hypertension, hypercholesterolemia, and diabetes (NIHCDP, 1985). For women, an increasing *body mass index* (BMI) has been shown to increase the relative risk of nonfatal myocardial infarction and fatal CHD (Manson, Colditz, Stampfer, et al., 1990; Manson, Willett, Stampfer, et al., 1995). The risk for CHD increases in middle aged and older women with abdominal obesity (Hanson, 1994).

Obesity is the result of nutritional intake exceeding energy expenditure. For every 1 kg reduction in weight there is an accompanying 2 mg/dl decline in total serum cholesterol (Dattilo & Kris-Etherton, 1992). Multiple tools can be used to assess obesity, including height-and-weight charts, BMI charts (BMI = weight [kg]/ height [m^2]), abdominal-girth measurements, and skinfold measurements. Assessment of abdominal or truncal obesity is especially important. Abdominal obesity is associated with adult-onset diabetes and CHD (Braunwald, 1992; Kannel, 1990) and is determined by dividing the diameter of the waist by the diameter of the hips. If the result is more than 0.85, abdominal obesity exists. For a normal person, waist diameter divided by hip diameter is .07 (Braunwald, 1992).

Sedentary Lifestyle/Acivity

An individual who does not engage in physical exercise has twice the risk of CHD as an active individual (Pate, Pratt, Blair, et al., 1995; Streff, 1987; Oberman, 1985). An estimated 40–80 % of adults in the United States are sedentary (Ward, Taylor, Ahlquist, et al., 1992). Multiple prospective epidemiologic studies have demonstrated the benefit of regular physical activity in slowing the atherosclerotic process, reducing coronary vasospasm, increasing fibrinolysis, improving insulin sensitivity and glucose tolerance, and increasing HDL levels (Paffenbarger, Hyde, Wing, et al., 1986; Kannel, Wilson, & Blair, 1985; Oberman, 1985; Leon, Connett, Jacobs, et al., 1987; Blair, Kohl, Paffenbarger, et al., 1989; Powell, Thompson, Caspersen, et al., 1987).

Assessment is problematic because physical activity is a multifaceted behavior for which there is no gold standard (Caspersen, Powell, & Christenson, 1985). Activity levels in three areas should be considered: occupational, leisure, and recreational. Exercise is defined as aerobic activity such as walking, running, biking, or swimming for at least 20 minutes, three to four times per week. Assessment of current activity levels includes determining if the individual currently exercises and if so, the type, frequency, and duration of exercise. An individual's definition of exercise may differ from the interviewer's: some individuals equate an active, busy life as "getting exercise." The Framingham Index of Physical Activity estimates energy expenditure in a 24-hour period (Kannel & Sorlie, 1979). A self-administered activity summary questionnaire may be used post cardiac events to establish a baseline of activity and measure progression (Sivarajan Froelicher, Kee, Newton, et al., 1994). A patient self-report tool, the *SF-36*, measures multiple aspects of health status, including patient perception of physical function, activity limitations, and impact of limitations on patient's quality of life. The tool can be completed before or after the history interview (Ware & Sherbourne, 1992).

In addition to activity level, assessment should address the multiple factors that can interfere with activity: functional limitations, intermittent claudication, concomitant pulmonary disease, orthopedic barriers, lack of social support, lack of time, fiscal barriers, and a belief system that does not value exercise (Streff, 1987). Chapter 8 addresses issues related to assessment and intervention in greater detail.

Smoking

Smoking is a major modifiable risk factor for CHD; smokers are two to three times more likely to die from coronary disease than non-smokers are (Stillman, 1995). The risk of sudden cardiac death increases five times for women and ten times for men who smoke (Freund, D'Agostino, Belanger, et al., 1992). In the United States, although the Risk Factor Surveillance Project indicated that smoking rates are down overall, minority populations and socioeconomic groups of people with less education and lower incomes have a higher rate of smoking (Holm & Penckofer, 1990).

In nonindustrialized nations, the risk factors of hyperlipidemia, obesity, and smoking are present more frequently in urban, economically affluent citizens. In contrast, in industrialized countries, although CHD is more common, many affluent well-educated citizens have adopted risk-factor modification behaviors, smoking less, reducing saturated-fat intake, and exercising more (Zevallos, Chiriboga, & Hebert, 1992). Chapter 7 contains a detailed discussion of behavioral and physiologic interventions for smoking cessation.

Several physiologic factors contribute to increased CHD risk. Carbon monoxide in cigarettes interferes with oxygen transportation, diminishing available supply (Benowitz, 1986). Nicotine increases myocardial oxygen demands by increasing heart rate. Nicotine has also been linked to coronary artery vasoconstriction and endothelial lining injury (Benowitz, 1993). Nicotine in cigarette smoke alters the metabolism of lipids, resulting in high levels of LDL and low levels of HDL (Henningfield & Nemeth-Coslett, 1988). Smoking also increases fibrinogen levels and promotes platelet aggregation and thrombus formation (Hanson, 1994).

Smoking risk is related to the dose and exposure time and can be reversed within 3 years (Sivarajan Froelicher, Berra, Stepp, et al., 1995, Ockene, Kuller, Svendsen, et al., 1990). Smoking cessation reduces risk and improves cardiac performance among all age groups, including individuals over age 55 (Hermanson, Omenn, Kronmal, et al., 1988). In women younger then 50, smoking is the most powerful risk factor for CHD development (Wenger, 1985).

Assessment should include the number of cigarettes smoked per day and the number of years the individual has smoked. Smoking history is often quantified as *pack years*. Previous attempts to quit and the present level of nicotine addiction are factors that help indicate the stage of readiness for stopping smoking and the interventions that would be most appropriate (Heatherton, Kozlowski, Frecker, et al., 1991; Prochaska & DiClemente, 1983). Several tools for focused assessment of nicotine addiction are available; the Fagerstrom Nicotine Addiction Scale or the Stanford Dependency Index can help the clinician identify the approach needed for smoking cessation (Fagerstrom, 1978; Killen, Fortman, Newman, et al., 1990). Individuals with severe nicotine dependency may require nicotine patch or gum therapy; others may require a social support group process.

Stress

Initiation of the neuroendocrine pathways may cause secretion of stress hormones, cortisone, catecholamines, and testosterone. The stress response may promote CHD via arterial lumen injury from high heart rates, elevated blood pressure, increased platelet aggregation, and lipid release (Kabat-Zin, 1992). Stress may precipitate a sudden cardiac death event (Gomez & Gomez, 1984). Mental stress may act as a trigger for myocardial ischemia in individuals with CHD (Rozanski, Bairey, Krantz, et al., 1988). Depression, a potential consequence of stress or a concurrent condition, can be an independent predictor of mortality in individuals who have sustained a myocardial infarction (Frasure-Smith, Lesperance, & Yalajic, 1993). Similarly, anger has been identified as a possible trigger for acute myocardial infarction (Mittleman, Maclure, Sherwood, et al., 1995).

Factors that buffer the effects of stress also affect physiologic function. The presence of social support after a myocardial infarction improves survival rates for both men and women (Berkman, Leo-Summers, & Horwitz, 1992). Factors that increase isolation include low socioeconomic status and limited education (Kaplan & Keil, 1993).

Stress assessment includes an individual's identification of stressors, reaction and coping mechanisms used, and the relationship of stressors to symptoms and support systems (Engler & Engler, 1995). Recent major life changes, both positive and negative, may contribute to an individual's perceived stress level and can be measured by the Schedule of Recent Life Changes instrument (Holmes & Rahe, 1967) and the Life Change Scale (Holmes & Masuda, 1972). Other assessment tools available include the Personal Stress Inventory (O'Donnell & Ainsworth, 1984), the State Trait Anxiety Inventory (Spielberger, 1983), and the Signs of Distress (Everly & Girdano, 1980).

Type A personality has been described as a behavior pattern in which the individual is driven to achieve, is competitive, needs recognition and advancement, displays a hurried preoccupation with time, has an intense ability to concentrate, and exhibits high levels of hostility (Friedman & Rosenman, 1974). Type A personality has been associated historically with increased risk of CHD, but some research has not supported this linkage (Shekelle, Hully, Neaton, et al., 1985; Shekelle, Gale, & Norusis, 1985; Ragland & Brand, 1988).

Historically, researchers have used the Jenkins Activity Survey (JAS) to measure Type A behavior (Jenkins, Rosenman, & Friedman, 1967; Jenkins, Rosenman, & Zyzanski, 1974). However, hostility, anger, aggression, and depression are now identified as the true risk factors for Type A behavior (Sivarajan Froelicher, Berra, Stepp, et al., 1995). Tools to measure these components vary. Hostility and cynicism have been measured using the Cook-Medley Hostility Scale, a subscale of the Minnesota Multiphasic Personality Inventory (MMPI) (Cook & Medley, 1954). Anger and aggression can be assessed by the Expression of Anger Scale (Spielberger, Johnson, Russell, et al., 1985). Screening for depression using the Beck Depression Inventory (BDI) or the Center for Epidemiologic Studies Depression Scale (CES-D) has been advocated (Beck, Steer, & Garbin, 1988; Burnam, Weeks, Leake, et al., 1991, Sivarajan Froelicher, Berra, Stepp, et al., 1995). The Self-Rating Depression Scale (SDS) is a quantitative 20-item tool available to measure depression (Zung, 1965).

CHD behavior pattern, stress, and coping styles can be measured with the Millon Behavioral Health Inventory (Millon, Green, & Meagher, 1982). The psychosocial questionnaire used in the MULTIFIT program at Stanford University is the result of a modification of multiple tools to measure depression, anger, anxiety, stress, alcohol use, and selected components of social support (Miller & Taylor, 1995). Chapter 10 contains a detailed discussion of stress management.

Alcohol Consumption

Assessment of alcohol consumption is important because extreme consumption may contribute to hypertension, cardiomyopathy, and dysrhythmias. Moderate alcohol intake (one to three drinks daily) may reduce the risk of acute thrombotic events by affecting platelet activity and vascular reactivity (Pasternak, Grundy, Levy, et al., 1996). When assessing alcohol intake, the clinician should bear in mind the high incidence of alcohol abuse and the tendency of some individuals to minimize their alcohol intake and their systemic response to alcohol in interviews. It may be helpful to also obtain data regarding behaviors and attitudes related to alcohol use.

Homocysteine

An individual who has symptoms of CHD but no apparent risk factors may have elevated blood and urine levels of the amino acid homocysteine and should be screened for this disorder. Homocystinemia is considered an independent risk factor for CHD (McLaughlin, Chesebro, & Fuster, 1996). The exact level that promotes premature coronary atherosclerosis and thrombogenesis is not known; however, normal serum levels are in the range of 4–17 μmol/L. Causes of elevated homocysteine may be genetic and nutritional, linked to a rare autosomal recessive disorder and inadequate levels of folate or B_{12} (Futterman & Lemberg, 1997).

Thrombogenic Factors

Several prothrombotic hemostatic factors have been identified that increase the risk of CHD, including fibrinogen, platelet aggregation, and Factor VII. Fibrinogen plays a significant role as a risk factor for the development of CHD (Kannel, D'Agostino, & Belanger, 1992; Ernst &

Resch, 1993). High fibrinogen levels promote platelet aggregation and plasma viscosity. Fibrinogen levels are elevated with smoking, inactivity, higher triglyceride levels (Hoeg, 1997), hypercholesterolemia, advanced age, obesity, oral contraceptive use, stress, and elevated leukocyte count (Ernst & Resch, 1993). Higher concentrations of fibrinogen are associated with an increased incidence of myocardial infarction (Thompson, Kienast, Pyke, et al., 1995), yet there is no universally accepted method for measuring fibrinogen (Ernst & Resch, 1993). Platelet aggregation is not routinely measured even though its role in thrombosis has been established. High coagulant levels of Factor VIIC are associated with increased risk of CHD (Pasternak, Grundy, Levy, et al., 1996). Elevated levels correlate with increased dietary fat intake and estrogen use (McLaughlin, Chesebro, Fuster, et al., 1996; Pasternak, Grundy, Levy, et al., 1996). Routine screening for prothrombotic disorders, however, is not recommended, nor is it cost effective (McLaughlin, Chesebro, Fuster, et al., 1996).

NURSING ASSESSMENT OF THE INDIVIDUAL

In the previous section, issues related to assessing individual CHD risk factors are addressed. However, true risk assessment involves assessment of all risk factors within the same time frame, with subsequent determination of overall risk. In addition, risk assessment should address issues that may affect risk-reduction interventions. These issues include motivation for behavioral change as well as barriers and facilitators for risk reduction.

Nursing assessment within the context of primary, secondary, and tertiary prevention focuses on risk-factor identification. Data may be obtained from (1) risk-appraisal instruments, (2) focused interviews, (3) evaluation of symptoms, (4) physical examination, and (5) diagnostic testing. The sequence in which these activities are performed is context-dependent.

In primary prevention, self-administered or nurse-assisted risk-factor assessment tools and focused interviews may be used. The settings may include primary care offices, community clinics, health fairs, occupational settings, or acute care settings. In acute care settings, it may be appropriate for the clinician to evaluate symptoms before doing anything else, whereas, in primary care settings during a routine checkup, it may be appropriate to identify risk factors first and obtain a biopsychosocial history. A comprehensive assessment will permit accurate interpretation of CHD risk-factor data and appropriate interventions within the context of the patient's physical and psychosocial circumstances.

RISK-APPRAISAL INSTRUMENTS

Many instruments are available to appraise CHD risk (Table 4–3). An individual's lifestyle, with its pattern of risk and health behaviors, can be evaluated using global approaches such as Gordon's framework of functional health patterns (Gordon, 1987). In contrast, Pender's (1987) clear, manageable cardiovascular risk-appraisal form is appropriate for individual assessment in community and occupational settings. It does not, however, include HDL cholesterol, which is currently recommended as part of a baseline screening.

The Framingham Heart Study's predictive chart for CHD also evaluates an individual's risk-factor pattern and estimates the probability for developing CHD within 5 and 10 years (Anderson, Wilson, & Odell, 1991). This chart may be applicable in both primary and acute care settings. Similarly, the American Heart Association's RISKO tool (1994) is simple and useful for individual risk screening in a community setting. In addition, multiple risk-assessment tools are available via computer software corporations, and projected risk may also be extrapolated from national population morbidity and mortality figures.

Accurate and precise prediction of disease by any tool is an unattainable goal (Schoenbach, 1987), but risk-appraisal instruments can be used by individuals to help them identify relative personal health risks. Limitations include lack of age-adjusted measures in many tools and varying validity of self-administered health status results and lifestyle questionnaires. But, risk-assessment tools can be effective in stimulating positive behavioral changes (Smith, McKinlay, & Thorington, 1987). Risk-factor screening is especially valuable when it identifies modifiable risk factors and guides specific interven-

TABLE 4–3 Cardiovascular Risk-Appraisal Tools

Tool	Description	Function
Risk-appraisal form (Pender, 1987)	15-item tool; may require some assistance to complete; primary prevention tool	Evaluates individual risk; includes women's unique risk factors; requires triglyceride measurement and percentage of fat in diet; does not include HDL and LDL
AHA risk-factor prediction kit (1991)	7-item tool; may require direction and assistance to complete; secondary prevention tool	Evaluates individual risk; secondary prevention component looks for expression of CHD and atrial fibrillation; EKG needed to determine whether left-ventricular hypertrophy is present; includes HDL levels; does not measure intensity of cigarette exposure; does not factor in heredity; includes no body weight or exercise component; source is Framingham Heart Study and Framingham Cohort Study population

tions, including information, education, counseling, and behavior modification. Interventions aimed at modifiable risk factors are most effective (Selig, 1991). Risk-factor profile information, with analysis of relative and attributable risk, should be communicated to the individual not as an absolute, but as an informational stepping-stone for behavior modification and lifestyle changes.

Focused Interview

The focused interview provides important information regarding the patient's biopsychosocial history. Patients seeking cardiac risk-factor evaluation have a variety of possible motivations. The concern, that motivated them to seek evaluation and care should be considered first (Seidel, Bale, Dains, et al., 1991). Indeed, the primary objective of a focused history interview is to identify these problems or concerns. Table 4–4 summarizes key data to be elicited during a focused interview. Awareness of cardiovascular risk, level of knowledge regarding the relationship of cardiovascular risk factors to CHD, and former attempts to modify risk behaviors should all be assessed (Fleury, 1992). (See Chapter 3 and 5 for more discussion of the key areas in Table 4–4).

Assessment of the individual's health belief system, locus of control, self-efficacy, and readiness for change may set the framework for risk-factor modification. Specific questions to address include

1 "Do you perceive that you are at risk of disease development and would benefit from changing behavior patterns" (Becker, Drachman, & Kirscht, 1974)?

2 "Are you aware of the relationship between behavior and risk for disease and the severity of the behavior" (Janz & Becker, 1984)?

3 "What are the obstacles to change or the supports in place to promote behavior change" (Bandura, 1986)?

4 "How confident are you of your ability to change behavior" (Bandura, 1977, 1986)?

5 "Have you contemplated making behavior changes, or have you made actual changes?"

Often a CHD event is the stimulus to moving an individual from contemplating behavior change to action. Thus, additional questions include

1 "Have you been successful in the past in modifying risk behaviors" (Prochaska, 1994)?

2 "Will you have a social support network as you attempt to modify risk factors?"

Finally, the patient's history provides a basis for subsequent diagnostic tests and interventions (Rossi & Leary, 1992).

TABLE 4–4 Key Data in Focused Interview

Conceptual Area	Key Data
Health-belief system	Awareness of risk factors; knowledge of risk factors and of their link to disease development; perception of risk and benefit from changing risk behaviors
Locus of control	Confidence in ability to change behavior
Self-efficacy	Supports or barriers for change
Readiness for change	Existence or absence of contemplation of change; history of attempts to change and degree of success

Existing Symptoms

CHD risk assessment frequently occurs within the context of an acute clinical event. The patient and clinicians must simultaneously address issues related to patient stabilization, prevention of complications, and CHD risk-factor modification. Therefore, the premise of this section of the chapter is that both the shorter-term and longer-term aspects of patient status must be addressed in CHD risk assessment.

CHEST PAIN. An individual's first evaluation for CHD may occur because of symptoms of chest pain or discomfort. These patients require immediate assessment. During initial assessment, the clinician should assume that an individual's chest pain is cardiac until proved to be something else (Colucciello, 1994; Merkley, 1994). Angina is a symptom of myocardial ischemia resulting from an imbalance between myocardial oxygen supply and demand. Prolonged ischemia may lead to myocardial necrosis and infarction. Chest pain resulting from myocardial infarction needs to be recognized immediately in order to initiate appropriate treatment. Upon recognition of myocardial infarction, the use of thrombolytic therapy or immediate primary coronary angioplasty to reperfuse and preserve myocardial tissue is now the standard of care for eligible patients in the United States (Gunnar, Bourdillion, Dixon, et al., 1990; Lambrew, Smith, Annas, et al., 1994; Futterman, Correa, & Lemberg, 1996).

Chest pain assessment should include the location, duration, radiation, type or quality, quantity, intensity, precipitating factors, aggravating factors, relieving factors, antecedent symptoms, and patterns such as stuttering or proximity to exercise. Chest pain resulting from angina is often located in the substernal area, with radiation to the arms—usually the ulnar aspect of the left arm—or the neck, shoulders, back, jaw, or teeth. The pain of angina is due to myocardial ischemia and is often described as dull or pressure-like—a weight on the chest or a squeezing, constricting, or burning sensation. When asked to describe the quality of the pain, individuals often comment, "It's not a pain, but an uncomfortable feeling."

Anginal discomfort can be rated from mild to severe on a pain scale of 0 to 10. It develops gradually and lasts typically 5 to 10 minutes, abating when the individual stops activity, rests, or takes nitroglycerin if prescribed (Fruth, 1991). The relationship of pain to activity or exercise should always be evaluated, as chest pain or shortness of breath that appears with exercise is characteristic of heart disease (Braunwald, 1992). Chronic, stable, activity-induced angina is predictable; patients will report no changed patterns over the previous 2 months (Fleury, 1992). Factors that increase myocardial oxygen demands and may precipitate anginal pain include physical activity, eating, emotional stress, extremes of temperature, fever, tachycardia, anemia, and hypoglycemia (Rutherford, Braunwald, & Cohn, 1988).

Various classification systems to quantify the severity of CHD exist. The Canadian cardiovascular classifications of angina can be used to describe mild, moderate, or severe angina based on activity (Campeau, 1976) (Table 4–5). The New York Heart Association functional classifications can also be used to determine the severity of heart disease via functional activity levels (see Table 4–5). Another system classifies patients' risk according to the type of chest pain, whether nonanginal or anginal, and if anginal, whether atypical, stable, progressive, or unstable (Table 4–6).

Unstable angina can occur without an increase in myocardial oxygen demand and is attributed to a temporary reduction in coronary artery blood supply (Falk, 1985). In unstable angina the plaque formation inside the coronary artery may rupture, causing partial thrombotic occlusion and platelet aggregation (Matrisciano, 1992). Unstable angina can occur at

TABLE 4–5 Angina Classifications

Canadian Classifications of Angina	New York Heart Association Functional Classifications
CLASS I. Prolonged exertion results in angina.	*CLASS I.* Patients have cardiac disease but no symptoms.
CLASS II. Walking longer than two blocks causes pain.	*CLASS II.* Patients have cardiac disease but are comfortable at rest; symptoms occur with ordinary activity.
CLASS III. Pain is experienced after less than two blocks of walking.	*CLASS III.* Patients have cardiac disease but are comfortable at rest; symptoms occur with less than ordinary activity.
CLASS IV. Pain occurs with minimal exertion or even at rest.	*CLASS IV.* Patients have cardiac disease, have pain even at rest, and are unable to perform any significant physical activity.

TABLE 4–6 Relative Risk Based on Anginal Characteristics

Characteristic	Points	One-Year Mortality (%)
Nonanginal pain	3	0.4%
Atypical angina	25	0.8%
Stable angina	41	1.3%
Progressive angina	46	1.5%
Unstable angina	51	1.7%

Based on 60-year-old patient with no comorbid conditions.
From Califf, R., Armstrong, P., Carver, J., D'Agostino, R., Strauss, W., (1996). Task force 5. Stratification of patients into high, medium and low risk subgroups for purposes of risk factor management. *Journal of the American College of Cardiology, 27*(5), 1007–1019. Used with permission from the American College of Cardiology.

rest or with minimal exertion. Individuals with unstable angina constitute 10% of all initial presentations of CHD (Califf, Armstrong, Carver, et al., 1996). The incidence of subsequent myocardial infarction following unstable angina is significant (Ambrose & Alexopoulos, 1989; Theroux, Ouimet, McCans, et al., 1988; Leeman, McCabe, Faxon, et al., 1988; Gotoh, Minamino, Katoh, et al., 1988; Gold, Johns, Lienbach, et al., 1987).

Chest pain resulting from myocardial infarction often occurs at rest and may be associated with other symptoms, such as diaphoresis, shortness of breath, nausea, vomiting, lightheadedness, anxiety, and sense of impending doom. This chest pain may be described as a pressure, tightness, aching, a heavy weight, constriction, vise-like sensation, burning, or indigestion type of pain. Myocardial infarction pain lasts longer than angina, typically exceeding 20 minutes. Myocardial infarction pain may be rated as mild to severe on a pain scale of 0 to 10, and it may gradually increase in intensity. Patients often expect that myocardial infarction pain must be severe. Rest does not relieve the pain.

The pain of myocardial infarction is often located substernally and can radiate to the throat, jaw, teeth, shoulders, arms, or back. It is not affected by position. Myocardial infarction often follows a circadian pattern, occurring most frequently in the early morning hours. It may be related to surges of catecholamine levels, which increase myocardial oxygen demands, coronary artery tone, and platelet aggregation, promoting thrombosis (Muller, Stone, Turi, et al., 1985; Levine, Pepe, Fromm, et al., 1992). Individuals, on average, delay seeking professional evaluation and treatment of chest pain for 2–4 hours. Delays are longer for blacks than for whites (Goldberg, Gurwitz, Yarzebski, et al., 1992; Gonzalez, Jones, Ornato, et al., 1992; Ell, Haywood, Sobel, et al., 1994). Differences in pain threshold, cultural norms, and psychological denial may affect an individual's report of pain (Schiro & Curtis, 1988).

The immediate differential diagnosis of chest pain should exclude other life-threatening causes such as cardiac tamponade, aortic dissection, pulmonary embolism, and esophageal rupture (Colucciello, 1994). Chest pain may also originate from the pleura, mediastinum, diaphragm, thoracic muscles, cervicodorsal spine, costochondral junctions, stomach, pancreas, and gallbladder (Braunwald, 1992). Noncardiac pain may be sharp, localized, of sudden onset, and affected by position changes.

OTHER SYMPTOMS. Patients may not report typical characteristic angina pain yet nevertheless be experiencing myocardial ischemia (Schiro & Grozinger Curtis, 1988). Symptoms other than chest pain may indicate CHD and the onset of myocardial infarction (Utretsky, Farguhar, Berezin, et al., 1977). For example, dyspnea may occur as an anginal equivalent caused by myocardial ischemia (Braunwald, 1992). Black patients have a lower incidence of chest pain and more frequently complain of dyspnea (Clark, Adams-Campbell, Maw, et al., 1989). Women and the elderly are more likely to have atypical symptoms of myocardial infarction (Peberdy & Ornato, 1992). Chest pain is the predominant symptom in the elderly; however, sometimes dyspnea, syncope, palpitations with exertion, fatigue, or change in mental status is the chief complaint (O'Rourke, Chatterjee, & Wei, 1987; Wei, 1984; Tresh, 1987; Wei & Gersh, 1987). In the Myocardial Infarction Triage and Intervention Trial (MITI), more than 40% of elderly patients over the age of 75 had atypical symptoms and no chest pain (Weaver, Litwin, Martin, et al., 1991).

Data from the Framingham Heart Study indicate that myocardial infarction can be recognized only retrospectively on electrocardiogram. Unrecognized, or "silent," myocardial infarction was found in a third of individuals experiencing myocardial infarction, frequently in diabetic men and hypertensive men and women (Kannel & Abbot, 1984). The population most at risk for silent ischemia are males with a family history of early CHD and with one or more of the major risk factors of hypertension, hyperlipidemia, cigarette smoking, and diabetes mellitus (Schiro & Grozinger Curtis, 1988).

The World Health Organization (WHO) diagnostic classifications of myocardial infarction combine clinical presentation, electrocardiographic changes, and laboratory data. This combination is used to determine if a myocardial infarction is definite, possible, or can be ruled out (Antman & Rutherford, 1986).

Physical Examination

Individuals experiencing chest pain may appear anxious, with cool, clammy skin and a clenched fist over the sternum. Examination of the skin may reveal *xanthelasma*, yellowish deposits of cholesterol on the eyelids. *Xanthomas*, cholesterol-filled nodules, may be found subcutaneously or over tendons, suggestive of hyperlipoproteinemia. Beading of the retinal artery found on fundoscopic exam and an arcus of light around the iris may indicate hypercholesteremia (Braunwald, 1992). Fundoscopic exam may also reveal arteriolar narrowing, arteriovenous nicking, hemorrhages, exudate, or papilledema suggestive of hypertension. Examination of the neck should include inspection of neck veins, assessment for an enlarged thyroid gland, and auscultation for carotid bruits. Elevated jugular venous pressure can occur with left-sided heart failure, elevated right jugular venous pressure with right ventricular infarct, or cardiac tamponade.

Examination of extremities should include evaluation of peripheral pulses and of the presence or absence of peripheral edema, capillary refill, and skin integrity.

Heart Assessment

Pulsations in the heart can be felt with the patient in the supine position or left lateral recumbent position. The apex is located medial and superior to the left midclavicular line, at the fifth intercostal space, and is felt as a brief outward motion of the left ventricle (Bates & Hokelman, 1987). The apex may also be the point of maximal impulse, usually the size of a quarter. A prominent pulsation or bulge in this area with lateral displacement may indicate left ventricular enlargement (Braunwald, 1992). Pain or tenderness on palpation may indicate costochondriasis as a source of chest pain.

In assessment of heart sounds, reversed or paradoxic splitting of S2 may indicate a condition that delays systole, including left bundle branch block, aortic stenosis, left ventricular disease, or uncontrolled hypertension (Guzzetta & Dossey, 1990). Third and fourth heart sounds originate in the ventricles and can be a signal of pathology. A third heart sound heard in children or young adults may be physiologic. The presence of an S3 early in diastole is due to early, rapid filling and may indicate congestive heart failure. An S4 heart sound is heard late in diastole or in the immediate presystolic time right before S1. Reduced left ventricular compliance, an elevated left ventricular end diastolic volume, left ventricular hypertrophy, and ischemic heart disease, including angina and myocardial infarction, can produce an S4 heart sound in adults.

Acute myocardial infarction with resulting ischemia to the papillary muscles supporting the mitral valve may cause a new mitral regurgitation murmur during systole. The patient may experience acute hemodynamic compromise with left ventricular failure and require immediate surgical intervention. Murmurs may be secondary to regurgitant or stenotic valves or to atrial or ventricular septal wall defects. The presence of a ventricular aneurysm from myocardial infarction may produce muffled heart sounds, with systolic and diastolic murmurs (Peeples, Fowkes, & Andreoli, 1987).

Individuals with acute myocardial infarction may experience alteration in blood pressure, either hypertension or hypotension (Webb, Adgey, & Pantridge, 1982). Patients with anterior myocardial infarctions may experience sympathetic excess, resulting in hypertension and tachycardia. In contrast, patients with inferior myocardial infarctions often demonstrate parasympathetic excess, with hypotension and bradycardia. Right ventricular infarction is frequently associated with inferior myocardial infarction (Andersen, Falk, & Nielsen, 1987) and can create increased right ventricular end diastolic volume and pressure, decreased right ventricular stroke volume, and decreased left ventricular cardiac output with subsequent hypotension.

Lung Assessment

Bibasilar crackles or rales may be present in the patient with increased left ventricular volume or pressure. In patients with bronchoconstrictive disease and in smokers, wheezes or rhonchi may be heard.

Diagnostic Tests

Screening tests for CHD are most effective when directed at individuals in higher risk categories (Lewy, 1980).

ELECTROCARDIOGRAM

In primary prevention, screening asymptomatic individuals with an electrocardiogram (EKG) is ineffective for reducing risk of CHD because the EKG may be normal until significant atherosclerosis is present (Detrano & Froelicher, 1987). An EKG screen should, however, be used in individuals who have multiple risk factors or who hold public safety roles.

The EKG is a noninvasive, inexpensive, immediately available tool to evaluate for myocardial ischemia, injury, or infarction. It is, therefore, the initial tool to evaluate chest discomfort, but it is diagnostic of myocardial infarction in only 60% of patients (Fisch, 1992). The remaining 40% of patients with myocardial infarctions have normal or nondiagnostic EKGs (Colucciello, 1994). Serial EKGs can increase the chances of detecting myocardial infarction to 95% (Fisch, 1992). Despite experiencing anginal discomfort, some patients exhibit no EKG abnormality. Abnormal EKG

findings are prevalent in the elderly (Gerber, 1990). The ability to compare prior EKGs helps in interpreting abnormal findings.

Myocardial cell damage and death begin within 20 to 40 minutes of occluded blood flow (Reimer, Lowe, Rasmussen, et al., 1977). EKG changes indicating myocardial ischemia include ST segment depression and T wave inversion. EKG changes indicating progressive ischemia leading to injury and infarction include hyperacute T wave changes, ST segment elevation over the area of injury, reciprocal ST depression, and, ultimately, Q waves. EKG changes indicating myocardial infarction may evolve over a matter of hours and days. The way in which the EKG appears will depend on when the patient is evaluated, the area of myocardium involved, and the extent of the infarct.

Myocardial infarctions can be classified as Q wave versus non–Q wave type, that is, with or without ST segment elevation. *Q wave myocardial infarctions* have a different EKG evolution, with ST segment elevation, reciprocal ST depression, and ultimate T wave inversions and Q waves the most common findings. *Non–Q wave myocardial infarctions* may produce no diagnostic EKG changes or only minor, subtle ST segment depression and thus require clinical signs and presence of CPK-MB isoenzyme to confirm the diagnosis (Smokler, 1992). Often there is less myocardial necrosis and therefore less creatine kinase enzyme elevation and heart failure with a non–Q wave myocardial infarction (Keller & Lemberg, 1994). In-hospital mortality is less with a non–Q wave infarct; however, patients may experience more postinfarction angina, signaling the risk of extending the myocardial infarction (Gibson, 1988; Berger, Murabito, Evans, et al., 1992).

The presence of left bundle branch block may mask ST segment changes, indicating acute myocardial infarction. Clinical prediction tools continue to be developed to assist in the diagnosis of myocardial infarction even in the presence of left bundle branch block (Sgarbossa, Pinski, Barbagelta, et al., 1996).

Left ventricular hypertrophy on EKG evidenced by repolarization changes, ST depression, and T wave inversion, along with increased voltage and large R waves in left precordial leads, may be an ominous sign of future clinical CHD expression (Kannel, 1990).

The results of the 26-year follow-up Framingham study revealed a sixfold greater increase in CHD for patients with left ventricular hypertrophy than for those without (Pekkanen, Linn, Heiss, et al., 1990).

ECHOCARDIOGRAPHY. When EKG evaluation is nondiagnostic, echocardiography may be used to detect wall motion abnormalities that may indicate ischemia and infarction. The echocardiographic examination can be used for patients with bundle branch block or with nondiagnostic ST-T wave changes. Echocardiography is also used to detect wall motion abnormalities of the ventricles, including akinesis, hypokinesis, and dyskinesis often found in the Q wave myocardial infarction (Gibson, 1988). The echocardiogram evaluates valve function and helps identify mitral valve prolapse or aortic stenosis as a potential cause of chest pain. Finally, left ventricular function as measured by ejection fraction is a powerful predictor of morbidity and mortality (Califf, Armstrong, Carver, et al., 1996).

STRESS TESTING. Exercise stress testing is a widely available diagnostic tool to check for the presence of CHD in high-risk individuals. The American College of Sports Medicine (1991) has outlined test indications for specific groups. *Sensitivity* refers to the ability of the test to identify those individuals with CHD. The sensitivity of an exercise stress test to identify single vessel disease ranges from 25% to 71% (Chaitman, 1992). With multiple-vessel disease, sensitivity increases, ranging from 40% to 100% (Gianrossi, Detrano, Mulvihill, et al., 1989; Detrano, Gianrossi, Mulvihill, et al., 1989). As a noninvasive indirect measure, an exercise stress test's sensitivity and specificity is influenced by gender and the degree of underlying disease. Men with atypical symptoms, asymptomatic men over 40 who are in specific occupations (pilots, firemen, policemen, bus or truck drivers, railroad engineers), and asymptomatic men over 40 who have two or more risk factors have clear and probable indications for the test. An exercise stress test may be indicated for a women with typical or atypical angina. The test is more likely to be falsely positive in a woman because of changes in ST segments produced by estrogen (Wingate, 1991).

A positive exercise tolerance test is defined as ST segment depression greater than 1 mm at 80 μsec after the J point, occurring in a horizontal and down-sloping fashion (Naccarelli, Nishikawa, & Giebel, 1987). The severity of underlying disease is suggested by the magnitude of ST segment depression, the level of exercise at which ST changes appear, and the persistence of changes into the recovery period of the test (Kattus, 1974; Goldschalger, Selzer, & Cohn, 1976; Goldman, Tselos, & Cohn, 1976). ST segment depression in five or more leads increases the probability of extensive disease (Chaitman, 1992). ST segment depression does not localize the area of myocardium that is ischemic; however, ST segment elevation with exercise is relatively specific for the area being viewed (Mark, Hlaty, Lee, et al., 1987).

The presence of angina with ST segment depression may indicate CHD during stress testing. Normal heart rate response to exercise should be a linear increase; systolic blood pressure rises, but the diastolic pressure should not rise (Franklin, 1995).

Individuals with intraventricular conduction defects, left ventricular hypertrophy, and widespread ST segment depression may be placed under stress using alternative imaging techniques. Perfusion imaging with thallium 201, or technetium Tc 99m sestamibi may reveal reversible perfusion defects or increased pulmonary uptake, indicating ischemia. Fixed defects indicate prior infarction. Individuals unable to exercise can be given pharmacologic agents for stress testing, including dipyridamole and adenosine. Dobutamine stress echocardiography is another alternative (Califf, Armstrong, Carver, et al., 1996).

SERUM MARKERS FOR MYOCARDIAL NECROSIS. Serum tests for myocardial necrosis may assist in defining infarction when the EKG is nondiagnostic. Cardiac enzymes released from damaged myocardial cells include *creatine kinase (CK)* and *CK-MB isoenzyme*. Total CK is located in skeletal and myocardial tissue, with CK-MB found predominantly in cardiac tissue. CK-MB is 100% sensitive and specific for identifying myocardial necrosis. CK and CK-MB appear in the non-reperfused patient 4–6 hours after symptoms, peaking in 14–18 hours and returning to normal within 2 days (Califf &

Ohman, 1992). Reperfusion with a thrombo-lytic agent causes the CK and CK-MB to be released earlier (Ishii, Nomura, Ando, et al., 1994). Elevation of CK-MB that is not due to myocardial necrosis may occur with chronic renal failure; surgery of prostrate or uterus; surgery or trauma to the small intestine, tongue, or diaphragm; strenuous exercise (such as marathon running); myocarditis; or cardiac surgery (Califf & Ohman, 1992).

Women have lower levels of CK and CK-MB than men. With small amounts of necrosis, levels of CK and CK-MB may not be high. In this situation the pattern of the CK-MB rise and fall should be considered, along with transient doubling of CK-MB (Clyne, Medeiros, & Marton, 1989; White, Grande, Califf, et al., 1985). Subforms of CK-MB, CK-MB-1 and CK-MB-2 are now able to be measured in some settings, their ratio being an early indicator of necrosis (Puelo, Guadagno, Roberts, et al., 1990).

Myoglobin is released after acute myocardial infarction more rapidly than CK-MB owing to its smaller molecular weight and may thus help identify myocardial necrosis earlier. Serum myoglobin levels rise quickly, reaching twice the normal levels within 2 hours and peaking within 4 hours. Myoglobin is not specific to the myocardium. False positive results may occur as a result of shock, trauma causing skeletal muscle injury, vigorous exercise, end-stage renal disease, open heart surgery, alcoholism, and electrical defibrillation (Brogan, Friedman, McCuskey, et al., 1994).

Cardiac troponin I (cTnI) is highly sensitive and specific for myocardial injury. Cardiac troponin I does not increase with chronic muscle injury, skeletal muscle injury, or chronic renal failure. Serum elevations begin within 4 hours of myocardial injury and persist for up to 5–9 days (Adams, Boder, Davila-Roman, et al., 1993).

Total serum *lactate dehydrogenase* is elevated in a variety of diseases, including myocardial infarction. Lactate dehydrogenase is elevated in the serum 12–18 hours after symptoms, peaks at 48–72 hours, and returns to normal within 6–10 days (Wolf, 1989). LDH measurements are helpful if myocardial infarction has occurred prior to the individual's presentation for evaluation. Lactate dehydrogenase isoenzyme 1 (LDH 1) is cardiac specific

and also increases within 10–12 hours, peaking at 48–72 hours, and returning to baseline within 10 days. When increased levels of LDH1 surpass LDH2 levels, a flipped pattern indicative of myocardial necrosis occurs (Apple, 1992).

CONCLUSION

In conclusion, CHD risk assessment is a detailed process that must be individually tailored to the patient's needs and health status. Risk assessment is especially important for patients being treated for acute CHD-related events. With increasingly shorter lengths of stay for patients in acute care facilities (Division National Cost Estimates, 1990), the assessment of risk and promotion of lifestyle change barely begins in the inpatient phase (Debusk, Miller, Superko, et al., 1994). Comprehensive risk assessment involves patient screening and profiling using one or more of the following: risk-assessment tools, focused interview, assessment of existing symptoms, physical examination, heart assessment, and diagnostic testing.

References

Adams, J., Boder, G., Davila-Roman, V., & Delmez, J., Apple, F., Ladenson, J., Jaffe, A. (1993). Cardiac troponin I: A marker with high specificity for cardiac injury. *Circulation, 88*(1), 101–106.

Ades, P.A., Huang, D., & Weaver, S.O. (1992). Cardiac rehabilitation participation predicts lower rehospitalization rates. *American Heart Journal, 123*, 916–921.

Ambrose, J.A., & Alexopoulous, D. (1989). Thrombolysis in unstable angina: Will the beneficial effects of thrombolytic therapy in MI apply to patients with unstable angina? *Journal of the American College of Cardiology. 13*, 1666–1671.

American College of Sports Medicines (1991). *Guidelines for Exercise Testing and Prescription*, 4th ed. Philadelphia: Lea & Febiger.

American Heart Association (1991). *1990 Heart and Stroke Facts, Statistics*. Dallas.

American Heart Association (1994). *1993 Heart and Stroke Facts, Statistics*. Dallas.

American Heart Association (1993). *Cardiovascular Disease in Women: Medical and Scientific Report*. Dallas.

American Heart Association (1994). *RISKO A Heart Health Appraisal*. Dallas.

American Heart Association (1997). *Heart and Stroke Facts: 1996 Statistical Supplement*. Dallas.

Andersen, H., Falk, E., & Nielsen, D. (1987). Right ventricular infarction: Frequency, size and topography in coronary heart disease, a prospective study comprising 107 consecutive autopsies from a coronary care unit. *Journal of the American College of Cardiology, 10*, 1223–1232.

Anderson, K., Wilson, P., & Odell, P. (1991). An updated coronary risk profile, a statement for health professionals. *Circulation, 83*, 356–362.

Antman, E.A., & Rutherford, J.D. (1986). *Coronary Care Medicine.* Hanover, Martinus Nijhoff Publishing.

Apple, F. (1992). Acute myocardial infarction and coronary reperfusion serum markers for the 1990s. *Clinical Chemistry, AJCP, 97*(2), 217–226.

Bandrau, A. (1977). Self-efficacy: Toward a unifying theory of behavior change. *Psychological Review, 84*, 191–215.

Bandrau, A. (1986). *Social Foundations of Thought and Action: A Social Cognitive Theory.* Englewood Cliffs, NJ: Prentice Hall.

Barrett-Connor, E., & Khaw, K. (1984). Family history of heart attacks as an independent predictor of death due to cardiovascular disease. *Circulation, 69*, 1065–1069.

Bates, B., & Hokelman, R. (1987). *A Guide to Physical Examination and History Taking*, 4th ed. Philadelphia: J.B. Lippincott.

Beck, A., Steer, R., & Garbin, M. (1988). Psychometric properties of the BDI: 25 years of evaluation. *Clinical Psychology Review, 8*, 77–100.

Becker, M., Drachman, R., & Kirscht, S. (1974). A new approach to explaining sick-role behavior in low-income populations. *American Journal of Public Health, 64*(3), 205–216.

Benowitz, N.L. (1986). Clinical pharmacology of nicotine. *Annual Review of Medicine, 37*, 21–32.

Benowitz, N.L. (1993). Smoking-induced coronary vasoconstriction: Implications for therapeutic use of nicotine. *Journal of the American College of Cardiology, 22*(3), 648–649.

Berger, C.J., Murabito, J.M., Evans, J.C., Anderson, K.M., & Levy, D. (1992). Prognosis after first myocardial infarction: Comparison of Q wave and non Q wave myocardial infarction in the Framingham heart study. *Journal of the American Medical Association, 268*, 1545–1560.

Berkman, L., Leo-Summers, L., & Horowitz, R. (1992). Emotional support and survival after myocardial infarction. *Annals of Internal Medicine, 117*(12), 1003–1009.

Blair, S.N., Kohl, H.W., Paffenbarger, R.S., Clark, D., Cooper, K., & Gibbons, L. (1989). Physical fitness and all-cause mortality, a prospective study of healthy men and women. *Journal of the American Medical Association, 262*(17), 2395–2401.

Braunwald, E. (1992). The physical examination. In Braunwald, E., *Heart Disease: A Textbook of Cardiovascular Medicine*, 4th ed., vol. 1. Philadelphia: W.B. Saunders.

Brogan, G., Friedman, S., McCuskey, C., Colling, D., Berrutti, L., Thode, H., & Bock, J. (1994). Evaluation of a new, rapid, quantitative immunoassay for serum myoglobin versus CK-MB for ruling out acute myocardial infarction in the emergency department. *Annals of Emergency Medicine, 24*(4), 665–671.

Burnam, M., Weeks, K., Leake, B., & Lansverk, J. (1991). Development of a brief screening instrument for detecting depressive disorders. *Medical Care, 26*, 775–789.

Califf, R., Armstrong, P., Carver, J., D'Agostino, R., & Strauss, W. (1996). Task force 5. Stratification of patients into high, medium and low risk subgroups for purposes of risk factor management. *Journal of the American College of Cardiology, 27*(5), 1007–1019.

Califf, R., & Ohman, E.M. (1992). The diagnosis of acute myocardial infarction. *Chest, 101*(14), 106S–115S.

Campeau, L. (1976). Grading of angina pectoris. *Circulation, 54*, 522–523.

Caspersen, C.J., Powell, K.E., & Christenson, G.M. (1985). Physical activity exercise and physical fitness: Definitions and distinctions for health-related research. *Public Health Report, 100*, 126–131.

Castelli, W.P. (1986). The triglyceride issue: A view from Framingham. *American Heart Journal, 112*, 432–437.

Castelli, W.P. (1988). Cardiovascular disease in women. *American Journal of Obstetrics and Gynecology, 158*(6), 1553–1560.

Cavender, J.B., Rogers, W.J., Fischer, L.D., Gersch, B.J., Coggins, C.J., & Myers, W.O. (1992). Effects of smoking on survival and morbidity in patients randomized to medical or surgical therapy in the Coronary Artery Surgery Study (CASS): 10-year follow-up CASS investigators. *Journal of the American College of Cardiology, 20*, 287–294.

Chait, A., Brunzell, J., Denke, M., Eisenberg, D., Ernst, N., Franklin, F., Ginsberg, H., Kotchen, T., Kuller, L., Mullis, R., Nichman, M., Nicolosi, R., Schaefer, E., Stone, N., & Weidman, W. (1993). Rationale of the Diet-Heart Statement of the American Heart Association. *Circulation, 88*(6), 3008–3029.

Chaitman, B. (1992). Exercise stress testing, In Braunwald, E., *Heart Disease: A Textbook of Cardiovascular Medicine*, 4th ed. Philadelphia: W.B. Saunders, pp. 161–179.

Clark, L., Adams-Campbell, L, Maw, M., Bridges, D., & Kline, G. (1989). Effects of race on the presenting symptoms of myocardial infarction. *Circulation, 80* (Suppl. II), 300.

Clyne, C, Mederiros, J., & Marton, K. (1989). The prognostic significance of immunoradiometric CK-MB assay (IRMA) diagnosis of myocardial infarction in patients with low total CK and elevated MB isoenzymes. *American Heart Journal, 118*(5), 901–906.

Colditz, G.A, Stampfer, M., Willett, W.C., Rozner, B., Speizer, F., & Hennekens, C. (1986). A prospective study of parental history of myocardial infarction and coronary heart disease in women. *American Journal of Epidemiology, 123*(1), 48–58.

Colucciello, S. (1994). Chest pain that isn't cardiac. Part I. *Emergency Medicine*, July, 71–79.

Cook, M., Medly, D. (1954). Proposed hostility and pharisaic-virtues scales for the MMPI. *Journal of Applied Psychology, 38*, 414–418.

Conti, C.R. (1993). Estrogen therapy for the prevention of coronary heart disease: What are the facts? *Clinical Cardiology*, 699–700.

Criqui, M. H., Froneck, A., Barrett-Connor, E., Klauber, M. Gabriel, & S., Goodman, D. (1985). Prevalence of peripheral arterial disease in a defined population. *Circulation, 71*(3), 510–515.

Cummins, R.O. (Ed.) (1994). Subcommittee on Advanced Cardiac Life Support 1991–1994. Committee on Emergency Cardiac Care. Community approach to ECC: Prevention and chain of survival. *Textbook of Advanced Cardiac Life Support.* Dallas: American Heart Association.

Dalen J.E., & Hickler, R.B. (1981). Oral contraceptives and cardiovascular disease. *American Heart Journal, 101*, 626–693.

Dattilo, A.M., & Kris-Etherton, P.M. (1992). Effects of weight on reduction of blood lipids and lipoproteins: A meta analysis. *American Journal of Clinical Nutrition, 56*, 320–328.

Davidoff, F. (1997). Blood sugar disease and nondisease. *Annals of Internal Medicine, 127*(3), 235–238.

Dawber, T.R. (1980). *The Framingham Study. The Epidemiology of Atherosclerotic Disease.* Cambridge: Harvard Press.

Debusk, R.F., Miller, N.H., Superko, R., Dennis, C.A., Thomas, R.J., Lew, H.T., Berger, W.E., Heller, R.S., Rompf, J., Gee, D., Kraemer, H.C., Bandura, A., Ghandour, G., Clark, M., Shah, R.V., Fischer, L., & Taylor, C.B. (1994). A case management system for coronary risk factor modification after acute MI. *Annals of Internal Medicine. 12*(9), 721–729.

Detrano, R., & Froelicher, V. (1987). A logical approach to screening for coronary artery disease. *Annals of Internal Medicine, 106*, 846–852.

Detrano, R., Gianrossi, R., Mulvihill, D., Lehmann, K., Dubach, P., Columbo, A., & Froelicher. W. (1989). Exercise-induced ST segment depression in the diagnosis of multi-vessel coronary disease: A meta analysis. *Journal of the American College of Cardiology. 14*(6), 1501–1508.

Division of National Cost Estimates, Office of the Actuary Department of Health and Human services. Health Care Financing Administration (HCFA) (1990). National health expenditures 1986–2000. In Lee, P.R., & Estees, C.L. *The Nation's Health*, 3rd ed. Boston: Jones and Bartlett Publishers, pp. 207–221.

Ell, K., Haywood, L., Sobel, E., DeGuzman, M., Boumfield, D., & Ning, J. (1994). Acute chest pain in African Americans: Factors in the delay in seeking emergency care. *American Journal of Public Health, 84*, 965–970.

Engler, M., & Engler, M. (1995). Assessment of the cardiovascular effects of stress. *Journal of Cardiovascular Nursing, 10*(1), 51–63.

Ernst, E., & Resch, K., L. (1993). Fibrinogen as a cardiovascular risk factor: A meta analysis and review of the literature. *Annals of Internal Medicine, 118*(12), 956–963.

Everly, G.S., & Girdano, D.A. (1980). *The Stress Mess Solution*. Bowie, MD: Brady Press.

Expert Survey Cardiology II: Forecast of Hospital Profitability Through and Beyond the Year 2000 (1994). Washington, DC: The Advisory Board Co.

Fagerstrom, K.O. (1978). Measuring the degree of physical dependence on tobacco smoking with reference to individualization of treatment. *Addictive Behavior, 3*(3), 235–241.

Fair, J., & Berra, K. (1995). Life-style changes and coronary heart disease: The influence of nonpharmacologic interventions. *Journal of Cardiovascular Nursing, 9*(2), 12–24.

Falk, E. (1985). Unstable angina with fatal outcome: Dynamic coronary thrombosis leading to infarction and or sudden death. *Circulation, 71*, 699–708.

Feinlieb, M., Garrison, R., Fabsitz, R., Christian, J.C., Hrobec, Z., Borhani, N., Kannel, W., Rosenman, R., Schwartz, J., & Wagner, J. (1977). The NHLBI twin study of cardiovascular disease risk factors: Methodology and summary of results. *American Journal of Epidemiology, 106*(4), 284–295.

Fisch, C. (1992). Electrocardiography and vectocardiography. In Braunwald, E., *Heart Disease: A Textbook of Cardiovascular Medicine*, Philadelphia: W.B. Saunders, pp. 116–160.

Fleury, J. (1992). Long-term management of the patient with stable angina. *Nursing Clinics of North America, 27*(1), 205–230.

Franklin, B., (1995). Diagnostic and functional exercise testing: Test selection and interpretation. *Journal of Cardiovascular Nursing, 10*(1), 8–29.

Frasure-Smith, N., Lesperance, F., & Yalajic, M. (1993). Depression following myocardial infarction: Impact on 6-month survival. *Journal of the American Medical Association, 270*(15), 1819–1825.

Freund, K.M., D'Agostino, R.B., Belanger, A.J., Kannel, W.B., & Stokes, J. (1992). Predictors of smoking cessation: The Framingham study. *American Journal of Epidemiology, 135*(9), 957–964.

Friedman, M., & Rosenman, R.H. (1974). *Type A Behavior and Your Heart*. New York: Knopf.

Frohlick, E., Grim, C., Labarthe, D., Maxwell, M., Perloff, D., Weidman, W., (1988). Recommendations for human blood pressure determination by sphygmomanometer. Report of special task force appointed by steering committee, AHA. *Circulation, 77*(2), 502A–514A.

Fruth, R. (1991). Differential diagnosis of chest pain. *Critical Care Nursing Clinics of North America, 3*(1), 59.

Futterman, L., Correa, L., & Lemberg, L. (1996). Thrombolysis or primary angioplasty? An ongoing controversy in the management of acute myocardial infarction. *American Journal of Critical Care, 5*(2), 160–167.

Futterman, L., & Lemberg, L., (1997). Homocysteine and coronary artery disease. *American Journal of Critical Care, 6*(1), 72–77.

Gerber, R.M. (1990). Coronary artery disease in the elderly. *Journal of Cardiovascular Nursing, 4*(4), 23–34.

Gianrossi, R., Detrano, R., Mulvihill, D., Lehmann, K., Dubach, P., Columbo, A., McArthur, D., & Froelicher, D. (1989). Exercise-induced ST depression in the diagnosis of coronary artery disease: A meta analysis. *Circulation, 80*, 87–98.

Gibson, R.S. (1988). Non Q wave myocardial infarction diagnosis, prognosis and management. *Current Problem in Cardiology, 13*(2), 8–72.

Gifford, R. (1993). *Fifth Report of the Joint National Committee on Detection, Evaluation and Treatment of High Blood Pressure*. National Institutes of Health, NHLBI (NIH publication no. 93-1088).

Gillum, R.F., & Grant, C.T. (1982). Coronary heart disease in black populations II: Risk factors. *American Heart Journal, 104*(4), 852–864.

Glanz, K. (1992). Nutritional intervention: A behavioral educational perspective. In I. Ockene & J. Ockene (Eds.), *Prevention of Coronary Heart Disease*. Boston: Little, Brown & Co., pp. 231–265.

Gold, H.K., Johns, J.A., Lienbach, R.C., Yasuda, T., Grossbard, E., Zusman, R., & Collen, D. (1987). A randomized, blinded, placebo-controlled trial of recombinant tissue type plasminogen activator in patients with unstable angina pectoris. *Circulation, 75*(6), 1192–1199.

Goldberg, R.J. (1992). Coronary heart disease: Epidemiology and risk factor. In I. Okene & J. Okene (Eds.), *Prevention of Coronary Heart Disease*, 1st ed. Boston: Little, Brown, & Co.

Goldberg, R.J., Gurwitz, J., Yarzebski, J., Landon, J., Gore, J., Alpert, J., Dalen. P., & Dalen, J. (1992). Patient delay and receipt of thrombolytic therapy among patients with acute myocardial infarction from a community-wide perspective. *American Journal Cardiology, 70*, 421–425.

Goldman, S., Tselos, S., & Cohn, K. (1979). Marked depth of ST segment depression during treadmill exercise testing: Indicator of severe coronary artery disease. *Chest, 69*, 729.

Goldschalger, N., Selzer, A., & Cohn, K. (1976). Treadmill stress tests as indications of presence and severity of coronary artery disease. *Annals of Internal Medicine, 85*, 277.

Gomez, G.E., & Gomez, E.A. (1984). Sudden death, biopsychosocial factors. *Heart and Lung, 13*, 389.

Gonzalez, E.R., Jones, L.A., Ornato, J.P., Bleecker G.G., & Strauss, M.J., (1992). Hospital delays and problems with thrombolytic administration in patients receiving thrombolytic therapy: A multicenter prospective assessment. Virginia Thrombolytic Study Group. *Annals of Emergency Medicine 21*, 1215–1221.

Gordon, M. (1987). *Nursing Diagnosis Process and Application*, 2nd ed. New York: McGraw-Hill.

Gordon, D.J., Probstfield, J.L., Garrison, R.R., Neaton, J.D., Castelli, W., Knoke, Jacobs, D., Bangdiwala, S., & Tyroler, A. (1989). High-density lipoprotein cholesterol and cardiovascular disease: Four prospective American studies. *Circulation, 79*, 8–15.

Gotoh, K., Minamino, T., Katoh, O., Hamano, Y., Fuki, S., Hori, M., Kusuoka, H., Mishima, M., Inoue, M., & Kamanda, T. (1988). The role of intracoronary thrombus in unstable angina: Angiographic assessment and thrombolytic therapy during ongoing anginal attacks. *Circulation, 77*, 526–534.

Gould, A., Rossouw, J., Santanello, N., Heyse, J., Ferberg, C. (1995). Cholesterol reduction yields clinical benefit: A new look at old data. *Circulation, 91(8)*, 2274–2282.

Grundy, S.M. (1986). Cholesterol and coronary heart disease: A new era. *Journal of the American Medical Association, 250*, 2849.

Grundy, S.M. (1993). *Second Report of the Expert Panel on Detection, Evaluation and Treatment of High Blood Cholesterol in Adults* (Adult Treatment Panel II). National Institutes of Health. NHLBI (NIH publication no. 93-3095).

Gunnar, R., Bourdillion, P., Dixon, D., Fuster, V., Karp, R., Kennedy, J., Klocke, F., Passamini, E., Betram, P., Rapaport, E., Reevws, T., Russell, R., Sobel, B., & Winters, W. (1990). ACC/AHA Task force report. Guidelines for the early management of patients with acute MI. *Journal of the American College of Cardiology, 16(2)*, 249–292.

Guzzetta, C., & Dossey, B. (1990). Cardiovascular assessment. In B. Dossey, C. Guzzetta, & C. Kenner. *Essentials of Critical Care Nursing: Body, Mind, Spirit*. Philadelphia: J.B. Lippincott.

Hanson, M. (1994). Modifiable risk factors for coronary heart disease in women. *American Journal of Critical Care, 3(3)*, 177–186.

Hayward, L.J. (1984). Coronary heart disease mortality, morbidity and risk in blacks. II: Access to medical care. *American Heart Journal, 108(3)*, 794–796.

Heatherton, T.F., Kozlowski, L.T., Frecker, R.C., & Fagerstrom, K.O. (1991). The Fagerstrom test for nicotine dependence: A revision of the Fagerstrom tolerance questionnaire. *British Journal Addiction, 86(9)*, 1: 119–121, 127.

Henningfield, J.E., & Nemeth-Coslett, R. (1988). Nicotine dependence: Interface between tobacco and tobacco-related diseases. *Chest, 93* (Suppl.), 37–55.

Hermanson, B., Omenn, G.S., Kronmal, R.A., & Gersh, B. (1988). Beneficial six-year outcome of smoking cessation in older men and women with coronary artery disease: Results from the CASS registry. *New England Journal of Medicine, 319(21)*, 1365–1369.

Heyden, S., Heiss, G., Bartel, A.G., & Hames, C. (1980). Sex differences in mortality among diabetics in Evans County, Georgia. *Journal of Chronic Disease, 33*, 265–273.

Hoeg, J. (1997). Evaluating coronary heart disease risk: Tiles in the mosaic. *Journal of American Medical Association, 277(17)*, 1387–1390.

Holm, K., & Penckofer, S. (1990). Coronary heart disease: Requisite knowledge for developing prevention strategies for the aging adult. *Progress in Cardiovascular Nursing, 5(4)*, 118–125.

Holmes, T., & Masuda, M. (1972). Psychosomatic syndrome. *Psychology Today*.

Holmes, T., & Rahe, R., (1967). The Social Readjustment Scale. *Journal of Psychosomatic Research, 11*, 213–218.

Hopkins, P., & Williams, R. (1986). Identification and relative weight of cardiovascular risk factors. *Cardiology Clinics. 4*, 3–31.

Hubert, H.B., Feinlieb, M., McNamara, P.M., & Castelli, W.P. (1983). Obesity as an independent risk factor for cardiovascular disease: A 26-year follow-up of participants in the Framingham Heart Study. *Circulation, 67*, 968–977.

Ishii, J., Nomura, M., Ando, T., Hasegawa, H., Kimura, M., Kurokawa, H., Iwase, M., Kondo, T., Wantanabe, Y., Hishida, H., Sotohata, I., & Mizuno, Y. (1994). Early detection of successful coronary reperfusion based on serum myoglobin concentration: Comparison with serum creatine kinase isoenzyme activity. *American Heart Journal, 128(4)*, 641–648.

Janz, N., & Becker, M., (1984). The health belief model a decade later. *Health Education Monograph, 11*, 1–47.

Jenkins, C.D., Rosenman, R.H., & Friedman, M. (1967). Development of an objective psychological test for the determination of coronary-prone behavior pattern in employed men. *Journal of Chronic Disease, 20*, 371–379.

Jenkins, C.D., Rosenman, R.H., & Zyzanski, S.J. (1974). Prediction of clinical coronary heart disease by a test for the coronary-prone behavior pattern. *New England Journal of Medicine, 290*, 1271–1275.

Kabat-Zin, J. (1992). Psychosocial factors: Their importance and management. In I. Ockene & J. Ockene (Eds.), *Prevention of Coronary Heart Disease*. Boston: Little, Brown & Co., pp. 299–333.

Kannel, W. (1987). New perspectives in cardiac risk factors. *American Heart Journal, 114(1)*, 213–219.

Kannel, W. (1990). Contribution of the Framingham study to preventive cardiology. *Journal of American College of Cardiology, 15(1)*, 206–211.

Kannel, W., Abbot, R. (1984). Incidence and prognosis of unrecognized myocardial infarction: An update of the Framingham study. *New England Journal of Medicine, 311*, 1144–1147.

Kannel, W., D'Agostino, R., & Belanger, A. (1992). Update on fibrinogen as a cardiovascular risk factor. *Annals of Epidemiology 2*, 457–466.

Kannel, W., Feinleib, M., McNamara, P., Garrison. R, & Castelli, W. (1979). An investigation of coronary heart disease in families: The Framingham Offspring study. *American Journal of Epidemiology, 110*, 281–290.

Kannel, W., & McGee, D. (1979). Diabetes anid cardiovascular disease: The Framingham study. *Journal of the American Medical Society, 241*, 2035–2038.

Kannel, W., McGee, D., & Gordon, T., (1976). A general cardiovascular risk profile: The Framingham heart study. *American Journal of Cardiology, 38*, 46–51.

Kannel, W., & Sorlie, P. (1979). Some health benefits of physical activity. The Framingham study. *Archives of Internal Medicine, 139*, 857–861.

Kannel, W., Wilson, P., & Blair, S. (1985). Epidemiological assessment of the role of physical activity and fitness in the development of cardiovascular disease. *American Heart Journal, 109(4)*, 876–885.

Kaplan, G., & Keil, J. (1993). Socioeconomic factors and cardiovascular disease: A review of the literature. *Circulation, 88(4)*, 1973–1998.

Kasl, S. (1984). Social and psychological factors in the etiology of coronary heart disease in black populations: An exploration of research needs. *American Heart Journal, 108(3)*, 660–668.

Kattus, A.A. (1974). Exercise electrocardiography: Recognition of the ischemic response, false positive and negative patterns. *American Journal of Cardiology, 33*, 721.

Keller, C., Fleury, J., & Bergstom, D. (1995). Risk factors for coronary heart disease in African American women. *Cardiovascular Nursing, 31*(2), 9–14.

Keller, K., & Lemberg, L. (1994). Q wave and non Q wave myocardial infarctions. *American Journal of Critical Care, 3*(2), 158–161.

Killen, J.D., Fortman, S.P., Newman, B., & Vardy, A. (1990). Evaluation of a treatment approach combining nicotine gum with self-guided behavioral treatments for smoking relapse prevention. *Journal of Clinical Counsel Psychology. 12*, 292–300.

Kirn, T.F. (1989). Research seeks to reduce toll of hypertension and other cardiovascular diseases in black population. *Journal of the American Medical Association, 261*, 195.

Kwiterovich, P.O., Coresh, J., Smith, H.H., Bachorik, P.S., Derby, C.A., & Pearson, T.A. (1992). Comparison of plasma levels of apolipoprotein B and A-1 and other risk factors in men and women with premature heart disease. *American Journal of Cardiology, 69*, 1015–1021.

Lambrew, C., Smith, M., Annas, G., & Bass, R. (1994). National Heart Attack Alert Program Coordinating Committee: 60 minutes-to-treatment working group. Emergency department rapid identification and treatment of patients with acute MI. *Annals of Emergency Medicine, 23*(2), 311–329.

Lavie C.J., Milani, R.V., & Littman, A.B. (1993). Benefits of cardiac rehabilitation and exercise training in secondary coronary prevention in the elderly. *Journal of the American College of Cardiology, 22*, 678–683.

Leeman, D.E., McCabe, C.A., Faxon, D.P., Lorel, B., Kellett, M., McCay, R., Varricchione, T., & Baim, D. (1988). Use of percutaneous transluminal coronary angioplasty and bypass surgery despite improved medical therapy for unstable angina pectoris. *American Journal of Cardiology, 61*, 38G–44G.

Leon, A.S., Connett, J., Jacobs D.R., & Rauramaa, R. (1987). Leisure-time physical activity levels and the risk of coronary heart disease and death: The Multiple Risk Intervention Trial. *Journal of the American Medical Association, 258*, 2388–2395.

Levin, L.A., Perk, J., & Hedlack, B. (1991). Cardiac rehabilitation: A cost analysis. *Journal of Internal Medicine, 230*, 427–434.

Levine, R.L., Pepe, P.E., Fromm, R.E., Curka, P.A., & Clark, P.A. (1992). Prospective evidence of a circadian rhythm for out-of-hospital cardiac arrest. *Journal of the American Medical Association, 267*, 2935–2937.

Lewy, R. (1980). *Preventive Primary Medicine: Reducing The Major Causes of Mortality.* Boston: Little, Brown & Co.

Manson, J., Colditz, G., Stampfer, M., Willett, W., Rosner, B., Monson, R., Spizer, F., & Hennekens, C. (1990). A prospective study of obesity and the risk of coronary artery disease in women. *New England Journal of Medicine, 322*(13), 882–889.

Manson J., Willett, W., Stampfer, M., Colditz, G., Hunter, D., Hankenson, S., Hennekens, C., & Speizer, F. (1995). Body weight and mortality among women. *New England Journal of Medicine, 333*(11), 677–685.

Mark, D.B., Hlatky, M.A., Lee, K.L., Harrell, F., Califf, R., & Pryor, D. (1987). Localizing coronary artery obstructions with the exercise treadmill test. *Annals of Internal Medicine, 106*(1), 53–55.

Martin, M.J., Hulley, S.B., Browner, W.S., Kuller, L.H., & Wentworth, D. (1986). Serum cholesterol, blood pressure and mortality: Implications from a cohort of 361,662 men. *Lancet, 2*, 933–936.

Matrisciano, L. (1992). Unstable angina: An overview. *Critical Care Nurse* (December), 30–40.

Matthews, K.A., Meilahn, E., Kuller, L.H., Kelsey, S., Caggiula, A., & Wings, R. (1989). Menopause and risk factors for coronary heart disease. *New England Journal of Medicine, 321*(10), 641–646.

McCance, K.L. (1983). Genetics: Implications for preventive nursing practice. *Journal of Advanced Nursing, 8*, 359–364.

McCauley, K. (1995). Assessing social support in patients with cardiac disease. *Journal of Cardiovascular Nursing, 10*(1), 73–80.

McLaughlin, M., Chesebro, J., & Fuster, V. (1996). Hypercoaguable states and cardiovascular disease. *ACC Current Journal Review* (May/June), 28–35.

Merkley, K. (1994). Assessing chest pain. *RN.*, 58–62.

Millar, D. (1992). Quantitative risk assessment: A tool to be used responsibly. *American Journal of Public Health Policy* (Spring), 5–13.

Miller, N.H., & Taylor, C.B. (1995). *Lifestyle Management for Patients with Coronary Heart Disease.* Champaign: Human Kinetics.

Millon, T., Green, C., & Meagher, R. (1982). *Millon Behavioral Health Inventory: Manual.* Minneapolis: National Computer Systems.

Mittleman, M., Maclure, M., Sherwood, J., Mulry, R., Tofler, G., Jacobs, S., Friedman, R., Benson, H., & Muller, J. (1995). Triggering of acute myocardial infarction onset by episodes of anger. *Circulation, 92*(7), 1720–1725.

Muller, J.E., Stone, P.H., Turi, Z.G., Rutherford, J., Czeisler, C., Parker, C., Poole, K., Passamani, E., Roberts, R., Robertson, T., Sobel, B., Willerson, J., & Braunwald, E. (1985). Circadian variation in the frequency of acute myocardial infarction. *New England Journal of Medicine, 313*(21), 1315–1322.

Murdaugh, C. (1990). Coronary artery disease in women. *Journal of Cardiovascular Nursing, 4*(4), 35–50.

Murdaugh, C., O'Rourke, R. (1988). Coronary heart disease in women: Special considerations. *Current Problems in Cardiology, 1*, 86–87.

Naccarelli, G.V., Nishikawa, A., Giebel, R., (1987). Patient assessment: Laboratory studies. In K. Andreoli, P. Zipes, A. Wallace, A., M. Kinney, & V. Fowkes, *Comprehensive Cardiac Care*, 6th ed. St. Louis: C.V. Mosby Co., pp. 58–81.

NDDG (1979). National diabetes data group classification and diagnosis of diabetes mellitus and other categories of glucose tolerance. *Diabetes, 28*, 1039–1057.

NIHCDP (1985). National Institutes of Health Consensus Development Conference statement: Health implications of obesity. February 11–13, 1985. *Annals of Internal Medicine, 103*, 1073–1077.

Nicolosi, R.J., & Schaefer, E.J. (1992). Pathobiology of hypercholesterolemia and atherosclerosis: Genetic and environmental determinants of elevated lipoprotein levels. In I. Ockene & J. Ockene (Eds.), *Prevention of Coronary Heart Disease.* Boston: Little, Brown and Co.

Oberman, A. (1985). Exercise and the primary prevention of cardiovascular disease. *American Journal of Cardiology, 55*, 10d–20d.

Ockene, J.K., Kuller, L.H., Svendsen, K.H., & Meilahn, E. (1990). The relationship of smoking cessation to coronary heart disease and lung cancer in the Multiple Risk Factor Intervention Trial (MRFIT). *American Journal of Public Health, 80*, 954–958.

O' Donnell, M.P., & Ainsworth, T.H. (Eds.) (1984). *Health*

Promotion in the Work Place. New York: Delmar Publishers.

Oldridge, N.B., Guyatt, G.H., Fischer, M.E., & Rimm, A.A. (1988). Cardiac rehabilitation after myocardial infarction: Combined experience of randomized clinical trials. *New England Journal of Medicine, 260*, 945–950.

Orchard, T. (1992). Intervention for the prevention of coronary heart disease in diabetes. In I. Ockene & J. Ockene (Eds.), *Prevention of Coronary Heart Disease.* Boston: Little, Brown & Co.

O'Rourke, R.A, Chatterjee, K., & Wei, J.Y. (1987). Coronary heart disease. *Journal of the American College of Cardiology, 10*(2), 52A–56A.

Paffenbarger, R.S., Hyde, R.T., Wing, A., & Hsieh, C.(1986). Physical activity, all-cause mortality, and longevity of college alumni. *New England Journal of Medicine, 314*(10), 605–613.

Pashkow, F. (1993). Issues in contemporary cardiac rehabilitation: A historical perspective. *Journal of the American College of Cardiology, 21*(93), 822–834.

Pasternak, R., Grundy, S., Levy, D., & Thompson, P. (1996). Task force 3. Spectrum of risk factors for coronary heart disease. *Journal of the American College of Cardiology, 27*(5), 978–990.

Pate, R., Pratt, M., Blair, S., Haskell, W., Macera, C., Bouchard, C., Buchner, D., Ettinger, W., Heath, G., King, A., Kriska, A., Leon, A., Marcus, B., Morris, J., Paffenberger, R., Patrick, K., Pollock, M., Rippe, J., Sallis, J., & Wilmore, J. (1995). Physical activity and public health. A recommendation from the Centers for Disease Control and Prevention and the American College of Sports Medicine. *Journal of the American College of Cardiology, 273*(5), 402–407.

Pearson, T., & Fuster, V. (1996). Twenty-Seventh Bethesda Conference. Matching the intensity of risk factor management with the hazard for coronary disease events. *Journal of the American College of Cardiology, 27*(5), 957–1047.

Pearson, T., McBride, P., Houston Miller, N., & Smith, S. (1996). Task force 8. Organization of Preventive Cardiology Services. *Journal of the American College of Cardiology, 27*(5), 1039–1047.

Peberdy, M., & Ornato, J.P. (1992). Coronary artery disease in women. *Heart Disease Stroke, 1*, 315–319.

Peeples, D., Fowkes, V., & Andreoli, K. (1987). Patient assessment: History and physical examination. In K. Andreoli, D. Zipes, A. Wallace, M. Kinney, & V. Fowkes (Eds.), *Comprehensive Cardiac Care.* 6th ed. St. Louis: C.V. Mosby Co., pp. 27–57.

Pekkanen, J., Linn, S., Heiss, G., Suchindran, C., Leon, A., Rifkind, B., & Tyroller, H. (1990). Ten-year mortality from cardiovascular disease in relation to cholesterol level among men with and without pre-existing cardiovascular disease. *New England Journal of Medicine, 322*(24), 1700–1707.

Pender, N. (1987). *Health Promotion in Nursing Practice,* 2nd ed. Norwalk, CT: Appleton and Lange.

PEPI (1995). Effects of estrogen or estrogen/progestin regimens on heart disease risk factors in postmenopausal women. The postmenopausal estrogen/ progestin interventions (PEPI) trial. *Journal of the American Medical Association, 273*(3), 199–228.

Powell, K., Thompson, P., Caspersen, C., & Kendrick, J. (1987). Physical activity and the incidence of coronary heart disease. *Annual Review of Public Health, 8*, 253–287.

Prochaska, J. (1994). Strong and weak principles for progressing from precontemplation to action based on 12 problem-solving behaviors. *Health Psychology, 13*, 47–51.

Prochaska, J.O., & DiClemente, C.C. (1983). Stages and processes of self-change of smoking: Toward an integrated model of change. *Journal of Consulting Clinical Psychology, 51*(3), 390–395.

Psaty, B.M., Heckbert, S.R., Atkins, D., Siscovick, D., Koepsell, T., Wahl, P., Longstreth, W., Weiss, N., Wagner, E., Prentice, R., & Furberg, C. (1993). A review of the association of estrogens and progesterone with cardiovascular disease in postmenopausal women. *Archives of Internal Medicine, 153*, 1421–1426.

Puelo, P.R., Guadagno, P.A., Roberts, R., Scheel, M., Marian, A., Churchhill, D., & Perryman, M. (1990). Early diagnosis of acute myocardial infarction based on assay for subforms of CPK-MB. *Circulation, 82*, 759–764.

Raglund, D.R., & Brand, R.J. 1988). Coronary heart disease in the Western Collaborative Group Study. *American Journal Epidemiology, 127*(3), 462–475.

Ratner, R. (1992). Review of diabetes mellitus. In Haire-Joshu, D. (Ed.), *Management of Diabetes Mellitus: Perspectives of Care Across the Life Span.* St. Louis: Mosby Year Book.

Reimer, K.A., Lowe, J.E., Rasmussen, M.M., & Jennings, R. (1977). The wave front phenomenon of ischemic cell death: I. Myocardial infarction size vs. duration of coronary occlusion in dogs. *Circulation*, 56, 786–794.

Remmell, P.S., & Benfari, R.C. (1980). Assessing dietary adherence in the Multiple Risk Factor Intervention Trial II. Food record rating as an indicator of compliance. *Jounal of the American Dietetic Association, 76*, 357–360.

Remmell, P.S., Gorder, D.D., Hall, L., & Tillotson, J.L. (1980). Assessing dietary adherence in the Multiple Risk Factor Intervention Trial I. Use of a dietary monitoring tool. *Journal of the American Dietetic Association, 76*, 351–356.

Report of the Expert Committee on the Diagnosis and Classification of Diabetes Mellitus (1997). *Diabetes Care, 20*, 1183–1197.

Roncaglioni, M., Santoro, L., D'Avanzo, B., Negri, E., Nobili, A., Ledda, A., Pietropaolo, F., Franzosi, M., La Vecchia, C., Feruglio, G., & Maseri, A. (1992). Role of family history in patients with myocardial infarction. An Italian case control study. GISSI-EFRIM investigators. *Circulation, 85*(6), 2065–2072.

Rossi, L., & Leary, E. (1992). Evaluating the patient with coronary artery disease. *Nursing Clinics of North America, 27*(1), 171–188.

Rozanski, A., Bairey, C., Krantz, D., Friedman, J., Resser, K., Morrell, M., Hilton-Chaflen, S., Hestrin, L., Bientendorf, J., & Berman, D. (1988). Mental stress and the induction of silent myocardial ischemia in patients with coronary artery disease. *New England Journal of Medicine, 318*(16), 1005–1011.

Rutherford, J.B., Braunwald, E., Cohn, P.F. (1988). Chronic ischemic heart disease. In E. Braunwald (Ed.), *Heart Disease: A Textbook of Cardiovascular Medicine.* Philadelphia: W.B. Saunders.

Schiro, A., & Grozinger Curtis, D. (1988). Asymptomatic CAD. *Heart and Lung, 17*(2), 144–149.

Schoenbach, V. (1987). Appraising health risk appraisal. *American Journal of Public Health, 77*(4), 409–411.

Scholtz, R.I., Rosenmann, R.H., & Brand, R.J. (1975). The relationship of reported parental history to the incidence of coronary heart disease in the Western Collaborative Study Group. *American Journal of Epidemiology, 102*, 350–356.

Semjos, C.T., Cleeman, J.I., Carroll, M.D., Johnson, C.L., Bachorik, D.S., Gordon, D.I., Burt, V.L., Brietal, R.R., Brown, C.D., Lippel, K., & Rifkind, B.M. (1993). Prevalence of high blood cholesterol among U.S. adults. *Journal of the American Medical Association, 23*, 3009–3014.

Seidel, H., Bale, J., Dains, J., & Benedict, G. (1991). *Mosby's Guide to Physical Examination* St. Louis: Mosby Year Book.

Selig, P. (1991). The prevention and screening of cardiovascular disease: An update. *Nurse Practitioner Forum, 2*(1), 14–18.

Sgarbossa, E., Pinski, S., Barbagelta, A., Underwood, D., Gates, K., Califf, R., & Wagner, G. (1996). Electrocardiographic diagnosis of evolving acute myocardial infarction in the presence of left bundle branch block. *New England Journal of Medicine, 334*(8), 481–487.

Shekelle, R.B., Gale, M., & Norusis, M. (1985). Type A behavior (Jenkins Activity Survey) and risk of recurrent coronary heart disease in the Aspirin Myocardial Infarction Study. *American Journal of Cardiology, 56*, 221–225.

Shekelle, R.B., Hully, S., Neaton, J., Billings, J., Borhani, N., Gerace, T., Jacobs, D., Lasser, N., Mittlemark, M., & Stamler, J. (1985). The Mr. Fit Behavior Pattern Study II. Type A behavior pattern and incidence of coronary heart disease. *American Journal Of Epidemiology. 122*(4), 559–570.

Sivarajan Froelicher, E., Berra, K., Stepp, C., Saxe, J., & Deitrich, C. (1995). Risk profile screening. *Journal of Cardiovascular Nursing, 10*(1), 30–50.

Sivarajan Froelicher, E., Kee, L., Newton, K.M., Lindskog, B., & Livingston, M. (1994). Return to work, sexual activity and other activities after acute myocardial infarction. *Heart and Lung, 23*, 423–435.

Smith, K. W., McKinlay, S., & Thorington, B. (1987). The validity of health risk appraisal instruments for assessing coronary heart disease risk. *American Journal of Public Health, 77*(4), 419–424.

Smokler, L.P. (1992). Clinical implications of non Q wave (subendocardial) myocardial infarctions. *Focus on Critical Care, 19*(1), 29–33.

Snowden, C., McNamara, P., Garrison, R., Feinlieb, M., Kannel, W., & Epstein, F. (1982). Predictive coronary heart disease in siblings: A multivariate assessment. The Framingham Heart Study. *American Journal of Epidemiology, 115*(2), 217–222.

Spielberger, C.D. (1983) *Manual of the State Trait Anxiety Inventory STAI Form Y.* Palo Alto, CA: Consulting Psychologists' Press.

Spielberger, C.D., Johnson, E., Russell, S., Crane, R., Jacobs, J., & Worden, T. (1985). The experience and expression of anger: Construction and validation of anger expression scale. *Anger and Hostility in Cardiovascular and Behavioral Disorders.* New York: Hemisphere McGraw-Hill.

Stadel, B.V. (1981). Oral contraceptives and cardiovascular disease. *New England Journal of Medicine, 305*, 672–677.

Stamler, J., Wentworth, D., & Neaton J. (1986). Is relationship between serum cholesterol and risk of premature death from coronary heart disease continuous and graded? Findings in 356,222 primary screens of the Multiple Risk Factor Intervention Trial (MRFIT). *Journal of the American Medical Association, 256*, 2823–2828.

Stampfer, M., & Colditz, G. (1991). Estrogen replacement therapy and coronary disease: A quantitative assessment of the epidemiologic evidence. *Preventive Medicine, 20*, 47–63.

Stampfer, M., Willett, W., Colditz, G., Speizer, F., & Hennekens, C. (1988). A prospective study of past use of oral contraceptive agents and risk of cardiovascular disease. *New England Journal of Medicine, 319*(20), 1313–1317.

Stillman, F. (1995). Smoking cessation for the hospitalized cardiac patient. Rationale for and report of a model program. *Journal of Cardiovascular Nursing, 9*(2), 25–36.

Stokes, J., Kannel, W., & Wolf, P.(1989). Blood pressure as a risk factor for cardiovascular disease: The Framingham Study, 30 years of follow-up. *Hypertension, 13*(Suppl. 1), IBl20.

Streff, M. (1987). Exercise in the prevention of coronary artery disease. *Journal of Cardiovascular Nursing, 1*(4), 42–53.

Swan, H., Gersh, B., Grayboys, T., & Ullyot, D.(1996). Task Force 7. Evaluation and management of risk factors for the individual patient (Case Management). *Journal of the American College of Cardiology, 27*(5), 1030–1039.

Theroux, P., Ouimet, H., McCans, J., Latour, J., Levy, G., Pelletier, E., Juneau, M., Stasiak, J., Deguise, P., Pelletier, G., Rinzler, D., & Waters, D. (1988). ASA heparin or both to treat acute unstable angina. *New England Journal Medicine, 319*(17), 1105–1111.

Thomas, S., & Liehr, P. (1995). Cardiovascular reactivity during verbal communication: An emerging risk factor. *Journal of Cardiovascular Nursing, 9*(2), 1–11.

Thompson, S., Kienast, J., Pyke, S., Haverkate, F., & Van De Loo, J.C. (1995). Hemostatic factors and the risk of myocardial infarction or sudden death in patients with angina pectoris. *New England Journal of Medicine, 332*(10), 635–641.

Tofler, G., Stone, P., Muller, J., Willich, S., Davis, V., Poole, W., Strauss, H., Willerson, J., Jaffe, A., Robertson, T., Passaman, E., & Braunwald, E. (1987). Effects of gender and race on prognosis after myocardial infarction: Adverse prognosis for women, particularly black women. *Journal of American College of Cardiology. 9*(3), 473–482.

Tresh, D.D. (1987). Atypical presentations of cardiovascular disorders in the elderly. *Geriatrics, 42*, 31–46.

Uber, L., & Uber, W. (1993). Hypertensive crisis in the 1990's. *Critical Care Nursing Quarterly, 16*(2), 27–34.

Utretski, B., Farguhar, B., Berezin, A., & Hood, W. (1977). Symptomatic myocardial infarction without chest pain: Prevalence and clinical course. *American Journal of Cardiology, 40*, 499–503.

Valle, B.K., & Lemberg, L. (1994). Estrogen replacement therapy in women: Prevention and treatment of CAD. *American Journal of Critical Care, 3*(5), 398–401.

Ward, A., Taylor, P., Ahlquist, L., Brown, D., Carlucci, D., & Rippe, J. (1992). Exercise intervention. In I. Ockene & J. Ockene (Eds.), *Prevention of Coronary Heart Disease.* Boston: Little, Brown & Co. pp. 267–298.

Ware, J.E., & Sherbourne, C.(1992). The MOS 36-item Short Form Health Survey (SF36). *Medical Care, 30*, 473–483.

Weaver, W., Litwin, P., Martin, J., Kudenchuk, P., Mynard, C., Eisenberg, M., Ho, M., Cobb, L., Kennedy, W., & Wirkus, M. M. (1991). Effect of age on use of thrombolytic therapy and mortality in acute myocardial infarction. *Journal of the American College of Cardiology, 18*(3), 657–662.

Webb, S.W., Adgey, A.A., & Pantridge, J.F. (1982). Autonomic disturbance at onset of acute myocardial infarction. *British Medical Journal*, 818, 89.

Wei, J.Y. (1984). Heart disease in the elderly. *Cardiovascular Medicine, 9*, 971–982.

Wei, J.Y., & Gersch, B.J. (1987). Heart disease in the elderly. *Current Problems in Cardiology, 12*(1), 1–65.

Wenger, N. (1985). Coronary disease in women. *Annual Review of Medicine, 36*, 285–294.

White, R.D., Grande, P., Califf, L., Palmeri, S., Califf, M., & Wagner, G. (1985). Diagnostic significance of minimally elevated creatine kinase MB in suspected acute myocardial infarction. *American Journal of Cardiology, 55*, 1478–84.

World Health Organization (1980). World Health Organization Expert Committee. *Second Report on Diabetes Mellitus* (Technical support series 646), Geneva.

Wingard, D.L., Barrett-Connor, E., Criqui, M.H., & Suarez, L. (1983). Clustering of heart disease risk factors in diabetics compared to non-diabetic adults. *American Journal of Epidemiology, 117*(1), 19–26.

Wingate, S. (1991). Women and heart disease: Implications for the critical care setting. *Focus on Critical Care, 18*, 212.

Wolf, P.L. (1989). Isoenzymes in myocardial disease. *Clinical Laboratory Medicine, 9*, 655–665.

Zevallos, J.C., Chiriboga, D., & Hebert, J.R. (1992). An international perspective on coronary heart disease and related risk factors. In I. Ockene & J. Ockene (Eds.), *Prevention of Coronary Heart Disease*. Boston: Little, Brown & Co., pp. 147–170.

Zung, W.(1965). A self-rating depression scale. *Archives of General Psychiatry, 12* 63–70.

CHAPTER 5

————
————
————
————
————
————
————
————
————
————
————
————
————

Communicating Risk to Patients

Michelle Fey
Nalini Jairath

Coronary heart disease (CHD) is the leading cause of death in the United States. Professional nurses are key members of the health-care team, and they share responsibility for educating clients in a variety of settings. Nurses are uniquely and powerfully situated to educate patients about the relationship of certain behaviors to CHD and to help them develop the skills required to make behavioral changes. Therefore, nurses, as well as other clinicians, play a major role in assisting people to change the health behaviors that place them at increased risk for CHD.

The initial phase in intervention for CHD risk reduction is communication of risk to the client. Furthermore, communication is an integral aspect of the counseling, client-education, and monitoring activities associated with risk-factor modification. Traditionally, communication of CHD risk has been performed in the relatively controlled environment of the clinician's office, clinic, or hospital. Now, however, risk-factor identification and communication of risk are being performed at health fairs and in other public settings, in part because of the greater availability and lowered cost of screening measures such as random cholesterol screening,

body-fat analysis, and so forth. As a result, communication of CHD risk may occur in potentially uncontrolled environments where no formal mechanisms for client follow-up exist. Another problem is that despite their importance, issues related to communication for reduction of CHD risk have been largely unexplored in the research, theoretical, and clinical literature. This chapter will address (1) the purpose of risk communication, (2) the process of risk communication, (3) barriers to effective risk communication, and (4) theoretical approaches pertinent to risk communication with individual clients and groups.

THE PURPOSE OF RISK COMMUNICATION

CHD risk communication is defined as the interchange and exchange of information between clinician and client about the nature, magnitude, and significance of CHD risk, as well as the strategies appropriate to control it. This definition draws upon general aspects of communication articulated by Briody (1984), Covello (1993), and Azjen & Fishbein (1980).

From the clinician's perspective, the purpose of CHD risk communication is to effect behavioral change leading to a decrease in the number or severity of CHD risk factors in the context of primary, secondary, or tertiary prevention. The client's perspective of the purpose may differ considerably from the clinician's and may emphasize comfort and support issues.

The benefits of good communication over time are well documented and include improved client satisfaction with care and enhanced physiologic outcomes. Clients in acute care settings rate communication as more important than technical competence (Del Mar, 1994; Kaplan, Greenfield, & Ware, 1989; and Epstein & Beckman, 1994). Some studies suggest that poor communication is associated with a greater likelihood of nonadherence to the health-care prescription (Francis, Korsch, & Morris, 1969; and Teasdale, 1993). Therefore, within the context of CHD risk, the communication process not only has the potential to influence behavior, but conceivably mortality and morbidity.

ETHICS OF RISK COMMUNICATION

Ethical considerations are central to CHD risk communication. Based on the fundamental principles of autonomy, beneficence, nonmaleficence, and justice, certain guidelines for CHD risk communication exist.

First, based on the principle of *autonomy*, clients have the right to self-determination, that is, to make their own decisions (Leddy & Pepper, 1993). Since knowledge is a precondition for informed decision making, clinicians are obligated to disclose all relevant information to clients about treatment and treatment alternatives.

Debate continues among clinicians about criteria for defining "relevant" information and about the appropriate emphasis, depth, and supportive evidence that should be presented. For example, as discussed in Chapter 12, controversy exists regarding the information that should be presented to clients about the role of antioxidant supplements. Our perspective is that all clients should be informed that promising new approaches such as antioxidant ther-

apy are being investigated. Then, for interested clients, the clinician should address the pros and cons of available approaches.

The second ethical guideline is based on the principle of *beneficence*, or the clinician's obligation to "do good." This means the clinician must always evaluate the relative risks versus benefits of interventions (Spivey, 1991; Strasser & Gallagher, 1994). When evaluating the risk-benefit ratio, the clinician should consider both the content and process of CHD risk communications. For example, interventional procedures for plaque reduction may be highly effective in the short term, and clients may not be interested in long-term considerations. However, since the underlying atherogenic processes will continue unless CHD risk factors are reduced, a detailed discussion of the need for CHD risk reduction is essential and consistent with the principle of beneficence.

The third guideline is based on the principle of *non-maleficence*, or the clinician's obligation to "do no harm." This means the clinician must not minimize, hide, or otherwise fail to communicate necessary risk information (Jonsen, 1991; Spivey, 1991). For example, when faced with a pattern of familial dyslipidemia, the clinician is obligated to attempt to inform other family members of their potential risk and assist them to obtain adequate testing, counseling, and other follow-up. Similarly, the clinician caring for clients with angina or myocardial infarction has an obligation to address the issue of CHD risk in the client's children. For minor children, CHD risk communication should occur with the client, spouse, guardian, or significant other.

The fourth principle, of *justice*, or "fairness," requires that all clients be given the same high-quality care irrespective of social conditions, economic status, personal attributes, or the nature of health problems (Leddy & Pepper, 1993). Justice necessitates that CHD risk communication by clinicians be equitable regardless of the client's circumstances. Furthermore, the clinician should expend the same degree of effort during CHD risk communication for all clients. From the societal perspective, the clinician is obligated to help achieve an equitable distribution of health information (Spivey, 1991). Despite potentially different priorities, homeless and affluent clients should both be evaluated for CHD risk, informed of their degree of risk, and counseled regarding risk-reduction strategies. The homeless client should receive at least equivalent effort, care, and concern as the affluent client.

Despite consensus regarding the importance of ethical principles, ambiguity in implementing these principles frequently exists in clinical settings. For example, the clinician may identify conflicts between the principles of autonomy and non-maleficence when caring for an adolescent client who smokes. Based on the principle of autonomy, the client has the right to smoke. Yet, the client may lack the emotional maturity to visualize a long-term future or to understand the potential damage of cigarette smoking. So, based on the principle of non-maleficence, the clinician may decide to use potentially coercive approaches such as forced attendance at smoking-cessation classes.

The constraints of the practice setting may make communication based on ethical principles problematic. For example, clients who undergo coronary artery bypass graft surgery may not be receptive to information regarding CHD risk communication prior to discharge because they are concerned with their immediate survival and not with a long-term future. Although, the principle of autonomy indicates that client must have access to information for informed decision making, the same principle requires that clinicians respect the client's right to refuse access. While suitable compromise is to provide information post discharge, mechanisms to provide clinicians with the necessary time and appropriate reimbursement for post-discharge counseling may be limited.

The state of knowledge regarding CHD and CHD risk reduction is complex, continuously evolving, and controversial. Clinicians may have varying degrees of sophistication in interpreting pertinent research and theoretical information. As discussed in Chapter 6, some clinicians adhere to the National Cholesterol Education Program (NCEP) guidelines regarding HDL cholesterol cut off points, or thresholds. However, in recognition that these cut off points may differ for women, some clinicians use different ones. Thus, even when ethical principles are adhered to, the content of CHD risk communications by clinicians may differ markedly.

In conclusion, basic ethical principles must be considered when structuring and analyzing CHD risk communication. Yet, the application of ethical principles to CHD risk communication may be difficult, and the subject has received little attention in the research and theoretical literature.

THE PROCESS OF RISK COMMUNICATION

CHD risk communication is most beneficial when the process is consciously structured. The process of communication may be conceptualized as having six basic components, or attributes, that should be considered prior to client contact: (1) the reason for the communication, (2) the sender, (3) the receiver, (4) the message, (5) the channel, and (6) feedback (Coutts & Hardy, 1985).

When identifying the *reason* for communication, the clinician may find it helpful to establish concrete, feasible goals prior to the initiation of communication (Baker, 1990; National Research Council, 1989). When applied to CHD risk, the clinician (the *sender*) communicates with the goal of helping the client (the *receiver*) modify behavior to effect CHD risk reduction. The content of the *message* may vary but typically includes identification of the client's risk for developing CHD or further complications of CHD, the existence of modifiable risk factors, and information about CHD risk-reduction strategies. Once the client is committed to reducing risk, communication may address issues that affect the client's ability to change behaviors. The *channel*, or communication medium, varies and may include conversation, printed literature, videotapes, and so on. *Feedback* from the client regarding the effectiveness of communication focuses on the degree to which the goal of CHD risk reduction has been achieved. Evaluation criteria may include demonstrable knowledge gain, verbalization of understanding, and, ultimately, objective data indicative of the risk reduction.

The conceptualization of the process of CHD risk communication presented in this chapter is based on general communication theory and, from our perspective, is inherently static. When planning and analyzing the communication process, we strongly recommend that the clinician also address the interactive nature of communication. Although most readers have already been formally exposed to salient aspects of verbal communication, nonverbal communication, and active listening as part of their clinical training, we will briefly review these aspects.

Verbal Communication

Ideally, risk communication uses language and concepts already understood by the client (National Research Council, 1989). Extrapolating from Bradley and Edinberg (1982), two basic types of language are pertinent to CHD risk communication: (1) the language of caring and (2) technical language. The *language of caring* addresses the clients' problems, prognosis, and progress and must always be used. *Technical language* addresses health-care terminology and helps ensure that clients receive "accurate" information about their health care. Technical language must be used judiciously. Tradeoffs exist between the client's legal and ethical right to know exact terminology and the client's need to truly understand the basis and nature of interventions. "Translation" of technical language into terms easily understood by the layperson can partially resolve these tradeoffs. In addition, providing translation and opportunities for the client to seek clarification of terminology can help to allay the client's fears and diffuse anxiety (Gregory & Cotler, 1994). Technical terms to be translated would include, for example, "risk factors, probability of disease progression, coronary artery disease, lipid reduction, triglyceridemia, hormone replacement therapy."

Nonverbal Communication

Whereas information on CHD risk reduction is conveyed through verbal, written, or audiovisual media, nonverbal communication explicitly addresses the affective components of communication. The clinician's nonverbal communication is important in establishing the trust and credibility necessary for effective CHD risk communication and in reinforcing messages communicated. In addition, the client's nonverbal communication helps the clinician assess the client's understanding of and receptiveness to the message, as well as the client's feelings and needs, thus providing the agenda for the next encounter.

Nonverbal communication exists whenever direct clinician-client encounters occur and is multidimensional in nature (Smith & Bass, 1979). In addition to facial expression, eye contact, body movements, and touch, the clinician should also consider spatial relationships when structuring and analyzing CHD risk communication. Typically, of the four zones of distance awareness used by adult North Americans, clinicians will find the personal zone of approximately 1/2 to 4 feet from arm's length most effective for therapeutic communications.

Active Listening

Listening is a major part of the communication process. *Active listening* involves the clinician focusing attention on the client's words and nonverbal cues. In addition, the clinician must interpret and often extrapolate from what is being said in order to understand the underlying message (Bradley & Edinberg, 1982; Smith & Bass, 1979). Del Mar (1994), Munn (1980), and Gregory and Cotler (1994) have all addressed the issue of active listening within the context of the clinician-client encounter. They conclude that, during active listening, the clinician must (1) want to listen, (2) be willing to suspend judgment and accept the client, (3) allow and encourage the client to express his or her feelings, and (4) be aware of personal feelings during the interaction, and integrate them into the conversation when appropriate (Munn, 1980).

Within the context of CHD risk communication, the clinician should be vigilant for indications of self-blame, low self-efficacy with respect to specific behaviors, denial of the severity of existing CHD or risk of developing CHD, lack of understanding of underlying concepts related to CHD risk reduction, and uncertainty regarding the meaning and implications of CHD in the client's life. In addition, as with all client encounters, the clinician should listen for evidence of anger, anxiety, and depression.

In conclusion, the process of communication is multifaceted and requires many skills.

"Good" communication may be characterized as being purposeful and focused, appropriate to the situation, timely, tactful, personal, clear, and precise (Smith & Bass, 1979). Whereas good communication of risk cannot always be expected to improve a situation, poor risk communication will nearly always make it worse (National Research Council on Risk, 1989).

Barriers to Effective CHD Risk Communication

Extrapolating from the general communication literature and our clinical experience, several major barriers to effective CHD risk communication exist. The first barrier is failure to choose an appropriate time frame and context for intervention. For example, during the early period following a myocardial infarction, clients are most receptive to concrete information directly relevant to current circumstances. They may be less interested in CHD risk reduction with its emphasis on long-term behavioral change immediately after an acute cardiac event.

The second barrier to effective CHD risk communication is equating knowledge gain with behavioral change such that issues related to the client's motivation for change and perceived self-efficacy are neglected. A common misconception about CHD risk communication is that with appropriate knowledge, the client will comply with risk-reducing behavior. In actuality, the relationship between education and adherence to clinician recommendations regarding various health issues has not been definitively determined (Burke & Dunbar-Jacob, 1995). Furthermore, even when knowledge results in attitudinal change, correlations between general attitudes and behavior are not very high (Baker, 1990). Therefore, knowledge and positive attitudes are more appropriately viewed as preconditions or resources for behavioral change.

Self-efficacy is regarded as a critical factor for modifying the effectiveness of knowledge gain in changing behavior. Self-efficacy increases with competence and mastery of skills in the initial phases, but specific communication may be necessary to bolster clients' confidence that they can ultimately change their behavior and maintain the changes. For a detailed discussion of the role of motivation and self-efficacy in changing behavior, see Chapter 3.

The third barrier to effective CHD risk communication is clinician failure to acknowledge the probabilistic nature of CHD risk when evaluating risk and subsequently communicating with clients. For example, a 20-year-old female who has a serum cholesterol of 250 mg/dl and has been smoking a pack of cigarettes per day for 3 years is at relatively low risk for developing CHD, primarily because of her age. However, CHD risk increases dramatically if the client continues smoking through menopause, and escalates even higher if she doesn't lower her serum cholesterol. To effectively address these factors, the clinician must help the client understand the probabilistic nature of risk, the progressive damage to the arterial system, and the inevitable increase of risk over time unless she stops smoking.

A fourth barrier to effective CHD risk communication is clinician failure to recognize the threshold beyond which communication may not influence behavior. As previously discussed, clients use probabilistic thinking when making decisions. Therefore, although communication can be used to alter clients' perceived susceptibility to CHD, ultimately clients take calculated risks and assume responsibility for their healthcare decisions (Harlem, 1977). Failure to acknowledge the client's right to make decisions, even ones deemed injudicious, can introduce anger and other counterproductive emotions into subsequent client-clinician communications.

The fifth barrier to effective communication is failure to address factors that impair the ability to assimilate information. Prochaska, Norcross, and DiClemente (1994) term these factors *perceptual blinders*. These investigators suggest people understand what they want to understand. Based on the communication and patient education literature, additional perceptual blinders may include learning disabilities, poor language skills, inattention or distraction, denial of illness, cognitive or sensory overload, and different values and health beliefs.

The sixth barrier to effective CHD risk communication is failure to acknowledge today's changing power relationships and dynamics of clinician-client relationships. Clients are beginning to understand that knowledge about health and illness is not the exclusive property of health professionals, and they are beginning to expect their questions to be answered as a right (Noble, 1991). Furthermore, with empowerment, clients may increasingly assume responsibility for making their own health-care decisions, including those associated with behavioral change. Therefore, during CHD risk communication, goals for behavioral changes, priority setting, and intervention strategies must be mutually negotiated and implemented.

Additional barriers to effective CHD risk communication exist in every clinician's practice. In identifying these barriers, we have found it helpful to consider the interfaces between clinicians, clients, and the environment. Barriers may also be detected using evaluation techniques in which the clinician may (1) identify a setting-specific critical path for his or her CHD risk communication, (2) determine the proportion of clients achieving certain benchmarks and clinical outcomes, (3) identify variances from the critical path, and (4) revise CHD risk communication patterns.

Suppose a clinician determines that following intervention, 90% of clients can identify strategies to decrease sedentary behavior, but only 20% subsequently change their behavior. Analysis of variances from the critical path indicates that 30% of the clients who do not change their behavior cite winter weather as a major contributory factor. In analyzing the situation, the clinician recognizes that one of the barriers to CHD risk communication has been a failure to identify client-specific strategies for decreasing sedentary behavior. As a result, the clinician modifies his or her clinical practice to address the way in which clients can adapt general activity guidelines to their specific situations.

THEORETICAL MODELS OF COMMUNICATION

Several models of communication exist, as well as models in which communication is an essential element. Although these models are at different levels of abstraction, and their successful application depends on the clinical context, they are useful tools for the clinician. Some approaches are especially useful for working

with individual clients; others can be used for broader-based approaches. Each of these models will be discussed and the implications for CHD risk communication addressed.

CHD Risk Reduction with Individual Clients

TRANSTHEORETICAL MODEL OF BEHAVIORAL CHANGE. Communication is an inherent component of interventions based on the widely used *transtheoretical model of behavioral change* (TTM). As discussed in detail in Chapter 3, based on the TTM, the process of CHD risk reduction involves six consecutive stages of change through which a client progresses: (1) precontemplation, (2) contemplation, (3) preparation, (4) action, (5) maintenance, and (6) termination. Interventions for risk reduction should be stage-appropriate. When mismatch between the stage and the selected intervention occurs, behavioral change may be adversely affected.

As discussed in Chapter 3, approximately 90% of clients fall within the first three stages, for which presentation of factual information regarding the need to change is a stage-appropriate intervention. As a result, communication of CHD risk may constitute one of the few health interventions applicable and beneficial to the majority of clients at high risk for CHD development or disease progression.

Extrapolating from the TTM, we recommend that the content communicated to clients should include (1) the existence of risk of CHD because of the presence of CHD risk factors, (2) their relative likelihood of developing a CHD-related disease that may require treatment and may ultimately result in their death, and (3) how CHD risk can be reduced by changes in lifestyle. This information should be communicated directly to the client in a neutral, nonjudgmental manner.

Research regarding the TTM also indicates that during the early stages of change, clients focus less upon the benefits, or "pros," of the behavioral change and more upon the drawbacks, or "cons." Accordingly, whereas the nurse should clearly delineate the benefits of CHD risk reduction, equal or greater emphasis should be used in dealing with the client's perceived "cons."

For example, the nurse could use the explanation shown in Box 5–1 when working with a client who has suffered an acute myocardial infarction and is receiving discharge preparation.

THEORY OF REASONED ACTION. The *theory of reasoned action* (TRA) is a decision model that incorporates the effects of both personal and social factors on behavior (Laschinger & Goldenberg, 1993). This theory states that a client's behavior is a function of his or her intention to perform the behavior (Pender & Pender, 1986). Behavioral *intention* is determined by the client's attitude toward the behavior and his or her subjective norms (Pender & Pender). *Attitude* refers to the person's judgment that performing the behavior is good or bad (Ajzen & Fishbein, 1980). *Subjective norms* encompass the client's perceptions about what important others expect him or her to do (Laschinger & Goldenberg). In general, people will intend to perform a certain behavior when they evaluate it positively and when they believe that important others think they should perform it (Ajzen & Fishbein). Therefore, the communication between the client and important others is a crucial consideration in intervention.

To effect behavioral change, the clinician could conceivably emphasize his or her legiti-

---

BOX 5–2 PATIENT EDUCATION EXAMPLE: THEORY OF REASONED ACTION

For five years, I have been your nurse practitioner. I care about you greatly and am really concerned that you are smoking. Smoking is very bad for your health and can ultimately kill you. It is imperative that you stop.

Mrs X, how do you feel about your husband's smoking? Are you willing to make your house a smoke-free house for the sake of your husband's health?

---

mate authority as a health professional and the importance of an ongoing clinician-client relationship. Furthermore, the clinician could enlist the support of the client's important others in communicating the need for behavioral change and supporting subsequent risk-reduction efforts. Although this approach is in marked contrast to the neutral approach consistent with the TTM, it may be appropriate in situations where rapid change is imperative. For example, Box 5–2 shows what a clinician could say, based on the TRA, in meeting with a smoker recovering from a myocardial infarction and his wife.

CHD Risk Reduction with High-Risk Groups

DIFFUSION THEORY. As described by Boutwell (1994), *diffusion theory* is a general communication theory that can be used for public health initiatives. The theory's underlying premise is that an intervention can be introduced and spread throughout a population using "diffusion" techniques. Involved communication media include television, radio, and written materials such as magazine or newspaper articles. Exposed individuals (i.e., recipients) will transmit the intervention received in a way that gradually diffuses, or permeates it throughout the target populations.

The degree of diffusion and consequent behavior change depends on each recipient's characteristics and the nature of the intervention. Diffusion is enhanced if a recipient perceives the intervention to be relatively advantageous, compatible with existing beliefs or ideas,

---

BOX 5–1 PATIENT EDUCATION EXAMPLE: TRANS-THEORETICAL MODEL

I'm really glad to hear that you are interested in learning about things you can do to make another heart attack less likely. We know that certain factors called "risk factors" give a person like you a greater chance of having heart disease. The good news is that many of these risk factors can be addressed so that your chance of having another heart attack is decreased. For example, you are a smoker. Smoking greatly increases the chance or risk of your having another heart attack. Stopping smoking will decrease the chance that you will have another heart attack.

It is possible to stop smoking. I am committed to helping you quit smoking when you are ready, or, at the very least, working with you so that you become ready to consider stopping.

and of manageable complexity. In addition, interventions are more diffusible if they are easy to communicate and explain, have low potential risk, are administered over a longer time frame, and have little inherent uncertainty.

Diffusion techniques have been successfully used in public health campaigns against risk factors such as smoking and sedentary behavior. The clinician could apply diffusion theory to risk-reduction strategies involving groups of clients or client-family clusters as indicated in Box 5–3.

LINKAGE APPROACH. The *linkage approach* posits that communication can be effected by linking, or connecting, a resource system such as that represented by the health-care professionals with a user system such as that represented by the health-care consumer. Although not a discrete theory with clear constructs, this approach bridges the gap between the emergence of new information and its diffusion. Linkages may be effected by incorporating new information into new or existing forums for patient communication and education (Padilla & Bulcavage, 1991). These forums may include broad-based community education, television, videotapes, radio, newspapers, and magazines. Box 5–4 gives an example.

BOX 5–3 PATIENT EDUCATION EXAMPLE: DIFFUSION THEORY

The diet of some adolescents is high in fat, placing these clients at risk for CHD over the long term unless their diet is modified. The school health nurses or dietician could devise an intervention targeting adolescents and their families and designed to (1) increase knowledge of the risk of high fat intake, (2) increase knowledge of the fat content of various foods, and (3) provide strategies for dietary fat reduction. Information could be disseminated through newsletters to the adolescents and their families, presentations at parent-teacher meetings, and in-class presentations to students. To increase the chances of success, the school nurse or dietician could decrease the complexity of information provided by restricting information on high-fat foods to a list of fast foods. The school nurse or dietician could increase the perceived advantage of switching to a lower-fat diet by emphasizing the relationship between high fat intake and obesity and possible linkages between diet and complexion.

BOX 5–4 PATIENT EDUCATION EXAMPLE: LINKAGE APPROACH

As discussed in detail in Chapter 14, new information is emerging regarding the role of hormone replacement therapy for postmenopausal women in reducing CHD risk. Client access to this new information is variable, so some women who might conceivably benefit from treatment may be unaware of its availability. Therefore, the clinician may choose to prepare a letter or handout for clients, present information at a health fair, or issue a news release or commentary about the issue.

SOCIAL POWER THEORY. The *social power theory* recognizes the potential influence of other people, groups, and societal forces on behavior (Padilla & Bulcavage, 1991). Behavioral change may be positively influenced by "healthy" group norms and communication of information regarding "acceptable," normative behavior. Although a detailed discussion of social power theory is beyond the scope of this chapter, communication of acceptable, normative behavior can dramatically change behavior. Box 5–5 suggests a possible application of this theory.

MCGUIRE'S PERSUASION MATRIX AND OTHER PERSUASION MODELS. The *persuasion matrix* views communication from the vantage point of persuasion. McGuire (1985) conceptualizes persuasion as a series of sequential steps. The success of each step is contingent on successful

---

BOX 5–5 PATIENT EDUCATION EXAMPLE: SOCIAL POWER THEORY

As a public health nurse in a poor community, you are concerned about the number of adolescents starting to smoke. Although you have tried various strategies, your clients view smoking as the "done" thing. In an attempt to reshape the general perception that smoking is acceptable, you ask well-known athletes to write letters for display indicating that smoking is not cool. You also use American Lung Association resources to emphasize the effect of smoking on physical appearance and breath. Finally, you arrange for teachers to replay a recent antismoking commercial by the U.S. Olympic Women's Soccer Team.

completion of preceding steps. The steps are (a) attention, (b) comprehension, (c) yielding, (d) retention, and (e) action. The outcome is behavioral change.

Several variables influence successful implementation of these steps. The variables that affect the *communicator*, or source (i.e., clinician), include credibility, power, and knowledge. The variables that affect the *message* include style, type of information, organization, and repetition. The *medium* by which a message is communicated is affected by the type of modality (i.e., printed material, videotape, conversation), verbal versus nonverbal, and the context in which the interaction occurs. Finally, variables that influence the *client* include personality, ability, demographics, motivation, and amount of participation (Boutwell, 1994). These variables constitute a ''matrix'' that the clinician must address during CHD risk communication.

The McGuire matrix model is one of several models of persuasive communication. These models assume that attitude change depends on knowledge gain; thus, communication is viewed from the perspective of transmission of knowledge. Such models are essentially unidirectional in that the clinician's stance is not subject to modification through persuasion. Persuasion models are useful when confusion exists regarding a CHD risk factor, requiring a particularly clear, direct, focused message, as in the situation described in Box 5–6.

INFERENTIAL MODEL. Communication is viewed as a problem-solving process in the *inferential model*. The variables influencing communication are similar to those in McGuire's persuasion matrix. However, in the inferential model, messages are viewed as inherently subjective, influenced both by the clinician's intention and inferences as well as the client's interpretation of these factors. (Teasdale, 1993). Therefore, when using persuasive communication, the communicator's thoughts must be ''coded'' into written or oral verbal communication, then ''decoded'' by the receiver (Teasdale, 1993). From our perspective, the main strength of this model is its emphasis on the need for the clinician to address discrepancies between messages sent and those received. Box 5–7 presents an example.

BOX 5–6 PATIENT EDUCATION EXAMPLE: PERSUASION MODELS

As an advanced-practice nurse running a weekly health clinic at a senior citizens' center, you encounter a large number of clients with CHD or a risk for CHD. Many of these clients have a high-fat diet and are reluctant to reduce fat intake. From their perspective, advice to severely reduce the intake of eggs, switch to skim milk, remove the skin and fat from meats is counter-intuitive. Their knowledge and beliefs date back to those of their youth when eggs, cream, and large, fatty portions of meat were believed to improve health. Furthermore, slight heaviness was associated with beauty and prosperity.

You structure an intervention based on McGuire's persuasion matrix. In order to ensure that client's "attend" to the message, you host an afternoon tea and social, open to all senior citizens. Flyers and invitations indicate that the topic will be "The More Things Change, the More They Stay the Same: A Few Words about Healthy Eating." You use nostalgia, memory, and the power of tradition to help with "comprehension." In addition to generic information about the need to reduce dietary fat and its benefits, your message focuses on traditional diets used in olden times. Using a historical perspective, you evoke a time when routine consumption of certain high-fat foods was a luxury. Clients remember their parents' stories of past times when farm children drank the whey of milk because the cream was sold for profit. They remember the war years and rationing of food. You introduce the idea that in these hardships, there were some good dietary aspects, and you explain that many of those aspects are now being reintroduced to diets because they were healthy. You suggest that, as in the past, certain high-fat foods should be viewed as a special treat, not for routine eating.

Gradually, you see clients "yielding" to the message. To facilitate "retention" and "action," you organize clients to prepare and use a cookbook of "heart healthy" recipes.

CONCLUSION

In conclusion, understanding the dynamics and complexities of CHD risk communication is essential. CHD risk communication requires adherence to ethical principles and planning and analysis of communications. The process of CHD risk communication may be conceptualized in different ways, but it always involves

BOX 5-7 PATIENT EDUCATION EXAMPLE: INFERENTIAL MODEL

During an annual health checkup, you note that a client's systolic blood pressure is elevated. After following the procedures articulated in Chapter 9 for ensuring that the blood pressure reading is not falsely elevated, you initiate a plan for blood pressure reduction. The first step is to communicate the increased CHD risk associated with elevated blood pressure, the need for change, and the importance of adhering to the proposed treatment regimen. Unfortunately, when you attempt to present this information to the client, she absolutely insists that she not be placed on medication. In analyzing the interaction, you see this discrepancy: From your perspective, the client must change her behavior for health reasons, and in refusing medication, she is being "non-compliant." However, from the client's perspective, the communication that she should be placed on medication means that her financial burden is dramatically increased for the rest of her life and that she is no longer a "healthy" person but a "sick" person.

both verbal and nonverbal communication, as well as active listening. Skills for CHD risk communication may be learned and should be continually refined. Several theoretical approaches are pertinent to understanding CHD risk communication. Selection of the appropriate approach depends on the clinical context and on particular clinician and client characteristics.

References

Azjen, I., & Fishbein, M. (1980). *Understanding Attitudes and Predicting Social Behavior*. Englewood Cliffs, NJ: Prentice-Hall.

Baker, F. (1990). Risk communication about environmental hazards. *Journal of Public Health Policy, 11*, 341–359.

Berger, E.S., & Hender, W.R. (1989). The expression of health risk information. *Archives of Internal Medicine, 149*, 1507–1508.

Boutwell, W.B. (1994). Theory-based approaches for improving biomedical communications. *Journal of Biomedical Communication, 21*, 2–6.

Bradley, J.C., & Edinberg, M.A. (1982). *Communication in the Nursing Context*. New York: Appleton-Century-Crofts.

Briody, M.E. (1984). The role of the nurse in modification of cardiac risk factors. *Nursing Clinics of North America, 19*, 387–395.

Burke, L.E., & Dunbar-Jacob, J. (1995). Adherence to medication, diet, and activity recommendations: From assessment to maintenance. *Journal of Cardiovascular Nursing, 9*, 62–79.

Cassel, E.J. (1985). *Talking with Patients*. Cambridge, MA: The MIT Press.

Conway, J.J. (1992). Communicating risk information in medical practice. *Radiographics, 12*, 207–214.

Coutts, L.C., & Hardy, L.K. (1985). *Teaching for Health: The Nurse as Health Educator*. Edinburgh, Scotland: Churchill Livingstone.

Covello, V.T. (1993). Risk communication and occupational medicine. *Journal of Occupational Medicine, 35*, 18–19.

Del Mar, C.B. (1994). Communicating well in general practice. *The Medical Journal of Australia, 160*, 367–370.

DiClemente, C.C., & Prochaska, J.O. (1982). Self-change and therapy change in smoking behavior: A comparison process of change in cessation and maintenance. *Addictive Behavior, 7*, 133–144.

Epstein, R.M., & Beckman, H.B. (1994). Health care reform and patient-physician communication. *American Family Physician, 49*, 1718–1720.

Fleury, M.L. (1984). *The Healing Bond*. Englewood Cliffs, NJ: Prentice-Hall, Inc.

Fiesta, J. (1994). Communication—Are you listening? *Nursing Management, 25* (9), 15–16.

Francis, V., Korsch, B.M., & Morris, M.J. (1969). Gaps in doctor-patient communication: Patients' response to medical advice. *The New England Journal of Medicine, 280*, 535–540.

Greene, M.G., Adelman, R.D., Friedmann, & Charon, R. (1994). Older patient satisfaction with communication during an initial medical encounter. *Social Science Medicine, 38*, 1279–1287.

Gregory, D.R., & Cotler, M.P. (1994). The problem of futility: III. The importance of physician-patient communication and a suggested guide through the minefield. *Cambridge Quarterly of Healthcare Ethics, 3*, 257–269.

Harlem, O.K. (1977). *Communication in Medicine: A Challenge to the Profession*. Basel, Switzerland: Karger.

Jonsen, A.R. (1991). Ethical considerations and responsibilities when communicating health risk information. *Journal of Clinical Epidemiology, 44*, (Suppl. 1), 69S–72S.

Kaplan, S.H., Greenfield, S., & Ware, J.E., Jr. (1989). Assessing the effects of physician-patient interactions on the outcomes of chronic disease. *Medical Care, 27* (Suppl. 3), S110–S127.

Keeney, R.L. (1994). Decisions about life-threatening risks. *The New England Journal of Medicine, 331*, 193–196.

Laschinger, H.K.S., & Goldenberg, D. (1993). Attitudes of practicing nurses as predictors of intended care behavior with persons who are HIV positive: Testing the Ajzen-Fishbein theory of reasoned action. *Research in Nursing & Health, 16*, 441–450.

Leddy, S., & Pepper, J.M. (1993). *Conceptual Bases of Professional Nursing*. Philadelphia: J.B. Lippincott.

McGuire, W. (1985). Attitudes and attitude change. In G. Lindzey & E. Aronson (Eds.), *The Handbook of Social Psychology*, 3rd ed. Reading, MA: Addison-Wesley.

Morgan, A.K. (1994). Client education experiences in professional nursing practice—A phenomenological perspective. *Journal of Advanced Nursing*, 792–801.

Munn, H.E., Jr. (1980). *The Nurse's Communication Handbook*. Germantown, MD: Aspen Systems Corporation.

National Research Council Committee on Risk Perception and Communication (1989). *Improving risk communication*. Washington, DC: National Academy Press.

Noble, C. (1991). Are nurses good patient educators? *Journal of Advanced Nursing, 16*, 1185–1189.

Ockene, I.S., & Ockene, J.K. (1992). *Prevention of Coronary Heart Disease*. Boston: Little, Brown & Co.

Padilla, G.V., & Bulcavage, L.M. (1991). Theories used in patient/health education. *Seminars in Oncology Nursing, 7*, 87–94.

Pender, N.J., & Pender, A.R. (1986). Attitudes, subjective norms, and intentions to engage in health behaviors. *Nursing Research, 35*, 15–18.

Prochaska, J.O., & DiClemente, C.C. (1992). *Stages of Change in the Modification of Problem Behaviors*. Sycamore, IL: Sycamore Publishing Co.

Prochaska, J.O., Norcross, J.C., & DiClemente, C.C. (1994). *Changing for Good*. New York: William Morrow.

Purtillo, R. (1990). *Health Professional and Patient Interaction*, 4th ed. Philadelphia: W.B. Saunders.

Shives, L.R. (1990). *Basic Concepts of Psychiatric-Mental Health Nursing*, 2nd ed. Philadelphia: J.B. Lippincott.

Smith, C.E. (1987). *Patient Education: Nurses in Partnership with Other Health Professionals*. Orlando, FL: Grune & Stratton.

Smith, V.M., & Bass, T.A. (1979). *Communication for Health Care Professionals*. Philadelphia: J.B. Lippincott.

Spivey, G.H. (1991) Health risk communication—A view from within industry. *Journal of Clinical Epidemiology, 44* (Suppl. 1), 63S–67S.

Stovsky, B. (1992). Nursing interventions for risk factor reduction. *Nursing Clinics of North America, 27*, 257–269.

Strasser, T., & Gallagher, J. (1994). The ethics of health communication. *World Health Forum, 15*, 175–177.

Teasdale, K. (1993). Information and anxiety: A critical appraisal. *Journal of Advanced Nursing, 18*, 1125–1132.

Thomas, S.A., & Liehr, P. (1995). Cardiovascular reactivity during verbal communication: An emerging risk factor. *Journal of Cardiovascular Nursing, 9*, 1–11.

SECTION II

INDIVIDUAL RISK FACTORS

CHAPTER 6

Dietary Factors*†

Susan R. Rossi
Satya S. Jonnalagadda
Penny M. Kris-Etherton

Dietary factors and their relationship to the lipid profile play a central role in coronary heart disease (CHD) risk reduction. The major modifiable risk factors for CHD are elevated blood *total cholesterol* (TC), elevated *low-density lipoprotein* (LDL) cholesterol, hypertension, and cigarette smoking (U.S. Department of Health and Human Services, 1993). Other risk factors include low levels of *high-density lipoprotein* (HDL) cholesterol (<35 mg/dl), diabetes mellitus, elevated *triglycerides* (TG), and overweight and obesity (U.S. Department of Health and Human Services, 1993). A high level of HDL cholesterol (>60 mg/dl) is protective against CHD and is counted as a negative risk factor (Table 6–1). The number of risk factors present,

together with LDL and HDL cholesterol levels, are considered in making treatment decisions.

With the advent of cost containment and massive restructuring of health-care delivery, nurses and other clinicians are being forced to assume a more active role in counseling patients with lipid abnormalities regarding the necessity to reduce dietary fat, LDL cholesterol, and caloric intake. The purpose of this chapter is to provide the clinician with a working understanding of the relationship between the lipid profile and CHD risk, the genetic forms of hyperlipidemias, and structural approaches to modifying diet for primary and secondary prevention. In addition, this chapter addresses the application of the *transtheoretical model* (TTM), discussed in Chapter 3, to reducing dietary fat. Our premise is that this detailed discussion will also assist the clinician in applying TTM strategies to modification of other CHD risk factors.

RELATIONSHIP BETWEEN LIPID PROFILE AND CHD RISK

As shown in Figure 6–1, the Multiple Risk Factor Intervention Study reported that mortality

---

*Material regarding the focus of dietary interventions was drawn from Table 1 in "Changing Addictive Behaviors: A Process Perspective" by C.C. DiClemente, 1993, *Current Directions in Psychological Science, 2*, (4), p. 102. Copyright 1993 by Cambridge University Press. Adapted with permission.

†Copies of Transtheoretical Model based dietary, weight control, smoking and exercise measures and papers associated with abstracts may be obtained from the University of Rhode Island, Cancer Prevention Research Center, Behavioral Sciences Center Building, Chafee Road, Kingston, RI 02881http://www.uri/research/cprc.

TABLE 6–1 Risk Status Based on Presence of CHD Risk Factors Other Than LDL Cholesterol

---

Positive Risk Factors
Age
    Male: ≥45 years
    Female: ≥55 years or experiencing premature
      menopause without estrogen replacement
      therapy
Family history of premature CHD (definite
    myocardial infarction or sudden death in
    father or other male first-degree relative before
    55 years of age or in mother or other female
    first-degree relative before 65 years of age)
Current cigarette smoking
Hypertension (≥140/90 mm Hg* or patient is on
    antihypertensive medication)
Low HDL cholesterol (<35 mg/dl*)
Diabetes mellitus
Negative Risk Factor†
High HDL-cholesterol (.60 mg/dl)

Note: *High risk,* defined as a net of two or more CHD risk factors, leads to more vigorous intervention. *Age* (defined differently for men and for women) is treated as a risk factor because rates of CHD are higher in the elderly than in the young, and in men than in women of the same age. *Obesity* is not listed as a risk factor because it operates through the other risk factors of *hypertension, hyperlipidemia, decreased HDL cholesterol,* and *diabetes mellitus,* but it should be considered a target for intervention. *Physical inactivity* is similarly not listed as a risk factor, but it too should be considered a target for intervention, and physical activity is recommended as desirable for everyone.

*Confirmed by measurements on several occasions.

†If the HDL cholesterol level is ≥60 mg/dl, subtract one risk factor (because high HDL cholesterol levels decrease CHD risk).

From U.S. Department of Health and Human Services (1993). *Report of the Expert Panel on Detection, Evaluation, and Treatment of High Blood Cholesterol in Adults (ATP II).* National Cholesterol Education Program. Bethesda, MD: National Heart, Lung, and Blood Institute (NIH Publication no. 93-3095).

increased when plasma total cholesterol (TC) levels were above 200 mg/dl and increased considerably when TC was above 240 mg/dl (U.S. Department of Health and Human Services, 1993). Furthermore, at the upper end of the curve, small changes in the TC level were associated with marked changes in CHD mortality. LDL is the major atherogenic lipoprotein, and decreasing LDL cholesterol reduces CHD risk (U.S. Department of Health and Human Services, 1993). Many intervention studies have shown that for every 1% decrease in TC (which usually represents a reduction in LDL

cholesterol), CHD risk is reduced 2–3%. Likewise, high levels of HDL cholesterol confer protection against CHD (Figure 6–2); for every 1 mg/dl decrease in HDL cholesterol, CHD risk increases 2–3% (Gordon, Probstfeld, Garrison, et al., 1989).

Even when LDL cholesterol levels are elevated, a high HDL cholesterol level is protective against CHD. Elevated plasma triglyceride (TG) levels are associated with an increased risk of CHD, especially when HDL cholesterol levels are low and LDL cholesterol levels are high. Desirable levels of lipids and lipoproteins to decrease CHD risk have been defined by the National Cholesterol Education Program. For adult men and women over age 20, TC should be below 200 mg/dl, LDL cholesterol below 130 mg/dl, HDL cholesterol above 35 mg/dl, and TG below 200 mg/dl. For patients with coronary disease, the optimal LDL cholesterol level is below 100 mg/dl.

EFFECTS OF DIET AND LIFESTYLE FACTORS ON CHD RISK FACTORS

Diet clearly can affect various CHD risk factors. A large body of evidence has shown that saturated fat and cholesterol raise TC LDL cholesterol levels, whereas monounsaturated and polyunsaturated fat lower them. The effect of unsaturated fats is especially pronounced when they are substituted for saturated fat in the diet.

Overweight and obesity raise TC and LDL cholesterol and TG levels and lower HDL cholesterol levels (Denke, Sempos, & Grundy, 1993). Overweight and obesity also increase the risk of both hypertension and diabetes (JNCV, 1993). Body weight that is distributed centrally (in the abdominal area) versus in the lower body area (in the hips and thighs) is associated with increased CHD risk because of adverse effects on plasma lipids and lipoproteins, blood pressure, and insulin resistance (Kannel, Cupples, Ramaswami, et al., 1991).

Exercise beneficially affects risk factors for CHD, principally by increasing HDL cholesterol levels and by facilitating weight control efforts. Because of their impact on CHD risk, diet and lifestyle practices form the basis of the recommendations that have been made for both the prevention and treatment of CHD. Specifically,

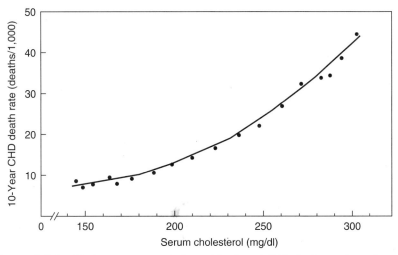

FIGURE 6–1   Relationship between serum cholesterol levels and CHD death rate. From *Report of the Expert Panel on Detection, Evaluation, and Treatment of High Blood Cholesterol in Adults (ATP II).* (1993). National Cholesterol Education Program, National Heart, Lung, and Blood Institute, U.S. Department of Health and Human Services, Bethesda, MD (NIH Publication no. 93–3095).

primary intervention efforts should emphasize decreasing saturated fat and cholesterol intake, achieving and maintaining an ideal body weight, participating in a program of regular physical activity, and smoking cessation.

Other dietary factors also shown to affect plasma lipids could be targets for special intervention with selected patients. These include soluble fiber, omega-3 fatty acids, antioxidants, folic acid, and alcohol in moderation (Anderson, Garrity, Wood, et al., 1992; Harris, 1997;

Hertog, Feskens, Hollman, et al., 1993; Steinberg, Pearson, & Kuller, 1992). *Trans* fatty acids (compared with unsaturated fatty acids) and large amounts of coffee and sodium (in some individuals) have been shown to adversely affect plasma lipids, lipoproteins, and blood pressure (JNCV, 1993; Kris-Etherton & Nicolosi, 1995). Interventions that also target these factors could lead to additional benefits beyond those achieved with Step-One and Step-Two diets (discussed later in this chapter).

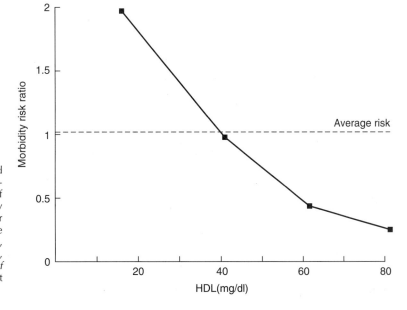

FIGURE 6–2   HDL-cholesterol and CHD risk—The Framingham Experience. Reprinted by permission of the publisher from "High density lipoprotein as a protective factor against coronary heart disease. The Framingham Study." Gordon, T., Castelli W. P., Hjortland, M. C., et al. (1996). *American Journal of Medicine, 62*:707–714. Copyright 1996 by Excerpta Medica Inc.

Collectively, diet and regular physical activity can favorably affect a number of major risk factors for CHD and hence significantly reduce CHD morbidity and mortality.

GENETIC FORMS OF HYPERLIPIDEMIA

Very dramatic elevations (above the 90th percentile) of plasma and LDL cholesterol levels are the result of genetic disorders of lipoprotein metabolism. These hyperlipidemias are initially classified on the basis of the predominant lipoprotein abnormality (Table 6–2). All immediate family members of patients with severe forms of hypercholesterolemia should undergo screening. The different genetic forms of hyperlipidemia as described by Grundy (1987) will now be discussed. The dietary components of treatment for genetic hyperlipidemias are discussed in a subsequent section.

Familial Hypercholesterolemia (Type IIa or High LDL Cholesterol, Normal TG)

Familial hypercholesterolemia (FH) is a heritable disease resulting from a series of mutations in the LDL receptor gene that results in a nonfunctional receptor. A person with the heterozygous form of FH (one in 500 individuals) has only half the number of LDL receptors, and as a result, clearance of LDL from the circulation is impaired. Cholesterol levels are usually 250–500 mg/dl. In contrast, in the homozygous individual (one in a million people) there is little or no LDL receptor activity, and plasma cholesterol levels are markedly elevated (700–1,200 mg/dl).

In heterozygote patients, the average age of onset of CHD is 45 in males and 55 in females, whereas homozygotes have more severe hypercholesterolemia and atherosclerosis (generally leading to myocardial infarction or death) in the first or second decade of life. For FH heterozygotes, a Step-Two diet combined with drug therapy can generally help achieve desirable LDL cholesterol levels. In marked contrast, homozygotes are unresponsive to aggressive dietary therapy. Typically, treatment of these patients involves extreme measures such as biweekly plasmapheresis to remove the excess LDL.

Severe Polygenic Hypercholesterolemia

Severe polygenic hypercholesterolemia is characterized by elevated LDL cholesterol levels (>220 mg/dl). The elevation in LDL cholesterol in these patients is less than that seen in FH heterozygotes. Tendon xanthomas are not observed in these patients. As would be expected, these patients are at high risk for premature disease. Treatment is essentially identical to that for individuals with heterozygous FH.

TABLE 6–2 Classification of Hyperlipidemias

Type	Lipoprotein Abnormality	Blood Lipids
Type I	↑ ↑ Chylomicrons	↑ ↑ ↑ Triglycerides ↑ Cholesterol
Type IIa	↑ ↑ LDL	↑ ↑ Cholesterol
Type IIb	↑ ↑ LDL, ↑ IDL, ↑ ↑ VLDL	↑ ↑ Cholesterol
Type III	↑ IDL, ↑ VLDL remnants	↑ ↑ Cholesterol ↑ Triglycerides
Type IV	↑ VLDL	↑ Cholesterol ↑ ↑ Triglycerides
Type V	↑ ↑ Chylomicrons, ↑ VLDL	↑ ↑ Triglycerides ↑ Cholesterol

From U.S. Department of Health and Human Services (1993). *Report of the Expert Panel on Detection, Evaluation and Treatment of High Blood Cholesterol in Adults (ATP II)*. National Cholesterol Education Program. Bethesda, MD: National Heart, Lung, and Blood Institute (NIH Publication no. 93-3095).

Familial Combined Hyperlipidemia

Familial combined hyperlipidemia (FCHL) is characterized by high TC, high TG, or both (above the 90th percentile). The defect in FCHL is due to hepatic overproduction of *very-low-density lipoprotein* (VLDL) and possibly other metabolic defects. Thus, these individuals have either (1) elevated LDL cholesterol with normal TG levels (Type IIa), (2) elevated LDL cholesterol with elevated TG levels (Type IIb), or (3) hypertriglyceridemia—that is, elevated VLDL levels (Type IV). In addition, they frequently have small, dense LDL, which is associated with increased risk of CHD. All types of FCHL cause premature death. Treatment includes a Step-Two diet, drug therapy, and management of other risk factors or conditions, which might entail weight loss, diabetes control, increased physical activity, or, in some patients, management of gout.

Familial Dyslipidemia

Patients with familial dyslipidemia have hypertriglyceridemia (above the 90th percentile) and low HDL cholesterol levels (below the 10th percentile). Approximately 15% of CHD patients have familial dyslipidemia along with other risk factors such as android obesity, insulin resistance, Type II diabetes, and hypertension. Frequently LDL cholesterol levels are elevated modestly in these patients. Lifestyle intervention to modify all risk factors, especially weight loss, is the most common treatment.

Familial Dysbetalipoproteinemia (Type III Hyperlipoproteinemia)

The relatively uncommon disorder of familial dysbetalipoproteinemia (Type III hyperlipoproteinemia) affects one in 5,000 persons in the United States. It is characterized by delayed catabolism of VLDL remnants, *intermediate-density lipoprotein* (IDL), and chylomicron remnants resulting from an abnormality in the structure of apolipoprotein E. It is usually associated with other risk factors such as age, obesity, hypothyroidism, diabetes, or other dyslipi-

demias. Blood TC levels in these individuals range from 300 to 600 mg/dl and TG from 400 to 800 mg/dl or higher. As a result, there is increased risk of premature atherogenic disease, including myocardial infarction, stroke, or peripheral vascular disease. Treatment of this condition includes weight reduction, control of hyperglycemia and diabetes, restriction of dietary saturated fat and cholesterol, and drug therapy.

PRIMARY AND SECONDARY PREVENTION OF CHD

This section describes the clinical guidelines for risk assessment and treatment in (1) patients at high risk but without established CHD (i.e., requiring primary prevention) and (2) patients with diagnosed CHD (i.e., requiring secondary prevention).

RISK ASSESSMENT AND TREATMENT GUIDELINES

Patients without Established CHD

The initial classification of the CHD risk status of a patient begins with the measurement of the TC and HDL cholesterol level. A desirable TC level is below 200 mg/dl, a borderline high TC is 200–239 mg/dl, and high TC is 240 mg/dl and above (Table 6–3). A desirable HDL cholesterol level is above 35 mg/dl. Initial treatment decisions are based on the TC and HDL

TABLE 6–3 Initial Classification Based on Total Cholesterol and HDL Cholesterol

Total Cholesterol	HDL Cholesterol
Desirable: <200 mg/dl	Low: <35 mg/dl
Borderline high: 200–239 mg/dl	
High: ≥240 mg/dl	

From U.S. Department of Health and Human Services (1993). *Report of the Expert Panel on Detection, Evaluation, and Treatment of High Blood Cholesterol in Adults (ATP II)*. National Cholesterol Education Program. Bethesda, MD: National Heart, Lung, and Blood Institute (NIH Publication no. 93-3095).

cholesterol levels and the presence of other risk factors (Figure 6–3).

Patients with a desirable TC and HDL cholesterol level should be given information about a healthy diet, recommended physical activity, and ways of reducing CHD risk factors (e.g., preventive medical care for cigarette smoking, hypertension, etc.). For these individuals, TC and HDL cholesterol levels should be checked again within 5 years. Patients with a borderline high TC level, an HDL cholesterol level of 35 mg/dl or above, and fewer than two risk factors also should receive information about healthy diet and lifestyle practices and be reevaluated in 1–2 years. Patients with a borderline high TC level, an HDL cholesterol level of less than 35 mg/dl, or with two or more risk factors, as well as patients with a high TC level, should undergo a fasting lipid and lipoprotein analysis to provide more information about TC, TG, HDL cholesterol, and LDL cholesterol.

For these higher-risk patients (i.e., those with elevated TC levels, low HDL cholesterol levels, or two or more risk factors), treatment decisions are based on LDL cholesterol levels (Figure 6–4). A desirable LDL cholesterol level is below 130 mg/dl. Borderline high risk is indicated by 130–159 mg/dl of LDL cholesterol and high risk by 160 mg/dl or more. Patients with a desirable LDL cholesterol level should be given information about healthy diet and lifestyle practices and preventive care (e.g., for hypertension) and followed up within 5 years.

Patients with a borderline-high-risk LDL cholesterol level and fewer than two risk factors should receive information about diet and other lifestyle practices and be reevaluated annually. Patients with a borderline-high-risk LDL cholesterol level and two or more risk factors, as well as patients with a high-risk LDL cholesterol level, should undergo a second LDL cholesterol analysis. Upon verification of a borderline-high-risk level of LDL cholesterol (with two or more risk factors) or a high risk of LDL cholesterol

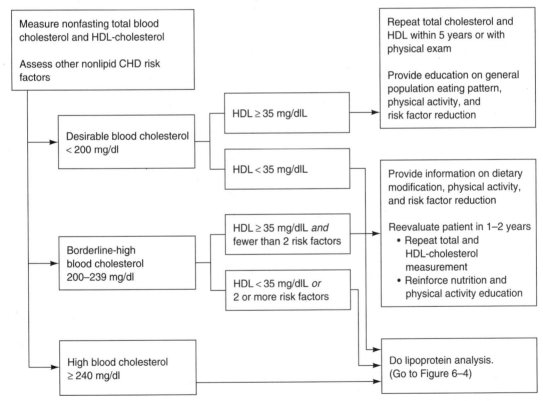

FIGURE 6–3 Primary prevention in adults without evidence of CHD: Initial classification based on total cholesterol and HDL-cholesterol. From *Report of the Expert Panel on Detection, Evaluation, and Treatment of High Blood Cholesterol in Adults (ATP II)*. (1993). National Cholesterol Education Program, National Heart, Lung, and Blood Institute, U.S. Department of Health and Human Services, Bethesda, MD (NIH Publication no. 93–3095).

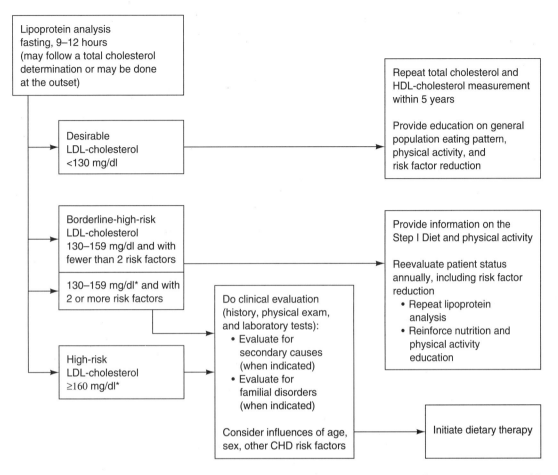

*On the basis of the average of two determinations. If the first two LDL-cholesterol tests differ by more than 30 mg/dL, a third test should be obtained within 1–8 weeks and the average value of three tests used.

FIGURE 6–4   Primary prevention in adults without evidence of CHD: Subsequent classification based on LDL-cholesterol. From *Report of the Expert Panel on Detection, Evaluation, and Treatment of High Blood Cholesterol in Adults (ATP II)*. (1993). National Cholesterol Education Program, National Heart, Lung, and Blood Institute, U.S. Department of Health and Human Services, Bethesda, MD (NIH Publication no. 93–3095).

(determined by averaging at least two values that do not differ by more than 30 mg/dl), patients should undergo a comprehensive clinical evaluation (including a history, physical examination, and basic laboratory tests). The purposes of the clinical evaluation are threefold: (1) to determine whether the elevated LDL cholesterol level is caused by a disease, diet, or a drug that can be changed; (2) to determine whether there is a genetic basis for the elevated LDL cholesterol level; and (3) to more comprehensively characterize the risk status of the patient, including the possible presence of CHD, in order to help guide treatment decisions. Following the clinical evaluation, patients follow an intensive lipid-intervention program.

Patients with Established CHD

Intensive intervention efforts are recommended for patients with established CHD. An LDL cholesterol level of more than 100 mg/dl is higher than ideal and is the criterion used to guide treatment decisions. A guide to comprehensive risk reduction for CHD patients has been described in which risk intervention is targeted to cigarette smoking cessation, lipid management, participation in regular physical activity, weight management, pharmacologic therapy, and blood pressure control (Figure 6–5). Implicit in these guidelines is the need for an individualized program of patient care and

Guide to Comprehensive Risk Reduction
for Patients With Coronary and Other Vascular Disease

Risk Intervention	Recommendations			
Smoking: Goal complete cessation	Strongly encourage patient and family to stop smoking. Provide counseling, nicotine replacement, and formal cessation programs as appropriate.			
Lipid Management: Primary goal LDL<100 mg/dl Secondary goals HDL>35 mg/dl; TG<200 mg/dl	Start AHA Step II Diet in all patients: ≤30% fat, <7% saturated fat, <200 mg/d cholesterol. Assess fasting lipid profile. In post-MI patients, lipid profile may take 4 to 6 weeks to stabilize. Add drug therapy according to the following guide:			

LDL<100 mg/dl	*LDL 100 to 130 mg/dl*	*LDL>130 mg/dl*	*HDL<35 mg/dl*
No drug therapy	Consider adding drug therapy to diet, as follows:	Add drug therapy to diet, as follows:	Emphasize weight management and physical activity. Advise smoking cessation. If needed to achieve LDL goals, consider niacin, statin, fibrate.

Suggested Drug Therapy

TG <200 mg/dl	*TG 200 to 400 mg/dl*	*TG >400 mg/dl*
Statin Resin Niacin	Statin Niacin	Consider combined drug therapy (niacin, fibrate, statin)

If LDL goal not achieved, consider combination therapy.

American Heart AssociationSM
Fighting Heart Disease and Stroke

Consensus Panel Statement
Preventing Heart Attack and Death

Physical Activity: Minimum goal 30 minutes 3 to 4 times per week	Assess risk, preferably with exercise test, to guide prescription. Encourage minimum of 30 to 60 minutes of moderate-intensity activity 3 or 4 times weekly (walking, jogging, cycling, or other aerobic activity) supplemented by an increase in daily lifestyle activities (eg, walking breaks at work, using stairs, gardening, household work). Maximum benefit 5 to 6 hours a week. Advise medically supervised programs for moderate-to high-risk patients.
Weight Management:	Start intensive diet and appropriate physical activity intervention, as outlined above, in patients >120% of ideal weight for height. Particularly emphasize need for weight loss in patients with hypertension, elevated triglycerides, or elevated glucose levels.
Antiplatelet Agents/ Anticoagulants:	Start aspirin 80 to 325 mg/d if not contraindicated. Manage warfarin to international normalized ratio=2 to 3.5 for post-MI patients not able to take aspirin.
ACE Inhibitors Post-MI:	Start early post-MI in stable high-risk patients (anterior MI, previous MI, Killip class II [S, gallop, rales, radiographic CHF]). Continue indefinitely for all with LV dysfunction (ejection fraction≤40%) or symptoms of failure. Use as needed to manage blood pressure or symptoms in all other patients.
Beta-Blockers:	Start in high-risk post-MI patients (arrhythmia, LV dysfunction, inducible ischemia) at 5 to 28 days. Continue 6 months minimum. Observe usual contraindications. Use as needed to manage angina, rhythm, or blood pressure in all other patients.
Estrogens:	Consider estrogen replacement in all postmenopausal women. Individualize recommendation consistent with other health risks.
Blood Pressure Control: Goal ≤140/90 mm Hg	Initiate lifestyle modification—weight control, physical activity, alcohol moderation, and moderate sodium restriction—in all patients with blood pressure>140 mm Hg systolic or 90 mm Hg diastolic. Add blood pressure medication, individualized to other patient requirements and characteristics (i.e., age, race, need for drugs with specific benefits) **if** blood pressure is not less then 140 mm Hg systolic or 90 mm Hg diastolic in 3 months **or** if *initial* blood pressure is >160 mm Hg systolic or 100 mm Hg diastolic.

ACE indicates angiotensin-converting enzyme; MI, myocardial infarction; TG, triglycerides; and LV, left ventricular.

FIGURE 6–5 Guide to comprehensive risk reduction for patients with coronary and other vascular disease. From Smith, S. C., Blair, S. N., Criqui, M. H., et al. (1995). Preventing heart attack and death in patients with coronary disease. *Circulation, 92,* 2–4. Reproduced with permission. *Circulation,* ©American Heart Association, Inc.

close monitoring and follow-up by a team of health-care providers.

Treatment Guidelines for Diet and Drug Therapy

Diet therapy is the first line of treatment for patients with elevated LDL cholesterol levels.

Table 6–4 presents the LDL cholesterol levels for which a formal program of dietary therapy would be initiated and drug treatment would be considered in patients with and without CHD. In addition, LDL goals are defined for each level. The initiation and goal levels are more stringent for patients with CHD than for those without CHD (a desirable LDL cholesterol level is 100 mg/dl). Similarly, CHD patients with

TABLE 6–4 Treatment Decisions Based on LDL Cholesterol

	Dietary Therapy	
	Initiation Level	*LDL Goal*
Without CHD and with fewer than two risk factors	≥160 mg/dl	<160 mg/dl
Without CHD and with two or more risk factors	≥130 mg/dl	<130 mg/dl
With CHD	>100 mg/dl	≤100 mg/dl
	Drug Treatment	
	Consideration Level	*LDL Goal*
Without CHD and with fewer than two risk factors	≥190 mg/dl*	<160 mg/dl
Without CHD and with two or more risk factors	≥160 mg/dl	<130 mg/dl
With CHD	≥130 mg/dl†	≤100 mg/dl

*In men under 35 years of age and premenopausal women with LDL cholesterol levels of 190–219 mg/dl, drug therapy should be delayed, except in high-risk patients such as those with diabetes.

†In CHD patients with LDL cholesterol levels of 100–129 mg/dl, the physician should exercise clinical judgment in deciding whether to initiate drug treatment.

From U.S. Department of Health and Human Services (1993). *Report of the Expert Panel on Detection, Evaluation and Treatment of High Blood Cholesterol in Adults (ATP II).* National Cholesterol Education Program. Bethesda, MD: National Heart, Lung, and Blood Institute (NIH Publication no. 93-3095).

two or more risk factors have a more stringent LDL goal than those with fewer than two risk factors (<130 VS <160 mg/dl). The goal levels for LDL cholesterol do not change with the type of therapy (i.e., dietary, drugs, or both). However, the initiation level for diet therapy is lower (by 30 mg/dl) than the consideration level for drug treatment in all patient categories.

Drug treatment decisions are based on the overall clinical profile of the patient. As a result, the current recommendation is that drug therapy be delayed in young men (under 35 years of age) and in premenopausal women who have only elevated LDL cholesterol levels. In addition, some patients with CHD who have an LDL cholesterol level of 100–129 mg/dl may be candidates for drug therapy. Thus, whereas all patients are candidates for dietary therapy, drug therapy decisions must be individualized and made on the basis of each patient's unique clinical condition.

Diet Therapy and Physical Activity

Dietary therapy is the first line of treatment for patients with elevated TC and LDL cholesterol levels as well as for patients with other lipid and lipoprotein disorders. It is generally recommended that the maximum daily amount of dietary fat be 30% or less of total daily calories (National Cancer Institute, 1987a; National Research Council, 1989; U.S. Department of Health and Human Services, 1991). Currently, only 14% of the population meets this recommended criterion (Murphy, Rose, Hudes, et al., 1992).

The Step-One and Step-Two diets (Table 6–5) are recommended and designed to progressively reduce intake of saturated fat and cholesterol and promote weight loss, if indicated. A program of regular physical activity (30 minutes each day of moderate-intensity activity such as brisk walking, or 30 minutes three times a week of higher-intensity activity such as running) is an essential component of nonpharmacologic therapy for the treatment of patients with high TC levels.

The Step-One diet recommends that (1) 8–10% of calories be obtained from saturated fat, (2) less than 300 mg of cholesterol be consumed per day, and (3) 30% or less of calories be obtained from total fat. The Step-Two diet recommends that (1) less than 7% of calories be obtained from saturated fat, (2) more than 200 mg cholesterol be consumed per day, and (3) 30% or less of calories be obtained from total fat. Unless the patient is already on it, the Step-One diet is recommended initially. (The Step-One diet is currently recommended for the

TABLE 6–5 Dietary Therapy for Patients with High Total Blood Cholesterol

Nutrient*	Step-One Diet	Both Step-One and Step-Two Diets	Step-Two Diet
Total fat		30% or less of total calories	
Saturated fatty acids	8–10% of total calories		Less than 7% of total calories
Polyunsaturated fatty acids		Up to 10% of total calories	
Monounsaturated fatty acids		Up to 15% of total calories	
Carbohydrates		55% or more of total calories	
Protein		Approximately 15% of total calories	
Cholesterol	Less than 300 mg/day		Less than 200 mg/day
Total calories		Amount necessary to achieve and maintain desirable weight	

*Calories from alcohol not included.

From U.S. Department of Health and Human Services (1993). *Report of the Expert Panel on Detection, Evaluation, and Treatment of High Blood Cholesterol in Adults (ATP II)*. National Cholesterol Education Program. Bethesda, MD: National Heart, Lung, and Blood Institute (NIH Publication no. 93-3095).

population at large.) Patients progress to the Step-Two diet if they have not met their LDL cholesterol goal on the Step-One diet. Patients initially on the Step-One diet can progress to the Step-Two diet, but patients with established CHD should skip the Step-One diet and begin immediately following the Step-Two diet. For many patients, the Step-Two diet represents an aggressive intervention, with saturated fat and cholesterol being reduced approximately 50% from the usual diet. Thus, these patients will benefit from nutrition counseling by a registered dietitian.

It is important to note that the Step-Two diet has no lower limit for saturated fat, cholesterol, and total fat, so for some patients these nutrients/dietary constituents can be progressively decreased far below the maximally recommended amount. A Step-Two diet that provides minimal amounts of saturated fat (<3% of calories), cholesterol (<100 mg/day) and total fat (<10% of calories) should be an option for highly motivated patients (e.g., those with cardiovascular disease or those receiving dietary therapy as a possible alternative to pharmacologic therapy). Together with other major lifestyle changes, this very aggressive low-fat diet has been shown to markedly lower TC and

LDL cholesterol levels and actually result in regression of atherosclerosis (Ornish, Brown, Scherwitz, et al., 1990).

Although this diet has been shown to be efficacious, it is a challenge for many patients because it requires major dietary and lifestyle changes. The very low-fat, very low-saturated-fat and low-cholesterol diet emphasizes the intake of low-fat breads, cereals, and other grain products, fruits, vegetables, legumes, and skim-milk dairy products. Meat, poultry, and fish are used sparingly (as a condiment, if at all), and consumption of fats and oils is markedly curtailed. Social activities and eating out can pose problems for many patients on this diet.

Weight reduction and physical activity are important aspects of therapy for patients with high TC (Dattilo & Kris-Etherton, 1992). Weight loss, if indicated, and physical activity will improve the plasma lipid and lipoprotein profile and favorably affect other CHD risk factors such as hypertension and diabetes. In addition, exercise and weight loss both increase HDL cholesterol levels.

For patients with elevated TG levels, a Step-One diet is recommended. Many patients with hypertriglyceridemia are overweight, so weight loss in these patients, even if they fail to achieve their ideal body weight, will lower and sometimes normalize TG levels. Thus, weight loss is an important component of the diet therapy for hypertriglyceridemic patients. Some patients are responsive to alcohol, and if these individuals consume it regularly, alcohol intake should be a primary target for intervention. Other patients may be responsive to dietary carbohydrate, and for these individuals a diet higher in total fat ($\approx$35% of calories) but still lower in saturated fat and cholesterol is indicated. These patients would benefit from a diet relatively high in monounsaturated fat that does not promote weight gain. Finally, in some clinical settings, under medical supervision, hypertriglyceridemic patients are treated with fish-oil supplements (13 g per day) (Harris, 1989). The triglyceride-lowering response that can be achieved in hypertriglyceridemic patients given fish-oil supplements is about 25%.

After initiation of a therapeutic diet, serum TC levels should be measured at 4–6 weeks and at 3 months. Serum TC correlates with the LDL cholesterol and is convenient and inexpensive to measure. In general, serum TC levels of 240 mg/dl and 200 mg/dl correspond to LDL cholesterol levels of 160 mg/dl and 130 mg/dl, respectively. If the TC goal is met, a lipoprotein analysis should be conducted to assure that the LDL cholesterol goal has been met.

Dietary therapy should be carried out for at least 6 months before initiating drug therapy, except in the case of patients with severe elevations in TC levels. For patients with CHD, a shorter period also is acceptable. Diet therapy is important for all patients, even those on drug therapy for whom a Step-One diet is recommended. After a 6-month period of diet therapy on a Step-One diet (or sooner, depending on the patient), if the TC and LDL cholesterol goals have not been achieved, patients generally should be referred to a registered dietitian. Patients then can progress to a Step-Two diet or try another trial on a Step-One diet (followed by progression to a Step-Two diet, if indicated).

Implementation of Step-One and Step-Two Diets

Dietary assessment is an important aspect of the treatment guidelines for patients with high TC levels. Specifically, knowing the habitual dietary practices of patients and monitoring their progress toward achieving the goals of the Step-One and Step-Two diets are essential components of the nutritional management of high-risk patients. Listed at the end of this chapter are some diet-assessment instruments that are easy and quick to use.

One popular food-frequency questionnaire used in clinical practice to assess adherence to a Step-One and Step-Two diet is MEDFICTS. This questionnaire assesses consumption practices of major sources of total fat, saturated fat, and dietary cholesterol. It is typically administered by a health professional and can be useful in teaching patients the principles of a cholesterol-lowering diet; foods within specific food groups are principally categorized according to amount of total fat (i.e., there are "high-fat" and "low-fat" food groupings).

Implementation of the Step-One and Step-Two diets is contingent upon estimating a patient's energy needs to maintain current weight. A simple method for estimating energy needs is to multiply current body weight by an average physical activity factor (Table 6–6). Thus, the energy requirements of a woman who weighs 55 kg and has a light activity level (e.g., 35 kcal/kg/day) are

$$55 \text{ kg} \times 35 \text{ kcal/kg/day} = 1,925 \text{ kcal/day}$$

Usual energy intake also can be estimated from a 24-hour recall, or food record, completed by the patient. Because of errors in dietary assessment methods, however, energy needs frequently are underestimated using this information. Achieving and maintaining desirable weight is a recommendation of both Step-One and Step-Two diets, and weight reduction is important for patients who are overweight or obese. A reasonable strategy for most patients who need to lose weight is to reduce calorie intake by 500 calories per day to achieve a gradual weight loss of ½–1 pound per week while increasing daily physical activity. A greater calorie restriction may be necessary for very obese patients.

In general, three approaches are used most often to implement Step-One and Step-Two diets: (1) counting grams of fat and saturated fat, (2) using the *exchange lists* from the Amer-

TABLE 6–6   Determination of Activity Factor

Level of Activity	Examples of Activity		Energy Expenditure (kcal/kg/day)
Very light	Seated/standing, driving, typing, cooking, ironing	Men	31
		Women	30
Light	Walking (2.5–3 mph), carpentry, house-cleaning, golf, sailing	Men	38
		Women	35
Moderate	Walking (3.5–4 mph), cycling, skiing, tennis, dancing	Men	41
		Women	37
Heavy	Walking with load uphill, basketball, football, mountain climbing	Men	50
		Women	44
Exceptional	Running, squash, handball, cross-country skiing	Men	58
		Women	51

Adapted from Mahan, L.K., & Escott-Stump, S. (Eds.) (1996). *Krause's Food, Nutrition and Diet Therapy*, 9th ed. Philadelphia: WB Saunders.

ican Heart Association (American Heart Association, 1988), and (3) applying relatively simple fat-reduction strategies to food choices. These approaches can be applied singly or in combination; two or even three can be used by one patient. Inherent in each of these strategies is initial and ongoing dietary assessment, goal setting, monitoring, evaluation, and, if indicated, modifying the treatment plan (e.g., changing the specific implementation strategy).

Frequent follow-up and monitoring visits are of great assistance to patients (especially in the early stages of their treatment programs) in achieving the goals of their prescribed diets. The initial phase of the dietary therapy program is critical to patients' overall success in making long-term dietary changes. It is essential that practitioners be available to answer questions and be prepared to consider a different dietary strategy (or a combination of strategies) if indicated for achieving dietary adherence.

The strategies described in the following text for implementing the Step-One and Step-Two diets are for patients who are at their desirable weight. Strategies 1 and 2 require identifying the appropriate calorie level for weight maintenance or weight loss. The application of the third strategy will result in reducing calories (mainly fat calories) in the diet. For patients who do not need to lose weight, weight maintenance is the goal; calories can be added back to the diet with high-carbohydrate foods.

STRATEGY 1: COUNTING GRAMS OF FAT AND SATURATED FAT (AND ACHIEVING RECOMMENDED CHOLESTEROL ALLOWANCE)

Just as calories can be counted, so can grams of fat. Table 6–7 lists the maximum daily intake of fat and saturated fat allowable in diets that provide 1,600–3,000 kcal. As most foods sold in the supermarket have grams of fat and saturated fat listed on the label, it is easy for patients to calculate their fat and saturated fat intake. Patients who choose to count grams of fat and saturated fat instead of calories will benefit from having resource books or booklets that provide this information on all types of foods, including those not required to have a nutrition label (e.g., fresh meat, fish, poultry, bulk foods) as well as those eaten in restaurants and other places away from home. To achieve the recommended cholesterol allowance, patients should also limit major food sources of dietary cholesterol. The predominant source of cholesterol in the diet of most Americans is egg yolk, which provides approximately 211 mg of cholesterol per yolk.

STRATEGY 2: USING EXCHANGE LISTS FROM AMERICAN HEART ASSOCIATION

Many individuals have used the AHA exchange lists to plan diets for weight loss or for managing conditions such as diabetes. They are famil-

TABLE 6–7 Maximum Daily Intake of Fat and Saturated Fat in Step-One and Step-Two Diets

	Total Calorie Level							
	1,600	**1,800**	**2,000**	**2,200**	**2,400**	**2,600**	**2,800**	**3,000**
Total fat, grams*	53	60	67	73	80	87	93	100
Saturated fat for Step-One, grams†	18	20	22	24	27	29	31	33
Saturated fat for Step-Two, grams**	12	14	16	17	19	20	22	23

Note: Average daily energy intake is 1800 kcal for women and 2500 kcal for men.

*Total fat of both diets = 30% of calories (estimated by multiplying calorie level of the diet by 0.3 and dividing the product by 9 kcal/g).

†Recommended intake of saturated fat is 8–10% of total calories for the Step-One diet and less than 7% for the Step-Two diet.

From U.S. Department of Health and Human Services (1993). *Report of the Expert Panel on Detection, Evaluation, and Treatment of High Blood Cholesterol in Adults (ATP II).* National Cholesterol Education Program. Bethesda, MD: National Heart, Lung, and Blood Institute (NIH Publication no. 93-3095).

iar with this approach and find it easy for meal planning. Table 6–8 lists the number of servings per day from food groups for Step-One and Step-Two diets for different calorie levels. (Guidelines for estimating energy needs were presented earlier.) When using this approach, patients still must be taught how to make appropriate food choices within each food group. In addition, many individuals are unaware of standard portion sizes and need guidance on estimating serving sizes.

STRATEGY 3: APPLYING FAT-REDUCTION TECHNIQUES TO MEAL PLANNING

Various fat-reduction techniques can be used to reduce total dietary fat, saturated fat, and cholesterol (Kristal, White, Shattuck, et al., 1992): (1) substituting low-fat foods for high-fat counterparts (e.g., skim milk for whole milk, lean meat for higher-fat meat); (2) reducing the quantity of high-fat foods; (3) replacing or augmenting high-fat foods with foods lower in fat

TABLE 6–8 Number of Servings per Day from Food Groups for Different Calorie Levels

Food Group	No. Servings for Different Calorie Levels in Step-One Diet				No. Servings for Different Calorie Levels in Step-Two Diet			
	2,500	**2,000**	**1,600**	**1,200**	**2,500**	**2,000**	**1,600**	**1,200**
Meat, poultry, and fish	1 (6 oz)	1 (6 oz)	1 (6 oz)	1 (6 oz)	1 (5 oz)	1 (5 oz)	1 (5 oz)	1 (5 oz)
Eggs (per week)	3	3	3	3	1	1	1	1
Dairy products	4	3	3	2	3	2	2	2
Fat	8	6	4	3	8	7	5	3
Bread, cereal, pasta, starchy vegetables	10	7	4	3	10	8	5	4
Vegetables	4	4	4	4	5	4	4	4
Fruit	5	3	3	3	7	4	3	3
Optional foods*	2	2	3	3	7	4	3	3

*Optional foods include fat-modified desserts, fat-free or low-fat sweets, and alcoholic beverages. If foods from this group are not used, add two portions from the "Bread, cereal, pasta, starchy vegetables" group plus one portion from the "Fat" group.

From US Department of Health and Human Services (1994). Step by step eating to lower your blood cholesterol. National Heart, Lung and Blood Institute. Bethesda, MD. NIH Publication No. 94-2920.

and with fruits, vegetables, and grains (e.g., legumes for red meat, fat-modified products for full-fat counterparts); and (4) changing food preparation techniques (e.g., broiling instead of frying).

Selective application of fat-reduction techniques provides flexibility in diet planning for individuals, especially with respect to a Step-One diet. Certain foods need not be eliminated as long as other dietary changes have been made, and patients frequently are surprised to find how often lean red meat can be included in a Step-One or Step-Two diet. Because of differences in the cuts and methods of preparation, not all types of red meats are as high in fat as dark meat poultry with skin. In general, removing the skin decreases the amount of total fat in a serving of chicken or turkey by 50%.

Choice of a single versus multiple strategies results in varying levels of dietary fat. Combining more than one technique—such as substituting lean meats and cheeses for higher-fat ones *plus* using skim milk instead of whole milk—can result in lowering total fat from 36% to about 28% of calories for men and from 37% to about 30% of calories for women. Use of additional fat-reduction techniques (such as substituting fat-modified products for higher-fat ones) could decrease total fat to less than 20% of calories, and calories could be reduced by as much as 350. Thus, extensive use of multiple fat-reduction techniques can significantly reduce total fat and saturated fat content of the diet. For most patients, however, these extreme dietary changes are not necessary.

Expected Response to Diet Therapy

Individual responsiveness to dietary change is highly variable. Clearly, some patients will experience appreciable decreases in TC and LDL cholesterol levels and others a modest or clinically insignificant decrease. The response to a cholesterol-lowering diet is affected by many factors, including dietary adherence, whether weight loss occurs, and the magnitude of the change in diet that is achieved. The variability of these factors explains in part the marked variability in patient response that is seen in clinical practice.

Although many patients are able to make

dietary changes initially, these changes often are not maintained. Some are unable to make changes even initially for various reasons, including failure to receive diet instruction, lack of understanding about implementation of a Step-One or Step-Two diet, and lack of motivation to change. Therefore, for many patients, the lack of a diet effect on blood cholesterol levels simply reflects noncompliance with the therapeutic diet. For those able to change from a typical American diet to a Step-One diet, an average TC lowering of 3–14% is expected. For individuals who also lose weight, an even greater TC lowering is expected, about 25%. And for individuals who make very large changes in their diets (e.g., very large decreases in saturated fat and cholesterol), still greater decreases in TC and LDL cholesterol levels can be achieved.

When compared with the average American diet, an average decrease in LDL cholesterol of 5–18% can be achieved on a Step-Two diet. Again, even greater decreases are possible (up to about 25%) when dietary saturated fat and cholesterol are minimal. The average reduction in TC that is expected in patients who switch from a Step-One to a Step-Two diet is an additional 3–7% depending on the degree to which saturated fat and cholesterol are restricted.

The decreases in TC levels that can be achieved with dietary therapy are less than those that typically occur in response to lipid-lowering drugs. Nonetheless, for all patients with elevated TC levels, diet is an important component of lipid-lowering therapy. For some patients, diet alone will decrease the risk of CHD and shift them to a treatment category that no longer requires drug therapy. Thus, with dietary therapy, many patients can avoid drug therapy and its associated side effects. Even for those who still must take drugs, a cholesterol-lowering diet is recommended and may decrease the drug dosage required and hence the side effects and cost of pharmacologic therapy.

DIETARY BEHAVIOR CHANGE

Cardiovascular health and quality of life can be dramatically improved when dietary behavior changes are instituted (Ornish, Brown, Scherwitz, et al., 1990). Consequently, dietary intervention has been recognized as an important tool for reducing CHD risk by both health-care professionals and the public. The previous portion of this chapter focused on dietary intervention as a part of clinical management guidelines for the prevention of CHD in patients at high risk for developing coronary disease or those experiencing a recurrent event. This section addresses a behavioral-change approach to dietary intervention for primary prevention of CHD in the population at large by means of reducing overall dietary fat consumption. Historically, research on this subject was mostly atheoretical in nature (Nitzke & Athens, 1987; Sims, 1987; Achterberg, Novak, & Gillespie, 1985; Brun & Rhoads, 1983; Johnson and Johnson, 1985; National Education Research Advisory Committee, 1987; Contento, 1983; Olson & Kelly, 1989). Today the gap between research and practice is smaller, but many clinicians still adopt a random, piecemeal, atheoretical approach to dietary intervention. For the most part, nurses and other health-care professionals continue to rely on a combination of strategies that emphasize dissemination of information along with cognitive/behavioral modification techniques aimed at developing skills to change dietary knowledge, attitudes, and behavior (Glanz & Mullis, 1988).

Specific interventions typically include self-monitoring, stimulus control, reward strategies, stress management, modeling, social support, and cognitive and behavioral strategies (Foreyt, 1989; Holli, 1988; Kayman, 1989). Cue-exposure approaches, goal setting, contracting, and problem-solving strategies are also commonly employed (Neale, Singleton, Dupius, et al., 1989; Wardle, 1990; White & Skinner, 1988).

Self-monitoring involves having the patient observe and keep track of his or her dietary behavior through the act of recording it in some form of written or electronic diary. Self-monitoring is a powerful strategy for reducing the risk of CHD through dietary behavior change, because it helps both the patient and the clinician become acutely aware of dietary behavior as it occurs. This is also useful because it illuminates ongoing problems and dietary patterns over time. The very act of recording dietary behavior often influences changes in the pattern of behavior. Of course, this reactivity can be a potential problem when the technique is primarily used for assessment purposes. But when used for therapeutic purposes, reactivity can be very helpful as a motivator for changing dietary behavior as well as adhering to the new dietary behavior that reduces the risk of CHD.

The well-documented behavioral principle of *stimulus control* involves the manipulation of environmental stimuli that trigger (i.e., "cue") unhealthy dietary behavior (Skinner, 1969). This approach generally involves having the patient use various cue-avoidance procedures, such as removing high-fat foods from the home, to help reduce exposure to the condition that may prompt unhealthy eating behaviors that increase the risk of CHD.

Reward strategies involve another fundamental behavioral principle known as *contingency management*. Reward strategies rely on the use of positive consequences valued by the patient as an incentive to change dietary behavior to reduce the risk of CHD. This simply means that a reward is given to motivate the patient to behave as expected. Rewards can be tangible in nature, such as receiving a free pass to the movies for adhering to a recommended diet for a week or more. Cognitive rewards like approval from others (e.g., being praised by a significant other for resisting a high-fat donut) are another form of contingency management. Patients can provide rewards for themselves or rely on others to furnish them.

Contracting is an activity sometimes used as an added incentive to reinforce a desired dietary behavior. *Contracts* are verbal or formal written agreements between people (e.g., the patient and the self, the significant other, or the clinician) that specify mutually agreed upon dietary behavior patterns. A reward is often offered as an incentive for adherence. For example, a patient who pays a fee as part of a program designed to enhance weight loss to lower the risk of CHD may receive money back if a certain amount of weight is lost over a specified amount of time. One of the problems with using contracts is that performance of the desired behavior tends to decrease when the incentive is removed (i.e., the contract expires) and relapse is a common occurence.

Goal setting is another commonly used technique to help patients change dietary behavior to reduce the risk of CHD. "Goals affect performance by directing attention, mobilizing effort, increasing persistence, and motivating strategy development'' (Locke, Shaw, Saari, et al., 1981). The act of setting a goal is more likely to produce dietary behavior change when objectives have been mutually agreed upon by the patient and the clinician. Success is also more likely under the following conditions (Locke, Shaw, Saari et al., 1981):

1. The patient has the ability to accomplish the goals.
2. Objectives are clearly and specifically stated rather than being vague and general in nature.
3. Feedback is provided about progress toward the goal.
4. Rewards are offered for achievement.
5. Support is provided.

Goal setting can be as simple as setting a date to begin the recommended dietary regimen to reduce dietary fat, cholesterol, and so forth, or as complex as creating a timetable with many specific objectives set for each day or week (e.g., substitute skim milk for whole milk, eat fish twice a week, eliminate red meat, limit salt, etc.).

Modeling is another strategy clinicians employ to help patients reduce their risk of CHD. Modeling often involves imitating healthy dietary behavior observed in others, but the patient may also perform the healthy behavior in order to act as a role model for others and thus inspire self-efficacy. For example, parents might choose to eat chicken or fish instead of red meat so that their children learn healthier eating patterns. In either case, modeling involves appraising the impact the problem dietary behavior has on others in the environment.

The concept of *social support* was elaborated on in some detail in Chapter 3 of this text (Rossi & Rossi, 1998). Whatever form social support takes (informational, emotional, material), providing assistance to both encourage and sustain dietary behavior change is an important tool the clinician can use to reduce the risk of CHD. Likewise, seeking, accepting, and utilizing help offered by others can motivate a patient to change dietary behavior. For example, the clinician can provide social support by encouraging the patient to talk about difficulties and feelings associated with making dietary changes.

Stress is a factor that can contribute to CHD risk (Thomas & Cohen, 1955). Consuming high-calorie, high-fat foods like chocolate, cookies, and ice cream as a response to stress are dietary behaviors many people use in an attempt to make themselves feel better. Consequently, many clinicians teach patients to use more appropriate coping mechanisms through *stress management* involving meditation, relaxation, or cognitive imagery techniques and engaging in physical activity.

By recommending substitution, reduction, augmentation, and alteration in food preparation, clinicians can design additional dietary interventions to help patients reduce their risk of CHD. The strategies presented here represent only a sampling of those employed by professionals to guide dietary intervention. Many dietary manuals, books, recipes, and listings of food products are available containing low-fat and reduced-cholesterol or cholesterol-free menus and other materials. Both the American Heart Association (1–800–AHA–USA1) and the American Cancer Society (1–800–4–CANCER) are good sources for detailed information and nutritional materials.

BEHAVIORAL PRINCIPLES OF DIETARY MODIFICATION

Reducing dietary fat consumption, decreasing cholesterol intake, controlling weight, and limiting sodium intake to control hypertension all play important roles in preventing CHD through dietary means. Unfortunately, knowledge does not automatically translate into action. A number of different theories and models of behavior change were explored in Chapter 3. Of these, it was concluded that the *transtheoretical model* (TTM) of behavior change offered the most promising future for primary prevention of CHD risk through behavior change. By systematically applying the TTM to dietary behavior change, clinicians can design more effective interventions for preventing CHD.

The TTM specifies that prior to intervening, the clinician should assess the patient's status in several areas: (1) motivational readiness to change dietary behavior (i.e., stage of change); (2) strategies, activities, or approaches the patient currently employs to limit dietary fat intake (i.e., processes of change); (3) the pros and cons of making a decision to reduce fat consumption; and (4) the amount of confidence or temptation the patient feels in different situations.

Clinician assessment of these parameters is important, because the results can be integrated to provide clinical guidelines for designing, implementing, monitoring, and evaluating the effectiveness of stage-matched dietary interventions, which can also be tailored to the individual. One study demonstrated that tailoring dietary fat-reduction interventions to stage produced a 23% decrease in total dietary fat scores compared with only 9% for the non-tailored group and 3% for controls (Campbell, DeVellis, Strecher, et al., 1994). By integrating additional key TTM constructs—such as the pros and cons of decisional balance, processes of change, self-efficacy, and temptation—in designing and implementing dietary interventions, clinicians can expect to have an even greater impact on CHD prevention.

In designing and implementing interventions to help patients reduce dietary fat consumption, the clinician needs to recognize that a large number of individuals are not ready to change. This means that in addition to reaching patients at every stage of change, clinicians need to be realistic about what can be accomplished in the short term and may have to be satisfied with helping patients move from one stage to the next, even if the action stage is not reached.

MOTIVATIONAL READINESS TO CHANGE

Clinicians involved in nutritional education can make more appropriate decisions about the content and mode of dietary intervention if an individual's readiness to learn is assessed first (Achterberg, 1988). Similarly, it is important for clinicians to recognize that they need to determine an individual's readiness to take action (Close, 1988). The stage of change in regard to reducing dietary fat consumption serves as an index of an individual's motivational readiness to change at any point in time. That is, the stage of change signals when a patient is ready to make changes. The stages

of change were discussed in detail in Chapter 3 (Rossi & Rossi, 1998), and descriptions for the five stages of change for dietary fat reduction were provided in Table 3–2 of Chapter 3 (Rossi & Rossi, 1998).

Several different algorithms have been used to stage people for dietary fat reduction (Barton, 1993; Contento, 1992; Curry, Kristal, & Bowen, 1992; Greene, Rossi, Reed, et al., 1994, Rossi, 1993; Rossi, Greene, Reed, et al., 1993). The algorithm currently recommended for use with dietary fat reduction is based on the individual's beliefs and intentions plus behavioral criteria for appropriately classifying people in the later stages of action and maintenance (Greene, Rossi, Reed, et al., 1994). The additional staging steps for action and maintenance are believed to enhance the consistency between staging and the implicit 30% of energy from fat that clinicians often employ as a criterion in practice for determining if intervention to reduce dietary fat consumption is warranted. The latest version of the assessment tool for staging dietary fat has been described in depth by Greene, Rossi, Reed, and co-workers (1994).

STRATEGIES/ACTIVITIES/ APPROACHES FOR LIMITING DIETARY FAT INTAKE

The overt and covert activities, strategies, and techniques individuals use to help themselves reduce dietary fat consumption are referred to as the *processes of change*. Processes can also be employed by clinicians to change the dietary behavior of patients. Stage-matched use of processes of change is extremely important in designing interventions, because appropriate process use helps to move people through the stages of change (Prochaska & DiClemente, 1984).

TTM-based dietary fat-reduction research has shown that people use at least 11 different processes of change in reducing dietary fat consumption (Rossi, 1993). As described in Chapter 3, processes of change can be experiential or behavioral in nature. *Experiential processes* have to do with thinking, feeling, or experiencing, whereas *behavioral processes* are concerned with the act of doing. Six experiential processes of change for dietary fat reduction identified by DiClemente (1993) are consciousness raising, dramatic relief, environmental reevaluation, self-reevaluation, self-liberation, and social liberation.

Consciousness raising involves increasing awareness that high-fat food consumption is a problem through information seeking, education, and feedback. Interventions often focus on observation, information dissemination, interpretation, and feedback (DiClemente, 1993).

Dramatic relief involves making affective use of a strong emotional reaction to events occurring in the environment as a means to change dietary behavior. Interventions can focus on experiencing and expressing feelings, creating emotional arousal, or role playing (DiClemente, 1993).

Environmental reevaluation has to do with the impact the dietary behavior has on others and involves reassessing how one's eating habits affect the personal and physical environment. Interventions may involve empathy training, role modeling, and enhancing awareness of the behavior's environmental impact (DiClemente, 1993).

Self-reevaluation is a process by which the individual reappraises the impact that engaging in the problem dietary behavior has on others in the environment. Interventions may involve examining, clarifying, or challenging values, beliefs, expectations, or self-image (DiClemente, 1993).

Self-liberation involves invoking willpower, affirming a commitment to change dietary behavior, or maximizing choice by using strategies that increase available options. Although self-liberation is usually a behavioral process for many problem areas, for dietary fat reduction, this process of change has been shown to be experiential in nature (Rossi, 1992). Interventions focus on decision making, making resolutions public, and enhancing awareness of choices.

Social liberation involves becoming sensitive to and concerned about changes in the environment that provide additional alternatives for changing dietary behavior. Interventions focus on empowerment, advocacy, or policymaking (DiClemente, 1993).

Five behavioral processes of change for dietary fat reduction are counterconditioning, helping relationships, interpersonal systems control, reinforcement management, and stimulus control.

Counterconditioning involves substituting a new or competing behavior for the problem dietary behavior. Interventions may involve relaxation, physical effort, desensitization, or affirmational thinking (DiClemente, 1993).

Helping relationships involve accepting and using the support of others to change dietary behavior. Interventions may include fostering trust in others or providing professional assistance, therapeutic alliances, or social support (DiClemente, 1993).

Interpersonal systems control includes avoiding other people who contribute to the problem dietary behavior or seeking out individuals who help decrease the problem. Interventions can involve avoiding or reducing social cues and restructuring social interactions.

Reinforcement management involves using positive consequences for changing the problem behavior, such as rewards by self or others as a means to increase the likelihood that dietary behavior change will occur. These interventions can involve reinforcement from others, self-reward, or contracts (DiClemente, 1993).

Stimulus control involves decreasing the likelihood that the problem dietary behavior will occur by removing cues or avoiding situations that trigger the behavior. These interventions involve modifying the environment (situations, places, and things) to exert control over cues (DiClemente, 1993).

Many health-care professionals already make use of many of these processes of change. For example, self-monitoring involves the processes of consciousness raising and self-reevaluation. Cue-exposure approaches and stimulus control involve the process of stimulus control and the concepts of situational temptation and self-efficacy. Reward strategies can be translated into the process of reinforcement management. Interventions that target situational temptation and confidence often involve managing stress. Modeling can be translated into the process of environmental reevaluation. Social support and problem-solving strategies are used in the process of helping relationships. Both goal setting and contracting can be translated into the process of self-liberation.

MAKING THE DECISION TO ENGAGE IN DIETARY BEHAVIOR CHANGE

Making the decision to change dietary behavior to reduce fat intake depends on the *pros* (benefits) and *cons* (costs) perceived by the individual. These two concepts represent the weight an individual gives to the positive and negative aspects of reducing dietary fat (Rossi, 1993). The pros and cons of reducing dietary fat consumption become clearer when thought of as reasons to cut down or not cut down on fat, respectively.

An example of a pro of reducing dietary fat consumption is that a significant other may disapprove when the individual eats too many high-fat foods. An example of a con of reducing dietary fat consumption is that foods that are high in fat are a quick way to satisfy an individual's hunger. Because these pros and cons are related to making the decision to cut down on dietary fat, it is more important for the clinician to focus on these particular concepts when working with patients who are in early stages of change (i.e., precontemplation, contemplation, preparation) than it is when working with people in the later stages of action and maintenance. Nevertheless, focusing on the pros of dietary fat reduction can also be useful for people in these later stages, as recalling benefits helps to reaffirm and sustain dietary change.

TEMPTATION TO EAT AND CONFIDENCE TO RESIST HIGH-FAT FOODS

Temptation and confidence are two concepts that become particularly important when intervening with patients who are in the later stages of change. *Temptation* represents an individual's overall tendency to be enticed to eat too many high-fat foods across different types of situations, whereas *confidence,* or *self-efficacy,* represents the overall confidence the individual feels that he or she can resist doing so.

Three situations have been identified as important with regard to both temptation and self-efficacy (Rossi, 1993). *Positive social situa-*

tions involve a positive feeling plus an implied or actual social situation. *Negative affective situations* involve feeling bad in a negative situation. *Difficult situations* involve situations in which it is difficult to obtain or prepare alternative low-fat foods. In general, temptation is high and self-efficacy low for people in the early stages of precontemplation, contemplation, and preparation, Self-efficacy becomes high and temptation decreases for those in the later stages of action and maintenance. Both positive social situations and difficult situations, however, have been found to be particularly troubling for people in the action stage.

TECHNIQUES FOR DIETARY MODIFICATION

Dietary interventions are targeted to match the patient's expected TTM profile for the pertinent stage of change. Although many TTM interventions are similar to those routinely used in practice, the intensity of the TTM intervention varies depending upon an individual's motivational readiness to change. An added benefit is that the clinician can use TTM-based assessment measures to tailor dietary interventions to the individual patient.

Using a Five-Step Program to Design Stage-Matched Dietary Interventions

A five-step program has been developed to help clinicians put the TTM into practice to reduce dietary fat intake for CHD prevention (Rossi, 1995). The steps include (1) considering the patient's stage of change and becoming familiar with characteristics of each stage, (2) considering the patient's TTM-based profile (i.e., stage-matched pros and cons, process use, temptation and confidence), (3) taking into account the task the patient needs to accomplish in a particular stage of change, (4) being prepared to deal with the major problems clinicians face in each stage, and (5) employing stage-matched guidelines to design dietary interventions for practice.

Table 6–9 illustrates how to apply the five-

TABLE 6-9 Summary of Five-Step Program by Stage for Dietary Fat Reduction

Step 1		Step 2		Step 3	Step 4	Step 5
Stage of Change	Description	Characteristics	TTM Profile	Patient's Task	Clinician's Major Problems	Stage-Matched Dietary Interventions
Precontemplation	Patients are not ready to reduce fat; do not consistently avoid high-fat foods; have no intention of doing so in the next 6 months.	Patients are unable or unwilling to make dietary changes; may be unaware that high dietary fat intake is a problem for them; may be in denial; may be demoralized.	*Pros & Cons:* Pros are low, and Cons are high. *Process Use:* These patients use processes the least. *Temptation* is high. *Confidence* is low.	Think about dietary fat; recognize it's a problem; personalize the problem.	Recruit patients for intervention; deal with patients' resistance to dietary behavior change; keep patients in intervention.	*Deal with feelings first:* • Overcome resistance. • Deal with denial. • Increase awareness of the problem. *Pros & Cons:* Raise pros and acknowledge cons. *Increase Process Use:* Emphasize CR, DR, SR, ER.
Contemplation	Patients are thinking about reducing fat.	Patients are ambivalent about cutting down on fat; think maybe they should cut down, but they don't want to.	*Pros & Cons:* Initially cons increase. Cons are higher than for PC. Later pros equal cons (i.e., decisional balance point). *Process Use:* These patients use processes more than precontemplators. *Temptation* is high.	Turn thoughts into behavior; make the decision to cut down on dietary fat.	Patients in this stage think too much; chronic contemplators substitute thinking about cutting down on fat for doing it.	Provide information about the problem. *Pros & Cons:* Tip the scales by raising the pros. *Increase Process Use:* Emphasize CR, SR, SL, SO, HR.
Preparation	Patients are ready to reduce dietary fat intake.	Patients are ready for change, have a plan, usually vague; are committed to changing their diet; have made a decision to cut down on dietary fat; are experimenting with their diet; most will attempt to reduce fat in next 6 months but fail.	*Pros & Cons:* Crossover occurs so pros outweigh cons. Pros are greater and cons are less than for contemplators. *Process Use:* These patients use processes more than contemplators do; Behavioral process use increases. *Temptation* is high in all three situations.* *Confidence* is low in all three situations.	Prepare for action; experiment to discover what works and what doesn't.	Patients in this stage want to decrease dietary fat but don't know how to go about it effectively; they may be inadequately prepared; they must be helped to learn from their mistakes.	Provide a detailed plan with choices. Include small steps. *Pros & Cons:* Strengthen and renew patient's commitment to cut down on dietary fat by emphasizing pros. *Increase Process Use:* Emphasize CR, SL, SO, HR, CC, SC. Make patients aware of the three tempting situations. Increase confidence.

Stage						
Action	Patients have consistently avoided high-fat foods for 6 months or less.	Patients have reduced dietary fat to desired level; whatever they are doing works well for them; they engage in lots of activity; they are in an unstable stage.	*Pros & Cons:* Pros decrease but remain high. Cons continue to decrease. *Process Use:* These patients use processes more than those in preparation. *Temptation* decreases, but positive social and difficult situations can be tempting. *Confidence* increases, but positive social and difficult situations can be a problem.	Stay in stage long enough to benefit from it; recycle quickly from relapse.	Patient may be inadequately prepared to cut down on fat; relapse is common.	Institute relapse prevention; help patients recycle quickly back into P or C if they relapse. *Pros & Cons:* Reinforce pros. *Increase Process Use:* Emphasize CR, SL, ER, HR, CC, SC, IP, RM. *Temptation:* Provide coping strategies for positive social and difficult situations. *Confidence:* Provide strategies for increasing confidence.
Maintenance	Patients have adopted a low-fat lifestyle, consistently avoiding high-fat foods for more than 6 months.	Patients' risk of relapse is low; they are in a dynamic yet stable stage; they have met the action criterion for more than 6 months.	*Pros & Cons:* • Pros decrease but remain higher than in contemplation stage. • Cons continue to decrease but remain lower than in precontemplation stage. *Process Use:* These patients continue to use processes; for most processes, use is greater than in action stage. *Temptation* is low. *Confidence* is high.	Consolidate gains made in previous stages; make low-fat eating a habit; accelerate to termination stage, if it exists.	Keep patient in maintenance stage; prevent relapses; accelerate movement to termination stage, if it exists.	Risk of relapse is low, but relapse prevention should be instituted when appropriate; help patients recycle quickly into P or C if they relapse. *Pros & Cons:* Can reinforce pros. *Continue Process Use:* Emphasize same processes as used in action stage CR, SL, ER, HR, CC, SC, IP. *Temptation:* Stress is often the problem. Institute stress management techniques if appropriate. *Confidence:* Provide strategies for reinforcing confidence.

PC = precontemplation
C = contemplation
P = preparation
A = action
M = maintenance

CR = consciousness raising
DR = dramatic relief
SR = self reevaluation
ER = environmental reevaluation
HR = helping relationships

CC = Counterconditioning
SC = Stimulus control
IP = Interpersonal systems control
SL = Self-liberation
RM = Reinforcement management

*The three situations are (1) positive social situations, (2) negative affective situations, and (3) situations in which it is difficult to substitute low-fat alternatives.

step program to design stage-matched dietary interventions for patients in any stage of change. The first step in applying the TTM to CHD prevention for patients at any stage of motivational readiness to change is to determine the patient's stage of change. Stages of change are listed in the first column of Table 6–9 and may be determined using the recommended stage-of-change algorithm for dietary fat reduction. Each stage of change is characterized with a brief description in the second column of the table. Clinicians will find it useful to keep the stage-of-change description in mind when dealing with patients in a particular stage.

Step 1 also involves understanding the characteristics of patients in a particular stage of change and is presented for patients in each stage in the third column of Table 6–9. This is a necessary and important part of designing effective dietary interventions. Being aware of the patient's stage-of-change characteristics helps the clinician orient the presentation of intervention material, because it provides insight into the patient's perspective of the problem.

The second step in applying the TTM to CHD prevention is to consider what is known about individuals in a particular stage of change. TTM profiles for patients in each stage of change are presented in the fourth column of Table 6–9. TTM-based research on dietary fat reduction has produced consistent stage-matched profiles for people in each stage of change for (1) the pros and cons (i.e., making the decision to engage in dietary behavior change), (2) the processes of change (i.e., using specific types of activities, strategies, and approaches to accomplish dietary change), and (3) the relationship between the temptation to eat high-fat foods and the self-efficacy (confidence) to resist. Profiles for each of these dimensions have been previously described and can be predicted according to the stage of change a patient is in. A patient's TTM profile may be determined using the model-based assessment tools for the pros and cons of decisional balance, processes of change, temptation, and confidence for dietary fat reduction.

The third step in applying the TTM to CHD prevention involves having the clinician focus on the task the patient needs to accomplish in a particular stage of change. The patient's task,

or main goal, varies depending on the stage of change and is presented in the fifth column of Table 6–9. It is important to help the patient focus on achieving this goal to facilitate dietary behavior change and progress toward the next stage.

The fourth step in applying the TTM to CHD prevention is concerned with the clinician and is presented in the sixth column of Table 6–9. It involves being prepared to deal with the major problems the clinician will have to face when intervening with patients in each stage of change.

The fifth step in applying the TTM to CHD prevention involves employing stage-matched guidelines to design dietary interventions for patients in each stage of change. Interventions vary and are designed and implemented based on patients' expected TTM profiles for their stage of change. Guidelines for focusing on the pros and cons and the temptation and confidence aspects as well as the processes that should be emphasized are included in the seventh column of Table 6–9.

Four points are particularly noteworthy regarding this step-based program. First, recommendations for stage-matched dietary intervention are currently based on cross-sectional data (Rossi, 1993) and are for *adults only*. Second, TTM-based research on dietary fat reduction has produced consistent stage-matched profiles for people in each stage of change in regard to (1) making the decision to engage in dietary behavior change, (2) using specific types of activities, strategies, and approaches to accomplish dietary change, and (3) understanding the relationship between the temptation to eat high-fat foods and the self-efficacy to resist. Third, the relationship between the pros and cons has been replicated in other TTM-based dietary research on decision making (Rossi, Greene, Reed, et al., 1993; Rossi, Greene, Reed, et al., 1994a). Finally, the relationship between process use and stage of change has been replicated in additional studies (Rossi, 1992; Rossi & Rossi, 1993; Rossi, Greene, Reed, et al., 1994b).

In the remainder of this chapter, the application of the five-step program for each stage of change will be discussed in detail. The subtle nuances of intervention at each stage will be highlighted and issues related to relapse and addressing temptation and confidence discussed.

Interventions for People Not Ready to Change Dietary Behavior: Precontemplation Stage

Patients who are not ready to reduce dietary fat consumption are in the *precontemplation* stage of change. Precontemplation tends to be a very stable stage in which individuals can linger for long periods of time. Precontemplators do not consistently avoid high-fat foods and have no intentions of doing so anytime in the future. They characteristically are unable or unwilling to change because of such factors as a general lack of awareness about the gravity of the problem of high fat consumption and a tendency toward denial (Prochaska & DiClemente, 1984). In addition, some patients in this stage of change may have tried to cut down on dietary fat in the past but failed, leaving them so demoralized that they feel dietary change is not possible for them.

For patients in this stage, the pros of reducing dietary fat intake are low, whereas the cons are high (Rossi, 1993). Consequently, the costs or hassles involved in cutting down on dietary fat appear to outweigh any potential benefits. Consistent with their lack of interest, precontemplators have been found to use the 11 processes of change much less than people in any of the other stages of change (Rossi, 1993). In the precontemplation stage, the temptation to eat high-fat foods is high, and confidence to resist them is low, whether in positive social situations, negative affective situations, or situations in which it is difficult to obtain or prepare low-fat alternatives (Ounpuu, Woolcott & Rossi, 1996; Rossi & Rossi, 1994; Rossi, Rossi, Greene, et al., 1994).

The patient task that clinicians must address is getting these patients to think about high dietary fat consumption. They need to recognize that high dietary fat intake not only constitutes a major health problem for people in general but, more importantly, affects them personally. The major problems facing the clinician in regard to these patients include recruitment, overcoming patient resistance, and, finally, sustaining patient interest (i.e., retention)

(Prochaska, 1992; Prochaska & DiClemente, 1984).

Intervention involves providing precontemplators with information and feedback. As they do not see the risk of high dietary fat intake as relevant, it is often very difficult for precontemplators to think of the benefits associated with reducing dietary fat intake. One effective decisional-balance exercise is to provide precontemplators with a list of reasons for changing their diet (i.e., pros) that counter reasons for not changing it (i.e., cons). Preliminary research indicates that interventions should focus on at least the four experiential processes of change: consciousness raising, dramatic relief, self-reevaluation, and environmental reevaluation, as previously described.

Interventions for People Thinking About Changing Dietary Behavior: Contemplation Stage

Patients who have not yet cut down on dietary fat intake but are seriously thinking about doing so sometime in the next 6 months are in the *contemplation* stage of change. Although considering change, as a group, contemplators are characteristically ambivalent. They think they should change, but they really don't want to (Prochaska & DiClemente, 1984). Thus, these patients are experiencing a battle of thoughts and feelings over making the decision to cut down on dietary fat consumption.

Initially the cons of changing dietary behavior are even higher for contemplators than for precontemplators, possibly because the negative aspects of changing may become more salient as patients weigh the costs and benefits of reducing dietary fat intake (Rossi, 1993). The pros, which are still low initially, rise later in the contemplation stage to approximately equal the cons. As this *decisional-balance point* is reached, the patient is ready to make a decision about reducing dietary fat intake (Prochaska & DiClemente, 1984).

Although their use of the processes of change is still low, contemplators tend to use more processes of change than precontemplators (Rossi, 1993). As with precontemplators, situational temptation remains high while confidence remains low (Ounpuu, Woolcott, &

Rossi, et al., 1996; Rossi & Rossi, 1994; Rossi, Rossi, Greene, et al., 1994).

During this stage, the task patients need to accomplish is to complete the decision-making process of committing themselves to reducing dietary fat. The major problem the clinician faces with people in this stage is that patients who are seriously considering reducing dietary fat consumption tend to think too much about it. *Chronic contemplators,* or people who linger in this stage, substitute thinking for action (Prochaska & DiClemente, 1984).

Because contemplators are already cognitively engaging in the change process, they can handle more information than precontemplators about the cardiovascular health problems associated with high dietary fat intake. Given the increase in cons in the beginning of this stage, the clinician should acknowledge the difficulties involved in making dietary changes (i.e., cutting down on fat intake is difficult but can be done). Given the ambivalence of these patients, the clinician also needs to increase pros by using such strategies as a decisional-balance exercise in which contemplators actively engage in generating a list of the pros and cons themselves and then determine which list is longer. If there are more cons than pros, the clinician assists the patient in generating additional pros until the pros outnumber the cons.

Process use by precontemplators focuses on experiential processes, but contemplators can begin to make use of some behavioral processes as well. The following specific processes of change may be emphasized: consciousness raising, self-reevaluation, self-liberation, social liberation, and helping relationships. Processes new to this stage, such as self-liberation, involve willpower, commitment, and choices.

Clinicians should design interventions that encourage the patient to think about how dietary changes could be made. Patients in this stage need reassurance that the professional helping them believes they can make changes if they try. The contemplator also needs support to make a commitment to reduce fat consumption. In addition, interventions should help patients become aware of low-fat alternative food choices. When operationalizing social liberation, dietary interventions should help the contemplator look around and take notice of changes in the environment that make it easier to cut down on fat. Similarly, in making use of the process of helping relationships, clinicians need to encourage contemplators to not only seek, but to accept, offered help from family members and friends in lowering fat consumption.

Interventions for People Ready to Change Dietary Behavior: Preparation Stage

Patients in the preparation stage of change are ready to reduce fat intake in the immediate future and generally have some kind of vague plan for reducing fat intake. Like precontemplators and contemplators, they do not consistently avoid high-fat food intake. Individuals in the preparation stage characteristically engage in a lot of experimentation. Most patients in this stage will attempt change in the next 6 months but fail unless adequately prepared.

In preparation, a crossover occurs so that the pattern of the pros and cons reverses, such that the pros begin to outweigh the cons (Rossi, 1993). As in previous stages, temptation remains high and confidence remains low in positive social situations, negative affective situations, and situations in which it is difficult to obtain or prepare low-fat alternatives (Ounpuu, Woolcott, & Rossi, 1996; Rossi & Rossi, 1994; Rossi, Greene, Reed, et al., 1994).

Patients in this stage of change need to find out what works for them through experimentation. When a strategy fails, the clinician needs to help the patient reframe the experience as a learning experience. It is important for patients to learn from mistakes rather than be discouraged by them.

The major problem the clinician faces is that although patients in preparation want to cut down on fat, they do not know how to go about it effectively. These patients need a detailed plan to help them change. In addition to providing choices to enlist patient cooperation, motivation, and put the patient in control, the clinician should include small steps toward dietary change in the detailed plan. For example, the clinician might offer a menu to consider trying.

When a patient shows enthusiastic signs of

being ready and motivated to change, clinicians often make the mistake of rushing into intensive, action-oriented behavioral-change strategies too soon. The risk of relapse then increases, because although cognitively motivated to change, patients in preparation are often inadequately prepared to do so in practice. Thus, the prudent clinician will encourage patients to choose one approach at a time, focusing on a single change for a week before adding another. This approach builds patients' confidence in their ability to make dietary changes and helps them find out what works for them.

Clinicians should also promote an increase in process use by designing interventions that emphasize the use of consciousness raising, self-reevaluation, self-liberation, social liberation, helping relationships, counterconditioning, and stimulus control. In counterconditioning, for example, the patient substitutes lower-fat foods for high-fat ones, such as using low-fat frozen yogurt in place of high-fat ice cream. As another example, in stimulus control, the patient uses cue reduction or avoidance, such as giving away leftover desserts lest they act as a trigger to temptation.

Although it is still desirable to bolster the pros in this stage of change, clinicians need to make patients in the preparation stage aware of the temptations they will face as they try out small changes. Clinicians also need to design interventions to increase patients' confidence to resist temptations in positive social situations, negative affective situations, and situations in which it is difficult to obtain or prepare low-fat alternatives. These interventions involve teaching patients to pay attention to and recognize specific triggers that may encourage them to eat high-fat foods. Patients should also be taught coping skills to help them deal with temptation in these situations and build confidence to resist high-fat foods. For example, patients who grab high-fat snacks like potato chips while watching TV could be coached to substitute pretzels or carrot sticks.

Interventions for People Changing Dietary Behavior: Action Stage

Patients in the *action* stage of change have recently reduced their fat intake and have consistently avoided high-fat foods for 6 months or less. Action tends to be a busy but unstable stage. One of the most important characteristics of people in this stage of change is that they have reduced fat intake to the desired target level or action criterion established by the clinician. The pros of change decrease but remain high, while the cons continue to decrease (Rossi, 1993). Process use is higher than in previous stages of change, reflecting the characteristic flurry of activity in this stage (Rossi, 1993). In sharp contrast to previous stages, temptation decreases and confidence increases (Ounpuu, Woolcott, Rossi, et al., 1996; Rossi & Rossi, 1994; Rossi, Rossi, Greene, et al., 1994). Difficult situations and, to a greater extent, positive social situations have been found to present a potential problem for the person in action (Rossi, 1993).

The patient's task for this stage is to stay in this stage long enough to derive benefit. Persistence for at least 6 months is required. Because action is a highly unstable stage, relapse is common and can be expected as part of the normal course of events. Relapse is a condition, not a stage of change and occurs only for patients in the action or maintenance stage of change. For relapse to occur, the desired *action* criterion behavior set by the clinician must have been reached. The major problems clinicians face relate to inadequate patient preparation and the problem of relapse. The clinician's role, aside from relapse prevention, is to help the individual recycle quickly. Returning the patient to the action stage is most desirable, but clinicians may have to settle for a return to the preparation or even contemplation stage.

Action is characterized by intense activity. Despite the clinician's own preferences, it is helpful to accept the nondetrimental strategies that the patient finds most effective. Whereas small steps are appropriate for preparation, the clinician who insists on small steps in this stage will hold patients back. Interventions involve helping the patient increase process use through consciousness raising, self-liberation, environmental reevaluation, helping relationships, counterconditioning, stimulus control, reinforcement management, and interpersonal systems control. There are a lot of processes to choose from, and it is important not to overwhelm people with too much information at one time.

Reinforcement management involves rewarding the healthy behavior of adopting lower-fat eating habits. Rewards administered by the clinician, patient, family, and so forth, may include praise, encouragement, a pat on the back, a spending spree, and such things. *Interpersonal systems control* involves either seeking the company of other individuals who eat lower-fat foods or avoiding those who encourage the patient to eat high-fat ones. Interventions also need to address temptations associated with positive social situations and difficult situations. Parties, events, or social gatherings where food will be present and times when it is a hassle to eat low-fat foods are prime examples of potential situations that can trigger temptation. Clinicians also need to focus on raising confidence to resist foods in those situations as well.

Interventions for People Maintaining Dietary Changes: Maintenance Stage

Patients in the *maintenance* stage have adopted a low-fat dietary lifestyle, having consistently avoided high-fat foods for more than 6 months. Research indicates that the risk of relapse is relatively low in this stage (Prochaska & DiClemente, 1984). Maintenance is a stable yet dynamic stage in which individuals need to continue using processes of change and remain vigilant (Redding, Rossi, Fava, et al., 1989; Rossi, 1993). Although both the pros and cons in maintenance decrease from action levels, the pros remain higher and the cons lower than in the precontemplation stage (Rossi, 1993). Process use remains high (Rossi, 1993). Temptation is low, and confidence is high (Ounpuu, Woolcott, Rossi, et al., 1996; Rossi & Rossi, 1994; Rossi, Rossi, Greene, et al., 1994).

The major task facing patients in the maintenance stage of change is to sustain lower-fat eating as a lifelong habit. Patients need to consolidate gains accomplished in the previous stage of change. The risk of relapse is very low in this stage (Prochaska & DiClemente, 1984). A possible sixth stage of change, *termination,* has been theoretically posed (Rossi & Rossi,

1998) and is described in Chapter 3. If a termination stage is validated, another potential task for patients will be to move toward that final stage.

The major problem facing the clinician in dealing with patients in the maintenance stage is to keep patients in this stage and prevent them from relapsing. Again, if the idea of a termination stage is valid, the clinician gains the additional task of helping patients toward that final stage.

Very preliminary work suggests that people who have been in maintenance for a year or less may be at higher risk for relapse than those who have been in maintenance longer than that (Rossi, 1993). TTM assessment tools can be very useful in predicting relapse. Pros and confidence scores that are lower, process use that is less, or temptation that is higher than it should be for people in this stage can alert the clinician that relapse is likely. Currently, many of the processes used in the action stage continue to be emphasized for use in maintenance in relapse (consciousness raising, self-liberation, environmental reevaluation, helping relationships, counterconditioning, stimulus control, and interpersonal systems control).

If relapse does occur, the clinician should help the patient recycle quickly. However, patients in this stage of change tend to be highly confident that they can resist eating favorite high-fat foods, and they tend to report that they are not tempted by such foods (Rossi & Rossi, 1994; Rossi, Greene, Reed, et al., 1994). When temptation does occur, stress is often the culprit, so stress management is an appropriate intervention. Boredom with lower-fat eating habits is also a problem for patients in this stage of change. Thus, clinicians may wish to broaden the diet and shift the emphasis from lower-fat eating to healthy eating in general. Interventions to increase dietary fiber and fruit and vegetable intake for patients in maintenance provides some novelty and may promote motivation to continue healthy dietary behavior.

CONCLUSION

Diet is the cornerstone of therapy for an elevated blood cholesterol. Cardiovascular health and quality of life can be dramatically improved when dietary behavior changes are instituted. Thus, dietary intervention has been recognized as an important tool for reducing CHD risk by both health-care professionals and the public. Two complementary approaches that represent a coordinated effort to reduce CHD were presented for dietary intervention in this chapter. The first focuses on nutritionally based primary and secondary clinical management guidelines for the prevention of CHD in patients at high risk for its development or its recurrence. The second, a behavioral-change approach to dietary intervention for primary prevention of CHD based on the TTM, can be used with patients at risk in the population at large; it focuses on reducing overall dietary fat consumption.

Acknowledgment

The authors wish to thank Kim Gans, Ph.D., MPH, LDN, Memorial Hospital Division of Health Education, and Stephanie Ounpuu, Ph.D., RD, University of Guelph, for their reviews and helpful comments on previous versions of this chapter.

RESOURCES TO ASSESS DIETARY ADHERENCE

A food-scoring tool to assess dietary adherence to a cholesterol-lowering diet is available from Dr. C. C. Tagney, Department of Clinical Nutrition, Rush-Presbyterian-St. Luke's Medical Center, 1742 West Harrison 502SSH, Chicago, IL 60612.

Other resources for assessing dietary adherence follow:

Peters, J. R., Quiter, E. S., Brekke, M. L., et al. (1994). The eating-pattern assessment tool: A simple instrument for assessing dietary fat and cholesterol intake. *Journal of the American Dietetic Association, 94,* 1008–1013.

Mitchell, D. T., Korslund, M. K., & Brewer, B. K. (1996). Development and validation of the Cholesterol-Saturated Fat Index (CSI) scorecard: A dietary self-monitoring tool. *Journal of the American Dietetic Association, 96,* 132–136.

Ammerman, A. S., DeVellis, B. M., Haines, P. S., et al. (1992). Nutrition education for cardiovascular disease prevention among low-income populations—Description and pilot evaluation of a physician-based model. *Patient Education and Counseling, 19,* 5–18.

Gans, K. M., Sundaram, S. G., McPhillips, J. B., et al.

(1993). Rate your plate: An eating-pattern assessment and educational tool used at cholesterol-screening and education programs. *Journal of Nutritional Education, 25,* 29–36.

References

Achterberg, C. L. (1988). Factors that influence learner readiness. *Journal of the American Dietetic Association, 88,* 1426–1428.

Achterberg, C. L., Novak, J. D., & Gillespie, A. H. (1985). Theory-driven research as a means to improve nutrition education. *Journal of Nutrition Education, 17,* 179–184.

American Heart Association. (1988). *Dietary Treatment of Hypercholesterolemia: A Handbook for Counselors.* Dallas.

American Heart Association. (1996). *Heart and Stroke Facts Statistics.* Dallas.

Anderson, J. W., Garrity, T. F., Wood, C. I., Whitis, S. E., Smith, B. M., & Oeltgen, P. R. (1992). Prospective, randomized, controlled comparison of the effects of low-fat and low-fat plus high-fiber diets on serum lipid concentrations. *American Journal of Clinical Nutrition, 56,* 887–894.

Barton, L., (1993). Evaluation of a nutrition education media program: The Nutrition Advisory column in the *Hamilton Spectator.* Unpublished masters thesis, University of Guelph.

Brun, J. K., & Rhoads (Eds.) (1983). *Nutrition Education Research: Strategies for Theory Building, Conference Proceedings.* Rosemont, IL: National Dairy Council and U.S. Department of Agriculture, pp. 49–67.

Campbell, M. K., DeVellis, B. M., Strecher, V. J., Ammerman A. S., DeVellis, R. F., & Sandler, R. S. (1994). Improving dietary behavior: The effectiveness of tailored messages in primary-care settings. *American Journal of Public Health, 84 (5),* 783–787.

Close, A. (1988). Patient education: A literature review. *Journal of Advanced Nursing, 13,* 203–213.

Contento, I. R. (1993). Toward a framework for theory building in nutrition education research. In J. K. Brun and A. F. Rhoads (Eds.), *Strategies for Theory Building: Conference Proceedings.* Rosemont, IL: National Dairy Council and U.S. Department of Agriculture, pp. 49–67.

Contento, I. R. (1992). Nutritional perspective on individual subject interventions. In M. M. Henderson, D. J. Bowen, K. K. De Roos (Eds.), *Promoting Dietary Change in Communities: Applying Existing Models of Dietary Change to Population Based Interventions.* Seattle, Fred Hutchinson Cancer Research Center, pp. 53–60.

Curry, S. J., Kristal, A. R., Bowen, D. J. (1992). An application of the stage model of behavior change to dietary fat reduction. *Health Education Research: Theory & Practice, 7,* 95–105.

DiClemente, C. C. (1993). Changing addictive behaviors: A process perspective. *Current Directions in Psychological Science, 2,* 101–106.

Dattilo, A. M., & Kris-Etherton, P. M. (1992). Effects of weight reduction on blood lipids and lipoproteins: A meta-analysis. *American Journal of Clinical Nutrition, 56,* 320–328.

Denke, M. A., Sempos, C. T., & Grundy, S. M. (1993). Excess body weight: An unrecognized contributor to high blood cholesterol levels in white American men. *Archives of Internal Medicine, 153,* 1093–1103.

Foreyt, J. P. (1989). Behavioral approaches for primary

prevention: Dietary modification. *Human Behavior and Cancer Risk Reduction: Proceedings of the Working Conference on Unmet Needs.* Atlanta, GA: American Cancer Society, November, pp. 86–87.

Glanz, K., & Mullis, R. M. (1988). Environmental interventions to promote healthy eating: A review of models, programs and evidence. *Health Education Quarterly, 15,* 395–415.

Gordon, D. J., Probstfeld, J. L., Garrison, R. J., Neaton, J. D., Castelli, W. P., Knoke, J. D., Jacobs, D. R., Bangdewala, S., & Tyroler, H. A. (1989). High-density lipoprotein cholesterol and cardiovascular disease: Four prospective American studies. *Circulation, 79,* 8–15.

Greene, G. W., Rossi, S. R., Reed, G. R., Willey, C., & Prochaska, J. O. (1994). Stages of change for reducing dietary fat to 30% of energy or less. *Journal of the American Dietetic Association, 94,* 1105–1110.

Grundy, S. M. (1987). Dietary therapy for different forms of hyperlipoproteinemia. *Circulation, 76,* 523–528.

Harris, W. S. (1997). n-3 fatty acids and serum lipoproteins: Human studies. *American Journal of Clinical Nutrition, 65*(5 Suppl.), 1645S–1654S.

Hertog, M. G. L., Feskens, E. J. M., Hollman, P. C. H., & Kromhout, D. (1993). Dietary antioxidant flavonoids and risk of coronary heart disease: The Zupthen elderly study. *Lancet, 342,* 1007–1011.

Holli, B. B. (1988). Using behavior modification in nutrition counseling. *Journal of the American Dietetic Association, 88,* 1530–1536.

Johnson, D. W., & Johnson, R. T. (1985). Nutrition education's future. *Journal of Nutrition Education, 17(2) (Suppl.),* 20–24.

Joint National Committee (1997). Sixth Report of the Joint National Committee on Prevention, Detection, Evaluation, and Treatment of High Blood Pressure. Bethesda, MD: National High Blood Pressure Education Program (NIH Publication no. 98-4080).

Kannel, W. B., Cupples, L. A., Ramaswami, R., Stokes, J. III, Kreger, B. E., & Higgins, M. (1991). Regional obesity and risk of cardiovascular disease: The Framingham study. *Journal of Clinical Epidemiology, 44,* 183–190.

Kayman, S. (1989). Applying theory from social psychology and cognitive behavioral psychology to dietary behavior change and assessment. *Journal of the American Dietetic Association, 89,* 191–193.

Kris-Etherton, P. M., & Nicolosi, R. J. (1995). *Trans* fatty acids and coronary heart disease risk. *International Life Sciences Institute, Technical Committee on Fatty Acids.* Washington, DC: ILSI Press, pp. 10–15.

Kristal, A. R., White, E., Shattuck, A. L., Curry, S., Anderson, G. L., Fowler, A., & Urban, N. (1992). Long-term maintenance of a low-fat diet: Durability of fat-related dietary habits in the Women's Health Trial. *Journal of the American Dietetic Association, 92,* 553–559.

Locke, E. A., Shaw, K. N., Saari, L. M., & Latham, G. P. (1981). Goal setting and task performance: 1969–1980. *Psychological Bulletin, 90,* 227–242.

Marcus, B. H., Eaton, C. A., Rossi, J. S., & Harlow, L. L. (1994). Self-efficacy, decision-making and stages of change: An integrative model of physical exercise. *Journal of Applied Social Psychology, 24,* 489–508.

Murphy, S. R., Rose, D., Hudes, M., & Viter, F. E. (1992). Demographic and economic factors associated with dietary quality for adults in the 1987–88 Nationwide Food Consumption Survey. *Journal of the American Dietetic Association, 92,* 1352–1357.

National Cancer Institute. (1987a). *Diet, Nutrition and Cancer Prevention: The Good News.* Bethesda, MD: Office of Cancer Communications. (NIH Publication no. 87-2878).

National Education Research Advisory Committee. (1987b). Nutrition education research: Announcement of a grant program. *Journal of Nutrition Education, 19,* 268–272.

National Research Council. (1989). Committee on Diet and Health. *Diet and Health.* Washington, D.C. National Academy Press.

Neale, A. V., Singleton, S. P., Dupius, M. H., & Hess, J. W. (1989). Correlates of adherence to behavioral contracts for cholesterol reduction. *Journal of Nutrition Education, 21,* 221–225.

Nitzke, S. A., & Athens, S. P. (1987). A snapshot summary of nutrition education research in progress. *Journal of Nutrition Education, 19,* 266–267.

Olson, C. M., & Kelly, G. L. (1989). The challenge of implementing theory-based intervention research in nutrition education. *Journal of Nutrition Education, 21,* 280–284.

Ornish, D., Brown, S. E., Scherwitz, L. W., Billings, J. H., Armstrong, W. T., Ports, T. A., McLanahan, S. M., Kirkeeide, R. L., Brand, R. J., & Gould, K. L. (1990). Can lifestyle changes reverse coronary heart disease? *Lancet, 336,* 129–133.

Ounpuu, S., Woolcott, D. M., & Rossi, S. R. (1996). Validation of a situational self-efficacy scale for dietary fat reduction (abstract). *Journal of the American Dietetic Association, 96,* A86.

Pennington, J. A. T. (1994). *Bowes & Church's Food Values of Portions Commonly Used,* 16th ed. Philadelphia: J.P. Lippincott.

Prochaska, J. O. (1992). A transtheoretical model of behavior change: Implications for diet interventions. In M. M. Henderson, D. J. Bowen, & K. K. DeRoss (Eds.), *Proceedings of the Conference on Promoting Dietary Change in Communities: Applying Existing Models of Dietary Change to Population-Based Interventions.* Seattle: Fred Hutchinson Cancer Center, pp. 37–49.

Prochaska, J. O. (1989). What causes people to change from unhealthy to health enhancing behavior? In C. C. Cummings & J. D. Floyd (Eds.), *Human Behavior and Cancer Risk Reduction: Overview and Report of a Conference on Unmet Research Needs.* Atlanta: American Cancer Society, pp. 30–34.

Prochaska, J. O., & DiClemente, C. C. (1984). *The Transtheoretical Approach: Crossing the Traditional Boundaries of Therapy.* Homewood, IL: Dow Jones/Irwin.

Redding, C. A., Rossi, J. S., Fava, J., Snow, M. G., Rossi, S. R., Prochaska, J. O., Velicer, W. F., & DiClemente, C. C. (1989). *Dynamic factors in the maintenance of smoking cessation: A naturalistic study.* Paper presented at the 10th annual meeting of the Society for Behavioral Medicine, April, San Francisco.

Rossi, J. S. (1992). *Common Processes of Change Across Nine Problem Behaviors.* Paper presented at the 100th annual convention of the American Psychological Association, August, Washington, DC.

Rossi, S. R. (1993). *Application of the Transtheoretical Model to Dietary Fat Reduction in a Naturalistic Environment.* Doctoral dissertation, University of Rhode Island (Dissertation Abstracts International, DA9421916).

Rossi, S. R., (1995). *Application of the Transtheoretical Model of Behavior Change to Dietary Intervention.* Workshop presented at the Annual Meeting of the Canadian Dietetic Association, June, Prince Edward Island, Canada.

Rossi, S. R., Ding, L., Rossi, J. S., Velicer, W. F., Greene, G. W., Fava, J., LaForge, R., Willey, C., & Levesque, D. (1996). Development of a measure for dietary fat intake in large-scale survey research. (Abstract). *Annals of Behavioral Medicine, 18*(Suppl.), 237.

Rossi, S. R., Greene, G. W., Reed, G., Prochaska, J. O., & Velicer, W. F. (1994a). Cross-validation of a decisional balance measure for dietary fat reduction (abstract). *Annals of Behavioral Medicine, 16*(Suppl.), 167.

Rossi, S. R., Greene, G. W., Reed, G., Prochaska, J. O., Velicer, W. F., & Rossi, J. S. (1993). A comparison of four stages of change algorithms for dietary fat reduction (abstract). *Annals of Behavioral Medicine, 15*(Suppl.), 62.

Rossi, S. R., Greene, G. W., Reed, G., Rossi, J. S., Prochaska, J. O., & Velicer, W. F. (1994b). Continued investigation of a process-of-change measure for dietary fat reduction (abstract). *Annals of Behavioral Medicine, 16*(Suppl.), 167.

Rossi, S. R., & Rossi, J. S. (1993). Processes of change for dietary fat reduction. *Annals of Behavioral Medicine, 15*(Suppl.), 62.

Rossi, S. R., & Rossi, J. S. (1994). Confirmation of a situational temptation measure for dietary fat reduction. *Annals of Behavioral Medicine, 16*(Suppl.), S168.

Rossi, S. R., & Rossi, J. S. (1998). Concepts and theoretical models applicable to risk reduction. In N. Jairath (Ed.), *Coronary Heart Disease and Risk Factor Management: A Nursing Perspective*. Philadelphia: Saunders, chapter 3.

Rossi, S. R., Rossi, J. S., Greene, G. W., Reed G., Prochaska, J. O., & Velicer, W. F. (1994). Development of a self-efficacy questionnaire for dietary fat reduction (abstract). *Annals of Behavioral Medicine, 16*(Suppl.), 168.

Rossi, S. R., Rossi, J. S., Prochaska, J. O., & Velicer, W. F. (1993). *Measurement Structure of a Decisional Balance Questionnaire for Dietary Fat Reduction*. Paper presented at the 101st annual convention of the American Psychological Association, August, Toronto, Ontario, Canada.

Rossi, J. S., Rossi, S. R., Velicer, W. F., & Prochaska, J. O. (1995). Motivational readiness to control weight. In D.B. Allison (Ed.), *Methods for the Assessment of Eating Behaviors and Weight-Related Problems*. Newbury Park, CA: Sage, pp. 381–424.

Sims, L. S. (1987). Nutrition education research: Reaching toward the leading edge. *Journal of the American Dietetic Association, 87*,(9)(Suppl.), 10–18.

Skinner, B. F. (1969). *Contingencies of Reinforcement: A Theoretical Analysis*. New York: Appleton-Century-Crofts.

Steinberg, D., Pearson, T. A., & Kuller, L. H. (1992). Davis Conference-Alcohol, and atherosclerosis. *Annals of Internal Medicine, 114,* 967–976.

Thomas, C. B., & Cohen, B. H. (1955). The familial occurrence of hypertension and coronary heart disease, with observations concerning obesity and diabetes. *Annals of Internal Medicine, 42,* 90–127.

U.S. Department of Health and Human Services (1991). *Healthy People 2000: National Health Promotion and Disease Prevention Objectives*. Washington, DC: U.S. Government Printing Office (DHHS Publication no. [PHS] 91–50212).

U.S. Department of Health and Human Services (1993). *Report of the Expert Panel on Detection, Evaluation, and Treatment of High Blood Cholesterol in Adults (ATP II)*. National Cholesterol Education Program. Bethesda, MD: National Heart, Lung, and Blood Institute (NIH Publication no. 93–3095).

Wardle, J. (1990). Conditioning processes and cue exposure in the modification of excessive eating. *Addictive Behaviors, 15,* 387–393.

White, A. A., & Skinner, J. D. (1988). Can goal setting as a component of nutrition education effect behavior change among adolescents? *Journal of Nutrition Education, 20,* 327–335.

CHAPTER 7

Smoking Cessation

Kathleen Hall Sims
Donna M. Zucker

Cigarette smoking is a major cause of morbidity and mortality in the United States, along with posing a major financial burden on the health-care industry. Reducing or eliminating smoking is of the utmost importance in reducing death and disease in the United States (U.S. Department of Health and Human Services, 1990). Basic nursing smoking interventions may facilitate cost-effective, successful smoking cessation and thus decrease the potential cost of health care and lack of productivity associated with smoking (Taylor, Houston-Miller, Killen, et al., 1990; Tesevat, 1992). This chapter illustrates the pathophysiologic and psychological effects of smoking and discusses research-supported behavioral modification techniques designed to promote adherence to smoking-cessation interventions. Although it is recognized that the use of spit and chew tobacco is on the rise nationally (Massachusetts Tobacco Control, 1995), this chapter focuses primarily on cigarette smoking. Our goal is to provide the nurse and other clinicians with tools to promote risk-factor management in smoking.

RELATIONSHIP BETWEEN SMOKING AND CORONARY HEART DISEASE RISK

Cardiovascular disease remains the leading cause of death and disability in the United States despite impressive declines in the past two decades (McBride, 1992). Cigarette smoking has been identified by the U.S. surgeon general as being the most important source of preventable morbidity and mortality, accounting for 435,000 deaths annually; 115,000 of those deaths are from coronary heart disease (CHD). In the United States this figure represents more annual deaths than from alcohol, cocaine, heroin, homicide, fires, car accidents, and AIDS combined (U.S. Department of Health and Human Services, 1990). Cigarette smoking has been strongly established as a major cause of atherosclerotic disease and is considered one of the major risk factors for CHD, making smoking cessation a national priority (U.S. Department of Health and Human Services, 1990).

Up to an estimated 30% of all deaths in the United States caused by CHD are attributed to cigarette smoking. In addition, smoking acts synergistically with other risk factors to substantially increase the risk for CHD. Smoking alone doubles the risk of heart disease; the risk is tripled for people age 45 to 65. When smoking is combined with either high blood pressure or elevated cholesterol, the risk of CHD is four times as high. When all three risk factors are present, the risk is eight times as high.

After 1–2 years of not smoking, the former smoker's risk of heart attack drops sharply and gradually returns to normal after about 10 years. Smokers are not the only ones affected by cigarette smoking. Involuntary smoking is identified as the third leading cause of preventable death in the United States (Lesmes & Donofrio, 1992) and is the attributed cause of 37,000 additional deaths from CHD annually (Glantz & Parmley, 1991).

The number of cigarettes smoked, or cumulative cigarette consumption, increases the risk of death and myocardial infarction, and no safe threshold for any amount of smoking has been identified (Rosenberg, Palmer, & Sharpiro, 1990; Pooling Project, 1978). Smoking reduces *high-density lipid* (HDL) protein levels and increases *low-density lipid* (LDL) protein levels (Willet, Green, Stampfer, et al., 1987).

Both men and women are equally affected by cigarette smoking in regard to the risk for heart disease. Women who smoke and are oral contraceptive users have a tenfold risk of CHD compared with nonusers (Petti & Wingred, 1978).

People who smoke are at greater risk of premature death than nonsmokers. And cigarette smoking brings economic loss as well as human suffering; it accounts for $22 billion in medical costs each year, with an additional $43 billion in lost production. Medicare and Medicaid alone pay out at least $4.2 billion annually to care for those who are ill from cigarette-related disease (McBride, 1992).

PATHOPHYSIOLOGIC EFFECTS OF SMOKING

The role of cigarette smoking in CHD development may be understood in terms of the patho-logic, physiologic, hematologic, and metabolic effects. Although a comprehensive exploration of these mechanisms is beyond the scope of this chapter, a summary of each of these effects follows.

Pathologic Effects

Smoking is clearly associated with the presence of atherosclerosis of the coronary arteries, small arteries of the myocardium, the aorta, and other vessels, as demonstrated in many autopsy and angiographic studies (U.S. Department of Health and Human Services, 1983; Davis, Shelton, Eigenberg, et al., 1985; U.S. Department of Health and Human Services, 1990). As discussed in Chapter 2, the process of atherosclerosis is complex, involving endothelial cell injury, endothelial smooth muscle cell proliferation, macrophage activity, foam cell development, lipid accumulation, and the development of plaques and plaque calcification. Smoking has a direct toxic effect on human endothelium. Nicotine may cause acute intimal injury to vascular endothelial cells (U.S. Department of Health and Human Services, 1983). The resultant smooth muscle proliferation may be influenced by several local mediators. Research indicates that smoking as few as two cigarettes doubles the number of circulating endothelial cells, causes the release of local stimulants to smooth muscle proliferation, and increases platelet adherence by over a hundredfold (Davis, Shelton, Eigenberg, et al., 1985; Pittilo, Clarke, Harris, et al., 1984).

Physiologic Effects

Inhalation of tobacco smoke and ingestion of nicotine affects the sympathetic nervous system, resulting in increases in heart rate, blood pressure, cardiac output, myocardial oxygen demand, and vasoconstriction. Vasoconstriction is caused by both systemic and local chemically induced effects (U.S. Department of Health and Human Services, 1983). For example, coronary artery spasm can be due to either local prostaglandin effects, platelet release of vasopressin, or systemic release of catecholamines (Scholl, Benacerraf, Ducimetiere, et al., 1986).

Carbon monoxide constitutes up to 6% of cigarette smoke and has a high affinity for binding to hemoglobin, elevating the carboxyhemoglobin levels, and reducing the oxygen-carrying capacity of the blood (Turner, McNichol, & Sillet, 1986; U.S. Department of Health and Human Services, 1983). Additionally, a 21% increased prevalence of ventricular premature beats has been documented on 2-minute electrocardiographic rhythm strips obtained from 10,119 men who smoked (Hennekens, Lown, Rosner, et al., 1980).

Hematologic Effects

The acute and chronic effects of cigarette smoke on the hematologic system contribute to the development of atherosclerotic lesions, thrombosis, and acute and chronic cardiovascular disease events. For example, smoking cigarettes acutely increases spontaneous aggregation of platelets, and chronic smoking adversely affects platelet activity and survival (Davis, Shelton, Eigenberg, et al., 1985; Folts, Gering, Lailby, et al., 1990; Nowak, Murray, Oates, et al., 1987).

Other hematologic factors, such as increased plasma viscosity and reduced red cell deformability and plasminogen levels that lead to thrombus formation, have been observed in smokers (Belch, McArdle, Burns, et al., 1984). Smoking partially inhibits the effects of aspirin on platelets by elevating catecholamines and increasing plasma viscosity, thus increasing the risk of thrombus formation (Belch, McArdle, Burns, et al., 1984; Folts, Gering, Lailby, et al., 1990). Levels of plasminogen that promote thrombolysis are lower in smokers, but levels increase after several years of smoking cessation (Wilhelmsen, Svardsudd, Korsan-Bengsten, et al., 1984; Belch, McArdle, Burns, et al., 1984). Therefore, the adverse hematologic effects of smoking can be reversed after smoking cessation.

Metabolic Effects

Metabolic factors that promote atherogenesis and changes in the lipoprotein distribution are associated with smoking. Smoking is associated with a significant reduction of HDL (U.S. Department of Health and Human Services, 1990). Conversely, an increase in HDL is seen after smoking cessation, with an expected rise after continued cessation of 6–8 mg/dl (Fortman, Haskell, & Williams, 1986; Stamford, Matter, Fell, et al., 1986). Smoking also has an indirect effect on cholesterol and triglyceride metabolism (Carney & Goldberg, 1984). Women who smoke have an earlier menopause and lower estrogen levels, which are considered to increase risk factors for cardiovascular disease (McBride, 1992).

The pathogenesis of CHD is extremely complex and is mediated by multiple mechanisms and etiologic factors. Clinical manifestations of CHD include myocardial infarction, angina pectoris, and sudden death (Munro & Cotran, 1988). Smoking appears to influence CHD progression in many ways. The exact components of cigarette smoke and tobacco that contribute to the development of CHD are unknown, although nicotine and carbon monoxide have been implicated (U.S. Department of Health and Human Services, 1983, 1990; Turner, McNichol, Sillett, et al., 1986). Tobacco smoke contains an estimated 4,000 known compounds, including some that are pharmacologically active, toxic, mutagenic, or carcinogenic (U.S. Department of Health and Human Services, 1989a).

PSYCHOPHYSIOLOGY OF CIGARETTE ADDICTION

Nicotine, one component of cigarette smoke, is currently identified as the active pharmacologic agent in tobacco that determines the addictive behavior of the cigarette smoker (U.S. Department of Health and Human Services, 1989b). The 1988 surgeon general's report concluded that tobacco meets the criteria for an addictive drug. Furthermore, the pharmacologic and behavioral processes that determine tobacco addiction are similar to those that determine addiction to drugs such as heroin or cocaine (U.S. Department of Health and Human Services, 1989b). Therefore, this discussion of the psychophysiology of cigarette addiction will focus primarily on nicotine addiction.

Nicotine addiction is characterized by (1) relative loss of control regarding use, (2) strength of addictive behavior, (3) occurrence of withdrawal signs and symptoms after abstinence, (4) increase in urge or craving to use the drug following abstinence, and (5) pressures to relapse despite completion of acute phases of nicotine withdrawal end within about 2 weeks after drug abstinence (Jarvik & Henningfield, 1988).

Pharmacology of Nicotine

When tobacco smoke is inhaled into the lungs, nicotine is easily absorbed into the systemic circulation and transported throughout the body because of its acid pH. Blood concentrations rise quickly during smoking and peak at the completion of cigarette smoking (Benowitz, 1992).

Benowitz (1992) describes the inhalation of nicotine via cigarette smoking as influencing the rate and pattern of delivery of the drug to the body organs. Inhalation results in rapid nicotine transfer into the arterial circulation and into the brain, which has specific receptor sites for the drug (U.S. Department of Health and Human Services, 1989a). Nicotine is estimated to take 19 seconds or less from the start of an inhalation to be delivered to the brain; this quick delivery to the brain means there is rapid behavioral reinforcement from smoking; moreover, the smoker can control the concentrations of nicotine in the brain by adjusting the depth and number of inhalations per minute (Benowitz, 1992).

Within 20–30 minutes of smoking, nicotine levels in the brain decline sharply as the nicotine is distributed by the systemic circulation. Nicotine is metabolized by the liver and excreted in the urine with a half-life of approximately 2 hours. As a result, nicotine accumulates during daily smoking, and its effects persist overnight (Benowitz, 1988). The net effect of these changes is that the smoker receives rapid behavioral reinforcement from nicotine and can regulate the amount of nicotine in the bloodstream.

Nicotine affects the nicotinic cholinergic receptor in the brain and other organs. Its effects appear to be predominately presynaptic; it facilitates the release of neurotransmitters such as acetycholine, norepinephrine, dopamine, and serotonin. Physiologic results of nicotine exposure include behavioral arousal and sympathetic neural activation. Resultant "positive" effects of smoking cigarettes cited by smokers include improved concentration, improved focus during task performance, and improved mood, demonstrated by reduced anger, tension, depression, and stress (Benowitz, 1992).

Nicotinic receptors have been found in greater numbers in the brains of smokers than in those of nonsmokers, suggesting that prolonged or repetitive exposure to nicotine results in neural adaptation. Over the course of a day, smokers develop tolerance to the behavioral arousal and cardiovascular effects of nicotine. Sensitivity to identified effects of nicotine is somewhat regained after nocturnal abstinence (Benowitz, 1992).

Most habitual smokers regulate the number of cigarettes per day, consuming 10–40 mg of nicotine per day to obtain the desired effects of cigarette smoking and to minimize withdrawal symptoms (Benowitz, 1992). Neuroadaption also results in nicotine withdrawal symptoms associated with abrupt smoking cessation. These symptoms include nicotine craving, restlessness, irritability, frustration, or anger, anxiety, impaired concentration, decreased heart rate, and increased appetite (Pomerleau, 1992). Withdrawal symptoms commonly reach maximum intensity 24–48 hours after cessation and gradually diminish in intensity over a period of 2 weeks.

Psychosocial Factors Supporting Smoking Behavior

The factors supporting smoking behavior have been examined from various perspectives. The role of nicotine in determining smoking behavior and tobacco addiction must be understood to effectively help a patient quit smoking (Haire-Joshu, Morgan, & Fisher, 1991). According to the 1990 surgeon general's report, "Smoking cessation is a dynamic process that begins with a decision to stop smoking and ends with abstinence from cigarettes maintained over a long period of time" (U.S. Department of Health and Human Services, p. 9, 1990). Smoking cessation is not an easy process and may require many attempts over a period of time.

The smoking-cessation process is often referred to as a *process of change* through *stages*. These stages may be influenced by a combination of social or environmental, psychological, and biologic factors. An interplay between intrinsic and biologic factors exists that reinforces the smoker's cigarette-smoking pattern. For example, the biologic potency of nicotine as a drug and the smoker's social, emotional, or environmental habits create a stronger smoking pattern, making it difficult for the smoker to quit.

Three physiologic processes help maintain cigarette smoking: (1) desire to avoid nicotine-withdrawal effects; (2) desire for the immediate peripheral and central effects of nicotine, such as arousal from the norepinephrine activity; and (3) anticipation of the conditioned reinforcement associated with the smoking (Pomerleau & Pomerleau, 1984; U.S. Department of Health and Human Services, 1986). The relative importance of these processes depends in part on the number of cigarettes and the content of nicotine and tar in the cigarettes.

Smoking is a learned behavior, the result of conditioning that is reinforced by the pharmacologic actions of nicotine, as well as an association between cues and anticipated effects of smoking and the resulting urges. Conditioning is an important element of drug addiction. However, conditioning develops only when the pharmacologic actions of the drug are combined with the behaviors. Nicotine is commonly seen as the primary reinforcer for cigarette smoking and the ritual components of smoking as the secondary reinforcers (Schneider & Jarvik, 1984). Conditioning loses its power without the active drug, but it is a major cause of relapse during the period of cessation. Other factors influencing drug addiction include personality and social setting.

Cigarette smoking is maintained by conditioning. Conditioned reinforcement from smoking a cigarette is understood as the association between cues to smoke and anticipated effects of smoking. Cues in the conditioning process include habitual associated behaviors such as drinking a cup of coffee or talking on the telephone. Resulting urges from these cues are another type of conditioning. Even unpleasant events become powerful cues to smoke, such as the irritability that a smoker may experience

from nicotine abstinence. Once smoking cessation has been achieved, symptoms such as a desire to smoke, especially during stressful situations, can persist for months or years (Benowitz, 1992).

Except for the first daily cigarette, most smoking behavior seems to be prompted by internal and external environmental cues rather than the need to terminate or avoid withdrawal (Pomerleau & Pomerleau, 1984). Daily rituals such as handling the cigarette one smokes create a powerful association with the effects of nicotine.

Smoking behaviors may be reinforced by family, friends, or peers; the fear of weight gain; stress; or depression. Former smokers who are married to a smoker, or have a lot of friends who smoke, are more likely to fail when trying to quit. Also, former smokers who work with smokers are less likely to maintain smoking cessation. The emotional influence of friends, family, and peers can diminish a smoker's ability to quit. Former smokers who are supported in their attempts to quit by friends and family are more successful. Those who are socially isolated because of divorce, health problems, and depression are more likely to continue to smoke (Bishop, Cook, Fisher, et al., 1985; Coppotelli & Orleans, 1985; House, Landis, & Umberson, 1988; Graham & Gibson, 1971; Mermelstein, Lichtenstein, & McIntyre, 1983; Shiffman, 1982; West, Graham, Swanson, et al., 1977).

Other Factors Supporting Smoking Behavior

People who experience a major depressive disorder smoke more frequently, and depressed smokers are less likely to quit than nondepressed smokers. Smokers enrolled in a smoking cessation program who were unsuccessful in attempts to quit had significantly higher pretreatment depression scores (Rausch, Nichinson, Lamke, et al., 1990). Other studies have demonstrated that smokers with a history of depression come to rely on the nicotine to prevent depressive episodes or the tobacco withdrawal syndrome that may cause depression (Anda, Williamson, Escobedo, et al., 1985; Covey, Glassman, & Stetner, 1990; Flanagan & Maany, 1982; Glassman, Helzer, Covey, et al., 1990; Hall, Tunstall, Rugg, et al., 1985).

Weight gain may also influence the persistence of smoking. Smokers weigh less than similar-aged nonsmokers. Smokers who quit often gain weight (Fisher, Haire-Joshu, Morgan, et al., 1990; U.S. Department of Health and Human Services, 1990). The average weight gain for a quitter is approximately 5 pounds; 3.5% may gain more than 20 pounds. The cause of weight gain is related to the normalization of metabolism and weight after smoking cessation; the notion that cessation causes a pathognomic weight gain is false. Sometimes the cause of weight gain after smoking cessation is due to increased appetite and hunger. The fear of weight gain is more common among women, because they are more likely than men to purposely use smoking to control their appetite and weight (Carney & Goldberg, 1984; Comstock & Stone, 1972).

In the acute phases of smoking cessation, individuals gain weight, and their reaction time may be impaired (Benowitz, 1992). These findings suggest that smoking-cessation efforts are more likely to be successful when nicotine addiction is addressed in conjunction with behavioral modification therapy.

BENEFITS OF SMOKING CESSATION

Cigarette smoking is the leading modifiable risk factor for CHD, and there is overwhelming evidence that smoking cessation reduces that risk substantially. Several studies have demonstrated the benefits of smoking cessation for the older adult (more than 60 years of age) as well as for younger and middle-age adults, for both primary and secondary prevention (Hermanson, Omenn, Kronmal, et al., 1988). One year of smoking cessation, or perhaps less, results in a reduction by one half or more of the excess risk associated with current smoking. It takes a number of years of smoking abstinence before a smoker's risk is reduced to that of a nonsmoker.

Smoking cessation after myocardial infarction is still beneficial. Whereas the former smoker's CHD risk is high relative to nonsmokers at baseline, it is decreased relative to smok-

ers who persist (U.S. Department of Health and Human Services, 1990). Unfortunately, the benefits of smoking cessation cannot be adequately explained in the literature because of the confounding effects of other risk factors in both primary and secondary prevention studies (Hermanson, Omenn, Kronmal, et al., 1988).

Theoretical Approaches

Theories of behavioral change have been detailed in Chapter 3. Theoretical approaches and concepts relevant to smoking cessation are derived from self-efficacy concepts, social learning theory, the health-belief model, and the transtheoretical (TTM), or stages-of-change model. According to principles of social learning theory, smoking is a learned behavior that can be unlearned. The individual needs to participate actively in learning behavior-changing skills. *Self-efficacy,* which is the degree to which individuals perceive they can be successful in making the behavior change, is very important. Self-efficacy increases with previous success with smoking cessation. Similarly, consistent with tenets of the health-belief model, it has been demonstrated that smokers will take action to change their smoking behavior if they believe (1) they are personally susceptible to a disease such as CHD or (2) the benefits of making the behavior change outweigh the costs of making the change.

The nurse and other clinicians can help patients develop the coping skills and attitudes necessary to help them quit. Setting small goals and rewards will increase a smoker's confidence in quitting smoking. According to the TTM, smoking cessation is a process of change that occurs in stages over a period of time (Ockene & Ockene, 1992a). This model is discussed in more detail in Chapter 3.

The stages of smoking include initial use, experimentation, and habitual use. The stages of cessation are precontemplation and contemplation of quitting, action, maintenance, and relapse. These stages of cessation occur over a period of time and in no specific order, and often different stages are repeated a number of times. The "stages-of-change" approach has been cited as perhaps the most important development in the past decade for smoking cessation (Prochaska & Goldstein, 1991).

The TTM as articulated by Prochaska and DiClemente (1984), suggests that smoking cessation may be viewed as a process of change that happens over a period of time. Most nurses and other clinicians think about smoking cessation as an overt and discrete event that involves changing a smoker into a nonsmoker. However, the average smoker experiences three to four serious quit attempts over a period of 7–10 years before successfully quitting (Prochaska & DiClemente, 1984). Therefore, the dichotomous classification of individuals as smokers or nonsmokers may represent an oversimplification of a complex process. Within the context of the TTM, clinicians such as advanced-practice nurses work with individuals to help them move through each stage in the smoking-cessation process. Furthermore, the stages-of-change component can guide the nurse in evaluating the best interventions to use.

The actual process of change is not linear but rather spiral. The smoker may relapse, and during relapse go to an earlier stage. Most smokers experience an *abstinence-violation effect,* in which negative feelings lead to a resistance against quitting smoking and return the individual to the precontemplation stage. (This effect is described in greater detail later in this chapter.) Fortunately, most smokers recycle back to the contemplation or preparation stages. Also fortunately, it has been found that whenever smokers recycle through a stage, they learn from their mistakes and can then try something different the next time around (Prochaska & Goldstein, 1991). Through accurate assessment of the smoker's stage and the use of stage-appropriate interventions, nurses and other clinicians can help current and former smokers move on to the next stage (Prochaska, DiClemente, Velicer, et al., 1985).

Based on the TTM, interventions for smoking cessation should be stage-specific. Suggestions follow:

1. For the *precontemplation* stage, assess perceptions regarding disease risk, vulnerability, and capability for change; provide continued personalized information on smoking and health; and correct misperceptions.
2. For the *contemplation* stage, provide support to attempt cessation and help to develop effective cessation strategies.
3. For the *ready-for-action* (i.e., *preparation*) stage, provide encouragement to set a quit date.
4. For the *action* and *maintenance* stages, promote the development of relapse-prevention skills and provide opportunities for the patient to ask for continued support.

Most smoking-cessation programs are designed for the smoker who is ready to take action, but many smokers may not be ready for action. Interventions will progress more smoothly when the nurse and smoker are focused on the same stage of change (Prochaska & Goldstein, 1991).

TECHNIQUES OF BEHAVIOR MODIFICATION

Smokers in the action stage of change need help in developing new skills related to smoking cessation. Behavior modification helps the smoker develop the skills and new behaviors necessary for success. Long-lasting results in behavioral change do not result merely from the information and personal support provided; the smoker often returns to smoking when the information is no longer remembered and the professional relationship is ended.

Clinicians can use one or more behavioral strategies based on the social learning theory concepts of self-efficacy, shaping, and behavioral self-management to help the smoker quit smoking. The health-care provider needs to understand why smokers smoke. Ockene and Ockene (1992b) have outlined five key strategies to help smokers take action: self-monitoring, stimulus control, incentives, substituting CHD-preventive behaviors, and contracts.

Self-Monitoring

Self-monitoring is used in most smoking-cessation programs, whether individual or group. As seen in Figure 7–1, it is helpful for smokers to keep records of the number of cigarettes smoked as well as the time, mood, activity,

	Time	Food and/or Alcohol	Relaxation	Work	Social/Recreational	Driving	Other (Please Describe)	Angry	Anxious	Bored	Depressed	Frustrated	Happy	Relaxed	Tired	Need Rating Most		Least
							NAME _____ DATE ,											
1																1	2	3
2																1	2	3
3																1	2	3
4																1	2	3
5																1	2	3
6																1	2	3
7																1	2	3
8																1	2	3
9																1	2	3
10																1	2	3

DATE is followed by DAY OF WEEK _____

Wrap this Pack Wrap around your pack of cigarettes and secure it with a rubber band. When you are about to take a cigarette, but before you actually put in in your mouth and light up: (1) enter the time of day; (2) check the activity you are doing; (3) check the word or words that best describe your feeling at the time; and (4) indicate how important that particular cigarette is to you at the time.   1. MOST IMPORTANT   2. ABOVE AVERAGE   3. LEAST IMPORTANT

FIGURE 7–1 Tobacco-use log: Pack wrap. From Massachusetts Tobacco Control Program (1995). Department of Public Health.

and desire level for each cigarette smoked. The record is kept for 1 week or more. This information is used to assess baseline smoking, treatment, and outcome (Schwartz, 1991). It helps smokers examine their smoking behavior, and such an examination may help them make changes in their smoking pattern (McFall, 1970).

Glasgow (1986) suggests that self-monitoring is useful if kept simple and short. If record keeping is too lengthy or complex, it will not be effective. The use of labels that can be wrapped around the cigarette packs is particularly effective.

Stimulus Control

Stimulus control is based on information from the smoker's record keeping that allows the smoker to identify situations and emotions that may trigger the craving for a cigarette. The smoker then can decide how to avoid those triggers and thus change behavior. For example, if a smoker always has a cigarette with an alcoholic drink, the smoker may decide to avoid alcoholic beverages (Ockene & Ockene, 1992b).

Incentives

Incentives are self-reward techniques that reinforce the performance of a specific behavior. Reward systems usually help maintain change more effectively than aversive ones (punishment). Rewards must be determined by the smoker and used often and repeatedly as needed (Ockene & Ockene, 1992b).

Substituting Behavior

Substituting CHD behavior with stress-reduction techniques, such as regular exercise, is helpful in reducing stress and relieving boredom. Stress, boredom, and increased relaxation are important reasons why smokers relapse. A walking program or other stress-reduction technique can be instituted with the help of the nurse.

Contracts

Contracts are useful tools in helping smokers keep their minds focused on smoking cessation and their plans to achieve it. The contract can include the plan (strategies for smoking cessation), quit date (timetable proposed), reasons for quitting, and a follow-up plan (Ockene & Ockene, 1992b).

Prescriptive Therapies

The nurse may supplement behavioral techniques with prescribed nicotine replacement. Knowledge about the advantages and disadvantages of nicotine replacement is essential when prescribing these therapies. Both behavioral and pharmacologic components are part of the complex of treating nicotine addiction. Nicotine replacement therapy provides a method similar to the pharmacologic treatment for other drug dependencies, allowing the smoker to obtain nicotine during the smoking-cessation effort (Jarvik & Henningfield, 1988).

When nicotine is given pharmacologically, either transmucosally (e.g., nicotine gum), or transdermally (e.g., nicotine patch), the drive to smoke may be reduced. Smokers may be able to reduce the number of cigarettes smoked even if they are not trying to stop smoking (Lucchesi, Schuster, & Emley, 1967). Pharmacologic nicotine enables smokers to lower their daily nicotine level while lessening tobacco withdrawal symptoms. This lessening of tobacco withdrawal symptoms allows the smoker to stay off cigarettes while learning how to deal with the psychological dependencies associated with smoking.

Over the years, the smoker has learned and become conditioned to respond to different triggers or cues to smoke. The triggers to smoke have been reinforced by the potent effects of nicotine. The smoker must therefore learn new behaviors and responses to long-established behaviors. However, we caution that the smoker is trading one addiction for another when using nicotine replacement and should plan to be on nicotine replacement therapy for at least 2–6 months in order to address this "new" addiction (Sachs & Leischow, 1991).

Additional Approaches

The focus of additional therapies includes nicotine replacement and the use of the medications such as antiadrenergic agents, anxiolytic agents, and antidepressants. The smoker who needs the most help is the heavy smoker who has a strong nicotine addiction, is not a self-changer, and will benefit from such prescriptive approaches (Robbins, 1993). Discussion of all new FDA-approved approaches to nicotine replacement therapy such as citric acid spray and nasal nicotine solution, a nicotine vapor, are beyond the scope of this chapter. However, specific approaches with more widespread application will be briefly addressed.

Nicotine fading is a technique that helps only with the physiologic dependence on nicotine. It fails to address the coping skills and relapse prevention necessary to achieve long-term abstinence. Therefore, it is primarily useful as an adjunct to other therapy. Nicotine fading is accomplished by changing to a lower-nicotine cigarette (fading) or cutting down on the number of cigarettes smoked *(tapering)*. The results from tapering have not been positive. As the smoker tapers his or her cigarettes, there is too much emphasis on the remaining cigarettes (Schwartz, 1987).

Medications used alone or in combination include lobeline, Restinil, silver acetate, methylphenidate, diazepam, hydroxyzine, lorazepam, amphetamines, meprobamate, phenobarbital, methamphetamine, methylscopolamine, various anticholinergics, and fenfluramine. Clinical trials of selected drugs have been studied from 1957 to 1977 in which cessation rates were based on self-report. Scopolamine had the highest success rate, 50% at 1 year, but those findings have not been replicable (Robbins, 1993).

SMOKING-CESSATION PROGRAMS

Overwhelming data supports the physiologic as well as the psychological addiction of smoking (Prochaska & Goldstein, 1991). Well-conducted trials are likely to provide answers to clinical questions, but gaps exist in predicting long-term maintenance of new behaviors. Smoking studies have created a new paradigm, or investigative model, for modern epidemiology in that observational studies may yield more of the "truth" than randomized trials (Susser, 1995).

A number of large community trials have shown some success with smoking-cessation interventions and support the following four conclusions: First, to bring about notable change in ingrained behavior and have the change pervade populations, time is needed to ignite and build a social movement at nongovernment levels. Second, once the movement is strong enough to induce policymakers to bring about formal policy change, change accelerates. Third, community intervention trials may fail the expectations of their sponsors; their seemingly small effects are compatible with those of nonexperimental interventions sustained continuously over the years. Fourth, community trials should not be abandoned, but a continued accumulation of knowledge is necessary to refine trials. There is much to learn about how to change group behavior to accomplish change at the population-based level. Social research is needed to understand how to bring about social change (Susser, 1995).

In the twenty-first century, smoking-cessation strategies will focus on a combination of the various modalities just mentioned (Prochaska & Goldstein, 1991). Despite research on multi-component-cessation programs that was encouraging initially, the majority of smokers entering these programs still return to smoking within 1 year (Schwartz, 1987; U.S. Department of Health and Human Services, 1986). A broad range of smoking-cessation programs is available, designed for personal or community use. The effectiveness of the programs depends on the individual seeking help. The most commonly used approaches are community and commercial programs, self-help programs, clinics and groups, hypnosis, and acupuncture.

Community Health Programs

A number of community programs have been developed to not only reduce smoking but also to reduce the risk of cardiovascular disease. The Stanford Three-Community Study was developed to determine whether community health education programs can reduce the risk of cardiovascular disease. This study used a mass media campaign consisting of television programming, radio spots, newspaper columns, advertising, billboards, and mailed messages.

Small-group meetings were held for 10 weeks to provide information on the harmful effects of smoking, advice on how to quit smoking, and instructions on self-control skills. The treatment group showed a 20–30% decrease in cardiovascular disease risk. A subgroup of smokers showed a 32% quit rate measured at 3 years after the program. In contrast, the control group had an increase in cardiovascular disease risk. It was concluded that group instruction with a mass media campaign was more successful than mass media alone in increasing community awareness of cardiovascular risk factors and in motivating and maintaining health behavior changes (Farquhar, Fortmann, Maccoby, et al., 1984).

Mass Media Campaigns

Mass media campaigns can increase motivation, but the combination of mass media campaigns and intensive individual instruction is more successful in smoking cessation and cardiovascular risk reduction. Outside factors, such as awareness of national antismoking campaigns, the death of a well-known person related to smoking, price increases in cigarettes, and new antismoking laws, are some of the many factors that can influence smoking cessation (Schwartz, 1987).

Self-Help Programs and Approaches

Many self-help programs can be an adjunct to individual follow-up with the nurse or group sessions such as cardiac rehabilitation programs. Using a self-help program such as *Freedom from Smoking* from the American Lung

Association or the *I Quit Kit* from the American Cancer Society is helpful. Self-help programs are used in adjunct with other programs such as cardiac rehabilitation, stress management, and with other behavioral techniques to help the patient become more successful at quit attempts. Hypnosis and acupuncture are ineffective alone, but perhaps would be beneficial with the use of adjunctive behavioral therapies (Schwartz, 1987). Patients often do not realize that they are responsible for the ultimate change in becoming a nonsmoker, and motivation must be present for success with either hypnosis or acupuncture.

As previously stated, most smokers quit on their own, but many use cessation programs at some point in time during their smoking years. Both individual and community-based programs have used a multicomponent approach that can be initially successful but not necessarily so in the long term.

ROLE OF ADVANCED-PRACTICE NURSE IN SMOKING CESSATION

In this section, we address the role of the *advanced-practice nurse* (APN) in smoking cessation. This role does not invalidate that of other nurses or clinicians. However, the APN's preparation in both the acute and primary care settings and expertise in case management confers substantial benefit. Areas in which APN expertise is currently used include management of cardiac risk factors such as hypertension and hyperlipidemia, in specialized clinics, and management of acute illness episodes in the hospital setting. Ongoing contact with patients during their hospitalization, as well as follow-up visits, affords the APN the opportunity to provide effective smoking-cessation assistance. In a climate of health-care reform, these are the major opportunities for the APN to provide cost-effective smoking-cessation interventions.

Empirical Evidence for Effectiveness of Nursing Intervention

Nurse-assisted interventions are designed to minimize physician burden and increase coun-

seling in primary care settings. These nursing interventions are associated with better cessation rates than are brief physician contacts alone (Hollis, Lichtenstein, Fogt, et al., 1993). Nurse-assisted interventions are helpful in increasing smoking-cessation rates both in acute and primary care settings (Rigotti, McKool, & Shiffman, 1994; Rice, Fox, Lepczyk, et al., 1994; Wewers, Bowen, Stanislaw, et al., 1994; Taylor, Houston-Miller, Killen, et al., 1990).

An example of a successful nurse-managed smoking intervention ($n = 173$) is the one structured and evaluated by Taylor and colleagues (1990). Patients were randomly assigned to usual care or an intervention program. The intervention was initiated in the hospital and maintained thereafter through telephone contact. The *Staying Free Manual* was given to patients to help them identify high-risk situations that could lead to relapse and develop skills to handle them. In addition to the manual, two audiotapes for home use were provided. One reviewed the major points of the manual, and the other described exercises for progressive muscle relaxation. The patients received counseling on how to cope with high-risk situations. Once discharged, the patients were followed up with a telephone call once a week for 2–3 weeks and monthly for 4 months.

Patients who were unable to stop smoking or had relapsed were able to meet with the nurse in the outpatient clinic. Nicotine replacement therapy was used in five of the patients to help with withdrawal symptoms. No intervention occurred after 6 months. A significant reduction in smoking rates at 1 year was reported for both groups. The intervention group had a 67% success rate of smoking cessation at the 1 year follow-up, compared with a 35% success rate in the usual-care group. This study demonstrates successful smoking cessation achieved through nursing interventions provided on an individual basis and delivered over the telephone. By providing a cost-effective approach, nurses can facilitate successful smoking cessation and decrease the potential cost to society and lost productivity associated with smoking (Taylor, Houston-Miller, Killen, et al., 1990).

To achieve effective smoking cessation, both psychological and physiologic factors must be addressed. Relief of withdrawal symptoms appears to be a vital component of effective smoking cessation, especially for the highly addicted smoker. The nurse can employ various smoking-cessation interventions to minimize the adverse effect of these withdrawal symptoms, as shown in Figure 7–2.

A Nursing Intervention Model

An example of an intervention model for smoking cessation suitable for APN use or modification by other clinicians is presented in Figure

WITHDRAWAL SYMPTOMS

Quitting smoking brings about a variety of symptoms associated with physical and psychological withdrawal. Most symptoms decrease sharply during the first few days of cessation, followed by a continued, but slower rate in decline in the second and third week of abstinence. For some people, coping with the withdrawal symptoms is like "riding a roller coaster"— there may be sharp turns, slow climbs and unexpected plunges. Most symptoms pass within 2–4 weeks after quitting.

SYMPTOM	CAUSE	AVERAGE DURATION	RELIEF
Irritability	Body's craving for nicotine is unsatisfied.	2–4 weeks	Take walks and hot baths; use relaxation techniques.
Fatigue	Nicotine is a stimulant, so discontinuing it causes fatigue.	2–4 weeks	Take naps; do not push yourself; use deep breathing.
Insomnia	Nicotine affects brain wave function and influences sleep patterns. Coughing and dreams about smoking are common.	1 week	Avoid caffeine after 6 PM; use relaxation techniques.
Cough, dry throat, nasal drip	Body is getting rid of mucus that has blocked airways and restricted breathing.	A few days	Drink plenty of fluids; try cough drops.
Dizziness	Body is getting extra oxygen.	1–2 days	Take extra caution in moving; change positions slowly.
Lack of concentration	Body needs time to adjust to not having constant stimulation from nicotine.	A few weeks	Plan workload accordingly; avoid additional stress during first few weeks.
Tightness in chest	Tension in chest may be created by body's need for nicotine, or tightness may be caused by sore muscles from coughing.	A few days	Use relaxation techniques, especially deep breathing.
Constipation, gas, stomach pain	Intestinal movement decreases for a brief period.	1–2 weeks	Drink plenty of fluids; add roughage to diet (i.e., fruits, vegetables, whole-grain cereals).
Hunger	Craving for cigarette can be confused with hunger pang, oral craving, desire for something in the mouth.	Up to several weeks	Drink water or low-calorie liquids; be prepared with low-calorie snacks.
Craving for a cigarette	Withdrawal from nicotine, a strongly addictive drug, produces craving.	Most frequent first 2–3 days; can happen occasionally for months or years	Wait out the urge; urges last only a few minutes. Distract yourself, exercise, go for a walk around the block.

FIGURE 7–2 Nicotine withdrawal symptoms and interventions to help minimize symptoms. From Massachusetts Tobacco Control Program (1995). Department of Public Health.

7–3. The *assessment* includes the smoker's present smoking status, stage of change, and nicotine dependency. The smoker's stage of change can quickly be assessed by asking the five questions shown in Table 7–1, which were developed by Prochaska and colleagues (Stillman, 1995). Physiologic nicotine addiction can be measured using either the Fagerstrom Tolerance Questionnaire or the modified version of the Horn-Russell Questionnaire shown in Figure 7–4 (Heatherton, 1991).

Once the APN has assessed the smoker's stage of change and nicotine dependency, it is appropriate to *advise* the smoker of the risk involved in continuing to smoke and the need to quit. This role provides an opportunity for the introduction of resources to help with smoking cessation, such as effective self-help materials and group or individual counseling. The APN should be aware that smoking cessation is a continuous process, so adequate follow-up and reassessment must be available. The unique position of the APN, as opposed to other clinicians, increases the chances of the APN being to help the smoker quit and avoid relapse.

Nursing Intervention Strategies

As noted in the model (see Figure 7–3), the advice provided by the APN is dictated by the smoker's stage of change. Following are suggestions for each stage:

During *precontemplation,* when the smoker has not decided to quit, useful interventions include distribution of self-help material and self-monitoring techniques such as record keeping. A follow-up phone call in 1 week and reassessment at the next scheduled visit is also warranted.

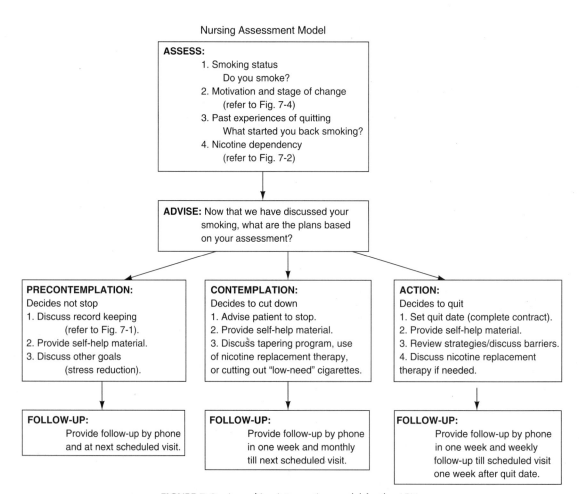

FIGURE 7–3 A smoking intervention model for the APN.

Table 7–1 Staging Algorithm
for Smoking Cessation

Instructions to Patient/Client: Select the group of statements that best describes your smoking behaviors.	
Stage	**Characteristic Responses**
Precontemplation	I smoke cigarettes or other tobacco products.
Contemplation	I am seriously considering stopping smoking within the next 6 months. I might have a specific plan to stop smoking in the next 30 days.
Preparation	I definitely have a specific plan to quit smoking in the next 30 days, and I have made a serious attempt to stop smoking in the past 12 months. This attempt lasted for at least 1 week. In the past 12 months, I might have made changes in my smoking behaviors such as switching brands and decreasing the amount smoked, etc.
Action	I stopped smoking within the past 6 months.
Maintenance	I have not smoked for the past 6 months.

Adapted from Prochaska, J.O., & DiClemente, C.C. (1983), Stages and processes of self-change of smoking: Toward an integrated model of change. *Journal of Consulting Clinical Psychology, 51*(3), 390–395.

During *contemplation,* when the smoker has decided to cut down but will not commit to a quit date, useful interventions include (1) advising the patient to think about a quit date and (2) providing material as mentioned in the precontemplation stage. Discussing techniques for helping the smoker get ready to quit is necessary. Examples of these techniques are tapering and nicotine replacement therapy. Keeping informed of the latest prescriptive therapies, using knowledge and clinical judgment such as that involved in assessment, and making a diagnosis are crucial in developing a plan for smoking cessation. Follow-up by phone should occur in 1 week and monthly until the next scheduled visit.

The *action* stage is the point in time when the smoker has decided to quit and will commit to a quit date. APNs should discuss what the smoker has tried in the past in order to determine what was successful and what was unsuccessful in previous quit attempts. It is also important to know the determinants of smoking for each individual and to understand the physiologic, psychological, and environmental influences that cause the smoker to smoke. Weight gain after cessation may result from a variety of changes, and it may be important to discuss what the smoker's perception of the causes of weight gain may be and then clarify these.

Stress reduction is necessary in the action stage. Smokers who are unable to quit are under higher stress levels than those who relapse but return to an earlier stage of change and eventually quit. The high rate of unsuccessful attempts to quit is partially attributable to stress; 56% of former smokers attribute their first slip to stress. However, former smokers do not differ from nonsmokers in their stress-coping skills. Apparently, some former smokers fail to use their coping skills in specific situations. Former smokers who do not have strategies for coping with temptations are more likely to relapse (Shiffman, 1982). In addition to stress-reduction techniques and smoking-cessation contracts, interventions that were used in the precontemplation and contemplation stages are useful in the action stage as well. Follow-up is necessary for at least the first year after a patient stops smoking, because this is the most likely time for relapse (Sachs & Leischow, 1991).

Maintenance is a stage of change not illustrated in the model. In this stage the APN should provide relapse-prevention skills and provide opportunities for the patient to ask for continued support. These interventions are warranted because of the high incidence of relapse. Marlatt and Gordon (1985) describe *relapse* as an "abstinence-violation effect." They outline this sequence following a slip: (1) negative affect leads to lowered self-confidence, which in turn leads to a smoking slip; (2) the slip, one or two cigarettes, leads to a further reduction in self-confidence; (3) further lowered self-confidence leads to the conclusion that the case is "hopeless," and the smoker abandons efforts to quit; and (4) too much emphasis placed on the single slip reinforces the smoker's belief that he or she is unable to quit (Marlatt & Gordon, 1980). It takes smokers many at-

Nicotine Dependency Assessment and Treatment

I. How to Assess Nicotine Dependency

    A. Ask the following questions:

		0 Points	1 Point	2 Points	3 Points	Score (Record)
1.	How soon after you wake do you smoke your first cigarette?	After 60 minutes	31–60 minutes	6–30 minutes	within 5 minutes	
2.	Do you find it difficult to refrain from smoking in places where it is forbidden, such as the library, theater, doctor's office?	No	Yes	—	—	
3.	Which would you hate most to give up?	All others	The first	—	—	
*4.	How many cigarettes do you smoke a day?	10 or less	11–20	21–30	31 or more	
5.	Do you smoke more frequently during the first hours after waking than the rest of the day?	No	Yes			
6.	Do you smoke when you are so ill that you are in bed most of the day?	No	Yes	—	—	
					TOTAL SCORE:	

How to Interpret Nicotine Dependency Score:

Score of 6 higher: Indicates high nicotine dependency and represents individuals who would be particularly likely to benefit from tapering and/or the prescription of nicotine replacement treatment therapy (gum or patch) to decrease nicotine withdrawal symptom as an adjunct to standard counseling.

Score of 5 or less: Suggest low to moderate nicotine dependency and represents individuals who may be less likely to require tapering and/or the prescription of nicotine replacement therapy (gum or patch). Standard counseling is most appropriate.

* **Key questions for brief assessment**

FIGURE 7–4 A revision of the Fagerstrom Tolerance Questionnaire. From Massachusetts Tobacco Control Program (1995). Department of Public Health.

tempts to quit, and they must learn from their slips and try again. With an understanding of relapse, the APN can effectively intervene with smokers and move them back on track.

CONCLUSION

The smoking-cessation techniques discussed offer a wide variety of approaches for both individual and group programs. A key component in the smoking-cessation plan is listening to the patient and identifying techniques that may be successful with that individual. An analysis of the literature suggests that no one method works for all patients. Accurate assessment of (1) why a smoker smokes, (2) experience of past quit attempts, (3) level of nicotine dependency, and (4) stage of change, can be completed by the APN regardless of the setting of clinical practice. It is necessary to try to help every smoker become successful at smoking cessation.

Comparison of success rates of specific programs and interventions is difficult. Many smoking studies used self-reporting without the validation of nonsmoking status by biochemical methods. Biochemical methods of validation of nonsmoking status such as carbon monoxide monitoring and saliva continine analysis have been shown to be more reliable than self-reporting (Schwartz, 1991). As the definition of success may vary across programs, comparison needs to be done carefully. As reported by Taylor and co-workers (1990), nursing telephone-contact support, with follow-up on an individual basis, can be highly successful.

The benefits of smoking cessation are of primary importance in both prevention and control of CHD, and nursing interventions can effectively assist patients to become aware of the negative consequences of smoking behavior. Willingness to intervene in smoking-cessation efforts requires that clinicians have adequate counseling, assessment, and intervention skills. By using specific approaches, nurses and other clinicians can gain confidence in their ability to intervene, and the outcomes of their intervention may then be more favorable. Furthermore, the APN has the ability to intervene and provide the appropriate smoking interventions for CHD patients across all settings and may thus have a unique and increasingly important role to play.

References

Anda, R. F., Williamson, D. F., Escobedo, L. G., Mast, E., Giovino, G., & Remington, T. (1985). Depression and the dynamics of smoking: A national perspective. *Journal of the American Medical Association, 264,* 1541–1545.

Belch, J. J., McArdle, B. M., Burns, P., Lowe, G. D., & Forbes, C. D. (1984). The effects of acute smoking on platelet behavior, fibrinolysis and hemorrheology in habitual smokers. *Thrombosis and Haemostasis, 51,* 6–8.

Benowitz, N. L. (1992). Cigarette smoking and nicotine addiction. *Medical Clinics of North America, 76*(2), 415–437.

Benowitz, N. L. (1988). Pharmacologic aspects of cigarette smoking and nicotine addiction. *New England Journal of Medicine, 319,* 1318–1330.

Bishop, D. B., Cook, T. L., Fisher, E. B., et al. (1985). *Grassroots Steering Committees in Worksite Smoking Cessation.* Paper presented at the Society of Behavioral Medicine, March, New Orleans.

Carney, R. M., & Goldberg A. P. (1984). Weight gain after cessation of cigarette smoking: A possible role for adipose-tissue lipoprotein lipase. *New England Journal of Medicine, 310,* 614–616.

Comstock, G. U., & Stone, R. W. (1972). Changes in body weight and subcutaneous fatness related to smoking habits. *Archives of Environmental Health, 24,* 271–276.

Coppotelli, H., & Orleans, C. T. (1985). Partner support and other determinants of smoking cessation mainte-nance among women. *Journal of Consulting and Clinical Psychology, 53,* 455–460.

Covey, L. S., Glassman, A. H., & Stetner, F. (1990). Depression and depressive symptoms in smoking cessation. *Comparative Psychiatry, 31,* 350–354.

Davis, J. W., Shelton, L., Eigenberg, D. A., Hignite, C. E., & Watanabe, I. S. (1985). Effects of tobacco and non-tobacco smoking on the endothelium and platelets. *Clinical Pharmacological Therapy, 37,* 529–533.

Farquhar, J. W., Fortmann, S. P., Maccoby, N., Haskell, W. L., Williams, P. T., Flora, J. A., Taylor, C. B., Brown, B. W., Solomon, D. S., & Hulley, S. B. (1984). The Stanford Five-City Project: An overview. In J. D. Matarazzo, N. Maccoby, S. M. Weiss, & J. A. Herd, et al. (Eds.), *Behavioral Health: A Handbook for Health Enhancement and Disease Prevention.* New York: Wiley & Sons, p. 1154.

Fisher, E. B., Haire-Joshu, E., Morgan, G. D., Rehberg, H., & Rost, K. (1990). Commentary on weight change following smoking cessation: The role of food intake and exercise. *Diabetes Spectrum, 3*(2), 95–97.

Flanagan, J., & Maany, I. (1982). Smoking and depression. *American Journal of Psychiatry, 139,* 541.

Folts, J. D., Gering, S. A., Lailby, S. W., Bertha, B. G., Bonebrake, F. C., & Keller, J. W. (1990). Effects of cigarette smoke and nicotine on platelets and experimental coronary artery thrombosis. In J. Diana (Ed.), *Tobacco Smoking and Atherosclerosis: Pathogenesis and Cellular Mechanisms.* New York: Plenum Publishing, pp 339–358.

Fortman, S. P., Haskell, S. L., & Williams, P. T. (1986). Changes in plasma high-density lipoprotein cholesterol after changes in cigarette use. *American Journal of Epidemiology, 124,* 706–710.

Glantz, S. A., & Parmley, W. W. (1991). Passive smoking and heart disease: Epidemiology, physiology, and biochemistry. *Circulation, 83,* 1–12.

Glasgow, R. E. (1986). Smoking. In K. Holroyd & T. Cree (Eds.), *Self-Management of Chronic Disease and Handbook of Clinical Interventions and Research.* Orlando, FL: Academic Press, p. 99.

Glassman, A. H., Helzer, J. E., Covey, L. S., Cottler, L. B., Stetner, F., Tipp, J. E., & Johnson, J. (1990). Smoking, smoking cessation, and major depression. *Journal of the American Medical Association, 264*(12), 1546–1549.

Graham, S., & Gibson, R. W. (1971). Cessation of patterned behavior: Withdrawal from smoking. *Social Science Medicine, 5,* 319–337.

Haire-Joshu, D., Morgan, G., & Fisher, E. B. (1991). Determinants of cigarette smoking. *Clinics in Chest Medicine, 12*(4), 711–725.

Hall, S. M., Tunstall, C., Rugg, D., Jones, R. T., & Benowitz, N. (1985). Nicotine gum and behavioral treatment in smoking cessation. *Journal of Consulting and Clinical Psychiatry, 53*(2), 256–258.

Heatherton, T. (1991). The Fagerstrom test for nicotine dependence: A revision of the Fagerstrom Tolerance Questionnaire. *British Journal of Addiction, 86,* 119–1127.

Hennekens, C. H., Lown, B., Rosner, B., Grufferman, S., & Dalen, J. (1980). Ventricular premature beats and coronary risk factors. *American Journal of Epidemiology, 112*(1), 93–99.

Hermanson, B., Omenn, G. S., Kronmal, R. A., & Gersh, B. J. (1988). Beneficial six-year outcome of smoking cessation in older men and women with coronary artery disease. Results from the CASS registry. *New England Journal of Medicine, 312,* 217–275.

Hollis, J. F., Lichtenstein, E., Fogt, T. M., Stevens, V. J., &

Biglan, A. (1993). Nurse-assisted counseling for smokers in primary care. *Annals of Internal Medicine, 118,* 521–525.

House, J. S., Landis, K. R., & Umberson, D. (1988). Social relationships and health. *Science, 241,* 540–545.

Jarvick, M. E., & Henningfield, J. E. (1988). Pharmacological treatment of tobacco dependence. *Pharmacology, Biochemistry & Behavior, 30*(1), 279–294.

Lesmes, G. R., & Donofrio, K. H. (1992). Passive smoking: The medical and economic issues. *The American Journal of Medicine, 93*(Suppl. 1A), 38s–42s.

Lucchesi, B. R., Schuster, C. R., & Emley, G. S. (1967). The role of nicotine as a determinant of cigarette smoking frequency in man with observations of certain cardiovascular effects associated with the tobacco alkaloid. *Clinical Pharmacology Therapy, 8,* 186–796.

Marlatt, G. A., & Gordon, J. R. (1980). Determinants of relapse: Implications for the maintenance of behavior change. In P. O. Davidson & S. M. Davidson, (Eds.), *Behavioral Medicine: Changing Health Lifestyles.* New York: Brunner/Mazel, pp. 410–452.

Marlatt, G. A., & Gordon, J. R. (Eds.) (1985). *Relapse Prevention: Maintenance Strategies in the Treatment of Addictive Behaviors.* New York: Guilford Press.

Massachusetts Tobacco Control (1995). Chew this over. In K. Pendell (Ed.), *Tobacco Awareness Program (TEG) and Tobacco Education Group (TAP) Training Manual.* Minneapolis, MN: Community Interventions Inc.

McBride, E. P. (1992). The health consequences of smoking. *Medical Clinics of North America, 76*(2), 333–350.

McFall, R. M. (1970). Effects of self-monitoring on normal smoking behavior. *Journal of Consulting and Clinical Psychology, 35,* 135.

Mermelstein, R., Lichtenstein, R., & McIntyre, K. (1983). Partner support and relapse in smoking cessation programs. *Journal of Consulting and Clinical Psychology, 51,* 465–466.

Munro, J. M., & Cotran, R. S. (1988). The pathogenesis of antherosclerosis: Atherogenesis and inflammation. *Laboratory Investigation, 58*(3), 249–261.

Nowak, J., Murray, J. J., Oates, J. A., & Fitzgerald, G. A. (1987). Biochemical evidence of a chronic abnormality in platelet and vascular function in healthy individuals who smoke cigarettes. *Circulation, 76,* 6–14.

Ockene, J., & Ockene, I. (1992a). Helping patients reduce their risk for coronary heart disease. In J. Ockene & I. Ockene (Eds.), *An Overview in Prevention of Coronary Heart Disease.* Boston: Little, Brown & Co., pp. 173–200.

Ockene, J., & Ockene, I. (1992b). Smoking intervention: A behavioral, educational, and pharmacologic perspective. In J. Ockene & I. Ockene (Eds.), *An Overview in Prevention of Coronary Heart Disease.* Boston: Little, Brown & Co., pp. 201–227.

Petti, D. B., & Wingred, J. (1978). Use of oral contraceptives, cigarette smoking, and risk of subarachnoid hemorrhage. *Lancet, 2,* 234–235.

Pittilo, R. M., Clarke, J. M., Harris, D., Mackie, I. J., Rowles, P. M., Machin, S. J., & Woolf, N. (1984). Cigarette smoking and platelet adhesions. *British Journal of Haematology, 58,* 627–632.

Pomerleau, O. F. (1992). Nicotine and the central nervous system: Biobehavioral effects of cigarette smoking. *Journal of American Medical Association, 93* (Suppl. 1A), 2s–7s.

Pomerleau, O. F., & Pomerleau, C. F. (1984). Neuroregulators and the reinforcement of smoking: Towards a biobehavioral explanation. *Neuroscience Biobehavioral Review, 8,* 503.

Pooling Project Research Group. (1978). Relationship of blood pressure, serum cholesterol, smoking habit, relative weight, and ECG abnormalities to incidence of major coronary events: Final report of the Pooling Project. *Journal of Chronic Disease, 31,* 201–306.

Prochaska, J. O., & DiClemente, C. C. (1984). *The transtheoretical approach: Crossing traditional boundaries of therapy.* Chicago: Dow Jones/Irwin.

Prochaska, J. O., DiClemente, C. C., Velicer, W. F., Ginpil, S., & Norcross, J. C. (1985). Predicting change in smoking status for self changers. *Addictive Behaviors, 10,* 395–406.

Prochaska, J. O., & Goldstein, M. G. (1991). Process of smoking cessation: Implications for clinicians. *Clinics in Chest Medicine, 12*(4), 727–735.

Rausch, J. L., Nichinson, B., Lamke, C., & Matloff, J. (1990). Influence of negative affect on smoking cessation treatment outcome: A pilot study. *British Journal of Addiction, 85,* 929–933.

Rice, V. H., Fox, D. H., Lepczyk, M., Siegreen, M., Mullin, M., Jarosz, P., & Templin, T. (1994). A comparison of nursing interventions in adults with cardiovascular health problems. *Heart and Lung, 23*(6), 473–486.

Rigotti, N., McKool, K., & Shiffman, S. (1994). Predictors of smoking cessation after coronary artery bypass graft surgery. *Annals of Internal Medicine, 120,* 287–293.

Robbins, A. (1993). Pharmacological approaches to smoking cessation. *American Journal of Preventative Medicine, 9*(1), 31–33.

Rosenberg, L., Palmer, J. R., & Sharpiro, S. (1990). Decline in the risk of myocardial infarction among women who stop smoking. *New England Journal of Medicine, 322,* 213–217.

Sachs, P. L., & Leischow, J. S. (1991). Pharmacologic approaches to smoking cessation. *Clinics in Chest Medicine, 12*(4), 769–791.

Schnieder, N. G., & Jarvik, M. E. (1984). Time course of smoking withdrawal symptoms as a function of nicotine replacement. *Psychopharmacology, 82,* 143–144.

Scholl, J. M., Benacerraf, A., Ducimetiere, P., Chabas, D., Brau, J., Chapelle, J., & Thery, J. L. (1986). Comparison of risk factors in vasospastic angina without a significant fixed coronary narrowing and non-vasospastic angina. *American Journal of Cardiology, 57,* 199–202.

Schwartz, J. L. (1987). *Review and Evaluation of Smoking Cessation Methods: The United States and Canada, 1978–1985.* Bethesda, MD: National Cancer Institute (Publication no. 87–2940).

Schwartz, J. L. (1991). Methods of smoking cessation. *Clinics in Chest Medicine, 12*(4), 737–753.

Shiffman, S. (1982). Relapse following smoking cessation: A situational analysis. *Journal of Consulting and Clinical Psychology, 50,* 71–86.

Stamford, B. A., Matter, S., Fell, R. D., & Papanek, P. (1986). Effects of smoking cessation on weight gain, metabolic rate, caloric consumption, and blood lipids. *American Journal of Clinical Nutrition, 43,* 486–494.

Stillman, F. A. (1995). Smoking cessation for the hospitalized cardiac patient: Rationale for and report of a model program. *Journal of Cardiovascular Nursing, 9*(2), 25–36.

Susser, M. (1995). The tribulations of trials-Intervention in communities (editorial). *American Journal of Public Health, 85*(2), 156–158.

Taylor, C. B., Houston-Miller, N., Killen, J. D., & DeBusk, R. F. (1990). Smoking cessation after acute myocardial infarction: Effects of a nurse-managed intervention. *Annals of Internal Medicine, 113,* 118–123.

Tesevat, J. (1992). Impact and cost-effectiveness of smoking interventions. *The American Journal of Medicine, 93*(Suppl. 1A), 43S–47S.

Turner, J. A., McNichol, M. W., & Sillett, R. W., (1986). Distribution of carboxyhaemoglobin concentrations in smokers and non-smokers. *Thorax, 41,* 25–27.

U.S. Department of Health and Human Services (1983). *The Health Consequences of Smoking: Cardiovascular Disease. A Report of the Surgeon General.* Atlanta: Centers for Disease Control (Publication no. 84–50204).

U.S. Department of Health and Human Services. (1986). *The Health Consequences of Involuntary Smoking: A Report of the Surgeon General.* Atlanta: Centers for Disease Control, chapter 1 (Publication no. 87–8398).

U.S. Department of Health and Human Services (1989a). *Smoking Tobacco & Health: A Fact Book.* Atlanta: Centers for Disease Control (Publication no. 87–8397).

U.S. Department of Health and Human Services. (1989b). *Reducing the Health Consequences of Smoking: 25 Years of Progress: A Report of the Surgeon General.* Atlanta: Centers for Disease Control (Publication no. 89–8411).

U.S. Department of Health and Human Services (1990). *The Health Benefits of Smoking Cessation, A Report of the Surgeon General, 1990.* Atlanta: Centers for Disease Control (Publication no. 90–8416).

West, D. W., Graham, S., Swanson, M., & Wilkinson G. (1977). Five-year follow-up of a smoking withdrawal clinic population. *American Journal of Public Health, 67*(6), 536–544.

Wewers, M. E., Bowen, J., Stanislaw, A. E., & Desimone, V. B. (1994). A nurse-delivered smoking cessation intervention among hospitalized postoperative patients—Influence of a smoking-related diagnosis. A pilot study. *Heart and Lung, 23*(2), 151–156.

Wilhelmensen, L., Svardsudd, K., Korsan-Bengsten, K., Larsson, B., Welin, L., & Tibblin, G. (1984). Fibrinogen as a risk factor for stroke and myocardial infarction. *New England Journal of Medicine, 311,* 501–505.

Willet W. C., Green, A., Stampfer, M. J., Speizer, F. E., Colditz, G. A., Rosner, B., Monson, R. R., Stason, W., & Hennekens, C. H. (1987). Relative and absolute excess risks of coronary heart disease among women who smoke cigarettes. *New England Journal of Medicine, 317(21),* 1303–1309.

CHAPTER 8

‒
‒
‒
‒
‒
‒
‒
‒
‒
‒
‒
‒
═
‒

Physical Activity

Lori Anne Lyne
Nalini Jairath

Sedentary behavior is a major risk factor for coronary heart disease (CHD), of similar magnitude to smoking, hypertension, and hypercholesterolemia (Berlin & Colditz, 1990; Powell, Thompson, Caspersen, et al., 1987). Conversely, increased physical activity reduces CHD risk and, unlike other risk-reduction strategies, has minimal side effects. Traditionally, clinicians have helped clients reduce CHD risk through prescription of formal exercise regimens. Now, however, based on epidemiologic data, clinicians are increasingly emphasizing the importance of generalized increases in physical activity, regardless of the duration or intensity of specific activities or exercises performed.

Advanced-practice nurses and nurses involved in risk-reduction, cardiac wellness, and cardiac rehabilitation programs play an increasingly important role in promoting exercise or increased activity as a CHD risk-reduction strategy. The purpose of this chapter is to provide these nurses and other clinicians with the necessary knowledge to assist clients in increasing their physical activity, prescribing and monitoring safe activity or exercise for CHD patients and those at risk for CHD because of sedentary behavior patterns. It is essential that the clini-

cian understand current controversies that affect clinical practice and form the underlying basis of patient responses to interventions. Accordingly, the physiology of exercise will be addressed throughout this chapter, and we will (1) briefly summarize the research establishing the relationship between physical activity, sedentary behavior, and CHD risk; (2) outline mechanisms for CHD risk reduction; and (3) discuss intervention strategies.

RELATIONSHIP AMONG PHYSICAL ACTIVITY, SEDENTARY BEHAVIOR, AND CHD RISK

Sedentary behavior has long been implicated as a risk factor for CHD. Landmark studies by Morris and others established that individuals in sedentary occupations were at greater risk for CHD than those in physically active occupations (Morris, Everitt, Pollard, et al., 1980; Morris, Heady, Raffle, et al., 1953). Epidemiologic research by Paffenbarger (1993) and others directly examined the effects of various activity levels on CHD morbidity and mortality. For example, in the Harvard alumni study (n =

10,000), men expending more than 3,500 kilocalories per week had 50% less risk of death from CHD than those expending less than 500 kilocalories per week. Furthermore, men who were previously active and became sedentary had a significantly increased risk. Conversely, the mortality rate was reduced for those who had previously led a sedentary lifestyle and became physically active during middle age (Paffenbarger, Hyde, Wing, et al., 1993).

Similarly, preliminary research suggests that an average expenditure of 2,200 kcal per week, or 5–6 hours of regular physical exercise, may be associated with regression of CHD (Hambrecht, Niebauer, Marburger, et al., 1993). A daily 30–60 minute brisk walk at the 10 MET (metabolic equivalent expenditure) intensity level for men and the 9 MET level for women has been reported to produce a plateau in mortality (Blair, Kohl, Paffenbarger, et al., 1989). One MET is defined as the individual's basal energy expenditure such that 10 METs corresponds to 10 times and 9 METs to nine times the basal energy expenditure.

Despite the importance of physical activity in CHD risk reduction, several issues remain unresolved. First, the time interval before increases in physical activity translate into reductions in CHD risk is unknown. Second, controversy has arisen regarding whether it is the amount of physical activity performed or actual physical fitness that reduces the risk for CHD. Third, in addition to the relationship that has been found between physical activity and CHD risk, a strong association has also been reported between physical fitness and CHD risk (Blair, Gibbons, Painter, et al., 1986). And, fourth, the vast majority of research is extrapolated from clinical trials examining the effect of highly structured exercise regimens; because of the narrow focus of such trials, the generalizability of such findings to physical activity accumulated throughout an individual's day may be questionable.

In conclusion, the research literature establishes a clear relationship between physical activity and CHD risk. Studies have demonstrated a strong inverse association between the level of activity and cardiovascular mortality and mortality from all causes (Haskell, 1994). The amount of physical activity required to achieve a reduction in mortality and decreased risk for

CHD is still being debated. Some epidemiologic studies indicate that people who are moderately active as compared with the least active, or least fit, have a significantly lower rate of CHD (Haskell, 1994). Based on this research, the Centers for Disease Control and Prevention and the American College of Sports Medicine recommend that adults should "accumulate" a minimum of 30 minutes of moderate intensity physical activity on most, if not all, days of the week (Pate, Pratt, Blair, et al., 1995).

Intervention studies to increase physical activity have methodologic limitations. The reliability and validity of diaries, activity monitors, and other methods of quantifying physical activity performed are questionable. In addition, pure experimental design research is not possible; random subject assignment to active or inactive lifestyles is unfeasible and ethically questionable. Furthermore, isolation of the unique contribution of physical activity to risk reduction is difficult, because subjects may have several CHD risk factors being concurrently addressed. Finally, because of issues in sampling, the generalizability of research findings to females, elderly, and clients of lower socioeconomic classes has not been established.

PROPOSED MECHANISMS FOR CHD RISK REDUCTION

Exercise regimens have been postulated to slow disease progression, delay the onset of morbid events (e.g., angina, myocardial infarction), and decrease mortality rates through several pathways. It is not known whether the same pathways account for the effects of increased physical activity or fitness upon CHD risk. Exercise may reduce CHD risk directly through improved functional capacity, decreased myocardial workload, increased thresholds for ventricular fibrillation, and enhanced fibrinolysis. It may also reduce risk indirectly by its effect on percentage of body fat, blood pressure, lipid profile, body composition, body fat distribution, regulation of glucose metabolism, and psychosocial function. Each of these risk-reduction mechanisms will be briefly discussed.

Improved Functional Capacity

With exercise, the sympathetic nervous system is activated and blood flow redistributed to the exercising muscle from systems that are not being used. The interaction of local metabolic and central autonomic nervous functions regulates the redistribution of blood and results in a decrease in systemic vascular resistance during increased intensity of exercise (Pate, Blair, Durstine, et al., 1991). Cardiac output, systolic blood pressure, and pulmonary ventilation increase to maintain adequate levels of oxygen to the exercising muscle.

In addition to short-term effects, exercise training results in longer-term improvements in *functional capacity,* that is, the ability of an individual to perform work. Functional capacity is typically expressed in terms of maximal oxygen consumption (V_{O2max}), MET level (i.e., the ratio of V_{O2max} divided by basal metabolic expenditure) and ergometric workload. Conceptually, V_{O2max} represents an individual's optimum capacity for using oxygen and aerobic metabolic processes to resynthesize *adenosine triphosphate* (ATP) and thus generate the internal energy required to perform work. Additional energy and work requirements would necessitate use of anaerobic metabolism, which results in increased lactic acid accumulation and fatigue (McArdle, Katch, & Katch, 1981).

Operationally, oxygen consumption (V_{O2} is the arithmetic product of cardiac output multiplied by the arteriovenous oxygen difference [A-V_{O2} difference]). The A-V_{O2} reflects the ability of the working muscle to extract oxygen from the blood (Juneau, Geneau, Marchand, et al., 1991). V_{O2max} is indirectly affected by (1) pulmonary ventilation, (2) oxygen diffusion between alveoli and pulmonary capillary blood, (3) cardiac performance, (4) redistribution of blood circulation to skeletal muscles, and (5) the working skeletal muscle's utilization and extraction of oxygen from the arterial blood (Pate, Blair, Durstine, et al., 1991).

Currently, exercise training is believed to improve maximum oxygen consumption (V_{O2max}) and functional capacity, primarily through peripheral adaptations. These adaptations include increases in the number and size of mitochondria in trained skeletal muscle (Juneau, Geneau, Marchand, et al., 1991; Todd, Wosornu, Stew-

art, et al., 1992). As a result of these increases, trained skeletal muscle is able to extract oxygen from the blood more efficiently, with widening of the A-V_{O2} difference and reduction of the exercise heart rate at any given workload (Juneau, Geneau, Marchand, et al., 1991).

Central adaptive mechanisms do not appear to contribute significantly to the exercise-related improvements in V_{O2max} and functional capacity. Exercise training has not been shown to increase coronary vessel size or the number of collaterals in humans (Juneau, Geneau, Marchand, et al., 1991). Yet, debate and investigation regarding the role of central adaptive mechanisms continues because of several observations regarding changes in cardiac parameters with exercise training. First, research indicates that after exercise training, stroke volume increases in patients who have undergone coronary artery bypass surgery (Kirken & Barnatt-Boyes, 1986). Second, prolonged aerobic training regimens have been associated with eccentric hypertrophy of the myocardium, typified by increased chamber size and left ventricular wall thickness as well as improved myocyte vasculature and myocardial function (Katz, 1992; Weber, 1988). Third, there is evidence of improved cardiac collateralization with exercise in animal models (Juneau, Geneau, Marchand, et al., 1991). Finally, concerns have been expressed that exercise regimens tested in myocardial infarction patients have been inadequate to spur the growth of collateral vessels (Ellestad, 1975; Wenger, 1977).

Decreased Myocardial Workload

With exercise training, decreases have been documented in blood pressure (BP), resting heart rate (HR), and submaximal HR (i.e., HR at less than the maximum workload tolerable). These decreases translate into a reduction in myocardial workload and an increase in the rate-pressure product. The *rate-pressure product* identifies the myocardial workload level at which myocardial ischemia occurs. In patients with stable angina, myocardial ischemia can be reproduced at a patient-specific rate-pressure product (i.e., specific HR × BP) (Blair, Kohl, Gordon, et al., 1992). Therefore, an increase in the rate-pressure product with exercise training is indirectly indicative of decreased myocardial workload over time.

Increased Ventricular Fibrillation Threshold and Enhanced Fibrinolysis

Lethal ventricular dysrhythmias are a primary cause of CHD mortality. Animal studies, mostly using rat models, suggest that exercise training may increase the electrical stability of the myocardium (Haskell, 1994). Thus, the threshold for ventricular fibrillation may be raised (Blair, Kohl, Gordon, et al., 1992). Confirmatory research in humans is required.

Short-term effects of exercise may also contribute to risk reduction. Mural thrombi are the underlying cause of approximately 90% of all myocardial infarctions (Blair, Kohl, Gordon, et al., 1992). Individual exercise sessions may reduce blood coagulability by decreasing blood platelet aggregability and adhesiveness over the next 1–2 days (Eichner, 1986; Sharkey, 1990). As a result, mural thrombi may be less likely to occur, although a dose-response relationship does not appear to exist. Paradoxically, exhaustive activity may potentially increase risk. Research indicates that exhaustive activity actually promotes a more rapid clotting time (Sharkey, 1990).

Reduced Blood Pressure

Exercise training independently reduces blood pressure in certain individuals with hypertension (Fletcher, Blair, Blumenthal, et al., 1992). Effective control of hypertension can result in a 20% reduction in cardiovascular mortality in patients who have had a myocardial infarction (Blumenthal, Emery, Madden, et al., 1991). Aerobic exercise training is associated with a decrease in systolic pressure and diastolic pressure of approximately 10 mm Hg in patients with mild hypertension and even more in some patients with hypertension secondary to renal insufficiency (Blair, Kohl, Gordon, et al., 1992; American College of Sports Medicine, 1993). Furthermore, endurance training results in a reduction in the natural rise of blood pressure

that occurs over time in individuals at high risk for becoming hypertensive. As discussed, even small decreases in blood pressure are associated with a reduced risk for CHD.

Improved Lipid Profile, Body Composition, and Body Fat Distribution

Meta-analysis of pertinent studies indicates that exercise training increases HDL cholesterol and significantly reduces total cholesterol, LDL cholesterol, and triglycerides in patients who have suffered myocardial infarction (Tran & Brammell, 1989). Although much higher levels of HDL cholesterol are frequently seen in individuals who perform extensive exercise, the amount of exercise necessary to elevate HDL cholesterol is not quantifiable because of marked variations in individual responses.

Some of the favorable effects of exercise on lipid metabolism are attributable to weight loss (Squires, Gau, Miller, et al., 1990). Weight is lost through increased energy expenditure coupled with reduced caloric intake. Exercise facilitates weight loss by counteracting the diet-related decline in resting metabolic rate (Leon, 1989). In addition, a combination of exercise and diet maintains lean body mass and may be associated with a long-term change in resting metabolic rate. Therefore, exercise may also be beneficial in maintenance of weight loss (Frey-Hewitt, Vranizan, Dreon, et al., 1990; Van Dale, Saris, & Ten Hoot, 1990).

An association also exists between abdominal, or central, obesity and increased cardiovascular risk (Larsson, Svardoudd, Welm, et al., 1984). Exercise appears to mobilize central subcutaneous fat (Blair, Kohl, Gordon, et al., 1992; Despres, Tremblay, Nadeau, et al., 1988). Schwartz, Shuman, and Larsen (1993) documented a loss of central fat in older men following intensive endurance training and subsequent weight loss. The role of body fat distribution in CHD development is of increasing interest.

Regulation of Glucose Metabolism

Several clinical trials indicate that exercise training improves glucose tolerance and enhances insulin sensitivity (Helmrich, Ragland, Leung, et al., 1991; Manson, Imm, Stampfer, et al., 1991; Manson, Nathan, Krolewski, et al., 1992; Schneider, Amorosa, Khachadurian, et al., 1984). Furthermore, the Nurses' Health Study demonstrated the effectiveness of physical activity in preventing or delaying the onset of non-insulin-dependent diabetes mellitus in women (Manson, Imm, Stampfer, et al., 1991).

Improved Psychological Function

Exercise training has been reported to reduce anxiety and depression in various patient populations (Raglin, 1990). Several studies have documented the positive effect of exercise on mental status. Exercise is associated with reduction in anxiety, tension, and CHD-prone behavior (Pauly, Palmer, Wright, et al., 1982; Sinyor, Seraganian, et al., 1983). As discussed in Chapter 10, reduction of anxiety and depression may reduce CHD risk.

In conclusion, exercise training can reduce CHD risk via several possible mechanisms that may occur concurrently. The strength of the research supporting each mechanism varies. Certainly the research clearly indicates that exercise training improves functional capacity and decreases myocardial workload in humans, but its role in increasing the threshold for ventricular fibrillation and facilitating collateral circulation is based on animal models. Furthermore, additional research is necessary to determine the extent to which the risk-reduction mechanisms for exercise training are similar to those for generalized increases in physical activity.

CLINICAL INTERVENTIONS FOR CHD RISK REDUCTION

In this section, we will address two different but compatible intervention approaches: (1) the traditional exercise training approach and (2) a stage-based approach to increasing physical activity.

Exercise Training

Exercise training has been traditionally used to decrease CHD risk in sedentary individuals. The regimen involves several steps: (1) client assessment and exercise tolerance testing, (2) risk stratification, (3) formulation of the exercise prescription, (4) implementation of the exercise prescription, and (5) monitoring. For additional guidelines and more detailed information regarding exercise training, the clinician is referred to statements by the American Association of Cardiovascular and Pulmonary Rehabilitation (1995), the American College of Cardiology (1997), and the American College of Sports Medicine (1991).

For patients with CHD-related clinical conditions, exercise training may occur within the context of *cardiac rehabilitation programs.* These programs are traditionally divided into three phases. Phase I occurs in the inpatient setting; the focus is on helping patients resume normal activities of daily living and minimize the effects of muscle deconditioning. Phase II programs are outpatient or home-based programs that address issues related to early recovery; the focus extends from helping patients resume normal life patterns to facilitating lifestyle change for CHD risk reduction. Phase III programs are community-based and address lifelong lifestyle changes. These programs may continue indefinitely; they target patients whose recovery from acute events is complete or nearly so.

Patient Assessment and Exercise Tolerance Testing

The purpose of patient assessment and exercise tolerance testing is to (1) determine the patient's functional capacity, (2) screen for existing CHD, and (3) identify the factors modifying or limiting the patient's response to exercise. Initially, the clinician conducts a focused interview, physical examination, flexibility and strength evaluation, and laboratory work. This assessment should include a resting 12-lead electrocardiogram. The patient should also be screened for health-related conditions such as diabetes and arthritis that necessitate both modification of the exercise prescription and more intensive monitoring. Key data to be evaluated include the individual's blood pressure and heart rate at rest and after exercise, ischemic ST segment changes, potentially lethal dysrhythmias, and the presence of angina. The anginal threshold should also be noted for patients with angina. Table 8–1 summarizes major contraindications to exercise. Briefly stated, patients with unstable angina, severe aortic stenosis, decompensated congestive heart failure, acute myocarditis, and uncontrolled cardiac dysrhythmias should not exercise until these problems are managed (Fletcher, Froelicher, Hartley, et al., 1990). Similarly, individuals with a blood pressure greater than 180/105 require pharmacologic therapy before an exercise program is initiated (American College of Sports Medicine, 1993).

Although *exercise tolerance testing* (ETT) typically follows patient assessment, not all patients referred to cardiac rehabilitation programs and other risk-reduction programs will have undergone an ETT. The American College of Sports Medicine (ACSM) (1995) does not currently recommend ETT for asymptom-

atic patients at risk for CHD based on the presence of two or more risk factors if they will only undergo moderate exercise (McConnell, 1996; American College of Sports Medicine, 1995). However, questions about the specificity and accuracy of the ACSM guidelines have been raised (Lowensteyn, Joseph, & Grover, 1997). Therefore, the clinician's own judgment regarding the need for ETT in asymptomatic patients should prevail.

ETT is used to determine the patient's functional capacity as measured by V_{O2max} heart rate, or MET level. V_{O2max} can be determined directly using open circuit spirometry. However, algorithms, nomograms, and other formulas for indirect estimation of V_{O2max} usually provide adequate information for exercise prescription.

In addition to functional capacity, the ETT may also help the clinician identify exercise-related dysrhythmias, ischemic changes, and the rate-pressure product at which myocardial ischemia is reproducible for patients with stable angina. Several test protocols exist, including the Bruce, Naughton, and Balke and Ware protocols (American College of Sports Medicine, 1991). The protocol used for the ETT must be carefully selected. Some protocols involving rapid speed/gradient increases may be accurate for diagnosis of CHD but less accurate for identification of functional capacity. Conversely, protocols with warm-up periods or slower increases in speeds/gradients may more accurately estimate functional capacity, but they may not stress the heart sufficiently for detection of ST segment or T wave abnormalities characteristic of CHD.

TABLE 8–1 Contraindications for Inpatient and Outpatient Cardiac Rehabilitation

- Unstable angina
- Resting systolic BP of more than 200 mm Hg or resting diastolic of more than 110 mm Hg (should be evaluated on a case-by-case basis)
- Orthostatic BP drop of more than 20 mm Hg with symptoms
- Critical aortic stenosis (peak systolic pressure gradient of more than 50 mm Hg with aortic valve orifice area less than 0.75 cm² in average size adult)
- Acute systemic illness or fever
- Uncontrolled atrial or ventricular dysrhythmias
- Uncontrolled sinus tachycardia (>120 beats/min)
- Uncompensated congestive heart failure
- Third-degree atrioventricular block (without pacemaker)
- Active pericarditis or myocarditis
- Recent embolism
- Thrombophlebitis
- Resting ST segment displacement of more than 2 mm
- Uncontrolled diabetes (resting blood glucose of about 400 mg/dl)
- Severe orthopedic problems that would prohibit exercise
- Other metabolic problems, such as acute thyroiditis, hypokalemia or hyperkalemia, hypovolemia, etc.

From ACSM Guidelines for Exercise Testing and Prescription, 5th ed. (1998). Philadelphia, Lippincott-Raven.

Risk Stratification

Once patient assessment and the ETT are completed, cases can be stratified according to the degree of risk for adverse events during exercise training. *Stratification* dictates the setting where exercise occurs and the degree of monitoring necessary. The estimated average risk of death is only 0.5 per 10,000 graded exercise tests. The risk of primary cardiac arrest during exercise in regular exercisers versus sedentary males is 21 versus 18 events per 100,000,000 person-hours (Pate, Blair, Durstine, et al., 1991). Thus, the overall risk of cardiac arrest or death from ETT is very low.

Risk stratification is based on the presence and nature of past and current coronary events such as myocardial infarction and angina. In addition, the patient's functional capacity and capacity for self-regulation and self-monitoring of exercise should be considered. Although several stratification approaches exist, we favor, because of its simplicity, an algorithmic approach integrating criteria by Pashkow, Greenland, and DeBusk. In our approach, the clinician initially decides whether the patient is at low risk or not. Patients with no CHD history are usually at low risk.

In addition, based on Pashkow (1993), low-risk patients include those who have a functional capacity of 7.5 MET or more at 3 weeks after a cardiac event and have no significant dysrhythmia, no left ventricular dysfunction, and no evidence of ischemia. These patients are suited for an unsupervised exercise program in their homes (Pashkow, 1993). Based on reinfarction rates and adherence, low-risk patients may also include those who have sustained an uncomplicated myocardial infarction 3 or more weeks earlier (DeBusk, Stenestrand, Sheehan, et al., 1990; DeBusk, Haskell, Miller, et al., 1985). Patients unable to monitor their heart rate need not be excluded from the low-risk group if use of alternative monitoring approaches, including transtelephonic monitoring, and *rating of perceived exertion* (RPE) is feasible.

The remaining patients are termed "at risk." These include patients with (1) resting complex ventricular dysrhythmias or exercise-induced ventricular dysrhythmias; (2) a previous cardiac arrest; (3) a drop in systolic blood pressure with exercise; (4) a post myocardial infarction course complicated by congestive heart failure, cardiogenic shock, and serious ventricular dysrhythmias; (5) a diminished ejection fraction of less than 30%; or (5) severe CHD with marked exercise-induced ischemia (>2 mm ST depression) (Greenland, 1991).

Patients at risk may be further differentiated into those at intermediate and those at high risk for exercise-related adverse events. Based on Pashkow's classification, intermediate-risk patients should participate in a supervised exercise program for a limited time, whereas high-risk patients must always exercise under supervision. Intermediate-risk patients are those who

have (1) a maximum oxygen consumption of less than 7.5 MET but greater than 4.5 MET 3 weeks after an ischemic event; (2) angina or evidence of ischemia with 1–2 mm ST segment depression with exercise, plus perfusion or wall motion abnormalities with stress; (3) a history of congestive heart failure or evidence of moderate left ventricular dysfunction; and (4) nonsustained ventricular dysrhythmias with late potentials on signal-averaged electrocardiograms. Intermediate-risk patients also include those who cannot self-monitor their exercise or who are unable to comply with exercise recommendations.

High-risk patients are those with (1) maximum oxygen consumption of less than or equal to 4.5 MET at a minimum of 3 weeks after the cardiac event, (2) exercise-induced hypertension of more than 15 mm Hg, (3) exercise-induced ischemia of more than 2 mm ST segment depression at low levels of exercise, or (4) a history of induced or spontaneous ventricular dysrhythmias (Pashkow, 1993).

Exercise Prescription

Following risk stratification, the clinician consults with the exercise physiologist and other pertinent members of the health-care team to determine the exercise prescription. An *exercise prescription* provides the patient with an exercise regimen of specified type (i.e., mode), intensity, duration, and frequency of exercise activity. Most exercise prescriptions for those with CHD or at high risk for it are based on the patient's medical condition, goals, and ETT-based maximum functional capacity.

In general, patients with the lowest initial fitness level demonstrate the greatest improvement with a cardiovascular exercise program. For example, a supervised exercise program after a myocardial infarction can result in a 15–25% increase in maximal capacity above what would occur spontaneously (Greenland & Chu, 1988). The exercise prescription is typically based on the ETT results. In the absence of ETT results, the clinician can titrate and gradually increase the intensity and duration of exercise using general guidelines such as articulated by McConnell (1996).

For all patients, a warm-up and cool-down

period of 5–10 minutes of stretching and lei-surely activity should be incorporated with each exercise session. The warm-up serves several functions. It gradually increases the heart rate and promotes enhanced circulation to the exer-cising muscle. It also promotes flexibility and reduces the chance for musculoskeletal injury. Finally, it prevents the electrocardiographic ab-normalities that have been seen in patients who, regardless of fitness level or age, perform sudden vigorous exercise without a warm-up period (Sharkey, 1990). Apparently, warm-up exercise decreases the risk for myocardial ische-mia and dysrhythmias through a gradual in-crease in coronary circulation (Ward, Malloy, & Rippe, 1987).

A cool-down period consisting of 5–10 minutes of gradual reduction in activity is also advocated. When exercise is terminated abruptly, preload will diminish owing to pooling of blood in the extremities. The heart rate will continue to increase such that imbalances be-tween myocardial oxygen supply and demand may occur, and ischemia and dysrhythmias may result (Ward, Malloy, & Rippe, 1987). Issues related to individualizing the exercise prescrip-tion will now be addressed.

Exercise Type/Mode

As previously discussed, exercise may involve both aerobic and anaerobic metabolic proc-esses. Cardiovascular benefits and risk reduc-tion are associated with regular aerobic exercise or exercise that involves aerobic metabolic proc-esses. Typically, aerobic exercise involves use of large muscle groups in sustained, rhythmic activity (Kattus, Brock, Bruce, et al., 1975). Examples of aerobic exercise include walking, swimming, cycling, cross-country skiing, and use of an upper body ergometer. The specific type of exercise prescribed depends on patient preference, involved muscle groups, functional capacity, and physical disabilities or limitations. Patient preference is always important because the patient is much more likely to adhere to a regular exercise regimen if it is enjoyable.

The clinician should also consider the in-volved muscle groups, because a major benefit of exercise training is the peripheral adaptation of the skeletal muscles used in training (Kay,

1991). Improved efficiency of the peripheral skeletal muscles in extracting oxygen from the blood results in a slower submaximal heart rate, decreased relative energy expenditure, and en-hanced ability to perform usual activities with less perceived exertion (RPE). Furthermore, training effects are specific to the individual muscle groups involved. For example, if a pa-tient has a job that requires substantial upper body work, upper body exercises should be emphasized.

Functional capacity, expressed in terms of the patient's V_{O2max} or MET level, determines the upper limit of exercise that a patient can safely tolerate. For example, although cross-country skiing is an excellent form of aerobic exercise using both upper and lower body ex-tremities, it should be reserved for the patient who is able to perform at a 7–8 MET level.

Physical disability or limitation may also dic-tate the type of exercise selected. A patient who is extremely overweight may benefit most from non-weight-bearing exercise such as sta-tionary cycling, whereas a patient at risk for osteoporosis would benefit from weight-bearing exercise. In addition to aerobic exercise, clini-cians and researchers are currently focusing on incorporation of adjunctive strength training, cross-training, and resistive exercise into exer-cise regimens. Although cross-training and strength training have been demonstrated to reduce the risk for musculoskeletal injury, none of these adjunctive exercise modes is known to reduce CHD risk. In addition, resistive training is not recommended as an isolated form of training in patients with hypertension (Ameri-can College of Sports Medicine, 1993).

Recommended Intensity, Frequency, and Duration

The ACSM's Guidelines for Exercise Testing and Training (American College of Sports Medi-cine, 1995), are commonly used in determining the intensity, frequency, and duration of exer-cise prescribed for CHD risk reduction. In gen-eral, the ACSM recommends that exercise be performed at an intensity of 60–90% of maxi-mum heart rate during ETT, for a duration of 20–60 minutes per session and at a frequency of 3–5 days per week. This intensity, duration, and frequency is deemed necessary for $V_{O_{2max}}$ to increase over time (i.e., for a cardiovascular training effect to be obtained). However, as previously discussed, exercise of lower intensity and duration may still be of benefit for CHD risk reduction. Therefore, it has been acknowleged that moderate exercise, between 40–60% of maximal capacity, may be appropriate for many people (Pate, Blair, Durstine, et al., 1991). Furthermore, clinicians are increasingly emphasizing that any increase in exercise or physical activity, regardless of intensity, is desirable.

The clinician may prescribe various intensity-duration combinations for CHD risk reduction. For example, assuming that the total work performed is equivalent, a lower-intensity workload, such as 50% of the predicted maximum, for a longer duration may be just as beneficial as the maximum. In addition, lower-intensity workloads diminish the risk for musculoskeletal injuries while they still promote weight loss and may increase adherence in the elderly patient. Similarly, intermittent exercise may be substituted for continuous exercise. DeBusk and co-workers (1990) reported similar improvements in physical fitness for patients exercising 30 minutes once a day, 5 days a week, and those exercising in three 10-minute sessions per day, 5 days per week, for 8 weeks (DeBusk, Stenestrand, Sheehan, et al., 1990).

In summation, the specific combination of intensity, frequency, and duration affects total energy expenditure and the benefit received. The total amount of activity, based on frequency and duration, performed at a moderate intensity level appears to be more important in promoting health than an increase in intensity (Haskell, 1994).

Monitoring

The parameters monitored during patient exercise sessions depend on the patient's risk stratification. For all patients, including those without diagnosed CHD, heart rate and symptoms should be monitored. Most patients can be taught to monitor their heart rate using a 10-second count. Heart rate can decelerate as quickly as 10 seconds after cessation of activity, so longer counts may be inaccurate (McCardle,

Zwiren, Magel, 1969). Pulse monitors can be used for patients who are unable to monitor their heart rate because of sensory deficits, atrial fibrillation, or other health conditions.

The energy requirements associated with activity and the patient's fitness level should be considered when interpreting the patient's heart rate response and other hemodynamic responses. Heart rate response is also affected by extraneous factors such as emotional status and extremes in temperature. During recovery, systolic blood pressure and heart rate decrease gradually as they return to baseline. For patients at moderate or high risk, we recommend that blood pressure be monitored if hypotensive or hypertensive blood pressure trends have been previously noted. An exercise-related fall in systolic blood pressure 15 mm Hg or more can be an ominous sign of exercise intolerance (Pashkow, 1993). This fall in blood pressure, which warrants termination of exercise, usually reflects severe left ventricular dysfunction from ischemia or congestive heart failure.

In addition to heart rate, we recommend that the clinician teach the patient to monitor sensations associated with exercise. *Perceived exertion*—that is, the patient's perception of his or her own exertion during exercise—is particularly useful. The majority of the research and clinical literature indicates that the Borg perceived-exertion scales can help in monitoring and regulating exercise intensity at different workloads (Ceci & Hassmen, 1991). Table 8–2 summarizes the numeric ratings that correspond to patients' verbal descriptions of exertion.

Ratings of perceived exertion (RPE) between 10 and 15 on a 15-point Borg scale

TABLE 8–2 Relationship between Verbal Descriptions of Perceived Exertion and Numeric Ratings on the Borg 15-Point Scale

Very, very light	7
Very light	9
Fairly light	11
Somewhat hard	13
Hard	15
Very hard	17
Very, very hard	19

Note: Borg scale ratings start at 6 and end at 20.

usually coincide with between 50–75% of the maximum MET for graded treadmill walking (Hanson, 1984). But caution must be used in interpreting RPE in several circumstances. First, the correlation between heart rate and RPE decreases with advancing age. Older patients report greater exertion than younger people at the same absolute workloads, possibly because of reduced heart rate variability and general lack of fitness (Hage, 1981). Second, one small study of 10 young adult men indicated that the RPE is less accurate is estimating heart rate at lower workloads (Smutok, Skrinar, & Pandolf, 1980). As cardiac patients are more likely to use lower workloads, Smutok and his associates (1980) caution that reliance on RPE alone could result in detrimentally high heart rates in the very circumstances where strict adherence to target heart rates is imperative. Finally, two studies raise questions about the reliability and validity of RPE during graded exercise testing (Whaley, Woodall, Kaminsky, et al., 1997; Whaley, Brubaker, Kaminsky, et al., 1997). Therefore, a combination of heart rate and RPE is most reflective of each patient's level of exertion.

Additional sensations that the patient should monitor and treat as indications for terminating the exercise session include chest discomfort, anginal type pain or sensations, anginal equivalents (if known), leg pain, severe shortness of breath, lightheadedness, palpitations, and excessive diaphoresis. Table 8–3 summarizes indications for terminating activity.

EXERCISE FOR SPECIAL AT-RISK POPULATIONS

Exercise prescription and monitoring for CHD risk reduction may need to be adapted for populations with concomitant health conditions or other factors that alter their physiologic response to exercise. These include patients (1) who are on beta blockers, (2) have congestive heart failure, (3) have received a cardiac transplant, (4) have diabetes mellitus, or (5) are of advanced age. Detailed discussions of each population are beyond the scope of this chapter. Therefore, only a brief presentation of the reasons why a population warrants special consideration, key differences in exercise training,

TABLE 8–3 Absolute and Relative Indications for Termination of an Exercise Test

Absolute Indications

- Acute myocardial infarction or suspicion of myocardial infarction
- Onset of moderate to severe angina
- Drop in systolic SBP with increasing workload accompanied by signs or symptoms or drop below standing resting pressure
- Serious dysrhythmias (e.g., second- or third-degree atrioventricular block, sustained ventricular tachycardia or increasing premature ventricular contractions, atrial fibrillation with fast ventricular response)
- Signs of poor perfusion, including pallor, cyanosis, or cold and clammy skin
- Unusual or severe shortness of breath
- Central nervous system symptoms, including ataxia, vertigo, visual or gait problems, or confusion
- Technical inability to monitor the electrocardiogram
- Patient's request

Relative Indications

- Pronounced electrocardiogram and changes from baseline (≥2 mm of horizontal or down-sloping ST segment depression, or ≥2 mm of ST segment elevation except in aVR)
- Any chest pain that is increasing
- Physical or verbal manifestations of severe fatigue or shortness of breath
- Wheezing
- Leg cramps or intermittent claudication (Grade 3 on a 4-point scale)
- Hypertensive response (systolic ≥260 mm Hg; diastolic ≥115 mm Hg)
- Less serious dysrhythmias, such as supraventricular tachycardia
- Exercise-induced bundle branch block that cannot be distinguished from ventricular tachycardia

From ACSM Guidelines for Exercise Testing and Prescription, 5th ed. (1998). Philadelphia, Lippincott-Raven.

and recommendations for exercise prescription follow.

Patients on Beta Blockers

Beta blockers reduce cardiac workload through inotropic and chronotropic effects. They are frequently administered to patients with hypertension or myocardial ischemia or those who have sustained a myocardial infarction. Beta blockers have been noted to increase exercise tolerance in patients with myocardial ischemia but decrease exercise tolerance in some patients with uncomplicated essential hypertension (Gordon & Duncan, 1991).

Beta blocker medication should not be interrupted, and the ETT should duplicate as much as possible the actual exercise conditions. Ideally, the ETT should be performed at the same time of the day and at the same time interval following beta blocker administration as would normally occur for exercise. Exercise intensity should be prescribed according to routine parameters. If the medication is discontinued, or if the patient is switched to a different medication, the ETT should be repeated, or RPE as opposed to heart rate should be used (Gordon & Duncan, 1991).

Patients with Congestive Heart Failure

With an increase in survival rates after myocardial infarction and an increase in the elderly population, congestive heart failure has become a common complication. Exercise benefits the patient with congestive heart failure in many ways such that isolating its unique benefit for CHD risk reduction is difficult. A 15–30% improvement in maximal exercise capacity has been reported for patients who have chronic heart failure and participate in either home exercise or cardiac rehabilitation programs (Coats, Adamopoulos, Radaelli, et al., 1992; Sullivan, Higginbotham, & Cobb, 1988). Resting heart rate, blood flow in the legs during submaximal exercise, and peripheral oxygen extraction have all been reported to increase during submaximal exercise while ejection fraction and left ventricular volumes remain unchanged (Keteyian, Brawner, & Schairer, 1997; Sullivan, Higginbotham, & Cobb, 1988).

Given its potential benefit, exercise is contraindicated only for (1) patients with congestive heart failure secondary to obstructive valvular disease such as aortic stenosis and (2) patients with active viral or autoimmune myocarditis (Coats, Adamopoulos, & Radaelli, 1992). Low ejection fraction is not an absolute contraindication to exercise. The correlation between maximal oxygen consumption and indices of resting cardiac function is poor (Fransciosa, Park, & Levine, 1981; Sziachcic, Massie, Kramer, et al., 1985). Therefore, patients with low ejection fractions have the potential to exercise and to benefit from exercise. Nevertheless, we recommend that heart rate and blood pressure be more frequently monitored during exercise in these patients and that monitoring be more extensive, because a poor ejection fraction will increase a patient's risk during exercise.

In formulating an exercise prescription, the clinician should specifically consider the underlying cause of the congestive heart failure, the ejection fraction, and the extent of muscle deconditioning. Studies of skeletal muscle metabolism, histology, and enzyme levels all indicate that muscle deconditioning is an important factor influencing the exercise prescription (Wilson & Mancini, 1993). Congestive heart failure causes diminished blood flow to the exercising skeletal muscle secondary to decreased cardiac output and decreased arteriolar vasodilatation. The mechanism for this decrease in arteriolar vasodilatation is unclear. Although increased fluid and sodium retention or increases in sympathetic activation and angiotensin may be contributory factors, various studies have failed to identify a relationship (Wilson & Mancini, 1993). Yet, indirect evidence is supportive. For example, angiotensin-converting enzyme (ACE) inhibitors have been shown to increase blood flow in the exercising leg (Drexler, Banhardt, Meinertz, et al., 1989; Meyer, Casadei, Coats, et al., 1991).

In general, based on the research, an aerobic exercise program at 60–80% of maximal heart rate, for 20–60 minutes depending on intensity, 3–5 days per week is recommended. Although of interest to clinicians, the effect of resistance training is only now receiving attention, and it cannot be conclusively recommended for use. Additional information from the literature on exercise testing and training in patients with congestive heart failure has been reviewed by Keteyian, Brawner, & Schairer (1997).

Patients with Cardiac Transplants

Patients who have undergone a cardiac transplant operation are usually extremely deconditioned owing to their limited functional capacity prior to surgery and continued inactivity after surgery. They often have complicated courses after surgery and require steroids to reduce the chance of rejection. Steroid myopathy can occur, with a clinical picture of increased muscle weakness and atrophy. Other side effects of steroid treatment are hypertension and osteoporosis (Squires, 1991).

The benefits of exercise training for cardiac transplant patients are similar to those in other patient populations. These include increased V_{O2max}, increased lean body mass, reduced blood pressure, reduced heart rate at submaximal workloads, and lowered resting heart rate (Squires, 1991).

Special considerations for cardiac transplant patients are related to the denervation of the heart that occurs during transplantation. As a result of denervation, exercise-related heart rate increases are due only to increased catecholamine secretion, not autonomic nervous system responses. Therefore, (1) heart rate does not increase as rapidly as in other patients, (2) maximal heart rate on graded exercise tests is lower than normal, and (3) the postexercise heart rate return to baseline is delayed. Consequently, we recommend that the warm-up and cool-down portions of the exercise session be prolonged.

Also, denervation in cardiac transplant recipients makes the accuracy of heart rate as an indirect estimate of oxygen uptake questionable. For this reason, such patients should regulate activity using endpoints such as RPE as opposed to target heart rate. Cardiac transplant patients have a lower V_{O2max} than normal owing to posttransplantation decreases in the exercise-induced ejection fractions for the right and left ventricle and the resting and exercise-induced fractions for the left ventricle.

Patients with Diabetes

Diabetes is an independent risk factor for CHD. Exercise may reduce CHD risk by facilitating greater control of diabetes mellitus and delaying the onset of insulin-dependent diabetes. Exercise is contraindicated for patients with serum glucose levels greater than 250–300 mg/dl and for patients with ketosis, because ketoacidosis may be exacerbated by exercise. In other diabetic populations, regular exercise improves glucose tolerance and increases insulin sensitivity.

Exercise in patients with insulin deficiency may be associated with increased hepatic production of glucose, decreased peripheral uptake of glucose, and decreased demand for glucose as a fuel substrate. An exercise-related exaggerated secretion of catecholamine and counterregulatory hormones may cause increased glycogenolysis (i.e., catabolism of glycogen to form glucose), gluconeogenesis (i.e., synthesis of glucose), and lipolysis (i.e., catabolism of fats) (Smith & Casso, 1988). The net result may be enhanced ketogenesis (i.e., formation of ketones) (Brown & Thompson, 1988).

Conversely, if insulin levels are high, production of hepatic glucose may be inadequate to match increased glucose uptake by the muscle. Up to 5 hours after exercise, hypoglycemia may then occur (Wallberg-Henriksson, 1989). This hypoglycemia may be due to reduced glycogenolysis and gluconeogenesis (Horton, 1988).

As a result, certain precautions need to be followed to prevent both hypoglycemia and ketosis. The American Diabetes Association's Position Statement (1990) recommends that the site of injection, amount of insulin, and carbohydrate intake be modified to prevent hypoglycemia. Blood glucose should initially be monitored before and after exercise and those values used for insulin prescription. Subcutaneous insulin should not be injected near the site of the working muscle. The patient should be involved in self-monitoring during exercise, should know the signs and symptoms of hypoglycemia, and should rehearse strategies to prevent or safely reverse hypoglycemic states. Special care must be used with diabetic patients on beta blocker medication, because they may not be able to experience these warning symptoms. In addition, patients must be taught to monitor themselves for any signs of increased redness, blisters, or skin breakdown, especially on the feet, ankles, and lower legs.

With respect to specific aspects of the exercise prescription, it has been recommended that the patient with non-insulin-dependent diabetes mellitus exercise five times per week at a lower intensity (40–60% functional capacity) but for a prolonged duration (40–60 minutes) to effect weight reduction (Pate, Blair, Durstine, et al., 1991). For insulin-dependent diabetics and those who do not require weight reduction, we recommend the previously discussed general guidelines for exercise prescription.

Elderly Patients

The elderly U.S. population continues to grow, and it is projected that 20% of all Americans will be older than 65 by the year 2030 (Abrams & Berkow, 1991). As discussed in previous chapters, age is an independent risk factor for CHD. Exercise has been reported to slow age-related decreases in maximal oxygen consumption (Limacher, 1994). In the elderly, dynamic exercise has also been shown to reverse the impaired cerebral circulation adjustment that can occur with rapid postural changes, and resistive training may reduce bone loss and reverse age-related skeletal muscle degeneration (Lowenthal, 1994). In addition, resistive training has the potential to improve skeletal muscle strength and endurance (American College of Sports Medicine, 1990). Even intellectual functioning may improve with regular exercise (Diesfeldt, 1977).

Despite the benefits of exercise training in the elderly patient, the complex interplay between the normal physiologic and sociocultural changes associated with aging affect the elderly patient's ability to exercise and his or her response to exercise. Furthermore, coexisting medical conditions may be associated with increased debility and deconditioning in these patients.

Normal physiologic changes associated with aging that may hinder the ability to exercise include (1) a decrease in V_{O2max} of approximately 10% per decade of age (Limacher, 1994), (2) a narrowed A-V_{O2} difference, (3) a reduction in the magnitude of the ejection fraction increase normally seen with exercise, (4) a lower peak heart rate, and (5) an increased dependence on the Frank-Starling mechanism to raise cardiac output, with corresponding decreased dependence on the heart rate.

Given these changes, the exercise prescription for the elderly patient should be modified in the following ways. Longer and modified warm-up and cool-down periods are necessary. Warm-up activities should emphasize flexibility and range of motion. The cool-down period should be more gradual and longer because the elderly patient is at greater risk for venous pooling, and a longer period of time is required for the heart rate to normalize (Wenger, 1994). The exercise mode and intensity should also be modified. Low-impact exercise such as walking is recommended to prevent musculoskeletal injuries. Upper body exercises and strength training should also be considered to minimize debility (Wenger, 1994). In the elderly patient who has poorly controlled hypertension or left ventricular dysfunction, strength training should be of light or moderate intensity with emphasis on the aerobic exercise component (Lowenthal, Kirschner, Scarpace, et al., 1994). Finally, for the elderly patient, the target exercise intensity should be reduced to 60–75% of maximum heart rate (Wenger, 1994).

The environment and monitoring procedures should also be adapted for the elderly patient. It is imperative that the clinician ensure that patients can self-monitor heart rate response to exercise. If not, a feasible substitute for self-monitoring should be prescribed. The elderly patient may be at greater risk for exercise-related injury, so the clinician should ensure that the patient is adequately dressed for exercise, with suitable footwear and protective clothing. As blood flow to the skin is diminished with aging, impairing the body's temperature regulation, the clinician should ensure that patients are adequately hydrated and that temperatures in the exercise environment are moderate (Lowenthal, Kirschner, Scarpace, et al., 1994; Wenger, 1994).

In conclusion, exercise training is an important strategy for assisting patients to reduce CHD risk. In conjunction with other members of the health-care team, the nurse potentially plays an important role in patient assessment, risk stratification, exercise prescription, and monitoring. Although exercise prescription and monitoring procedures must be individualized for each patient, certain populations warrant particular consideration. These include patients on beta-blocker medication, patients with congestive heart failure, cardiac transplant patients, diabetic patients, and the elderly. Debate continues as to whether women should be identified as a special population with respect to exercise training.

STAGE-BASED APPROACH TO INCREASING PHYSICAL ACTIVITY

In the previous section the traditional approach of decreasing sedentary behavior through exercise training was discussed. These formal exercise training programs do not meet the needs of certain patients, such as those lacking transportation to exercise facilities, those who are severely debilitated and thus do not meet program admission criteria, and those who qualify for limited health-care reimbursement. Only 50% of patients who join an exercise program continue their exercise programs beyond 6–12 months (Carmody, Senner, Malinow, et al., 1980; Oldridge, 1988). Commonly cited reasons include complexity, inconvenience, duration of the regimen, lifestyle change required, side effects, cost, and required skills (Carmody, Fey, Pierce, et al., 1982; Eraker, Kirscht, Becker, et al., 1984).

Various approaches have been used to address specific reasons for "noncompliance" or "nonadherence" with respect to an exercise regimen. These include (1) education; (2) spousal and familial involvement; (3) an incremental approach to change, using small, achievable goals; and (4) behavior modification strategies such as cueing, self-monitoring, modeling, social support, and reinforcement (Becker, 1987; Burke & Dunbar-Jacob, 1995; Greene, 1987; Taylor, Bandura, Ewart, et al., 1985). Categorizing patients as compliant or noncompliant is problematic in that noncompliance does not necessarily result in sedentary behavior, but rather suggests a poor fit between the exercise regimen and the patient.

As the exercise regimen is a strategy for helping patients reduce sedentary behavior, not a primary endpoint in itself, clinicians are increasingly recognizing that a more global approach to changing sedentary behavior in the entire population at risk for CHD is necessary.

Several cardiac rehabilitation programs are using the *transtheoretical model* (TTM), as described in Chapter 3, to restructure their intervention approach. Although the way in which these programs are operationalized differs, most programs are based on the premise that behavioral change, such as increasing activity levels and decreasing sedentary behavior, is most effective when interventions are appropriate for the patient's readiness to change.

Patient Assessment

In TTM-based approaches, the assessment parameters associated with the process of behavioral change are (1) stage of change; (2) *decisional balance*, or the relative importance of factors promoting and inhibiting the desired change; (3) processes or strategies used or anticipated as being helpful for behavioral change; and (4) perceived *self-efficacy*, or the capability of performing the desired behavioral change. As discussed in the subsequent sections, TTM-based instruments exist to measure these parameters with respect to "exercise behavior." However, despite adequate reliability and construct validity, the generalizability and appropriateness of these instruments for clinical practice as opposed to research has not always been satisfactorily established. Therefore, the clinician may wish to adapt these questionnaires to the clinical setting or develop interview approaches to elicit the specific information desired.

STAGE OF CHANGE. Marcus, Rakowski, and Rossi (1992) have developed a reliable and valid questionnaire to measure the patient's stage of change with respect to *exercise behavior*. This questionnaire is short and clinically useful. The patient answers six questions regarding intent to exercise within the next 6 months. Based on responses, the stage of change a patient is in can be determined. *Precontemplators* do not exercise and do not intend to start exercising in the next 6 months. *Contemplators* do not presently exercise but plan to begin in the next 6 months. *Preparers* exercise, but not regularly. *Actors* have exercised regularly for less than 6 months. *Maintainers* have exercised regularly for 6 months or longer. Analogously, the clinician could use a similar questionnaire and staging approach to assess the patient's stage of change with respect to increasing activity.

DECISIONAL BALANCE. Assessment of decisional balance provides information regarding the factors that encourage the patient to adopt, or discourage the patient from adopting, a desired behavior. Based on Marcus, Rossi, and Selby's (1992) research, in general, patients in the earlier stages of change tend to give more credence to the discouraging factors, or "cons," and less to the encouraging factors, or "pros." In the later stages, this decisional balance changes, with pros given more credence. The decisional-balance questionnaires adequately map the construct and allow identification of common pros and cons. The clinician may want to use open-ended questions to identify the unique pros and cons of a given patient.

PROCESSES OF CHANGE. The processes of change can be assessed through questioning the patient about which strategies or approaches she or he perceives as useful for change. Although validated and sensitive questionnaires to determine the processes of change exist, their usefulness and transferability to clinical practice has not been established. The research indicates that patients use at least 10 processes of change during initiation and maintenance of an exercise program, with the relative importance of specific processes of change and their frequency of use depending on the patient's stage of change (Marcus, Rossi, & Selby, 1992). For example, patients in the precontemplation stage use the processes of change less often than those in other stages. Patients in the preparation stage use more behavioral processes than those in the contemplation stage. Those in the action stage use both behavioral and experiential processes more than those in the preparation stage. Those in the maintenance phase use less experiential processes of change than other patients.

SELF-EFFICACY. Self-efficacy theory is based on the assumption that a patient's perceived ability to perform a given behavior directly affects the actual capability to perform that behavior (Bandura, 1986). Hence, self-efficacy is a predictor of future change in behavior. Self-efficacy has been positively correlated to the stage in the change (Marcus, Selby, Niaura, et al., 1992). The clinician can use various questionnaires to assess self-efficacy. Although not based on the TTM, the Cardiac Exercise Self-Efficacy questionnaire (Hickey, Owen, & Froman, 1992) is clinically easy to administer, yields concrete information, and is short.

Patient Intervention

The degree of rigor and consistency in applying the TTM constructs varies among intervention programs. In general, the clinician adapts TTM-based interventions to the patient's stage of change by (1) changing the relative importance placed on addressing "pros" and "cons" of increased activity, (2) assisting the patient to use those processes of change that the patient has identified as potentially helpful, and (3) restricting detailed teaching and counseling regarding specific behavior modification strategies to patients who are in the action stage of change. Thus, for patients in the precontemplation stage, the clinician would simply reiterate the message that increased physical activity improves health; then, when the patient is more interested in change, the clinician will help in any manner possible. Conversely, for the patient in the action stage of change, the clinician would use all available resources to assist the patient to enroll in a cardiac rehabilitation program or other suitable exercise regimen and would emphasize patient-identified benefits of increased activity. In addition, the clinician would discuss processes of change, such as the use of imagery, that might help the patient increase physical activity. Because use of stage-based programs to modify sedentary behavior is relatively new, little is known about their success rate, nor have they been critically evaluated in the clinical or research literature. Nonetheless, given the limitations of conventional approaches and the potential to increase patient adoption of a more healthy lifestyle, stage-based approaches represent a promising area of intervention.

CONCLUSION

The importance of regular exercise in reducing the risk for CHD is well documented. Emphasis on health promotion and prevention sets new standards for exercise prescription. Increased physical activity is associated with a reduction in overall mortality. Evidence is supportive of a sedentary patient improving health through an increase in activity level. With reduced intensity and more flexibility in the type of physical activity allowed, more patients may be willing to adhere to an increase in the amount of physical activity performed. The exact amount of physical activity required is still unclear, and the search for the most effective method to promote adherence continues. Further research is imperative. Research needs to be expanded to substantiate the role of exercise in reducing the risk for women.

References

Abrams, W. B., & Berkow, R. (Eds.) (1991). *The Merck Manual of Geriatrics.* Rahway, NJ: Merck & Co., Inc.

Ades, P. A., Waldmann, M. L., Polk, D. M. & Coflesky, J. T. (1992). Referral Patterns and Exercise Response in The Rehabilitation of Female Coronary Patients Aged > 62 Years. *American Journal of Cardiology, 69,* 1422–1425.

Ainsworth, B. E., Haskell, W. L., Leon, A. S., Jacobs, D. R., Montoye, H. J., Sallis, & Paffenbarger, R. S. (1993). Compendium of Physical Activities: Classification of Energy Costs of Human Physical Activities. *Medicine and Science in Sports and Exercise, 25*(1), 71–80.

American College of Sports Medicine (1991). *Guidelines for Exercise Testing and Prescription,* 5th ed. Philadelphia: Lea & Febiger.

American Association of Cardiovascular and Pulmonary Rehabilitation (1995). *Guidelines for Cardiac Rehabilitation Programs, 2nd ed.* Champagne, IL: Human Kinetics.

American College of Sports Medicine Position Stand (1993). Physical activity, physical fitness, and hypertension. *Medicine and Science in Sports and Exercise, 25*(10), i–x.

American College of Sports Medicine Position Stand (1994). Exercise for patients with coronary artery disease. *Medicine and Science in Sports and Exercise, 26*(3), i–v.

Anderson, J. M. (1991). Rehabilitating elderly cardiac patients. *Western Journal of Medicine, 154*(5), 573–578.

Anonymous (1990). On Bed Resting in Heart Failure. *Lancet, 52,* 41–50.

Bandura, A. (1986). *Social Foundations of Thought and Action: A Social Cognitive Theory.* Englewood Cliffs, NJ: Prentice Hall.

Becker, M. H. (1987). Improving patient compliance to prescribed therapy. *Cardiovascular Reviews and Reports, 8,* 57–59.

Berlin, J. A., & Colditz, G. A. (1990). A meta-analysis of physical activity in the prevention of coronary heart disease. *American Journal of Epidemiology, 132*(4), 612–628.

Blair, S. N., Gibbons, L. W., Painter, P., Pate, R., Taylor, C. B., & Will, J. (Eds.) (1986). *Guidelines for Exercise Testing and Prescription.* Philadelphia: Lea & Febiger.

Blair, S. N., Kohl, H. W., Gordon, N. F., & Paffenbarger, R. S. (1992). How much physical activity is good for health? *Annual Review of Public Health, 13,* 99–126.

Blair, S. N., Kohl, H. W., Paffenbarger, R. S., et al. (1989). Physical fitness and all-cause mortality: A prospective study of healthy men and women. *Journal of the American Medical Association, 262,* 2395–2401.

Blumenthal, J., Emery, C. H., Madden D. J., Coleman, R. E., Riddle, M. W., Schniebolk, S., Cobb, R. R., Sullivan M. J., & Higginbotham, M. B. (1991). Effects of exercise training on cardiorespiratory function in men and women over 60 years of age. *American Journal of Cardiology, 67,* 633–639.

Brown, S. P., & Thompson, W. R. (1988). The therapeutic role of exercise in diabetes mellitus. *The Diabetes Educator, 14,* 202–206.

Burke, L., & Dunbar-Jacob, J. (1995). Adherence to medication, diet, and activity recommendations: From assessment to maintenance. *Journal of Cardiovascular Nursing, 9*(2), 62–79.

Butler, R. M., & Goldberg, L. (1989). Exercise and prevention of coronary heart disease. *Primary Care, 16*(1), 99–114.

Caird, F. I., Andres, G. R., Kennedy R. D. (1973). Effect of posture on blood pressure in the elderly. *British Heart Journal, 35,* 527–530.

Carmody, T., Fey, S. G., Pierce, D. K., Connor, E., Matarazzo, J. D. (1982). Behavioral treatment of hyperlipidemia: Techniques, results, future directions. *Journal of Behavioral Medicine, 5,* 91–116.

Carmody, T., Senner, J., Malinow, L., Matarazzo, J. (1980). Physical exercise rehabilitation: Long-term drop-out rate in cardiac patients. *Journal of Behavioral Medicine, 3,* 163–169.

Ceci, R., & Hassmen, P. (1991). Self-monitored exercise at three different RPE intensities in treadmill vs. field running. *Medicine and Science in Sports and Exercise, 23*(6), 732–738.

Coats, A. J. S. (1993). Exercise rehabilitation in chronic heart failure. *Journal of American College of Cardiology, 22*(Suppl. A), 172A–177A.

Coats, A., Adamopoulos, S., Radaelli, A., et al. (1992). Controlled trial of physical training in chronic heart failure. *Circulation, 85,* 2119–2131.

DeBusk, R. F., Haskell, W. L., Miller, N. H., et al (1985). Medically directed at home rehabilitation soon after clinically uncomplicated acute myocardial infarction. New model for patient care. *American Journal of Cardiology, 55,* 251–257.

DeBusk, R. F., Stenestrand, U., Sheehan, M., & Haskell, W. L. (1990). Training effects of long versus short bouts of exercise in healthy subjects. *American Journal of Cardiology, 65,* 1010–1013.

Despres, J. P., Tremblay, A., Nadeau, A., Bouchard, C. (1988). Physical training and changes in regional adipose tissue distribution. *Acta Medica Scandinavia, 723*(Suppl.). 205–212.

Diesfeldt, H. (1977). Improving cognitive performance in psychogeriatric patients: The influence of physical exercise. *Age and Aging, 6,* 58–64.

Dishman, R. K. (1989). Determinants of physical activity and exercise for persons 65 years and older. In W. W. Spirduso & H. M. Eckert, (Ed.), *Physical Activity and Aging,* Champaign, IL: Human Kinetics Publishers, pp. 140–162.

Dishman, R. K. (1994). Motivating Older Adults to Exercise. *Southern Medical Journal, 87*(5), S79–S82.

Drexler, H., Banhardt, U., Meinertz, T., Wollschlager, H., Lehmann, M., & Just, H. (1989). Contrasting peripheral short-term and long-term effects of converting enzyme inhibition in patients with congestive heart failure: A double-blind, placebo-controlled trial. *Circulation, 79,* 491–502.

Eichner, E. (1986). Coagulability and rheology: Hematologic benefits from exercise, fish and aspirin: Implications for athletes and non-athletes. *Physician and Sports Medicine, 14*, 102–110.

Ellestad, M. H. (1975). *Stress Testing: Principles and Practice.* Philadelphia: F. A. Davis Company.

Eraker, S. A., Kirscht, J. P., Becker, M. H. (1984). Understanding and improving patient compliance. *Annals of Internal Medicine, 100*, 259–268.

Fentem, P. H. (1992). Exercise in prevention of disease. *British Medical Bulletin, 48*(3), 630–650.

Fletcher, G. F., Blair, S. N., Blumenthal, J., et al. (1992). Benefits and recommendations for physical activity programs for all Americans. A Statement for health professionals by the Committee on Exercise and Cardiac Rehabilitation of the Council on Clinical Cardiology, American Heart Association. *Circulation, 86*, 340–344.

Fletcher, B. J., Dunbar, S. B., Felner, J. M., Jensen, B. E., Almon, L., Cotsonis, G., & Fletcher, G. F. (1994). Exercise testing and training in physically disabled men with clinical evidence of coronary artery disease. *American Journal of Cardiology, 73*, 170–174.

Fletcher, G. F., Froelicher, V. F., Hartley, L. H., Haskell, W. L. & Pollock, M. L. (1990). Exercise standards: A statement of health professionals from the American Heart Association. *Circulation, 82*, 2286–2322.

Folta, A., & Metzger, B. L. (1989). Exercise and functional capacity after myocardial infarction. *IMAGE: Journal of Nursing Scholarship, 21*(4), 215–219.

Franscioa, J. A., Park, M., Levine, B. (1981). Lack of correlation between exercise capacity and indexes of resting left ventricular performance in heart failure. *American Journal of Cardiology, 47*, 33–39.

Frey-Hewitt, B., Vranizan, K. M., Dreon, D. M., Wood, P. D. (1990). The effect of weight loss by dieting and exercise on resting metabolic rate in overweight men. *International Journal of Obesity and Related Metabolic Disorders, 14*, 327–334.

Froelich, J. P., Lakatta, E. G., Beard, E., et al. (1978). Studies of sarcoplasmic reticulum function and contraction duration in young adult and aged rat myocardium. *Journal of Molecular and Cellular Cardiology, 10*, 427.

Froelicher, V. (1988). Cardiac rehabilitation. In W. Parmley & K. Chatterjee (Eds.), *Cardiology*. Philadelphia: J. B. Lippincott, pp. 1–17.

Gerstenblith, G., Frederickson, J., Yin F. C., et al. (1977). Echocardiographic Assessment of a Normal Aging Population. *Circulation, 56*, 273–278.

Gibbons, R. J., Balady, G. S., Beasley, J. W., Bricker, J. T., Duvernoy, W. F., Foelicher, V. F., et al. (1997). ACC/AHA guidelines for exercise testing: executive summary. A report of the American College of Cardiology/American Heart Association Task Force on Practice Guidelines (Committee on Exercise Testing). *Circulation, 96*(1), 345–354.

Glass, S. C., Knowlton, R. G., & Becque, M. D. (1992). Accuracy of RPE from graded exercise to establish exercise training intensity. *Medicine and Science in Sports and Exercise, 24*(11), 1303–1307.

Gordon, N. F., & Duncan, J. J. (1991). Effect of betablockers on exercise physiology: Implications for exercise training. *Medicine and Science in Sports and Exercise, 23*(6), 668–676.

Green, L. W. (1987). How physicians can improve patients' participation and maintenance in self-care. *Western Journal of Medicine, 147*, 346–349.

Greenland, P. (1991). Efficacy of supervised cardiac rehabilitation programs for coronary patients: Update 1986–1990. *Journal of Cardiopulmonary Rehabilitation, 11*, 197–203.

Greenland, P., & Chu, J. S. (1988). Efficacy of cardiac rehabilitation services with emphasis on patients after myocardial infarction. *Annals of Internal Medicine, 109*, 650–663.

Hage, P. (1981). Perceived exertion: One measure of exercise intensity. *The Physician and Sports Medicine, 9*(9), 136–143.

Hambrecht, R., Niebauer, J., Marburger, C., Grunze, M., Kalberer, B., Hauer, K., Schlierf, G., Kubler, W., & Schuler, G. (1993). Various intensities of leisure-time physical activity in patients with coronary artery disease: Effects on cardiorespiratory fitness and progression of coronary atherosclerotic lesions. *Journal of American College of Cardiology, 22*, 468–477.

Hanson, P. (1984). Clinical exercise testing. In R. Strauss (Ed.), *Sports Medicine*. Philadelphia: W. B. Saunders, pp. 13–40.

Hanson, P., & Nagle, F. (1987). Isometric exercise: Cardiovascular responses in normal and cardiac populations. *Cardiology Clinics, 5*(2), 157–170.

Haskell, W. (1994). Health consequences of physical activity: Understanding and challenges regarding dose-response. *Medicine and Science in Sports and Exercise, 26*(6), 649–660.

Hedback, B., Perk, J., & Wodlin, P. (1993). Long-term reduction of cardiac mortality after myocardial infarction: 10-year results of a comprehensive rehabilitation programme. *European Heart Journal, 14*, 831–835.

Helmrich, S. P., Ragland, D. R., Leung, R. W., et al. (1991). Physical activity and reduced occurrence of non-insulin-dependent diabetes mellitus. *New England Journal of Medicine, 325*, 147–152.

Hickey, M. L., Owen, S. V., & Froman, C. T. (1992). Instrument development: Cardiac diet and exercise self-efficacy. *Nursing Research, 41*(6), 347–351.

Horton, E. (1988). Exercise and diabetes mellitus. *Medical Clinics of North America, 72*, 1302–1321.

Jasnoski, M. L., Holmes, D. S. (1978). Influence of initial aerobic fitness, aerobic training and changes in aerobic fitness on personality functioning. *Psychosomatic Research, 25*, 553–556.

Juneau, M., Geneau, S., Marchand, C., Brosseau, R. (1991). Cardiac rehabilitation after coronary bypass surgery. In D. D. Waters, M. G. Bourassa, & A. N. Brest (Eds.), *Care of the Patient with Previous Coronary Bypass Surgery*. Philadelphia: F. A. Davis Company, pp. 25–42.

Kannel, W. (1976). Blood pressure and the development of cardiovascular disease in the aged. In F. Caird, J. Dahl, & R. Kennedy R. (Eds.), *Cardiology in Old Age*. New York: Plenum Press, pp. 143–175.

Kattus, A., Brock, L., Bruce, R., Fox, S., Haskell, W., Hellerstein, H., Naughton, J., Parmley, L. Taylor, H., & Zohman, L. (Eds.) (1975). *Exercise Testing and Training of Individuals with Heart Disease or at High Risk for Its Development: A Handbook for Physicians*. Dallas: American Heart Association.

Katz, Arnold M. (1992). *Physiology of the Heart*, 2nd ed. New York: Raven Press.

Kay, G. L. (1991). Athletic Participation after Myocardial Revascularization: Possibilities and Benefits. *Clinics in Sports Medicine, 10*(2), 371–389.

Keteyian, S. J., Brawner, C. A., & Schairer, J. R. (1997). Exercise testing and training of patients with heart failure due to left ventricular systolic dysfunction. *Journal of Cardiopulmonary Rehabilitation, 17*(1), 19–28.

Kirken, J. W., & Barnatt-Boyes, B. G. (1986). *Cardiac Surgery*. New York: Wiley & Sons.

Kowal, D. M., Patton J. F., Vogel J. A. (1978). Psychological states and aerobic fitness of male and female recruits before and after basic training. *Aviation Space and Environmental Medicine, 49*, 603–606.

Larsson, B., Svardoudd, K., Welm, L., Wilhelmsen, L., Bjorntorp, P., & Tibblin, G. (1984). Abdominal adipose tissue distribution, obesity and risk of cardiovascular disease and death: 13-year follow-up of participants in the study of men born in 1913. *British Medical Journal, 288*, 1401–1404.

Lazarus, B., Cullinane, E., & Thompson, P. D. (1981). Comparison of the results and reproducibility of arm and leg exercise tests in men with angina pectoris. *American Journal of Cardiology, 47*, 1075–1079.

Leon, A. S., Connett, J., Jacobs, D., & Rairamma, R. (1987). Leisure-time physical activity levels and risk of coronary heart disease and death. *Journal of American Medical Association, 258*, 2388–2395.

Leon, A. S. (1989). The role of physical activity in the prevention and management of obesity. In A. J. Ryan & F. L. Allman (Eds.), *Sports Medicine*. San Diego: Academic Press, pp. 593–646.

Limacher, M. C. (1994). Aging and cardiac function: Influence of exercise. *Southern Medical Journal, 87*(5), S13–S16.

Lowensteyn, I., Joseph, L., & Grover S. (1997). Who needs an exercise stress test? Evaluating the New American College of Sports Medicine Risk Stratification Guidelines. *Journal of Cardiopulmonary Rehabilitation, 17*(4), 253–260.

Lowenthal, D. T., Kirschner, D. A., Scarpace, N. T., Pollock, M., & Graves, J. (1994). Effects of exercise on age and disease. *Southern Medical Journal, 87*(5), S5–S12.

Malloy, M. J. (1993). Effects of exercise on coronary atherosclerotic lesions. *Journal of the American College of Cardiology, 22*(2), 478–479.

Manson, J. E., Imm, E. B., Stampfer, M. J., et al. (1991). Physical activity and the incidence of non-insulin-dependent diabetes mellitus in women. *Lancet, 338*, 774–778.

Manson, J. E., Nathan, D. M., Krolewski, A. S., et al. (1992). A prospective study of exercise and incidence of diabetes among U.S. male physicians. *Journal of the American Medical Association, 268*, 63–67.

Marcus, B. H., Rakowski, W., & Rossi, J. S. (1992). Assessing motivational readiness and decision making for exercise. *Health Psychology, 11*(4), 257–261.

Marcus, B. H., Rossi, J. S., & Selby, V. C. (1992). The stages and processes of exercise adoption and maintenance in a worksite sample. *Health Psychology, 11*(6), 386–395.

Marcus, B. H., Selby, V. C., Niaura, R. S., & Rossi, J. S. (1992). Self-efficacy and the stages of exercise behavior change. *Research Quarterly for Exercise and Sport, 63*(1), 60–66.

McArdle, W. D., Katch, F. I., & Katch, V. L. (1981). *Exercise Physiology: Energy, Nutrition, and Human Performance*. Philadelphia: Lea & Febiger.

McCardle, W. D., Zwiren, L., & Magel, J. R. (1969). Validity of postexercise heart rate as means of estimating heart rate during work of varying intensities. *Research Quarterly for Exercise and Sport, 40*, 523–528.

McConnell, T. R. (1996). Exercise prescription. When the guidelines do not work. *Journal of Cardiopulmonary Rehabilitation, 16*(1), 34–37.

Meyer, T. E., Casadei, B., Coats, A. J. S., et al. (1991). Angiotensin-converting enzyme inhibition and physical training in heart failure. *Journal of Internal Medicine, 230*, 407–413.

Miers, L. J., & Arnold, R. (1990). The cardiovascular response to exercise in the patient with congestive heart failure. *Journal of Cardiovascular Nursing, 4*(3), 47–58.

Miles, D. S., Cox, M. H., & Bomze, J. P. (1989). Cardiovascular responses to upper body exercise in normals and cardiac patients. *Medicine and Science in Sports and Exercise, 21*(5), S126–S131.

Morris, J. N., Heady, J. A., Raffle, P., Roberts, C. G., & Parks, J. W. (1953). Coronary heart disease and physical activity of work. *Lancet, 2*, 1053–1120.

Morris, J. N., Everitt, M., Pollard, R., Chave, S., & Semmance, A. (1980). Vigorous exercise in leisure-time: Protection against coronary heart disease. *Lancet, 2*, 1207–1210.

O'Connor, G. T., Buring, J. E., Yusuf, S., Goldhaber, S. Z., & Olmstead, E. M., Paffenbarger, R. S., & Hennekens, C. H. (1989). An overview of randomized trials of rehabilitation with exercise after myocardial infarction. *Circulation, 80*, 234–244.

Oldridge, N. B. (1988). Cardiac rehabilitation exercise programme: Compliance and compliance-enhancing strategies. *Sports Medicine, 6*, 42–55.

Paffenbarger, R. S., Hyde, R. T., Wing, A., Lee, I. M., Jung, D. L., & Kampert J. B. (1993). The association of changes in physical activity level and other lifestyle characteristics with mortality among men. *New England Journal of Medicine, 328*, 538–545.

Pashkow, F. J. (1993). Issues in contemporary cardiac rehabilitation: A historical perspective. *Journal of American College of Cardiology, 21*, 822–834.

Pate, R. R., Blair, S. N., Durstine, J. L., Eddy, D. O., Hanson, P., Painter, P., Smith, L. K., & Wolfe, L. A. (Eds.) (1991). *Guidelines for Exercise Testing and Prescription*. Philadelphia: Lea & Febiger.

Pauly, J. T., Palmer, J. A., Wright, C. C., & Pfeiffer, G. J. (1982). The effect of a 14-week employee fitness program on selected physiological and psychological parameters. *Occupational Medicine, 24*, 457–463.

Powell, K. E., Thompson, P. D., Caspersen, & C. J., Kendrick, J. S. (1987). Physical activity and the incidence of coronary heart disease. *Annual Review of Public Health, 8*, 253–287.

Prochaska, J. O., & DiClemente, C. C. (1983). Stages and processes of self-change in smoking: towards an integrative model of change. *Journal of Consulting and Clinical Psychology, 51*, 390–395.

Raglin, J. S. (1990). Exercise and mental health. Beneficial and detrimental effects. *Sports Medicine, 9*, 323–329.

Rossi, P. (1992). Physical training in patients with congestive heart failure. *Chest, 101*(5), 350S–353S.

Sackett, D. L. (1976). The magnitude of compliance and noncompliance. In D. Sackett, et al. (Eds.), *Compliance with Therapeutic Regimens*. Baltimore: Johns Hopkins University Press, p. 9.

Schneider, S. H., Amorosa L. F., Khachadurian, A. K., et al. (1984). Studies on the mechanism of improved glucose control during regular exercise in Type II (non-insulin dependent) diabetes. *Diabetalogia, 26*, 355–360.

Schwartz, R. S., Shuman, W. P., Larson, et al. (1993). The effect of intensive endurance exercise training on body fat distribution in young and older men. *Metabolism, 40*, 545–551.

Sharkey, B. J. (1990). *Physiology of Fitness*, 3rd ed., Champaign, IL: Human Kinetics Books.

Shaw, L. (1981). Effects of a prescribed supervised exercise program on mortality and cardiovascular morbidity in patients after a myocardial infarction: The National Exercise and Heart Disease Project. *The American Journal of Cardiology, 48*, 39–46.

Sinyor, D., Seraganian, P., et al. (1983). Aerobic fitness level and reactivity to psychosocial stress: Psychological, biochemical and subjective measures. *Psychosomatic Medicine, 45*, 205–216.

Smith, L. K. (1991). Exercise training in patients with impaired left ventricular function. *Medicine and Science in Sports and Exercise, 23*(6), 654–660.

Smith, L., & Casso, M. (1988). Exercise and the intensively treated IDDM patient. *The Diabetes Educator, 14*, 510–515.

Smutok, M., Skrinar, G. S., & Pandolf, K. H. (1980). Exercise intensity: Subjective regulation by perceived exertion. *Archives of Physical Medicine and Rehabilitation, 61*, 569–574.

Spurway, N. C. (1992). Aerobic exercise, anaerobic exercise and the lactate threshold. *British Medical Bulletin, 48*(3), 569–591.

Squires, R. W., Gau, G. T., Miller, T., Allison T., & Lavie, C. J. (1990). Cardiovascular Rehabilitation: Status, 1990. *Mayo Clinic Proceedings, 65*, 731–755.

Squires, R. W. (1991). Exercise training after cardiac transplantation. *Medicine and Science in Sports and Exercise, 23*(6), 686–694.

Stephens, T., Craig, C. L. (1990). The well-being of Canadians: Highlights of the 1985 Campbell's Survey. Ottawa: Canadian Fitness and Lifestyle Institute.

Stewart, K. J., & Kelemen M. H. (1989). Introduction to the symposium: Resistive weight training: a new approach to exercise for cardiac and coronary disease prone populations. *Medicine and Science in Sports and Exercise, 21*(6), 667–668.

Sullivan, M. J., Higginbotham, M. B., & Cobb, F. R. (1988). Exercise training in patients with severe left ventricular dysfunction: Hemodynamic and metabolic effects. *Circulation, 78*, 506–515.

Superko, H. R. (1991). Exercise training, serum lipids, and lipoprotein particles: Is there a change threshold. *Medicine and Science in Sports and Exercise, 23*(6), 677–685.

Sziachcic, J., Massie, B. M., Kramer, B. L., Topic, N., & Tubau, J. (1985). Correlations and prognostic implications of exercise capacity in chronic congestive heart failure. *American Journal of Cardiology, 55*, 1037–1042.

Taylor, C. B., Bandura, A., Ewart, C. K., Miller, N. H., & Debusk, R. F. (1985). Exercise testing to enhance wives' confidence in their husband's capability soon after clinically uncomplicated myocardial infarction. *American Journal of Cardiology, 55*, 635–638.

Thompson, P. (1988). The benefits and risks of exercise training in patients with chronic coronary artery disease. *Journal of American Medical Association, 259*, 1537–1540.

Thompson, W. G. (1994). Exercise and health: Fact or hype? *Southern Medical Journal, 87*(5), 567–574.

Todd, I., Wosornu, D., Stewart, I., & Wild, T. (1992). Cardiac rehabilitation following myocardial infarction: A practical approach. *Sports Medicine, 14*(4), 243–259.

Topp, R. (1991). Development of an exercise program for older adults: Pre-exercise testing, exercise prescription and program maintenance. *Nurse Practitioner, 16*(10), 16–28.

Tran, S. V., & Brammell, H. L. (1989). Effects of exercise training on serum lipid and lipoprotein levels in post-MI patients. A meta-analysis. *Journal of Cardiopulmonary Rehabilitation, 9*, 250–255.

Van Dale, D, Saris, W., & Ten Hoot, F. (1990). Weight maintenance and resting metabolic rate 18–40 months after a diet-exercise treatment. *International Journal of Obesity and Related Metabolic Disorders, 14*, 347–359.

Van Dixhoorn, J., Duivenvoorden, H. J., & Pool, J. (1990). Success and failure of exercise training after myocardial infarction: Is the outcome predictable? *Journal of the American College of Cardiology, 15*, 974–982.

Wallace, P. G., Brennan, P. J., & Haines, A. P. (1987). Are general practitioners doing enough to promote healthy lifestyles? Findings of the Medical Research Council's General Practice Research Framework Study on Lifestyle and Health. *British Medical Journal, 294*, 940–942.

Wallberg-Henriksson, H. (1989). Acute exercise: Fuel homeostasis and glucose transport in insulin-dependent diabetes mellitus. *Medicine and Science in Sports and Exercise, 21*, 356–361.

Ward, A., Malloy, P., & Rippe, J. (1987). Exercise prescription guidelines for normal and cardiac populations. *Cardiology Clinics, 5*, 197.

Weber, J. R. (1988). Left ventricular hypertrophy: Its prime importance as a controllable risk factor. *American Heart Journal, 116*, 272–279.

Wenger, N. K. (1977). Does exercise training enhance collateral circulation? In J. Kellerman & H. Denolin (Eds.), *Critical Evaluation of Cardiac Rehabilitation*. Basel: Karger, pp. 143–195.

Wenger, N. K. (1989). Rehabilitation of the patient with coronary heart disease. *Postgraduate Medicine, 85*(5), 369–380.

Wenger, N. K. (1993). Modern coronary rehabilitation. *Postgraduate Medicine, 94*(2), 131–136.

Wenger, N. K. (1994). Guidelines for exercise training of elderly patients with coronary artery disease. *Southern Medical Journal, 87*(5), S66–S69.

Whaley, M. H., Brubaker, P. H., Kaminsky, L. A., & Miller, C. R. (1997). Validity of rating perceived exertion during graded exercise testing in apparently healthy adults and cardiac patients. *Journal of Cardiopulmonary Rehabilitation, 17*(4), 261–267.

Whaley, M. H., Woodall, M. T., Kaminsky, L. A., & Emmett, J. D. (1997). Reliability of perceived exertion during graded exercise testing in apparently healthy adults. *Journal of Cardiopulmonary Rehabilitation, 17*(1), 37–42.

Wilson, J. R., & Mancini, D. M. (1993). Factors contributing to the exercise limitation of heart failure. *Journal of the American College of Cardiology, 22*(Suppl. A), 93A–98A.

CHAPTER 9

Blood Pressure Regulation

Debra Lee Servello

A high percentage of people will develop hypertension (HTN) at some point during their lives. Approximately 50–58 million Americans have elevated blood pressure and are at risk for coronary heart disease (CHD) (Joint National Committee V, 1993). HTN is so widespread in the United States that it is often considered to be at epidemic proportions (Salazar, 1995). About 20% of the adult population aged 18–74 years has HTN (Kannel, 1996).

Although the serious consequences of high blood pressure can be prevented in those who seek early treatment, long-term control of this disease continues to be a major problem, and the rate of improvement in control rates has slowed during the past decade (Joint National Committee VI, 1997). The etiology of HTN is unknown; the disease is generally asymptomatic; there is no cure for it; and treatment is generally lifelong (May, Young, & Wiser, 1992). The ultimate aim of investigators is to discover the etiology of this chronic, usually incurable disorder and thus be able to prevent its occurrence (Lenfant, 1996).

The focus in this chapter is the assessment and management of HTN and its role in CHD. Management is broken down into three areas: lifestyle modification, pharmacologic management, and patient education. The goal of this chapter is to give clinicians a better understanding of the prevalence of HTN, its relationship to CHD, and strategies for controlling it. This chapter also provides advanced-practice nurses and others with a comprehensive knowledge base and tools for the management of HTN. The detail and length of this chapter reflect the extensive knowledge base regarding hypertension, the third risk factor in the deadly triad that includes elevated LDL cholesterol levels and smoking. An overview of HTN and its relationship to CHD now follows.

HYPERTENSION AND CORONARY HEART DISEASE

HTN is the most prevalent and recognized modifiable risk factor for CHD, as demonstrated in epidemiologic studies (Burt, Whelton, Roccella, et al., 1995; Kannel, 1996; Joint National Committee VI, 1997). HTN is also a risk factor for cerebral vascular accidents, congestive heart failure, renal insufficiency, and peripheral vascular disease (McAbee, 1995). The incidence of CHD among individuals with HTN is equal to all the other adverse outcomes combined (Kannel, 1996). In addition, many risk factors associated with HTN are also risk factors for CHD. Smoking, elevated serum choles-terol, increased body weight, diabetes mellitus, emotional stress, and sedentary lifestyle are all risk factors associated with HTN and CHD (Kaplan, 1995; Somova, Connolly, & Diara, 1995; SHEP Cooperative Research Group, 1991).

Clinical trials show that lowering blood pres-sure by about 12–20 mm Hg systolic and 5–6 mm Hg diastolic reduces the relative risk of CHD by about 15% and of stroke by about 40% (Sackett, 1996). This reduction in risk is seen regardless of the initial blood pressure and the absolute risk for CHD. The reduction in risk occurs usually within 2½ years (Sackett, 1996).

Severe HTN may directly damage arterioles and cause atherosclerosis. It is important to recognize that in a complex multifactorial proc-ess such as atherosclerosis, no single factor, including HTN, is sufficient to produce CHD, stroke, peripheral artery disease, or heart fail-ure (Kannel, 1996). HTN is only one of the many risk factors involved in atherogenesis. It is not sufficient treatment to single out HTN for control, disregarding the other risk factors (Kannel, 1996).

The prevalence of HTN increases with age, and HTN is more common in African Ameri-cans than in whites (McAbee, 1995). In young adulthood and early middle age, HTN is more prevalent in males than in females; however, after menopause, the opposite is true (McAbee, 1995). Regional differences in blood pressure exist, with the highest incidence in the south-eastern part of the United States. Both elevated diastolic blood pressure (DBP) and systolic blood pressure (SBP) are associated with an increased risk of morbidity and mortality (Joint National Committee VI, 1997). The long-term risks of developing CHD increase proportion-ally with blood pressure.

DEFINITION OF BLOOD PRESSURE

HTN is simply defined as a cardiovascular disease characterized by elevation of blood pressure above arbitrary values considered "normal" for people of similar racial and envi-ronmental background (May, Young, & Wiser, 1992). *Blood pressure* is determined by the

pumping action of the heart *(cardiac output)* and the tone of the arteries *(peripheral resis-tance)*. The predominant control mechanisms are the central nervous system and the renal pressor system. Extracellular fluid volume con-tributes to blood pressure through increased preload and resultant increased cardiac output (Callahan, 1991). HTN is ascribed to an abnor-mality of any of these mechanisms (Kaplan, 1994).

Although HTN has been defined as a distinct disease for 100 years, authorities continue to debate the dividing line between normal and elevated blood pressure. For many years, HTN was frequently diagnosed by DBP alone, with no consideration of SBP to guide treatment decisions (Vidt, 1993). Data now confirm that elevated SBP has great importance in determin-ing cardiovascular risk (Moser, 1996). Data from the Framingham study suggest that even borderline elevation of SBP with a normal DBP may be a risk factor for CHD (Littenberg, 1995). Presently, both DBP and SBP values are used to identify individuals at risk for CHD (Neaton & Wentworth, 1992). The World Health Organization (WHO), the International Society of Hypertension (ISH), and the Sixth Joint National Committee on Detection, Evalu-ation, and Treatment of Hypertension (JNC VI), now use both the SBP and DBP in defining HTN (Joint National Committee VI, 1997; Zan-chetti, 1993).

HTN can be defined as sustained average blood pressure levels above 140/90 mm Hg in adults (Joint National Committee VI, 1997). Although the traditional terms "mild HTN" and "moderate HTN" are still used by WHO/ISH (Chalmers, 1993), these terms fail to convey the impact of high blood pressure on the risk of CHD and are being replaced by the JNC VI "stages" as seen in Table 9–1. "High-normal" identifies individuals at increased risk of devel-oping HTN and experiencing cardiovascular in-cidents such as CHD (Moser, 1993). Further-more, all stages of HTN are associated with increased risk of nonfatal and fatal CHD. The higher the blood pressure is, the higher the risk. Stage 1, previously called mild, is the most common stage of high blood pressure (Joint National Committee VI, 1997).

Even though we know that controlling HTN will reduce the risk of CHD, reports from the

TABLE 9–1 Classification of Blood Pressure for Adults, with Follow-up Recommendations Based on Risk Group

Category (Stages of mm Hg)	Blood Pressure	Risk Group A*	Risk Group B†	Risk Group C**	Follow-up Recommendations
Optimal	<120 systolic and <80 diastolic				
Normal	<130 systolic and <85 disastolic				Recheck in 2 years
High-normal	130–139 systolic or 85–89 disastolic	Lifestyle modification	Lifestyle modification	Drug therapy	Recheck in 1 year
Hypertension Stage 1	140–159 systolic or 90–99 diastolic	Lifestyle modification (up to 12 months)	Lifestyle modification (up to 6 months)	Drug therapy	Confirm within 2 months
Hypertension Stage 2	160–179 systolic or 100–109 diastolic	Drug therapy	Drug therapy	Drug therapy	Evaluate or refer to source of care within 1 month
Hypertension Stage 3	≥180 systolic or $n \geq$ 110 diastolic	Drug therapy	Drug therapy	Drug therapy	Evaluate or refer to source of care immediately or within 1 week depending on clinical situation

*No risk factors, no target organ disease or clinical cardiovascular disease.
†At least one risk factor, not including diabetes; no target organ disease or clinical cardiovascular disease.
**Target organ disease or clinical cardiovascular disease or diabetes, with or without risk factors.
Based on Joint National Committee on Detection, Evaluation, and Treatment of High Blood Pressure (1997). The Sixth Report of the Joint National Committee (JNC VI). *Archives of Internal Medicine, 157*, 2412–2446.

Third National Health and Nutrition Examination Survey indicate that many patients are not being treated effectively. Only 68% of people with HTN know that they have the disease. Only 53% are being treated with drugs, and only 24% have SBP of less than 140 mm Hg and DBP of less than 90 mm Hg (Joint National Committee VI, 1997).

In 95% of cases, HTN is of unknown cause and labeled "essential," "idiopathic," "benign," or "primary." Presently the gene for angiotensinogen is considered the strongest candidate for a role in causing essential HTN (MacFadyen & Prasad, 1995). Environmental factors that increase the incidence of HTN include obesity, stress, high sodium intake, and alcohol consumption of greater than 1 ounce per day (Kaplan, 1995).

Secondary HTN occurs in about 2% of the hypertensive population. The most common causes of secondary HTN are renal artery stenosis, renal parenchymal disease, adrenal aldosteronism, pheochromocytoma, thyroid disorders, medication, excessive alcohol use, and drug abuse. Oral contraceptives, steroids, nonsteroidal anti-inflammatory drugs, nasal decongestants, cold suppressants, cyclosporin, erythropoietin, tricyclic antidepressants, and monoamine oxidase inhibitors can also cause secondary HTN (Hutchins, 1995).

SIGNS AND SYMPTOMS OF HYPERTENSION

Generally, HTN is asymptomatic until well advanced and is thus termed "the silent killer." Blurred vision, headache, temporary loss of vision, dizziness, lethargy, or transient paralysis are signs of severe HTN (O'Donnell, 1990). Increased agitation, confusion, and change of mental status may also be present. Headaches characteristically occur in the morning and diminish as the day progresses. Nosebleeds may also occur. Flushing of the face is common, but it is not a definitive sign of hypertension.

Manifestations of *target organ disease* include cardiac, cerebrovascular, peripheral vascular, renal, and retinal changes. Electrocardiograms may reveal evidence of left ventricular hypertrophy or CHD. The patient may have experienced transient ischemic attacks or cerebrovascular accident. One or more of the major pulses may be absent. A funduscopic exam may reveal hemorrhages or exudates and, in patients with severe target organ disease, papilledema (Ferri, 1995). Table 9–2 lists manifestations of target organ disease.

RATIONALE FOR TREATMENT

MacMahon and co-workers (1990) analyzed observational studies relating DBP level to the incidence of stroke and CHD. The overall results demonstrated a direct, continuous, and independent association between DBP and CHD. The lower the DBP was (70–110 mm Hg), the lower the risks of stroke and CHD. No direct extrapolation to DBP levels below 70

TABLE 9–2 Manifestations of Target Organ Disease and Clinical Cardiovascular Disease

Organ System	Manifestations
Cardiac	Myocardial infarction, angina, or previous myocardial revascularization; left ventricular hypertrophy or "strain" based on electrocardiography or echocardiography; left ventricular dysfunction or cardiac failure
Cerebrovascular	Transient ischemic attack or stroke
Peripheral arterial	Absence of one or more major pulses in extremities (except for dorsalis pedis) with or without intermittent claudication; aneurysm
Renal	Serum creatinine of 130 μmol/L (1.5 mg/dL) or more; proteinuria (1+ or greater); microalbuminuria
Retinopathy	Hemorrhages or exudates, with or without papilledema

Based on Joint National Committee on Detection, Evaluation, and Treatment of High Blood Pressure (1993). The Fifth Report of the Joint National Committee (JNC V). *Archives of Internal Medicine, 153,* 154–183; Joint National Committee on Prevention, Detection, Evaluation, and Treatment of High Blood Pressure (1997). The Sixth Report of the Joint National Committee (JNC VI). *Archives of Internal Medicine, 157,* 2412–2446.

mm Hg is available, but indirect evidence is provided by populations in South America and New Guinea, where the average DBP is only 62–66 mm Hg and the rates of CHD and stroke are extremely low (Intersalt Cooperative Research Group, 1988).

Even among individuals considered to be normotensive, moderate reduction in blood pressure may still be necessary, especially for those with other risk factors, such as advanced age, family history of CHD, smoking, diabetes, and peripheral vascular disease (MacMahon, Peto, et al., 1990). The combined results of various studies, including the Multiple Risk Factor Intervention Trial and the Framingham Heart Study, the Chicago Heart Association study, and the Western Electric and People's Gas studies, demonstrate that in previously normotensive individuals, as DBP increases so does the risk of stroke and CHD (Neaton & Wentworth, 1992; MacMahon, Peto, et al., 1990; Dyer, 1975). A small decrease in blood pressure has the potential to produce substantial reduction in cardiovascular risk (McAbee, 1995). Therefore, comprehensive programs focusing on primary prevention of HTN and behaviors known to be associated with HTN are needed (Salazar, 1995).

ASSESSMENT OF THE HYPERTENSIVE PATIENT

The goal of assessment is threefold (1) to determine whether a secondary cause for the elevation in blood pressure is present; (2) to assess target organ disease; and (3) to assess other cardiovascular risk factors (Hutchins, 1995). A complete assessment of the hypertensive patient should include medical history, complete physical examination, and baseline laboratory tests. Chapter 4 contains more specific information regarding nursing assessment.

Medical/Health History

A complete medical/health history needs to be obtained for all individuals being assessed for hypertension as a CHD risk factor. This history should include (1) family history of HTN, CHD, stroke, cardiovascular disease, diabetes mellitus,

and dyslipidemia; (2) patient history of symptoms of cardiovascular disease, cerebrovascular disease, renal disease, diabetes mellitus, dyslipidemia, or gout; (3) duration of elevated blood pressure; (4) history of weight gain and of smoking or other tobacco use; (5) dietary assessment, including sodium intake, alcohol use, and intake of cholesterol and saturated fats; (6) previous treatment for HTN, including effectiveness and side effects of the medications; (7) symptoms suggesting secondary HTN (i.e., abdominal or flank pain or masses, tremors, sweating, pallor, orthostatic hypotension, tachycardia); (8) psychosocial and environmental factors contributing to stress (i.e., family, work, education level); (9) current medications, including over-the-counter, prescription, and illicit drugs; (10) sexual function or dysfunction, especially if related to medication; and (11) financial concerns (Joint National Committee VI, 1997; O'Donnell, 1990).

Physical Examination

The initial physical examination includes (1) two or more blood pressure readings, with verification in both arms; (2) height and weight; (3) funduscopic examination for arteriolar narrowing, arteriovenous nicking, hemorrhages, exudates, or papilledema; (4) examination of the neck for carotid bruits, distended neck veins, or enlarged thyroid; (5) examination of the heart for increased rate and size, clicks, murmurs, arrhythmias, or third and fourth heart sounds; (6) examination of the abdomen for bruits over abdominal aorta, iliac, and femoral arteries, enlarged kidneys, masses, or abnormal abdominal aortic pulsation; (7) examination of the extremities for diminished or absent peripheral arterial pulsations, bruits, edema or other evidence of peripheral vascular disease or ischemia; and (8) neurologic assessment, including cranial nerves, (especially cranial nerves II and III), pupils, visual fields, and gait (Joint National Committee VI, 1997; O'Donnell, 1990).

MEASURING BLOOD PRESSURE. Blood pressure can be highly labile; therefore, a single abnormally high reading is of little significance in predicting long-term outcomes. Hypertension is best diagnosed by averaging blood pressure measurements obtained during three or more clinical visits. An average of several high blood pressure measurements are predictive of increased cardiovascular morbidity and mortality (May, Young, & Wiser, 1992).

Blood pressure needs to be measured in such a manner that the values obtained are representative of the patient's usual level (World Health Organization, 1993). Suggestions for obtaining an accurate blood pressure measurement include (1) seating the patient for 5 minutes prior to measurement; (2) keeping the patient's arm bare and held at heart level; (3) ensuring that the patient not smoke or consume caffeine within 30 minutes of the measurement; (4) using a cuff of proper size, with the bladder nearly or completely encompassing the arm, to prevent artificially high readings in obese individuals; (5) using either a mercury sphygmomanometer or a recently calibrated aneroid manometer or validated electronic device; (6) applying the cuff smoothly and firmly, with the midpoint of the bladder placed directly over the brachial artery; (7) measuring blood pressure in both arms to determine any variations; (8) recording both SBP (Phase 1 Korotkoff sound) and DBP (Phase 5 Korotkoff sound); and (9) averaging two or more readings, each separated by 2 minutes (Joint National Committee VI, 1997).

Differences between blood pressure measured at home and blood pressure measured in the clinic are causing debate over the definition of "mildly" elevated blood pressure. A phenomenon called *white coat hypertension* is commonly seen in clinical practice, but its pathogenesis and prognosis remain relatively unknown (Kuwajima, Miyao, Uno, et al., 1994). White coat HTN is diagnosed when the elevation in arterial blood pressure is limited to the clinical setting (MacFadyen & Prasad, 1995; Martin, Phillips, & Krakoff, 1994). White coat HTN has been estimated to be present in approximately one quarter of patients with newly diagnosed mild to moderate HTN (Hoeghlm, Kristensen, Madsen, et al., 1992).

White coat HTN must be differentiated from true HTN, because incorrect treatment can cause excessive reduction in blood pressure with consequent ischemia of vital organs. Ambulatory blood pressure is shown to be a better predictor of clinical outcome than a blood pressure value obtained in the clinical setting

(Hoeghlm, Kristensen, Madsen, et al., 1992). The development of home blood pressure measurement equipment makes the determination of blood pressures convenient and affordable, aiding in the correct differential diagnosis of white coat HTN versus true HTN. Whereas finger monitoring is inaccurate, ambulatory blood pressure monitoring holds considerable promise. Although no single factor can be used as a marker of white coat HTN, ambulatory monitoring will help avoid the incorrect diagnosis of essential HTN (Joint National Committee VI, 1997). At the time of this writing, no long-term studies have established the stability over time of white coat HTN.

Compared with clinic/office-based blood pressure readings, those of ambulatory monitoring are more closely correlated with indicators of target organ damage in hypertensive patients (Joint National Committee VI, 1997). Additional advantages of ambulatory blood pressure monitoring include the ability to obtain several blood pressure measurements every day, the ability to obtain readings at home or at work, the simplicity of performance, the cost effectiveness, and the patient's potentially improved adherence to treatment. The disadvantages of ambulatory blood pressure readings are possible inaccurate measurements, patient resistance to instructions, and patient anxiety over recording frequent blood pressure readings (Kriesand & Cohen, 1996). Not every individual is a good candidate for ambulatory blood pressure monitoring. Some may become overanxious about elevated readings. Others may adjust their medications without consulting their clinician in an attempt to lower their blood pressure (Kriesand & Cohen, 1996).

Laboratory Tests

Laboratory tests are used to determine the severity of cardiovascular disease, identify target organ damage, and identify possible causes of secondary HTN. They are also necessary to obtain baseline values prior to initiating therapy. Tests include urinalysis, complete blood count, blood glucose, blood urea nitrogen (BUN), creatinine, potassium, calcium, uric acid, cholesterol, and triglyceride levels. Elevated BUN and creatinine levels and sediment in the urinalysis may indicate renal disease. Hypokalemia may be indicative of primary aldosteronism or diuretic use. Elevated glucose or cholesterol levels may indicate coexisting diseases such as diabetes or dyslipidemia (Kaplan, 1995). Optional laboratory tests include creatinine clearance, microalbuminuria, blood calcium, uric acid, fasting triglycerides, low-density lipoprotein (LDL) cholesterol, glycosylated hemoglobin, thyroid-stimulating hormone, limited echocardiography and a 24-hour urine test for protein. A 24-hour urine test will also enable proper evaluation of a sodium-restricted diet and assessment of potential abnormalities in renal function (Joint National Committee VI, 1997).

An electrocardiogram is valuable for the initial assessment of cardiac rate and rhythm and for identifying left ventricular strain patterns, ischemia, and hypertrophy. It is particularly valuable because a high proportion of individuals with HTN experience "silent," or unrecognized, myocardial infarctions (Kannel, 1996). A chest x-ray and echocardiography exam are also used for detection of left ventricular hypertrophy (Ferri, 1995).

MANAGEMENT OF HYPERTENSION

The treatment goal for HTN is the prevention of cardiovascular morbidity and mortality associated with the disease and control of blood pressure with the least invasive means available (Joint National Committee VI, 1997). Morbidity and mortality resulting from cardiovascular disease increase linearly with higher SBP and DBP (May, Young, & Wiser, 1992). Furthermore, early detection and treatment of other cardiovascular risk factors are key to the treatment of persons with HTN (Hutchins, 1995).

Antihypertensive therapy reduces the rate of CHD, renal failure, stroke, congestive heart failure, and death that results from untreated HTN (Kaplan, 1994). Similar to the controversy over the threshold pressures that define HTN, the threshold pressures for initiation of treatment are also under debate. The risk-benefit ratio must be considered such that treatment does more good than harm (Rose, 1980). WHO/ISH (1993) recommends starting treatment

when DBP is 95 mm Hg or more. JNC V (1993) recommends starting treatment when DBP is 90 mm Hg or more, especially when associated risk factors are present. The British Hypertension Society, the Canadian Hypertension Society, and practitioners in Germany recommend starting treatment when DBP is consistently greater than 100 mm Hg (Weiland, Keil, Spelsberg, et al., 1991). It is noteworthy that this 10 mm Hg difference in opinion accounts for more than half of the entire hypertensive population in the United States. Over 20 million Americans are being treated who might not be treated in other countries (Kaplan, 1992).

Individuals with associated cardiovascular risk factors such as smoking, dyslipedemias, diabetes mellitus, physical inactivity, and obesity, are at a significantly higher risk of developing CHD when accompanied by HTN. The American approach is based upon JNC VI (1997) recommendations for risk stratification and intervention based on blood pressure level, severity of target organ damage, and presence of other risk factors such as smoking, diabetes, and dyslipidemia (see Table 9–1).

In the past, the goal of therapy was to lower blood pressure to a level close to normal without excessive side effects (Kaplan, 1992). Decreasing DBP too much may actually increase the risk of CHD by lowering diastolic perfusion pressure in the coronary circulation. The *J-curve hypothesis* postulates that CHD risk falls with DBP reduction until cardiac perfusion becomes inadequate, then rises with further reduction of DBP (Fletcher & Bulpitt, 1992). This concern is most relevant to the hypertensive patient with preexisting CHD that mandates a more conservative approach to antihypertensive therapy (Kaplan, 1992). However, some clinicians contend that the concern over the J-curve is unfounded (MacFadyen & Prasad, 1995).

In the next sections of this chapter, the two components of HTN management, lifestyle modification and pharmacologic therapy, will be addressed.

Lifestyle Modifications

Lifestyle modification is the cornerstone of HTN treatment and the least costly therapy. It minimizes treatment risk to the individual, is low in cost, and is effective in lowering blood pressure and decreasing the risk of other cardiovascular events. This therapy deserves greater emphasis in the management of HTN. It also helps control blood pressure, reduces other risk factors for CHD (Kaplan, 1993), and may provide a positive example for family members.

The lifestyle changes of reducing weight, limiting alcohol intake, engaging in regular physical activity/exercise, and restricting sodium intake are endorsed as effective strategies for controlling blood pressure by both JNC VI (1993) and WHO/ISH. JNC VI (1997) further recommends maintaining adequate dietary potassium, calcium, and magnesium, as well as reducing the intake of saturated fat and cholesterol. The remaining lifestyle changes of dietary change, smoking cessation, and stress reduction may possibly influence blood pressure control. In this section, current evidence regarding the exact relationship between HTN and these lifestyle changes as well as JNC VI (1997) recommendations are addressed. JNC VI (1997) recommendations are given special emphasis because they are evidence-based and represent consensus within the U.S. health community regarding appropriate intervention on both the individual and the patient population level.

WEIGHT REDUCTION. HTN is more common in overweight individuals, and a large proportion of hypertensives are obese. Excess body weight is strongly correlated with increased blood pressure. Conversely, a decrease in body weight correlates with a decrease in blood pressure (Corrigan, Raczynski, Swencionis, et al., 1991). Weight reduction significantly decreases blood pressure in hypertensive people who are 10% above their ideal body weight (Langford, Blaufos, Oberman, et al., 1991). Significant decreases in blood pressure can occur with only a moderate reduction in weight (Kaplan, 1994). Obesity is highly prevalent in the United States and especially among African Americans and Hispanics (McAbee, 1995).

Weight loss is believed to be an effective nonpharmacologic approach in the management of HTN (McAbee, 1995; Jeffrey, 1991). JNC VI (1997) and WHO/ISH (1993) both recommend it. However, the relationship be-

tween weight reduction, HTN control, and CHD risk is not well understood. Reduction in saturated fat, rather than caloric restriction, may be responsible (Fair & Berra, 1995).

As discussed in Chapter 6, increased weight is associated with increased risk of CHD. The Framingham Heart Study reported an association between obesity and an increased incidence of stroke and CHD (Kannel, 1990). In the Dietary Intervention Study of Hypertension, participants in the weight-loss group were significantly more likely to maintain blood pressure reductions without medication than participants in the low-sodium/high-potassium dietary group (Cunningham, 1987). Furthermore, MacMahon, MacDonald, Bernstein, and co-workers (1985) found that an average weight loss of 7.3 kg, or approximately 15 lb, is as effective as the drug metoprolol in reducing DBP and SBP. The mean effect of a 1 kg, or 2.2 lb, loss in weight was a decrease in SBP by 1.6 mm Hg and in DBP by 1.3 mm Hg. Yet, despite having the knowledge that obesity is a contributing factor to HTN and that losing weight may result in lowered blood pressure, patients often find the process of dietary change difficult. The reader is referred to Chapter 6 for detailed information about strategies to promote weight loss and dietary change.

Weight reduction in obese hypertensive people also enhances the blood pressure lowering effect of antihypertensive agents and can significantly reduce the risk factors for CHD (Corrigan, Raczynski, Swencionis, et al., 1991). Accordingly, all obese hypertensive patients need to be started on an individualized weight-loss program that includes calorie restriction, monitored weight loss, and regular exercise. With the exception of those with target organ disease or clinical cardiovascular disease (Risk Group C), overweight individuals with Stage 1 HTN should apply weight-reduction and other lifestyle modifications for at least 3–6 months before resorting to pharmacologic therapy. If a pharmacologic agent is to be added, the weight-loss program should nevertheless be continued (Corrigan, Raczynski, Swencionis, et al., 1991; Joint National Committee VI, 1997).

It is noteworthy that conflicting evidence regarding the importance of weight reduction alone in lowering blood pressure exists. In some cases, even with weight reduction, HTN may be insufficiently controlled. Fagerberg, Berglund, Anderson, and co-workers (1991) found that weight reduction in obese males with HTN, without other interventions, did not have a clinically significant antihypertensive effect. However, sodium restriction together with weight reduction lowered blood pressure significantly.

DIETARY FATS. Evidence shows that dietary fat may play a role in blood pressure. An increase in the polyunsaturated-to-saturated fat ratio and a decrease in fat consumption may decrease blood pressure (Joint National Committee VI, 1997). Conflicting evidence and much controversy regarding the role of dietary fats is seen in the literature, and JNC VI (1997) does not address the polyunsaturated-to-saturated ratio.

SODIUM RESTRICTION. A large volume of literature exists on the relationship between HTN and sodium intake. However, data on the effectiveness of reducing sodium intake as a means of controlling blood pressure is not nearly as convincing as that regarding the effectiveness of weight reduction. Although many studies involving various human and animal populations have linked sodium intake to HTN, a close correlation between salt intake and HTN has not been identified. These findings may partially reflect the effect of other nutrients, such as potassium, calcium, saturated fats, or the total caloric intake.

Controlled studies show mixed results. Cunningham (1987) notes the Dietary Intervention Study in Hypertension examined the effectiveness of weight loss and sodium restriction on blood pressure reduction. Among non-overweight subjects who had a sodium-restricted diet, 78% had a demonstrable reduction in blood pressure. The impact of dietary sodium on blood pressure varies. Only 30–50% of individuals with HTN respond to sodium restriction; therefore, sodium restriction is not recommended for every patient with HTN (Laragh & Pecker, 1983). In general, African Americans and older individuals are more sensitive to changes in their dietary sodium (Flack, Ensrud, Mascioli, et al., 1991; Grobbee, 1991; Kaplan 1994). People whose blood pressure decreases with low sodium intake are called *salt-sensitive*.

Blood pressure may be controlled by sodium restrictions alone in some individuals with Stage 1 HTN. For those who still need pharmacologic

therapy, the medication requirements may be decreased (Joint National Committee VI, 1997). Simply changing food purchases and preparation can reduce sodium intake and, in turn, decrease the patient's blood pressure. Sodium restriction can be beneficial in other ways, too. When individuals are more aware of their sodium intake, they tend to decrease their total calorie intake, thereby enhancing weight loss. Also, individuals may tend to eat less "junk" food (Stuart, Friedman, & Benson, 1993). Although disagreement regarding the usefulness of sodium restriction exists, moderate sodium restriction has not been associated with any adverse consequences (Stuart, Friedman, & Benson, 1993). Therefore, JNC VI (1997) recommends sodium-restricted diets for both the prevention and management of HTN. WWHO/ISH (1993) recommends a sodium intake of no more than 5 g per day to effectively lower blood pressure in some patients, whereas JNC VI (1997) recommends a sodium intake of no more than 2.4 g per day.

Although adherence to sodium-restricted diets is possible, it may be difficult given that the average American ingests 6–12 grams of sodium per day (McAbee, 1995; Stuart, Friedman, & Benson, 1993; Intersalt Cooperative Research Group, 1988). To help reduce the patient's sodium intake, it is helpful to obtain a minimum of a 3-day diet history. Patients should be asked how often they eat out, and they should form a diet plan with a dietitian if available. Patients should also be instructed on how to read food labels, how to plan their meals, and how to modify food preparation.

Individuals fail to adhere to a low-sodium diet for a number of reasons, including (1) perceived blandness of low-salt food, (2) clinicians' lack of enthusiasm in prescribing a low-sodium diet, (3) perceived complexity and difficulty of dietary change, and (4) cultural norms promoting ingestion of "fast food" with a very high salt content (Dahl, 1972). Goal setting that involves the clinician, dietitian, and patient will help overcome these barriers. Specific guidelines for increasing adherence are discussed later in this chapter.

DIETARY POTASSIUM, CALCIUM, AND MAGNESIUM INTAKE. Potassium deficiency may be a cause of increased blood pressure (Intersalt Cooperative

Research Group, 1988), but clinical trials of dietary potassium supplements for patients with mild HTN are not convincing about the role of potassium. No significant data are available on the short-term or long-term effects of potassium supplements on blood pressure. Relatively few studies have focused on the effects of increased dietary potassium on blood pressure because of the risks associated with untreated potassium imbalance. These risks include potentially lethal cardiac arrhythmias. Therefore, even if potassium supplements lower blood pressure, they are too hazardous for routine use in the treatment of HTN. In addition, difficulty exists devising a diet that controls potassium intake and does not affect sodium intake (Cunningham, 1987).

In many epidemiologic studies, an inverse relationship between calcium and HTN exists. Calcium deficiency is noted to be associated with an increase in blood pressure. An increased calcium intake may lower blood pressure, but its overall effect is minimal (Hamet, Mongeau, Lambert, et al., 1991). Magnesium intake may also have an inverse effect on blood pressure (Joint National Committee VI, 1993). An increase in dietary magnesium may decrease blood pressure, but no convincing data exist to justify increasing dietary magnesium in order to lower blood pressure.

Given these findings, daily vitamin and mineral supplements may be used unless contraindicated, and the amount of processed and fast foods should be decreased because of their high sodium and low potassium levels. At present, JNC VI (1997) recommends "adequate intakes" of dietary calcium and magnesium, with daily potassium intake of approximately 90 μmol.

ALCOHOL INTAKE. Excessive alcohol consumption increased blood pressure, and a reduction in alcohol intake is associated with a decrease in blood pressure (Klatsky, 1996). The positive relationship between alcohol and blood pressure is more evident for SBP than DBP (Potter & Beevers, 1984). Potential mechanisms for the relationship include a direct pressor effect of alcohol on the vessel wall, a sensitization of resistance vessels to pressor substances, stimulation of the sympathetic nervous system, and increased production of adrenocorticoid hormones (McAbee, 1995).

Initially, alcohol causes a moderate decrease in blood pressure, but continued consumption of more than 1 oz of ethanol per day results in a dose-dependent rise in blood pressure (Kaplan, 1995). Therefore, many clinicians recommend decreasing alcohol consumption in the hypertensive patient to less than 1 oz per day, which is equivalent to 2 oz of hundred-proof whiskey, 8 oz of wine, or 24 oz of beer (Kaplan, 1994). Although a significant increase in blood pressure may be seen with initial withdrawal of alcohol in a heavy drinker, this effect is reversed within a few days.

In promoting decreased alcohol consumption, the clinician must be aware of the individual patient's needs. Alcohol may be a coping mechanism for many. Others may find it difficult in social situations to change their drinking style. With encouragement, patients who are not alcohol-dependent may be able to change their drinking habits. It is important to make them aware of the relationship between alcohol and HTN (Wallace, Cutler, & Haines, 1988).

Obtaining a detailed history of current and past alcohol consumption is important for the clinician in determining the patient's alcohol dependency. Some questions to ask are

1 "Have your family or friends ever objected to your drinking?"
2 "Do you feel that you drink too much?"
3 "Have your family or friends ever said that you have had too much to drink?"

If any of these questions are answered positively, the patient should be referred for counseling (Stuart, Friedman, & Benson, 1993).

Studies show that an excessive intake of alcohol can also cause resistance to antihypertensive therapy, decreased adherence to lifestyle modifications and pharmacotherapy, and occasionally increased incidence of refractory HTN (Potter & Beevers, 1984). No health-related reason exists to advocate abstinence for most people who drink a moderate amount of alcohol, but for those individuals who abuse alcohol, moderation should be aggressively pursued (Kaplan, 1995). Hypertensive individuals who drink more than 1 oz of ethanol per day will probably see a decrease in their blood pressure after moderation of their alcohol intake. Even if their blood pressure stays high, they will decrease the risk of the numerous other consequences of excessive alcohol intake (Kaplan, 1995). JNC VI (1997) and WHO/ISH (1993) both recommend a reduction in alcohol consumption in an attempt to lower blood pressure.

TOBACCO USAGE. Studies show no clinically significant association between the use of tobacco and HTN. Acute nicotine consumption raises the blood pressure. However, in the chronic smoker, blood pressure levels and the incidence of HTN are not increased because of habituation. Furthermore, smoking cessation has not been shown to decrease blood pressure. In fact, when smokers stop smoking, they may experience a small increase in blood pressure, possibly secondary to an increase in weight.

Nicotine adversely affects the metabolism of antihypertensive medications. Studies show that hypertensives who smoke require higher doses of propranolol to achieve similar reduction in blood pressure than those who do not smoke (Joint National Committee IV, 1986). Furthermore, smoking is a major cardiovascular risk factor. While smoking, patients experience rises in blood pressure that may prevent them from receiving the full benefits of antihypertensive therapy (Joint National Committee VI, 1997). In addition, smokers have a greater risk of developing heart disease and have a higher incidence of death, malignant hypertension, and subarachnoid hemorrhage (Stillman, 1995). Chapter 7 contains detailed strategies for the clinician to use in facilitating smoking cessation in patients.

PHYSICAL ACTIVITY AND EXERCISE. Interest in physical activity as a therapeutic modality to lower blood pressure is longstanding. JNC VI (1997) recommends regular aerobic exercise to facilitate weight control and help decrease blood pressure. WHO/ISH suggests mild, not strenuous, exercise for sedentary people. As with many of the previously discussed factors, the role of exercise in achieving lower blood pressures has been inconclusive. Some evidence supports the antihypertensive effect of regular aerobic exercise, but findings are not clinically significant. In addition, research designs of many relevant studies are flawed. Sample sizes are sometimes small, pre-exercise baseline data minimal or absent, or intervening factors—such as weight loss and dietary

changes—poorly controlled (Kaplan, 1994). Regular exercise enhances weight loss, which in turn decreases blood pressure, but no direct effect of exercise on blood pressure has been documented.

HTN appears to be less prevalent in more physically active adults (Miller, 1995). A study by Blair, Kohl, Barlow, and Gibbons (1991) demonstrated a lower death rate in hypertensive men who were physically fit than in normotensive men who were unfit. These observations are important, because the goal of antihypertensive treatment is not only to control HTN, but to prevent related mortality and morbidity. Chapter 8 contains a detailed discussion of the use of exercise for CHD risk reduction. With respect to the hypertensive patient, it is extremely important that the clinician recognize the effect of some antihypertensive drugs on exercise response. Nonselective beta blockers, and to a lesser degree beta-1-selective blockers, impair exercise tolerance (Gordon & Scott, 1994). The clinician and the patient should be aware of the potential interactions of any medication and exercise and take any precautions that are necessary. In individuals with left ventricular hypertrophy, the intensity and vigor of exercise should be restricted to prevent further cardiac damage (Jacober & Sowers, 1995).

RELAXATION. Stress can acutely raise blood pressure and may contribute to HTN. Despite the belief of many clinicians that repeated or prolonged exposure to stressful stimuli might contribute to chronic HTN (Sollek & Lee, 1989), the role of stress management in treating patients with HTN remains uncertain. A comprehensive review of the literature shows a decrease in blood pressure when a patient is exposed to relaxation training. But few controlled studies exist, and the observed effects may reflect (1) patients' apprehension and (2) pre-intervention increases in blood pressure associated with the physical act of measuring blood pressure (Jacob, Chesney, & Williams, 1991). Therefore, the research literature does not support the use of relaxation therapies or biofeedback for definitive treatment or prevention of HTN (Podszus & Grote, 1996; Joint National Committee VI, 1997). It is possible, though, that relaxation therapy could indirectly influence HTN by helping to reduce the anxiety, depression, and hostility associated with behavioral change (Stuart, Friedman, & Benson, 1993).

Pharmacotherapy

With the exception of patients with Stages 2 and 3 HTN or those in any stage of HTN accompanied by target organ disease or clinical cardiovascular disease (i.e., JNC VI Risk Group C), initiation of drug therapy should occur only after a lifestyle-modification program has been established. The decision to initiate pharmacologic treatment depends on (1) severity of the high blood pressure, (2) presence of risk factors, (3) evidence of target organ disease, (4) existence of other disease conditions, and (5) benefits already achieved by lifestyle modification.

Five major classes of drugs are used to reduce blood pressure: diuretics, beta blockers, alpha blockers, calcium channel blockers, and angiotensin-converting enzyme (ACE) inhibitors. Each provides antihypertensive coverage, but each differs in its effects on other major CHD risk factors and on associated conditions such as diabetes, angina pectoris, stroke, and heart failure (World Health Organization, 1993). The average blood pressure drop induced by each of the different categories of drugs is similar, although the blood pressure response of individual patients to the drugs may differ markedly. In long-term clinical trials, only beta blockers and diuretics have been definitively shown to reduce the risk of CHD and strokes in hypertensives. Long-term controlled trials to demonstrate the efficacy of the remaining drug classes in decreasing morbidity and mortality are still being conducted at the time of this writing (Kannel, 1996; Joint National Committee VI, 1997). Therefore, JNC VI (1997) recommends only diuretics and beta blockers as the first-line agents in the treatment of HTN unless contraindicated or unless special indications for use of other drugs exist. In contrast, WHO/ISH recommends several classes of first-line agents, including diuretics, beta blockers, ACE inhibitors, and calcium antagonists (Chalmers, 1993). By the year 2002, data from the ongoing Antihypertensive Lipid-Lowering Heart At-

tack Trial should resolve any controversy regarding the relative abilities of various drug classes to reduce CHD and its complications (Davis, Cutler, Gordon, et al., 1996).

The major classes of pharmacologic agents used in the treatment of HTN along with dosages, side effects, contraindications, and considerations for special populations, are summarized in Table 9–3. Because of the complexity of dosing regimens, the large number of ongoing clinical trials, and the evolving understanding of pharmacologic management, this chapter merely presents an overview of pharmacologic management. Clinicians should refer to original sources, the JNC VI (1997) report itself, health databases, and the World Wide Web for more detailed, updated information when prescribing antihypertensive medications.

DIURETICS. Diuretics are widely used as first-line antihypertensive agents. They have been shown to be clearly effective in the prevention of cardiovascular morbidity and mortality, especially for fatal and nonfatal strokes. Unfortunately, diuretics may cause a variety of unwanted effects, especially in larger doses. Some of the unwanted effects include potassium depletion, reduced glucose tolerance, ventricular ectopic beats, and impotence. The negative effects of diuretics may be reduced or avoided by lower doses that provide all of the antihypertensive effects but minimize the metabolic effects of the higher doses (Kaplan & Gifford, 1996). Even at low dosages, diuretics have been shown to be effective in decreasing blood pressure as well as lowering cardiovascular morbidity and mortality (SHEP Cooperative Research Group, 1991). Another advantage of using diuretics is the lower cost in comparison with other antihypertensives. Diuretics are also effective as ancillary treatment to enhance the effects of other antihypertensive medications. Potassium depletion may be avoided by combining diuretics with potassium-sparing drugs or ACE inhibitors (World Health Organization, 1993).

BETA BLOCKERS. Beta blockers are used effectively as first-line agents for the treatment of HTN and reduction of cardiovascular morbidity and mortality (McVeigh, Flack, & Grimm, 1995; Collins, Peto, et al., 1990). A wide variety of beta blockers is available. Some have cardioselective properties; others have partial agonist, alpha-blocking, or vasodilator properties.

Beta blockers have not been shown to be effective in the primary prevention of myocardial infarctions. They are effective in the reduction of recurrent fatal and nonfatal coronary events in patients with a previous myocardial infarction, and they improve survival rates (World Health Organization, 1993; Goldstein, 1989). Moreover, beta blockers are especially useful in hypertensive patients with exertional angina or tachyarrhythmias.

In many instances, though, beta blockers should be avoided. The potential for these medications to cause heart block or worsen bradycardia makes them dangerous, and they are contraindicated for patients with sick sinus syndrome or other bradyarrhythmias. Beta blockers are also contraindicated for patients with congestive heart failure because they tend to exacerbate it secondary to their negative inotropic effect. Another problem with beta blockers is that they may worsen claudication in patients with peripheral vascular disease (Bloomfield, Pearce, & Cross, 1993). As bronchospasm is a side effect of beta blockers, they should be avoided in patients with obstructive airway diseases. They should also be used with caution in individuals with insulin-dependent diabetes, because they may mask the symptoms of hypoglycemia (Hutchins, 1995).

ACE INHIBITORS. ACE inhibitors are effective in lowering blood pressure, are generally well tolerated, and reduce cardiovascular morbidity and mortality in patients with congestive heart failure and low ejection fraction after myocardial infarction (SOLVD Investigators, 1992). Studies have not shown the clinical significance of ACE inhibitors in the reduction of HTN-related morbidity and mortality. ACE inhibitors are effective for individuals with diabetes mellitus or with congestive heart failure resulting from left ventricular systolic dysfunction (Kaplan, 1996). Possible adverse effects include persistent cough and, on rare occasions, angioedema. ACE inhibitors should be avoided for women of child-bearing potential and are contraindicated in the second half of pregnancy owing to an increased rate of fetal and neonatal death. Otherwise the safety profile of ACE inhibitors is satisfactory (Hutchins, 1995; World Health Organization, 1993).

CALCIUM ANTAGONISTS. Calcium antagonists are divided into three classes: phenylalkylamines, dihydropyridines, and benzothiazepines. All are effective in lowering blood pressure. Verapamil and diltiazem reduce morbidity and mortality in patients after myocardial infarction when heart failure and left ventricular dysfunction are absent (World Health Organization, 1993). Side effects may include headache, tachycardia, flushing, ankle edema, and constipation (Hutchins, 1995).

Calcium antagonists are more likely to be effective in the elderly and in African Americans, both of whom are reportedly less responsive to beta blockers than other population groups (May, Young, & Wiser, 1992). As with many of the newer classes of antihypertensives, the effect of calcium antagonists upon the incidence of cardiovascular events in hypertensive populations has not been studied sufficiently (World Health Organization, 1995).

Pahor, Guralnik, Corti, and co-workers (1995) found that the risk of cardiac mortality was significantly higher with the use of nifedipine than with other antihypertensive agents tested. The increased mortality with the short-acting calcium antagonists occurred primarily among patients who had suffered a recent myocardial infarction (Davis, Cutler, Gordon, et al., 1996). Until these results can be further evaluated, the Food and Drug Administration warns to use extreme caution in prescribing short-acting nifedipine for the treatment of HTN (Townsend & Kimmel, 1996).

ALPHA-ADRENERGIC BLOCKING AGENTS. Alpha-adrenoceptor blocking agents may be effective in reducing high blood pressure and have relatively few side effects (Kaplan, 1994). Hypotension, a complication of this class of drugs, is particularly undesirable in the elderly population. Dosages should be titrated carefully in the older patient. Unfortunately, based on controlled, clinical studies, alpha blockers do not result in clinically meaningful reductions of blood pressure (WHO/ISH, 1993). However, they may be a valuable adjunct for hypertensive patients who are attempting to discontinue cigarette smoking, because some of the symptoms of nicotine withdrawal may be blunted by de-

TABLE 9-3 Oral Antihihypertensive Drugs

Drug	Trade Name	Usual Dose Range: Total mg/d* (Frequency per Day)	Selected Side Effects and Comments*
Calcium antagonists			
Nondihydropyridines			
Diltiazem hydrochloride	Cardizem SR	120–360 (2)	Conduction defects; worsening of systolic dysfunction; gingival hyperplasia
	Cardizem CD, Dilacor XR Tiazac	120–360 (1)	Nausea, headache
Mibefradil dihydrochloride (T-channel calcium antagonist)	Posicor	50–100 (1)	No worsening of systolic dysfunction; contraindicated with terfenadine (Seldane), astemizole (Hismanal), and cisapride (Propulsid)
Verapamil hydrochloride	Isoptin SR, Calan SR	90–480 (2)	Constipation
	Verelan, Covera-HS	120–480 (1)	
Dihydropyridines			
Amlodipine besylate	Norvasc	2.5–10 (1)	
Felodipine	Plendil	2.5–20 (1)	
Isradipine	DynaCirc	5–20 (2)	
	DynaCirc CR	5–20 (1)	
Nicardipine hydrochloride	Cardene SR	60–90 (2)	
Nifedipine	Procardia XL, Adalat CC	30–120 (1)	
Nisoldipine	Sular	20–60 (1)	
Angiotensin-converting enzyme inhibitors			Common side effects: Cough; rare side effects: angiodema, hyperkalemia, rash, loss of taste, leukopenia
Benazepril hydrochloride	Lotensin	5–40 (1–2)	
Captopril (G)	Capoten	25–150 (2–3)	
Enalapril maleate	Vasotec	5–40 (1–2)	
Fosinopril sodium	Monopril	10–40 (1–2)	
Lisinopril	Prinivil, Zestril	5–40, (1–2)	
Moexipril	Univasc	7.5–15 (2)	
Quinapril hydrochloride	Accupril	5–80 (1–2)	
Ramipril	Altace	1.25–20 (1–2)	
Trandolapril	Mavik	1–4 (1)	

188

Drug	Brand name	Dosage range (frequency)	Selected side effects
Angiotensin II receptor blockers			Angioedema (very rare); hyperkalemia
Losartan potassium	Cozaar	25–100 (1–2)	
Valsartan	Diovan	80–320 (1)	
Irbesartan	Avapro	150–300 (1)	
Betaxolol hydrochloride(s)	Korlone	5–20 (1)	
Bisoprolol fumarate(s)	Zebeta	2.5–10 (1)	
Carteolol hydrochloride (II)	Cartrol	2.5–10 (1)	
Metoprolol tartrate (G)(s)	Lopressor	50–300 (2)	
Metoprolol succinate(s)	Toprol XL	50–300 (2)	
Nadolol (G)	Corgard	40–320 (1)	
Peributolol sulfate (II)	Levatol	10–20 (1)	
Pindolol (G) (II)	Visken	10–60 (2)	
Propranolol hydrochloride (G)	Inderal	40–480 (2)	
	Inderal LA	40–480 (1)	
Timolol maleate (G)	Blocadren	20–60 (2)	Postural hypotension; bronchospasm
Combined alpha and beta blockers			
Carvedilol	Coreg	12.5–50 (2)	
Labetalol hydrochloride (G)	Normodyne, Irandate	200–1200 (2)	
Direct vasodilators			Headaches; fluid retention; tachycardia
Hydralazine hydrochloride (G)	Apresoline	50–300 (2)	Lupus syndrome
Minoxidil (G)	Loniten	5–100 (1)	Hirsutism

*These dosages may vary from those listed in the *Physicians' Desk Reference*, 51st ed, which may be consulted for additional information. The listing of side effects is not all-inclusive, and side effects are shown·for the class of drug except where noted for individual drug (in parentheses); clinicians are urged to refer to the package insert for a more detailed listing.

(G) = generic drug available.
± = also acts centrally.
s = cardioselective.
II = intrinsic sympathomimetic activity.

Based on Joint National Committee on Detection, Evaluation, and Treatment of High Blood Pressure (1993). The Fifth Report of the Joint National Committee (JNC V). *Archives of Internal Medicine, 153*, 154–183; Joint National Committee on Prevention, Detection, Evaluation, and Treatment of High Blood Pressure (1997); The Sixth Report of the Joint National Committee (JNC VI). *Archives of Internal Medicine, 157*, 2412–2446.

creasing adrenergic activity (May, Young, & Wiser, 1992). Another benefit of alpha-adrenergic blocking agents is that they are the only antihypertensive agents to have beneficial effects on both serum lipid levels and glucose metabolism (Kaplan & Gifford, 1996).

CENTRALLY ACTING AGENTS. Centrally acting agents are effective in the treatment of HTN and in reducing cardiovascular events associated with HTN. Many of these agents are used in combination with diuretics. Centrally acting agents, especially methyldopa, have been shown to be clinically effective in the treatment of HTN in pregnancy (National High Blood Pressure Education Program, 1990). Side effects include a higher incidence of drowsiness, sedation, dry mouth, fatigue, and orthostatic dizziness than found for other classes of antihypertensives (Hutchins, 1995; Joint National Committee VI, 1997).

VASODILATORS. Vasodilators are effective in decreasing blood pressure. As a large portion of hypertensive patients have increased systemic vascular resistance, a logical approach to the treatment of HTN is to use a drug that lowers blood pressure by direct dilation of the arterial bed (May, Young, & Wiser, 1992). But monotherapy with this class of drugs is difficult because of side effects like tachycardia, headache, and sodium and water retention (World Health Organization, 1993). Adding a diuretic or a beta blocker increases the antihypertensive effects and reduces the side effects (May, Young, & Wiser, 1992).

COMBINATION THERAPY. Combinations of different groups of drugs are more effective than single agents. Combination therapy minimizes side effects by encouraging the use of medications in lower doses (World Health Organization, 1993). Two-drug and sometimes three-drug combinations are frequently required in order to achieve the full goal of antihypertensive therapy in all hypertensive patients. After reducing the blood pressure to an acceptable level and stabilizing the maintenance dose, the clinician can simplify the patient's therapy by substituting a combination tablet. Combination capsules or tablets may be appropriate for many hypertensive patients. Combination preparations are convenient, cost-effective, and effective in increasing patient adherence. A simpler therapy may help the individual be more adherent.

PRINCIPLES OF PHARMACOLOGIC THERAPY

Initial Therapy

The JNC VI risk group and blood pressure stage determines when antihypertensive medications should be started (see Table 9–1). For patients in Risk Group C—that is, those with target organ disease (TOD) or clinical cardiovascular disease (CCD)—antihypertensive medication should be immediately started in patients with high-normal blood pressure and Stages 1, 2, and 3 of HTN. For Risk Group A (no risk factors, no TOD/CCD) and Risk Group B (at least one risk factor but no TOD/CCD), antihypertensive medications are not started for high-normal blood pressure but are started (1) after failure of lifestyle modification for Stage 1 HTN and (2) immediately in patients with Stage 2 or Stage 3 HTN. Lifestyle modification may be tried for up to 12 months in Risk Group A and up to 6 months in Risk Group B (Joint National Committee VI, 1997).

In initial antihypertensive therapy, monotherapy with a first-line agent, typically diuretics or beta blockers, is used. To protect the patient from adverse reactions, initial treatment should be at the lowest therapeutic dose, even if this dose does not control the HTN completely. Increases to the next dosage level should occur only after several weeks. It may take several months to gain complete control over the HTN.

After 1–3 months, if the blood pressure control is inadequate and the patient is not experiencing any significant side effects, a change should be made in therapy. Before proceeding to the next step in treatment, the clinician should address possible reasons for the inadequate effect such as (1) suboptimal drug levels, (2) inappropriate combinations of medications, (3) drug interactions, (4) secondary HTN, (5) volume overload, (6) obesity, (7) alcohol use, and (8) nonadherence.

JNC VI (1997) recommends (1) starting with a low dose of a long-acting once-daily drug, (2) titrating the dose (i.e., increasing the dose of the first drug toward maximal levels) with a possibility of low-dose combinations, (3) substituting medication from another class if no response or side effects occur, and (4) adding a second drug from another class if response is inadequate but the drug is well tolerated. Figure 9–1 diagrams the JNC VI's (1997) recommended treatment algorithm.

The approach to treatment of Stage 3 HTN is similar to that for Stage 1 and Stage 2. For Stage 3 it may be appropriate to add a second or third medication *earlier* than would be the case for the first two stages to permit rapid control of HTN. In addition, it may be appropriate to start therapy with more than one agent (Joint National Committee VI, 1997).

Follow-Up

After pharmacologic therapy has been initiated, the patient needs to be seen at regular intervals until the blood pressure levels are controlled. Achieving and maintaining decreases in blood pressure requires ongoing patient follow-up. Gradual and careful lowering of the blood pressure will minimize side effects and complications and improve adherence. Individuals in Stages 1 and 2 HTN should be seen within 1–2 months of the initiation of therapy. Target organ disease, risk factors, and abnormal laboratory tests are important considerations in determining the frequency of follow-up visits. Once the blood pressure has stabilized, subsequent visits should occur at 3–6-month intervals (Joint National Committee VI, 1997). The time interval for implementing follow-up recommendations based on the stage of HTN is indicated in Table 9–1.

For each follow-up visit, blood pressure should be measured, side effects monitored, and quality of life evaluated. Patient education should be an important feature. Medication adherence should be assessed and reinforced. The importance of lifestyle modifications, particularly smoking cessation, weight control, limiting alcohol, and physical exercise should be emphasized to the patient and assistance with lifestyle changes provided.

Step-Down Therapy

After a patient has been stabilized on medication therapy for approximately 1 year, the clinician should consider decreasing the dosage or the number of antihypertensive medications while maintaining lifestyle modifications. Generally, complete cessation of the antihypertensive medication is not indicated. A slow and progressive reduction of medication may be successful, especially in individuals who are adhering to lifestyle modifications. Patients whose drugs are discontinued should be followed regularly, because blood pressure can rise again to hypertensive levels (Joint National Committee VI, 1997).

Treatment for Resistant Hypertension

HTN should be considered resistant if the patient's blood pressure cannot be decreased to below 140/100 by an adequate treatment with a triple-drug regimen, including a diuretic, at maximal or near maximal doses. For older patients with isolated systolic HTN, SBP of 160 mm Hg is a more appropriate threshold (Joint National Committee VI, 1997). The clinician should rule out other causes, such as nonadherence and drug interactions, before labeling the patient as having resistant HTN. Although resistant HTN is difficult to treat, even suboptimal decreases of blood pressure will be beneficial in decreasing morbidity and mortality.

General Pharmacologic Treatment Considerations

The choice of initial drug therapy for an individual hypertensive patient is a challenge for the clinician. Considerations in choosing a medication are duration of efficacy, cost, side effects, drug interactions, and demographic characteristics applying to the patient, as well as concomitant diseases that might be adversely affected by medication.

DURATION OF EFFICACY. JNC VI (1997) recommends an ideal drug regimen of once-daily dosing to achieve 24-hour efficacy. At the end of

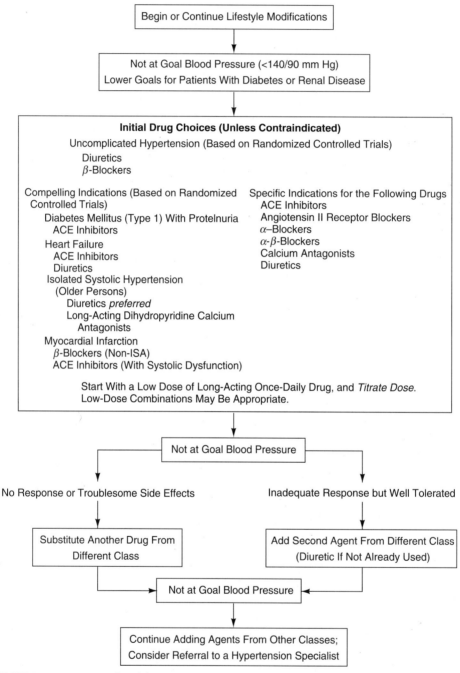

FIGURE 9–1   Treatment algorithm. "Response" means that the patient achieved goal blood pressure or is making considerable progress toward this goal.
ACE = angiotensin converting enzyme.
Adapted with permission from Joint National Committee on Detection, Evaluation, and Treatment of High Blood Pressure (1997). The Sixth Report of the Joint Committee on Detection, Evaluation, and Treatment of High Blood Pressure (JNC VI). *Archives of Internal Medicine, 157,* 2412–2446.

the 24-hour period, 50% of the maximum effect should persist. Once-daily formulations may be more costly on a per-pill basis but may be more cost-effective overall, encourage better adherence, result in consistent and stable blood pressure control, and protect against sudden death, myocardial infarction, and stroke associated with rapid blood pressure increases with morning rising.

COST. Although far from negligible, the cost of treating HTN is considerably less than the cost of treating the effects of untreated HTN. Over the life span of treatment, costs are high because antihypertensive medications must typically be used for several decades; these agents do not remove the cause or causes of HTN but merely lower blood pressure on a daily basis (Mancia & Giannattasio, 1996). Furthermore, the incidental cost of office visits, laboratory tests, and time lost from work for follow-up should also be considered. When cost is a prominent factor in nonadherence, the clinician should prescribe less expensive generic or combination drugs and avoid medications requiring frequent laboratory studies and follow-up visits. Keeping the costs as low as possible makes it easier for individuals to adhere to therapy (Elliott, 1996).

SIDE EFFECTS. Antihypertensive medications have numerous side effects, and symptomatic side effects are difficult to predict (see Table 9–3). Some medications may impair mental acuity. Beta blockers may reduce exercise tolerance or impair sexual function. Sexual dysfunction, weakness, dry mouth, and diarrhea appear in a significant number of hypertensive patients treated with a variety of medications (Kaplan, 1994). It is important to (1) structure pharmacologic therapy to minimize side effects, (2) encourage patients to report side effects and (3) assure patients that if one drug causes problems, substitutions will be made if possible (Bloomfield, Pearce, & Cross, 1993). JNC VI (1997) indicates that combinations of certain drug formulations may increase efficacy while decreasing the probability of dose-dependent side effects.

DRUG INTERACTIONS. The major groups of drugs used in the treatment of hypertension have the potential for various drug interactions, as outlined in Table 9–4. Some drug interactions are beneficial in that they potentiate the antihypertensive effects or reduce the adverse symptoms or side effects. In general, drug interactions, whether beneficial or adverse, can be predicted (Laragh & Brenner, 1990).

DEMOGRAPHICS. Neither race, age, nor gender provides significant reason to avoid any medication, especially if it is needed for concomitant diseases. Generally, the African-American population is more responsive to diuretics and calcium antagonists than to beta blockers or ACE inhibitors. The elderly are usually more responsive to all classes of medications and more susceptible to adverse effects. Gender does not appear to have an effect on drug responsiveness.

HYPERTENSION IN SPECIAL POPULATIONS

Race and Ethnicity

HTN among the African-American population is a major health problem in the United States (Kaplan, 1994). HTN develops at an earlier age in these individuals, and the disease is more severe than in white populations. The earlier onset, higher incidence, and greater severity of HTN in African Americans is accompanied by an increase in nonfatal and fatal stroke, heart disease deaths, and end-stage renal disease. Lifestyle modifications are particularly important for this racial group because of its high incidence of salt sensitivity, obesity, and cigarette smoking. Moreover, control of obesity is particularly important because of a higher incidence of non-insulin-dependent diabetes mellitus (Joint National Committee VI, 1997).

Diuretics are the first-choice medications in the absence of any concomitant diseases that would prohibit their use. Drugs that stimulate the renin-angiotensin mechanism, such as beta blockers and ACE inhibitors, are less effective in reducing blood pressure among African Americans than among whites because of the generally lower levels of plasma renin activity seen in the black population (Kaplan, 1995). Calcium antagonists, alpha-1-receptor blockers and alpha-beta blockers are as effective in

TABLE 9–4 Selective Drug Interactions with Antihypertensive Therapy

Drug	Increased Antihypertensive Effect	Decreased Antihypertensive Effect	Effects on Other Drugs
Diuretics	Thiazides combined with furosemide	NSAIDs; cholestyramine; colestipol	May increase lithium levels; may make it more difficult to control dyslipidemia and diabetes
Beta blockers	Cimetidine; quinidine; food (hepatically metabolized beta blockers)	NSAIDs; rifampin; phenobarbital; smoking	When combined with diltiazem or verapamil, may have an additive sinoatrial and atrioventricular node depressant effect
ACE inhibitors	Chlorpromazine; clozapine	NSAIDs; antacids	Hyperkalemia with potassium supplements; may increase lithium levels
Calcium antagonists	Cimetidine; ranitidine; grapefruit juice	Combinations of rifampin-verapamil; carbamazepine-diltiazem and verapamil; phenobarbital and phenytoin-verapamil	May elevate serum levels of digoxin, carbamazepine, prazosin, quinidine, theophylline, and cyclosporine
Alpha blockers	Concomitant antihypertensive drug therapy		

Based on Joint National Committee on Detection, Evaluation, and Treatment of High Blood Pressure (1993). The Fifth Report of the Joint National Committee (JNC V). *Archives of Internal Medicine, 153,* 154–183; Joint National Committee on Prevention, Detection, Evaluation, and Treatment of High Blood Pressure (1997). The Sixth Report of the Joint National Committee (JNC VI). *Archives of Internal Medicine, 157,* 2412–2446.

blacks as they are in whites. However, more blacks require multidrug therapies and more powerful agents because of the greater severity of HTN among them (Joint National Committee VI, 1997; Kaplan, 1994). As indicated in Chapter 15, few studies are available on other racial or ethnic differences in response to antihypertensive medications.

Children

An underlying cause of HTN can usually be identified in children, so more thorough screening is appropriate in them. Children who have a slight or periodic elevation frequently exhibit other risk factors for cardiovascular disease (Task Force on Blood Pressure Control in Children, 1987). All clinicians who care for children older than 3 years of age should routinely check blood pressure once a year, especially if the child has a hypertensive parent. As with adults, the appropriate sized cuff must be used and

more than one blood pressure reading obtained. In infants it may be necessary to use a Doppler apparatus to obtain an accurate blood pressure.

A risk-factor assessment should be completed on any child with an elevated blood pressure, including family history and evaluation for obesity, improper diet, and inadequate physical activity. In adolescents, the use of alcohol, cocaine, and other addictive substances should be considered as possible causes of blood pressure elevation (Kaplan, 1994). Laboratory studies for the young patient are similar to those for the adult.

Treatment depends on the cause, complications, and severity of the HTN. Therapeutic goals are to decrease blood pressure without causing adverse effects that would impair normal growth and development. Lifestyle modification is the initial treatment, but it may be inadequate for severe HTN or when a demonstrated cause is seen. Weight reduction in obese children lowers blood pressure in most cases.

Antihypertensive therapy should be reserved for children with significantly elevated blood pressure levels, those who do not respond to lifestyle changes, and those with target organ disease. Medications used for adults are also effective in children, but doses should be lower. In addition, ACE inhibitors and angiotensin II receptor blockers should not be used in pregnant or sexually active girls because of teratogenic effects (Joint National Committee VI, 1997). Physical activities, especially exercise, should not be restricted in children with uncomplicated HTN. Exercise may be helpful in prevention and relief of HTN. Chapter 12 contains additional information about childhood HTN.

Women

The prevalence of HTN in men and women is approximately equal. As elderly women outnumber elderly men, and hypertension is more common and deadly in the elderly than in the general population, more women than men will eventually suffer from a cardiovascular event secondary to HTN (Kaplan, 1994). Contributory factors for HTN in women may differ from those in men in terms of their magnitude and prevalence, and certain risk factors are unique to women. Although gender differences in response to therapy have also been reported, little research on antihypertensive therapy in women exists (Lewis, 1996). Therefore, the use of different management approaches for men and women cannot be supported.

Key gender differences exist in response to weight reduction and medications. Overweight women are particularly susceptible to HTN. Unfortunately, women tend to have greater difficulty losing weight than their male counterparts (Lewis, 1996). Women appear to have a greater lowering of blood pressure in response to a reduction in salt intake than men do (Lewis, 1996). Beta blockers tend to be less effective in women than in men. Calcium channel blockers are effective, but the long-term safety of the short-acting agents (e.g., nifedipine) has not been confirmed (Lewis, 1996). Although women tend to report more side effects from medications than men, placebo-controlled studies are needed to validate whether the differences are in the frequency of reporting or the actual occurrence of side effects. In addition, women are exposed to two hypertension-inducing mechanisms specific to their gender: pregnancy and the use of oral contraceptives (Kaplan, 1995).

PREGNANCY. Whereas a small percentage of women enter pregnancy with preexisting HTN, it develops in a larger number during pregnancy. In most normal pregnancies the blood pressure is lower than normal in the first and second trimester and returns to the pre-pregnancy state in the third trimester. This change in blood pressure makes it difficult to differentiate pregnancy-induced HTN from preexisting HTN. HTN that develops after the 20th week of gestation, accompanied by proteinuria and edema, is probably preeclampsia, especially if a family history of preeclampsia is present (Kaplan, 1994).

Calcium channel blockers should be avoided during the last trimester of pregnancy because they may inhibit uterine contraction (Lewis, 1996). They may also potentiate the effect of the magnesium sulfate commonly used to treat eclampsia and contribute to dangerous hypotension (Joint National Committee VI, 1997). ACE inhibitors should also be avoided during pregnancy because of the potential for birth defects associated with their use (Lewis, 1996). When parenteral administration is necessary, hydralazine hydrochloride is recommended (Joint National Committee VI, 1997).

HYPERTENSION AND ORAL CONTRACEPTIVES. Women who are taking oral contraceptives may experience a small increase in their blood pressure, usually staying within the normal range. Many of the studies pertaining to HTN and oral contraceptives involved a higher dose of oral contraceptives than is currently used; therefore, the incidence of induced HTN is probably lower today than what was previously reported (World Health Organization, 1993). The risk of HTN appears to increase with age, duration of oral contraceptive use, and possibly with increased body mass. Women over the age of 35 who smoke should be encouraged to quit smoking. If unable or unwilling to stop smoking, they should be discouraged from using oral contraceptives. Postmenopausal estrogen replacement therapy does not cause HTN and can be safely given to hypertensive women (Kaplan, 1995).

In counseling women taking oral contraceptives, the risk of HTN should be weighed against the risk of pregnancy. If HTN develops, women should be advised to stop taking oral contraceptives. Blood pressure should return to normal within a couple of months. If the risk of pregnancy is considered to be greater than the risks of Stage 1 HTN, and other contraceptive methods are unsuitable, it may be necessary to continue the oral contraceptive. Lifestyle modifications and antihypertensive medications should then be used to normalize the blood pressure. Patients may be prescribed a 6-month supply of oral contraceptives to allow semiannual blood pressure monitoring and evaluation (Joint National Committee VI, 1997).

Elderly

HTN poses a much greater risk factor for cardiovascular events in the elderly than in younger people (World Health Organization, 1993). Elevated pulse pressure (i.e., SBP − DBP) relative to SBP or DBP may be a more important indicator of cardiovascular risk (Joint National Committee VI, 1997). Studies such as the Systolic Hypertension in the Elderly Program (SHEP) (SHEP Cooperative Research Group, 1991) and the Swedish Trial in Old Patients with Hypertension (STOP-Hypertension) (Dahlof, Lindholm, Hansson, et al., 1991) evaluated active antihypertensive therapy in the elderly and found a significant reduction in the incidence of fatal and nonfatal cardiovascular events and a reduction in morbidity and mortality with therapy.

The initial goal of therapy is to decrease the SBP to less than 140 mm Hg, with an SBP of less than 160 mm Hg as an intermediate goal (Joint National Committee VI, 1997). Generally, goals for DBP in the older population are similar to those for the general population. Older individuals may be more sensitive to volume depletion than younger individuals and hence more susceptible to hypotension. Elderly people also have more problems with antihypertensive medications because of various age-related changes such as (1) loss of baroreceptor responsiveness, increasing a propensity to pos-

tural HTN; (2) decreases in myocardial contractility; (3) decreases in body fluid volume; (4) decreases in renal excretory capacity; and (5) an inability to remember doses (Kaplan, 1995). Consequently, antihypertensive medications should be initiated in smaller doses and spaced at longer intervals. The initial dose should be roughly half the normal starting dose. Thiazide diuretics with or without beta blockers reduce mortality and morbidity in elderly hypertensive patients (Joint National Committee VI, 1997).

Drugs have a tendency to cause orthostatic hypotension in the elderly. For this reason, the clinician needs to obtain the patient's orthostatic blood pressure in both the standing and the supine (or seated) positions; and antihypertensives, especially those that amplify postural hypotension, should be used with caution in the elderly population (Joint National Committee VI, 1997; Dahlof, Lindholm, Hansson, et al., 1991). These drugs include peripheral adrenergic blockers, alpha blockers, and high-dose diuretics. Central alpha-2 agonists that could contribute to cognitive dysfunction should likewise be used carefully (Joint National Committee VI, 1997).

Hypertensives with Concomitant Diseases

HTN is frequently associated with other medical diseases and chronic conditions. Ideally, drug therapy for these patients should be simple, effective, and have no adverse effects on any coexisting diseases (Houston, 1993). If possible, the fewest number of drugs should be given to achieve a favorable impact on as many problems as possible. Antihypertensive medications may worsen some diseases while being beneficial to others. For example, beta blockers may worsen asthma, diabetes, and peripheral ischemia but are beneficial for angina pectoris, migraine headaches, and certain dysrhythmias (Bloomfield, Pearce, & Cross, 1993).

By selecting an antihypertensive medication that will also treat concomitant disease, it may be possible to simplify therapy and decrease treatment costs. The JNC VI (1997) report addresses the respective merits of various medications for specific clinical situations. Because of the complexity of this information and the evolving nature of our understanding of treatment issues, the reader is referred directly to this source material.

It is noteworthy that the target blood pressure varies in certain populations. For example, for patients with renal parenchymal disease, the target blood pressure may range from 130/85 to 125/75 depending on the extent of proteinurea (Joint National Committee VI, 1997).

HYPERTENSIVE CRISIS: EMERGENCIES AND URGENCIES

The most common cause of hypertensive crisis is withdrawal from antihypertensive medications (Varon & Fromm, 1996). Other causes include acute glomerulonephritis, collagen vascular diseases, drug abuse, head trauma, malignant disease, preeclampsia and eclampsia, and renovascular hypertension. Differentiating hypertensive crises into hypertensive emergencies and hypertensive urgencies is important in formulating a therapeutic treatment plan (Zampaglione, Pascale, Marchisio, et al., 1996). *Hypertensive emergencies* are situations requiring immediate reduction in the blood pressure to prevent or limit target organ disease. Examples include hypertensive encephalopathy, intracranial hemorrhage, acute left ventricular failure with pulmonary edema, dissecting aortic aneurysm, eclampsia or severe hypertension associated with pregnancy, unstable angina pectoris, and acute myocardial infarction. Common presenting signs are chest pain, dyspnea, and neurologic deficits (Zampaglione, Pascale, Marchisio, et al., 1996).

In contrast, *hypertensive urgencies* are situations requiring a reduction in blood pressure within 24 hours. These situations are associated with accelerated or malignant hypertension. Common presenting signs are headache, epitaxis, faintness, arrhythmias, vertigo, and agitation (Zampaglione, Pascale, Marchisio, et al., 1996).

Treatment of any hypertensive crisis begins with accurate history taking and physical examination. The history focuses on assessment of end-organ dysfunction and symptoms, with the goal of identifying a cause. The physical examination starts with the basic "ABCs" (airway, breathing, and circulation) and is followed by assessment of mental status and level of consciousness (Varon & Fromm, 1996). A funduscopic exam and laboratory studies are aimed at identifying target organ disease. Elevated blood pressure alone, without evidence or symptoms of target organ disease, rarely requires emergency therapy. Indeed, overly aggressive intervention can cause renal or myocardial ischemia as well as cerebral hypoperfusion. Initially, mean arterial pressure should be reduced by no more than 25% up to 2 hours. Over a 2- to 6-hour time frame, the target blood pressure is 160/100 mm Hg.

As addressed in detail in JNC VI (1997), a wide variety of medications exists for treating hypertensive emergencies. These medications include vasodilators and adrenergic inhibitors. The dosing regimens and onset of action vary markedly.

PATIENT EDUCATION

The goals of patient education are to (1) facilitate compliance and adherence, (2) improve understanding of the specific treatment and general treatment goals, (3) enhance blood pressure control, (4) reduce HTN-related morbidity and mortality, (5) correct misconceptions, and (6) enhance family support. Studies have demonstrated the positive effects of HTN education on the long-term control of blood pressure.

Patient education should address the following issues: (1) the patient's current and target blood pressure, (2) the need for lifelong treatment, (3) the potential lack of symptoms and attendant risks of elevated blood pressure, (4) the diagnosis and treatment of HTN, (5) the need to follow the prescribed treatment, (6) suggested methods of positive reinforcement and encouragement for achieving goals, (7) the method of blood pressure self-monitoring, (8) lifestyle modifications and medications (using both oral and written approaches), and (9) the consequences of nonadherence (i.e., CHD, stroke, renal disease).

Patients need both written and verbal information about their medications. Facts all individuals should know include (1) names of all medications, including prescribed and over-the-counter medications; (2) allergies to medications and foods; (3) the significance of medication expiration dates; (4) proper storage methods for medications, including use of refrigeration and protection from sunlight, heat, and so on; (5) the dangers of taking nonprescribed medications; (6) possible side effects of prescribed medications; and (7) the need to inform clinicians if a problem arises or if medications are not affordable.

Drug Interactions with Other Drugs and Agents

Patients with HTN need to be educated about nonprescription drugs and other agents that may affect their blood pressure, specifically adrenergic agents, nonsteroidal anti-inflammatory drugs (NSAIDs), ethanol, and sodium (Bradley, 1991). Relevant information should be presented to patients in a way they can understand, including the common names of over-the-counter medications.

Adrenergic agents found in nonprescription decongestants, bronchodilators, and vasoconstrictors include phenypropanolamine, ephedrine, pseudoephedrine, and phenylephrine. Some preparations cause blood pressure elevation in normotensive and hypertensive patients. Our understanding of these drug interactions is poor because of confounding variables and poor data-collection methods in existing research. However, adrenergic agents in hypertensive patients should be avoided (Bradley, 1991). NSAIDs such as ibuprofen may elevate blood pressure if taken in maximum over-the-counter doses for more than a few days. The ethanol and sodium chloride content of nonprescription drugs taken in recommended doses does not appear to increase blood pressure (Bradley, 1991).

ADHERENCE

Nonadherence to lifestyle modifications and to pharmacologic therapy contributes to inadequate blood pressure control (Kjellgren, Ahlner, & Saljo, 1995). Poor adherence to medications and diet also leads to increased morbidity and mortality, increased medical costs, and increased costs to society secondary

to lost wages and productivity. Nonadherence would be of only minor concern if it were not so common or if it were limited only to medical conditions that were self-limiting or minor in nature (Urquhart, 1996). Unfortunately, a third or more of individuals adhere poorly to prescribed medication regimens regardless of the disease or prognosis (Urquhart, 1996). More than 50% of the nearly 2 billion prescriptions written annually for treatment of various conditions are taken incorrectly by patients (Burke & Dunbar-Jacob, 1995). An estimated 16–50% of hypertensives discontinue their antihypertensive medications within the first year of therapy (Flack, Novikov, & Ferrario, 1996). Among those who continue with long-term therapy, a substantial number frequently miss doses.

The reasons most often cited for nonadherence are complexity of medical therapy, inconvenience, duration of the treatment, side effects, cost of treatment, and skills needed for implementation of the treatment (Burke & Dunbar-Jacob, 1995). Factors that influence adherence to treatment can be broken down into three categories: patient and disease factors, characteristics of therapy, and nature of patient-clinician interaction (Solleck & Lee, 1989).

Patient and Disease Factors in Nonadherence

Patient-related factors in nonadherence stem primarily from health values and beliefs (Solleck & Lee, 1989). In addition, many hypertensive patients are unaware of the definition, possible causes, and therapy for HTN. Many hypertensive patients are asymptomatic and thus less likely to seek and follow treatment. Moreover, the diagnosis carries economic and social threats that may inhibit people from accepting it, such as loss of work, loss of insurance, or diminished sexual potency (Kaplan, 1994). Nonadherence is seen in all groups, without preference for age, gender, socioeconomic status, culture, disease, or therapy. Every hypertensive individual has the potential for nonadherence to the prescribed regimen of treatment.

Characteristics of Therapy That Influence Adherence

As discussed earlier, cost and side effects influence patient adherence. In addition, the complexity and length of the treatment regimen affect adherence. As also previously discussed, complexity can be reduced by using combination formulations of drugs or drugs requiring less frequent administration. Unfortunately, treatment for HTN is lifelong, and motivation decreases with time (Haynes, Sackett, Gibson, et al., 1976).

Patient-Clinician Interaction and Adherence

Establishing a good clinician-patient relationship can improve the patient's adherence with treatment. Time must be given to explain the importance of the therapy, including its benefits and potential problems. The clinician can help the patient incorporate the prescribed routine into his or her everyday activities.

Assessment of Adherence and Intervention

ASSESSMENT. Nonadherence to pharmacologic interventions can be manifest as overdosing, underdosing, erratic dosing, or simply not having the prescription filled. Similarly, nonadherence to lifestyle interventions may be manifest by overeating, insufficient activity, or failure to restrict sodium intake, and so on. In general, adherence improves just prior to an appointment with the clinician. The clinician may assess adherence using self-report measures, biologic measures, pill counts, and pharmacy refills. *Self-report* measures provide the most depth but are subject to measurement errors. *Biologic measures* determine only if the individual is adhering to therapy close to the time of the testing. *Pill counts* and *pharmacy refills* cannot be used to tell if the patient is taking the medication properly. Therefore, none of these methods fulfills the criteria of being valid, reliable, and practical while not affecting the behavior being measured.

Self-report measures are inexpensive and easily administered but are extremely vulnerable to overestimation bias. Questionnaires, interviews, and daily diaries are some of the commonly used methods of self-report. The usefulness of structured *questionnaires* may be limited by their lack of comprehensiveness, reliability, validity, and generalizability to specific patient populations. In contrast, *interviews* are easy to conduct in the office setting or over the phone. Errors occur because of inaccurate patient responses designed to avoid offending the clinician, inaccurate patient recall, nonrepresentative time frames, and the inability to measure all dimensions of behavior of concern (Burke & Dunbar-Jacob, 1995). Questions that may be helpful in determining sources of error include: "How often do you exercise? What time do you take your medications? When did you last take your medications? Did you suddenly stop them?"

Daily diaries are inexpensive, permit collection of detailed information, and limit the need for accurate recall of past events and behaviors. Yet, reporting still may be inaccurate. The clinician should instruct the patient on the proper way to record the information to minimize deliberate and nondeliberate reporting errors. Patients often are influenced by the act of recording their intake and therefore change their dietary habits on the days of recording (Burke & Dunbar-Jacob, 1995).

Several biologic tests are used to determine adherence, including drug screens, 24-hour urine samples, and urine dipsticks. *Drug screens* can be costly and tend to identify only those individuals who have followed their prescribed treatment close to the time of the measurement. Drug screens cannot determine the level of adherence to therapy (Burke & Dunbar-Jacob, 1995). The *24-hour urine sample* can be used to determine sodium intake. The random measurement of sodium level can be a positive incentive for the patient to stay on a sodium-restricted diet. Sodium intake can also be estimated by dietary records, if kept accurately, but most people fail to record all sources of sodium in the diet (Stuart, Friedman, & Benson, 1993).

Pharmacy refills and pill counts provide relatively effective, "low tech" measurements of adherence. For *pharmacy refills*, adherence is estimated from the number of days beyond the estimated refill date. One of the drawbacks to pharmacy refills is that patients do not always refill their medications at the same pharmacy. *Pill counts* consist of counting the number of pills remaining from a prescription over a defined period of time and subtracting the number of pills that should have remained. However, pill counts tend to overestimate adherence. Computerized encoder caps to identify the times the bottles are being opened and permit comparison with projected times hold promise for the future.

INTERVENTION. No single technique has been identified for improving adherence, but several interventions, when used in combination, appear to have merit (Dunbar-Jacob, Dwyer, & Dunning, 1991). These interventions include patient education, phone call and mail reminders, monitoring of adherence, mobilization of social supports, planning for rewards, patient-clinician contracts, worksite care, home visits, and group sessions. Some ways to improve adherence include (1) assessing the individual's understanding of the diagnosis and encouraging questions, (2) providing simple written instructions on dosage and side effects, (3) using material appropriate for the individual's reading/comprehension level, (4) using other media (videotapes, interactive computer programs), (5) informing the patient of the blood pressure level measurement at each visit, (6) simplifying the regimen by using antihypertensive medications that can be taken once or twice daily, (7) using weekly pill boxes, (8) encouraging the patient to be an active participant in developing the plan of therapy, (9) encouraging the patient to self-monitor blood pressure at home and maintain a blood pressure record, (10) reviewing the patient's progress on each successive visit, (11) expressing a willingness to alter medication to avoid undesirable side effects, (12) encouraging the patient to express concerns and problems with therapy, (13) encouraging the patient to contact the clinician with any questions or problems, (14) increasing attention provided to the nonadherent individual by scheduling visits more frequently and by referring the patient to other support systems, (15) providing praise for the patient's success in achieving blood pressure reductions, (16) promoting social support, (17) encouraging families to be involved in blood pressure control and to provide daily reinforcement to the patient, and (18) minimizing costs by prescribing nonformulary drugs and watching for hidden costs necessitated by laboratory tests, potassium supplements, and follow-up.

CONCLUSION

HTN is a major CHD risk factor. This chapter has presented a detailed discussion of the many issues related to the assessment and management of HTN. The cornerstone of treatment is accurate patient assessment that identifies risk factors, recognizes target organ disease, establishes the diagnosis of HTN as primary or secondary, and defines the course of treatment. HTN may be controlled through lifestyle modifications, pharmacologic therapy, and patient education. Many areas require further research. Studies are presently looking at the effects of the newer antihypertensives and their effect on reduction of cardiovascular morbidity and mortality compared to diuretics and beta blockers. Developments in genetic research may help clarify which hypertensive patients are at greater risk for developing cardiovascular disease and are in greatest need of early treatment. Research results may eventually lead to the discovery of a genetic basis of HTN and a cure.

References

Alderman, M.H. (1992). Which antihypertensive drugs first—and why! *JAMA, 267,* 2786–2787.

Applegate, W.B. (1992). Hypertension in the elderly. *Consultant, 32*(10), 39–40.

Blair, S.N., Kohl, H.W., Barlow, C.E., & Gibbons, L.W. (1991). Physical fitness and all-cause mortality in hypertensive men. *Annals of Medicine, 23,*307–312.

Bloomfield, R., Pearce, K., & Cross, H. (1993). Hypertension: Choosing therapy when coexisting disease confounds the choice. *Consultant, 33*(7), 69–79.

Bradley, J.G. (1991). Nonprescription drugs and hypertension: Which ones affect blood pressure? *Postgraduate Medicine, 89*(6), 195–207.

Burke, L.E., & Dunbar-Jacob, J. (1995). Adherence to medication, diet, and activity recommendations: From assessment to maintenance. *Journal of Cardiovascular Nursing, 9*(2), 62–79.

Burt, V.L., Whelton, P., Roccella, E.J., Brown, C., Cutler, J.A., Higgins, M., Horan. M.J., & Labarthe, D. (1995). Prevalence of hypertension in the U.S. adult population. Results from the Third National Health and Nutrition

Examination Survey, 1988–1991. *Hypertension, 25*(3), 305–313.

Callahan, M. (1991). High blood pressure. *The Lippincott Manual of Nursing Practice.* New York: J. B. Lippincott.

Chalmers, J. (1993). Round table 2. First-line drugs: The position of the World Health Organization–International Society of Hypertension. *Journal of Hypertension, 11*(Suppl. 5), S381–S383.

Collins, R., Peto, R., et al. (1990). Blood pressure, stroke, and coronary heart disease: Part 2, short-term reductions in blood pressure: Overview of randomized drug trials in their epidemiological context. *Lancet, 335,*827–838.

Corrigan, S.A., Raczynski, J.M., Swencionis, C., & Jennings, S.G. (1991). Weight reduction in the prevention and treatment of hypertension: A review of representative clinical trials. *American Journal of Health Promotion, 5*(3), 208–214.

Cunningham, S.G. (1987). Nonpharmacologic management of high blood pressure. *Cardiovascular Nursing, 23*(4), 18–22.

Cutler, J.A., MacMahon, S.W., & Furberg, C.D. (1989). Controlled clinical trials of drug treatment for hypertension: A review. *Hypertension, 13*(Suppl. I), I36–I44.

Dahl, L.K. (1972). Salt and hypertension. *American Journal of Clinical Nutrition, 25,*231–244.

Dahlof, B., Lindholm, L.H., Hansson, L., Schersten, B., Ekbom, T., & Wester, P.O. (1991). Morbidity and mortality in the Swedish trial in old patients with hypertension (STOP-Hypertension). *Lancet, 338,*1281–1285.

Davis, B.R., Cutler, J.A., Gordon, N., et al. (1996). Rationale and design for the antihypertensive and lipid-lowering treatment to prevent heart attack trial (ALLHAT). *American Journal of Hypertension, 9,*342–360.

Dunbar-Jacob, J., Dwyer, K., & Dunning, E.J. (1991). Compliance with antihypertensive regimen: a review of the research in the 1980s. *Annals of Behavioral Medicine 13*(1): 31–38.

Dyer, A.R. (1975). An analysis of the relationship of systolic blood pressure, serum cholesterol, and smoking to 14-year mortality in the Chicago People's Gas Company Study. *Journal of Chronic Disease, 28,* 20–31.

Elias, M.F., Wolf, P.A., D'Agostino, R.B., Cobb, J., & White, L.R. (1993). Untreated blood pressure level is inversely related to cognitive functioning: The Framingham Study. *American Journal of Epidemiology, 138*(6), 353–364.

Elliott, W.J. (1996). The costs of treating hypertension: What are the long-term realities of cost containment and pharmacoeconomics? *Postgraduate Medicine, 99*(4), 241–248, 251.

Fagerberg, B., Berglund, A., Anderson, O.K., Berlung, G., & Wilstrand, J. (1991). Cardiovascular effects of weight reduction versus antihypertensive drug treatment: A comparative, randomized, 1-year study of obese men with mild hypertension. *Journal of Hypertension, 9*(5), 431–439.

Fair, J.M., & Berra, K. (1995). Lifestyle changes and coronary heart disease; the influence of nonpharmacological interventions. *Journal of Cardiovascular Nursing 9*(2): 12–24.

Ferri, F. (1995). *Practical Guide to the Care of the Medical Patient.* St. Louis: Mosby.

Flack, J.M., Ensrud, K.E., Mascioli, S., Launer, C.A., Svendsen, K., Elmer, P.J., & Grimm, R.H. (1991). Racial and ethnic modifiers of the salt-blood pressure response. *Hypertension, 17*(Suppl. I), I115–I121.

Flack, J.M., Novikov, S., & Ferrario, C. (1996). Benefits of adherence to antihypertensive drug therapy. *European Heart Journal, 17*(Suppl. A), 16–20.

Fletcher, A.E., & Bulpitt, C.J. (1992). How far should blood pressure be lowered? *New England Journal of Medicine, 326,* 251–254.

Friedman, R., Stuart, E., & Benson, H. (1994). Non-pharmacologic adjuncts to therapy. In S.P. Cooke & E.D. Frohlich (Eds.), *Current Management of Hypertension and Vascular Diseases.* Philadelphia: Mosby Yearbook.

Goldstein, S. (1989). Review of β-blocker myocardial infarction trials. *Clinical Cardiology, 12*(III), 54–57.

Gordon, N.F., & Scott, C.B. (1994). Exercise guidelines for patients with high blood pressure: An update. *Journal of Cardiopulmonary Rehabilitation, 14*(2), 93–96.

Grobbee, D.E. (1991). Methodology of sodium sensitivity assessment: The example of age and sex. *Hypertension, 17*(Suppl. I), I109–I114.

Hamet, P., Mongeau, E., Lambert, J., Bellavance, F., Daignault-Gelinas, M., Ledoux, M., & Whissell-Cambiotti, L. (1991). Interactions among calcium, sodium, and alcohol intake as determinants of blood pressure. *Hypertension, 17*(Suppl. I), I150–I154.

Haynes, R.B., Sackett, D.L., Gibson, E.S., Taylor, D.W., Hackett, B.C., Roberts, R.S., & Johnson, A.L. (1976). Improvement of medication compliance in uncontrolled hypertension. *Lancet, 1*(7972), 1265–1268.

Hoegholm, A., Kristensen, K.S., Madson, N.H., & Svendsen, T.L. (1992). White coat hypertension diagnosed by 24-h ambulatory monitoring. Examination of 159 newly diagnosed hypertensive patients. *American Journal of Hypertension, 5*(2), 64–70.

Houston, M.C. (1993). The management of hypertension and associated risk factors for the prevention of long-term cardiac complications. *Journal of Cardiovascular Pharmacology, 21*(Suppl. 2), S2–S13.

Hutchins, L. (1995). Drug therapy for hypertension and hyperlipidemia. *Journal of Cardiovascular Nursing, 9*(2), 37–55.

Intersalt Cooperative Research Group. (1988). Intersalt: An international study of electrolyte excretion and blood pressure. Results for 24-hour urinary sodium and potassium excretion. *British Medical Journal, 287,* 319–328.

Jacob, R., Chesney, M., & Williams, D. (1991). Relaxation therapy for hypertension: design effects and treatment effects. *Annals of Behavioral Medicine, 13*(1): 5–15.

Jacober, S.J., & Sowers, J.R. (1995). Exercise and hypertension. *JAMA, 273*(24), 1965.

Jeffrey, R.W. (1991). Weight management and hypertension. *Annals of Behavior Medicine, 13*(1), 18–21.

Joint National Committee on Detection, Evaluation, and Treatment of High Blood Pressure (1986). Nonpharmacological approaches to the control of high blood pressure. *Hypertension, 8,* 444–467.

Joint National Committee on Detection, Evaluation, and Treatment of High Blood Pressure. (1993). The Fifth Report of the Joint National Committee (JNC V). *Archives of Internal Medicine, 153,* 154–183.

Joint National Committee on Prevention, Detection, Evaluation, and Treatment of High Blood Pressure. (1997). The Sixth Report of the Joint National Committee (JNC VI). *Archives of Internal Medicine, 157,* 2412–2446.

Kannel, W.B. (1990). CHD risk factors: A Framingham study update. *Hospital Practice, 25*(7), 119–127.

Kannel, W.B. (1993). Hypertension as a risk factor for cardiac events—Epidemiological results of long-term studies. *Journal of Cardiovascular Pharmacology, 21*(Suppl. 2), S27–S37.

Kannel, W.B. (1996). Blood pressure as a cardiovascular risk factor: Prevention and treatment. *Journal of the American Medical Association, 275*(20), 1571–1576.

Kannel, W.B. (1996). Cardioprotective and antihypertensive therapy: The key importance of addressing the associated coronary risk factors (The Framingham experience). *American Journal of Cardiology, 77*(6), 6B–11B.

Kaplan, N. (1992). The appropriate goals of antihypertensive therapy; neither too much nor too little. *Annals of Internal Medicine, 116*(8): 686–690.

Kaplan, N.M. (1991). Managing hypertension. *Hospital Practice, 26*(Suppl. 2), 26–30.

Kaplan, N.M. (1993). Introduction: Is hypertension a metabolic disease? *American Heart Journal, 125*(5), 1485–1487.

Kaplan, N.M. (1994). *Clinical Hypertension,* 6th ed., Philadelphia: Williams & Wilkins.

Kaplan, N.M. (1994). Ethnic aspects of hypertension. *Lancet, 344*(8920), 450–452.

Kaplan, N.M. (1995). *Management of Hypertension,* 6th ed., Durant, OK: Essential Medical Information Systems, Inc.

Kaplan, N.M. (1995). The treatment of hypertension in women. *Archives of Internal Medicine, 155*(6), 563–567.

Kaplan, N.M. (1995). Alcohol and hypertension. *Lancet, 345*(8965), 1588–1589.

Kaplan, N.M., & Gifford, R.W. (1996). Choice of initial therapy for hypertension. *Journal of the American Medical Association, 275*(20), 1577–1580.

Kjellgren, K.I., Ahlner, J., & Saljo, R. (1995). Taking antihypertensive medication—Controlling or co-operating with patients? *International Journal of Cardiology, 47*(3), 257–268.

Klatsky, A. (1996). Alcohol and hypertension. *Clinica Chimica Acta, 246*(1–2), 91–105.

Kriesand, R., & Cohen, I. (1996). Home blood pressure monitoring. *American Family Physician, 54*(2), 538–540.

Kuwajima, I., Miyao, M., Uno, A., Suzuki, Y., Matsushita, S., & Kuramoto, K. (1994). Diagnostic value of electrocardiography and echocardiography for white coat hypertension in the elderly. *American Journal of Cardiology, 73*(16), 1232–1234.

Langford, H.G., Davis, B.R., Blaufos, M.D., Oberman, A., Wassertheil-Smoler, S., Hawkins, M., & Zimbaldi, N. (1991). Effect of drug and diet treatment of mild hypertension on diastolic blood pressure. *Hypertension, 17,* 210–217.

Laragh, J.H., & Brenner, B.M. (Eds.) (1990). *Hypertension: Pathophysiology, Diagnosis, and Management.* New York: Raven Press.

Laragh, J.H., & Pecker, M.S. (1983). Dietary sodium and essential hypertension: Some myths, hopes and truths. *Annals of Internal Medicine, 98*(P2), 735–743.

Lenfant, C. (1996). High blood pressure: Some answers, new questions, continuing challenges. *Journal of the American Medical Association, 275*(20), 1604–1606.

Lewis, C.E. (1996). Characteristics and treatment of hypertension in women: A review of the literature. *American Journal of the Medical Sciences, 311*(4), 193–199.

Littenberg, B. (1995). A practice guideline revisited: Screening for hypertension. *Annals of Internal Medicine, 122*(12), 937–939.

MacFadyen, R.J., & Prasad, N. (1995). Current issues in hypertension research and therapy. *British Journal of Hospital Medicine, 53*(7), 335–343.

MacMahon, S.W., MacDonald, G.S., Bersnstein, L., Andrews, G., & Blascket, R.B. (1985). Comparison of weight reduction with metoprolol in treatment of hypertension in young overweight patients. *Lancet, 1,* 1233–1236.

MacMahon, S., Peto, R., et al. (1990) Blood pressure, stroke, and coronary heart disease. Part 1, prolonged differences in blood pressure: Prospective observational studies corrected for the regression dilution bias. *Lancet, 335,* 765–774.

Mancia, G., & Giannattasio, C. (1996). Benefit and costs of anti-hypertensive treatment. *European Heart Journal, 17*(Suppl. A), 25–28.

Martin, K., Phillips, R.A., & Krakoff, L.R. (1994). Persistent white coat hypertension. *American Journal of Hypertension, 7*(4, Pt 1), 368–370.

May, D.B., Young, L.Y., & Wiser, T.H. (1992). Applied therapeutics. *AAOHN Journal, 43*(6): 306–312.

McAbee, R. (1995). Primary prevention of hypertension: A challenge for occupational health nurses. *AAOHN Journal, 43*(6), 306–312.

McVeigh, G.E., Flack, J., & Grimm, R. (1995). Goals of antihypertensive therapy. *Drugs, 49*(2), 161–175.

Miller, N.H. (1995). Physical activity: One approach to the primary prevention of hypertension. *AAOHN Journal, 43*(6), 319–326.

Moser, M. (1996). Management of Hypertension, Part I. *American Family Physician, 53*(7), 2295–2303.

Moser, M. (1993). A critique of The Fifth Joint National Committee Report on Detection, Evaluation and Treatment of High Blood Pressure. *Journal of Hypertension, 11* (Suppl. 5), S381–S383.

National High Blood Pressure Education Program— Working Group on High Blood Pressure in Pregnancy. (1990). Working group report on high blood pressure in pregnancy. *American Journal of Obstetrics and Gynecology, 163,* 1689–1712.

Neaton, J.D., & Wentworth, D. (1992). Serum cholesterol, blood pressure, smoking, and death from coronary heart disease. *Archives of Internal Medicine, 152,* 56–64.

O'Donnell, M.E. (1990). Assessment of the patient with malignant hypertension. *Dimensions in Critical Care Nursing, 9*(5), 280–286.

Pahor, M., Guralnik, J.M., Corti, M.C., Foley, D.J., Carbonin, P., & Havlik, R.J. (1995). Long-term survival and use of antihypertensive medications in older persons. *Journal of American Geriatric Society, 43,* 1191–1197.

Podszus, T., & Grote, L. (1996). Stress management in hypertension. *Journal of Hypertension, 14*(4), 419–421.

Potter, J.F., & Beevers, D.G. (1984). Pressor effect of alcohol in hypertension. *Lancet, 1,* 119–122.

Prochaska, J.O., DiClemente, C.C., & Norcross, J.C. (1994). *Changing for Good.* New York: Morrow and Co.

Prochaska, J.O., DiClemente, C.C., & Norcross, J.C. (1992). In search of how people change. *American Psychologist, 9,* 1102–1114.

Rose, G. (1980). Epidemiology. In A.J. Marshall & D.W. Barritt (Eds.), *The Hypertensive Patient.* Kent, England: Pitman Medical, pp. 1–21.

Sackett, D.L. (1996). Guidelines for managing raised blood pressure. *British Medical Journal, 313,* 64–65.

Salazar, M.K. (1995). Dealing with hypertension: Using theory to promote behavioral change. *AAOHN Journal, 43*(6), 313–318.

SHEP Cooperative Research Group. (1991). Prevention of stroke by antihypertensive drug treatment in older persons with isolated systolic hypertension. *Journal of the American Medical Association, 265,* 3255–3264.

Sollek, M.V., & Lee, K.A. (1989). High blood pressure. In S.L. Underhill, S.L. Woods, E.S. Froelicher, & C.J. Halpenny (Eds.), *Cardiac Nursing,* 2nd ed. Philadelphia: J. B. Lippincott, pp. 814–857.

SOLVD Investigators. (1992). Effect of enalapril on mortality and the development of heart failure in asymptomatic patients with reduced left ventricular ejection fraction. *New England Journal of Medicine, 327,* 685–691.

Somova, L.I., Connolly, C., & Diara, K. (1995). Psychosocial predictors of hypertension in black and white Africans. *Journal of Hypertension, 13*(2), 193–199.

Stillman, F.A. (1995). Smoking cessation for the hospitalized cardiac patient: Rationale for and report of a model program. *Journal of Cardiovascular Nursing, 9*(2), 25–36.

Stuart, E.M., Friedman, R., & Benson, H. (1993). Promoting nonpharmacologic interventions to treat elevated blood pressure. *Behavioral Science Learning Modules.* Geneva, Switzerland: Division of Mental Health: World Health Organization, pp. 1–42.

Task Force on Blood Pressure Control in Children (1987). Report of the second task force on blood pressure control in children—1987. *Pediatrics, 79,* 1–25.

Townsend, R., & Kimmel, S. (1996). Calcium channel blockers and hypertension: 1. New trials. *Hospital Practice,* 31(7): 125–128, 133–136,

Urquhart, J. (1996). Patient non-compliance with drug regimens: Measurement, clinical correlates, economic impact. *European Heart Journal, 17 (Suppl. A),* 8–15.

Varon, J., & Fromm, R.E. (1996). Hypertensive crisis: The need for urgent management. *Postgraduate Medicine, 99*(1), 189–200.

Vidt, D.G. (1993). Hypertension: A new classification system helps you better define risk. *Consultant, 33*(5), 53–61.

Wallace, P., Cutler, S., & Haines, A. (1988). Randomized controlled trial of general practitioner intervention in patients with excessive alcohol consumption. *British Medical Journal, 297,* 663–668.

Weiland, S.K., Keil, U., Spelsberg, A., Hense, H.W., Härtel, U., & Gefeller, O. (1991). Diagnosis and management of hypertension by physicians in the Federal Republic of Germany. *Journal of Hypertension, 9,* 131–134.

World Health Organization/International Society of Hypertension. (1993). 1993 guidelines for the management of mild hypertension: Memorandum from a World Health Organization/International Society of Hypertension meeting. *Journal of Hypertension, 11,* 905–918.

Zampaglione, B., Pascale, C., Marchisio, M., & Cavallo-Perin, P. (1996). Hypertensive urgencies and emergencies. Prevalence and clinical presentation. *Hypertension, 27*(1), 144–147.

Zanchetti, A. (1992). What blood pressure should be treated? *Clinical Investigative Medicine, 70*(Suppl. 1), S2–S6.

Zanchetti, A. (1993). Round table 2: World Health Organization–International Society of Hypertension versus United States guidelines on hypertension treatment: Similarities and differences. *Journal of Hypertension, 11* (Suppl. 5), S380.

CHAPTER 10

———
———
———
———
———
———
———
———
———
———
———
———
═══

Stress Management

Susan L. Kozicz
Aggie Casey

Stress and a variety of psychosocial factors that contribute to coronary heart disease (CHD) have received considerable attention because a large percentage of CHD cases cannot be attributed to traditional risk factors (Eliot, 1988). Scientific evidence is emerging that psychosocial factors such as depression, hostility, and low levels of social support can increase CHD risk. The rate of cardiovascular rehospitalization and recurrent events 6 months postdischarge is significantly higher in "psychologically distressed" versus "nondistressed" patients (Allison, Williams, Miller, et al., 1995). Additionally, research suggests that comprehensive lifestyle changes, including cognitive and behavioral interventions aimed at interrupting and modifying the stress response, can prevent, control, and even reverse the atherosclerotic process (Gould, Ornish, Kirkecide, et al., 1992; Ornish, Brown, Schewitz, et al., 1990).

Current thinking is that regardless of the specific factor involved, the relationship between psychosocial factors and CHD is partly explained by a common pathway associated with the stress response. Furthermore, at the level of treating the individual patient, the common pathway is most frequently addressed in inter-

ventions. Studies suggest that a comprehensive stress management program, including relaxation training and cognitive therapy, can be effective in modifying stress and thus decreasing cardiovascular reactivity (Nunes, Frank, & Kornfeld, 1987; Mendes de Leon, Powell, & Kaplan, 1991).

The purpose of this chapter is to review current conceptualizations of stress and its relationship to CHD, identify psychosocial factors that can result from stress and increase CHD risk, and provide a brief overview of stress management strategies.

STRESS

Stress has been conceptualized from both the physiologic and psychological perspectives. Within the context of CHD risk reduction, an understanding of both perspectives and the relationship between them is essential. *Physiologic stress* is typically defined as the nonspecific response of the body to any demand (Selye, 1974). Current research suggests the physiologic stress response is triggered when a person perceives a threat or danger to his or her wellbeing and is unable to cope effectively with the demand. This definition is adapted from the work of Lazarus and Folkman (1984). Lazarus and Folkman's *transactional theory* of stress and coping further expands upon Selye's work to provide a theoretical framework in which to better understand how stress affects one's health.

Lazarus's (1966) *stress-coping theory* views stress as a transaction between the individual and his or her environment, thus recognizing the differences in how individuals perceive and respond to stress. According to *cognitive primacy theory,* the patient's interpretation of the environment is the primary determinant in the elicitation of the stress response. Therefore, the *interpretation* of the event rather than the event itself determines whether or not the event is perceived as a threat (Roseman, 1984).

Psychosocial stressors are perceived as such because of *cognitive appraisal* (Lazarus & Folkman, 1984), which includes both a primary and secondary appraisal. According to Lazarus (1966), *primary appraisal* is when one first perceives a threat to one's wellbeing. Stress results when a transaction between a person and the environment is considered overwhelming, and the person does not perceive himself or herself to have adequate resources to cope with it. This primary appraisal leads to a concurrent *secondary appraisal,* which is an evaluation of what can be done to reduce the threat. Coping options are then identified and available resources determined.

Individuals' responses vary under comparable conditions because cognitive processes, mediating factors, and coping mechanisms are unique to each individual. The individual's central role as an active participant in the perception and management of the stressors is key to applying Lazarus's theory in stress management programs.

Physiologic Stress Response

A *stressor* is a stimulus that provokes a stress response. The two types of stressors are biogenic and psychosocial (Girdano & Everly, 1986). *Biogenic stressors* initiate a stress response without any cognitive interpretation. Biogenic stressors such as coffee, tea, and am-

phetamines act directly through a biochemical pathway to cause a stress response (Everly, 1989). *Psychosocial stressors,* as previously mentioned, are determined by the individual's cognitive appraisal of the event. These stressors, too, elicit a stress response (Lazarus & Folkman, 1984). The resultant physiologic stress response refers to a constellation of adjustments.

The exact mechanism by which the stress response is related to CHD is unclear. Current research suggests no single hormone or system is responsible for the stress response (Everly, 1989). Rather, a complex and interrelated network exists that includes the autonomic, hormonal, and immune systems.

The perception of a threat initiates a cascade of biochemical events originating from the central nervous system. As depicted in Figure 10–1, the three major pathways involved in the stress response include the *autonomic nervous system* (ANS), *musculoskeletal system* (MSS), and *psychoneuroendocrine system* (PNE). The limbic system is responsible for the integration of thoughts and emotions in general, and homeostasis is regulated by the hypothalmic part of the limbic system (Wells-Federman, Stuart, Deckro, et al., 1995).

The activation of the stress response begins with a perceived stress. This response was originally described as "fight or flight" by Cannon in 1914. The stressor is recognized by the cerebral cortex, which stimulates the hypothalamus to activate the sympathetic branch of the ANS. At this point, two potent neurotransmitters, epinephrine and norepinephrine, are secreted from the adrenal medulla and peripheral nerve endings into the systemic circulation, where they are carried to their respective target organs (Everly & Sobelman, 1987).

Activation of these neuroendocrine hormones includes increased arterial blood pressure, diminished renal blood flow, increased cardiac output, increased contraction of the MSS, increased triglyceride levels, increased cholesterol levels, and diminished blood flow to the skin and gastrointestinal system (Everly & Sobelman, 1987, p. 24).

As indicated in Figure 10–1, the stress response affects the MSS through neural messages transduced via motor pathways and activation of the sympathetic nervous system. The

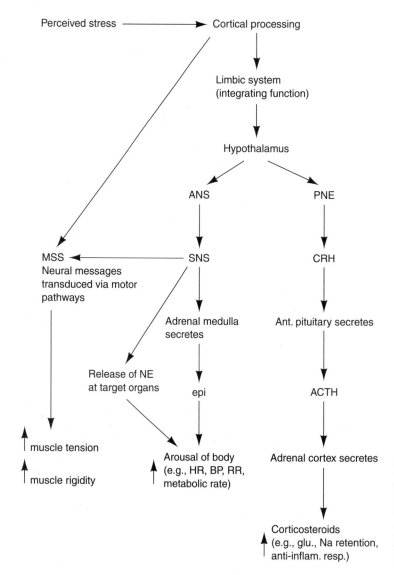

FIGURE 10–1 Physiologic stress response. Adapted with permission from Wells-Federman, C., Stuart, E., Deckro, J., Mandle, C., Baim, M. and Medich, C. (1995). The mind-body connection: The psychophysiology of many traditional nursing interventions. *Clinical Nurse Specialist, 9*(1), 59–66.

MSS responds with increased muscle tension and increased muscular rigidity, which can increase chronic painful conditions (Well-Federman, Stuart, Deckro, et al., 1995).

As indicated in Figure 10–1, the PNE pathway of the stress response involves the hypothalamic-pituitary-adrenocortical system. Upon stimulation of the limbic system, impulses descend to the hypothalamus and trigger the secretion of *corticotropin-releasing hormone* (CRH). This hormone stimulates the anterior portion of the pituitary to secrete *adrenocorticotropic hormone* (ACTH), which stimulates the adrenal cortex to secrete corticosteroids. Corticosteroids affect immune function by increasing glucose levels, increasing sodium re-

tention, and altering lipid metabolism. Although an acute stress response can initially boost immune function, chronic stress eventually decreases immune function (Wells-Federman, Stuart, Deckro, 1995).

Stress Response and CHD

The multisystem physiologic responses to stress described in the previous section may promote the development of CHD. Researchers have hypothesized that excessive cardiovascular reactivity to psychologic stress may provide the physiologic link between psychological factors and CHD (Glass, 1977; Goldband, Katkin, &

Morell, 1979; Krantz & Manuck, 1984). The activation of neuroendocrine hormones that is associated with the stress response raises both heart rate and blood pressure. Increased heart rate and blood pressure may in turn promote intimal injury through hemodynamic forces such as turbulent blood flow and shear stress on the endothelium. The sympathetic activation results in coronary artery pressure surges and tone increases, contributing to plaque rupture and thrombus formation. Catecholamines can also modify metabolism and permeability of the arterial wall, reducing oxygen uptake and influencing platelet aggregation and thus promoting the development of atherosclerosis (Teplitz & Siwik, 1994).

A pathophysiologic mechanism linking depression and CHD has yet to be established. Current research suggests changes in autonomic balance and platelet function are two potential pathophysiologic mechanisms. Changes in sympathetic-parasympathetic balance in depressed patients who have sustained a myocardial infarction may place them at risk for fatal arrhythmias. Research suggests that serotonin, which plays a major role in depression, also influences thrombogenesis. Catecholamines and serotonin are relatively weak agonists of platelet aggregation by themselves but amplify aggregation responses of platelets to other thrombogenic agents. Evidence suggests this response is enhanced in depressed patients and may make them more susceptible to thrombogenic events (Frasure-Smith, Lesperance, & Talajic, 1993).

Studies of the etiologic role of psychological stress as related to CHD have demonstrated that hostility and cardiovascular reactivity correlate positively with CHD (Vitaliano, Russo, Bailey, et al., 1993). Mental stress has been shown to increase heart rate, blood pressure, and myocardial demand (Muller, Tofler, & Stone, 1989). However, this area of research requires further investigation. A better understanding of the mechanism linking psychological stress and CHD will facilitate the development of innovative preventive strategies.

PSYCHOSOCIAL FACTORS IN CHD

Thus far in this chapter, the relationships among stress, the physiologic stress response, and CHD have been addressed. As previously discussed, the cumulative effect of frequent invocations of the stress response and pathway activation (i.e., cardiovascular reactivity) is believed to contribute to the development of CHD. In addition to stressful life events, three psychosocial factors related to the stress response (hostility, depression, and low levels of social support) have been identified as correlates or risk factors for CHD. These psychosocial factors may be exacerbated by stressful situations. In this section, these factors will be discussed, with special emphasis on their relationship to CHD development, the quality of supportive evidence of that relationship, and the unanswered questions that warrant further investigation.

Type A Behavior/Hostility

Type A behavior pattern (TABP) is a construct characterized by hard-driving, achievement-oriented behavior, excessive job involvement, time urgency, aggressiveness, competitiveness, and impatience (Dembroski & Costa, 1987). Three major prospective studies, the Western Collaborative Group Study, the Framingham Heart Study, and the French-Belgian Cooperative Group Study, led to the confirmation of TABP as an independent risk factor for CHD. These studies indicated that Type A men had twice the incidence of CHD as did Type B men (Rosenman, Brand, Jenkins, et al., 1975).

Other studies, including the Aspirin Myocardial Infarction Study and the Multiple Risk Intervention Trial, reported no relationship between TABP and recurrent cardiac events (Matthews & Haynes, 1986). In light of conflicting research regarding the risk status of global TABP, scientific research has focused on subcomponents of the multifaceted TABP, including hostility and anger (Dembroski, MacDougall, Williams, et al., 1985).

When data from the Multiple Risk Intervention Trial were reevaluated to assess subcomponents of TABP, Dembroski and colleagues (1989) reported that hostility showed a significant association with CHD incidence, independent of traditional risk factors. Hostility is defined as the tendency to experience anger, irritability, and resentment in response to everyday events or the tendency to react to these events with expressions of antagonism, disagreeableness, rudeness, surliness, criticalness, and uncooperativeness (Dembroski, MacDougall, Williams, et al., 1985).

In the Western Electric Study (Shekelle, Gale, Ostfeld, et al., 1983), CHD events increased with higher hostility scores over a 10-year period. Barefoot, Dahlstrom, and Williams (1983) reported a predictive relationship between hostility and CHD over a 25-year period in a sample of physicians. Similarly, in a 25-year study of 118 law students, Barefoot and colleagues (1989) reported that higher hostility scores predicted higher all-cause mortality.

Investigators for the Determinants of Myocardial Infarction Onset Study reported that episodes of anger are capable of triggering the onset of an acute myocardial infarction (Mittleman, Maclure, Sherwood, et al., 1995).

Nunes, Frank, and Kornfeld (1987) conducted a meta-analysis on interventions for TABP and suggested that a combination of treatment techniques, including stress management, is most effective in reducing TABP and risk of CHD. Similarly, in the Recurrent Coronary Prevention Project, patients who received counseling for TABP in addition to cardiac counseling after experiencing a myocardial infarction had a 44% lower recurrence rate after 3 years than those who received cardiac counseling alone (Mendes de Leon, Powell, & Kaplan, 1991).

Nurses and other clinicians frequently identify characteristics of TABP or its subcomponents in patients during routine interactions. Patients are often aware of their tendency toward hostility or anger but may not understand the adverse effect on their health. Nurses can help patients identify and acknowledge these characteristics and educate them about available interventions. Specific relaxation techniques and cognitive behavioral techniques will be described later in this chapter.

Depression

The prevalence of depression among patients with a recent diagnosis of CHD/myocardial infarction is estimated to be as high as 30% (Carney, Rich, TeVelde, et al., 1988; Forrester,

Lipsey, Teitelbaum, et al., 1992; Frasure-Smith, Lesperance, & Talajic, 1995). During the first year postdischarge, depression is common and largely unrelated to medical factors (Lesperance, Frasure-Smith, & Talajic, 1996). Depression in patients who have suffered myocardial infarctions is associated with an increased 6-month and 18-month mortality, greater than the mortality rate attributed to such clinical factors as heart failure or extent of CHD (Pasternak, 1996).

The Diagnostic and Statistical Manual of Mental Disorders, Revised Fourth Edition (DSM-IV) (American Psychiatric Association, 1994) defines *depression* as a mood disturbance, including either loss of pleasure in all or most activities or lack of reactivity to usual pleasurable stimuli, and sadness combined with three or more of the following symptoms: depression that is regularly worse in morning, early-morning awakening, marked psychomotor retardation or agitation, significant anorexia or weight loss, excessive or inappropriate guilt, and distinct quality of depressed mood. In major depression, these symptoms cause significant functional impairment and represent a change from previous functioning.

History of depression prior to an initial cardiac event is a risk factor for depression following a myocardial infarction (Frasure-Smith, Lesperance, & Talajic, 1995). Evidence suggests that biochemical changes associated with an initial bout of depression may permanently alter transmitters and receptors, thereby making an individual more susceptible to subsequent depressive episodes (Post, 1992).

In a number of studies, depression after a myocardial infarction was a significant predictor of mortality. In the Cardiac Arrhythmia Pilot Study, patients with myocardial infarctions accompanied by significant ventricular arrhythmias and high levels of depressive symptoms had an increased 1-year risk of mortality or cardiac arrest, even after other risk factors were controlled (Ahern, Gorkin, Anderson, et al., 1990). Furthermore, a study by Frasure-Smith (1991) found that patients with high levels of anxiety and depression were significantly more likely to die of cardiac causes over the subsequent 5 years.

In a follow-up study, Frasure-Smith and colleagues (1993) reported that patients suffering from a major depression had three to four times the risk of dying within 6 months. In one study, even when left ventricular dysfunction, previous myocardial infarction, and CHD severity were controlled for, major depression, depressive symptoms, anxiety, and a history of major depression significantly predicted cardiac events (Carney, Rich, Freedland, et al., 1988; Frasure-Smith, Lesperance, & Talajic, 1995). Similarly, in a quantitative review of studies examining the relationship between CHD and depression, Friedman and Booth-Kewley (1987) found the effects of depression to be comparable to those of other major risk factors.

Because depression affects a large percentage of people with CHD, and because it has such a negative impact on morbidity and mortality, screening and treatment for depression in this population is essential. Frequently, symptoms of depression after myocardial infarction are attributed to the patient's physical condition and consequently left untreated (Freeland, Lustman, Carney, et al., 1992). Depression may go untreated because health-care providers are more concerned with urgent medical issues or because they lack expertise in psychiatric diagnosis. In addition, some antidepressants have cardiotoxic effects, making providers reluctant to prescribe them. But without treatment, depression in these patients becomes chronic, especially in patients with a previous history of depression (Schleifer, Macari-Hinson, Coyle, et al., 1989).

Interventions for psychological distress have been shown to decrease mortality after myocardial infarction (Frasure-Smith & Prince, 1985). In the Ischemic Heart Disease Life Stress Monitoring Program, patients were interviewed in the hospital and followed monthly by telephone to assess their psychological symptoms. If they were found to demonstrate significant psychological symptoms, a home visit with the nurse was made, which included providing a supportive environment and acting as a liaison. A major aspect of this program was evaluation of the role of stress monitoring in a nursing intervention program. The resultant study demonstrated a significant reduction in stress scores and a 1-year reduction in cardiac-related mortality by almost 50%, as a result of stress monitoring (Frasure-Smith & Prince, 1989).

Studies indicate people with no close friends or significant other are more likely to be depressed following a myocardial infarction. This fact suggests that interventions focusing on increasing social support may be helpful in decreasing depression and subsequent cardiac events after myocardial infarction (Frasure-Smith, Lesperance, & Talajic, 1993). However, additional research is needed to develop and evaluate appropriate interventional strategies for this population.

Routine screening of all cardiac patients for depression as part of a comprehensive admission and discharge assessment, with one of a number of instruments available, would facilitate early diagnosis and intervention. As nurses and other clinicians may not always be familiar with the use of psychological instruments, it is important for them to develop a collegial relationship with the departments of psychiatry or behavioral medicine in the inpatient or outpatient setting. By identifying patients with symptoms of depression, nurses can facilitate appropriate referrals for further evaluation.

Social Support

Current research consistently demonstrates an association between low levels of social support and adverse health outcomes (Orth-Gomer, Rosengren, & Wilhelmsen, 1993). Five large prospective studies, summarized by House, Landis, & Umberson (1988), reported significant associations between low levels of social support and a severalfold increase in all-cause mortality.

As discussed in Chapter 3, social support is a multidimensional concept that is not easy to define. Holahan, Moos, Holahan, and Brennan (1997) reported preliminary research linking social support and stressors to the construct of social context. Their research also examined negative and positive aspects of social relationships. Based on the current research, *social support* can be described as the interactive process in which one receives emotional or functional aid from one's social network (Tolsdorf, 1976).

Norbeck (1981) developed an instrument to define social support. The functional properties measured were *affect* (feeling loved and respected), *affirmation* (having a supportive confidante), and *aid* (having help if needed). *Social network* may be defined as the web of identified relationships that a person has and the characteristics of those relationships (Bowling, 1991). Both the number of social networks and the quality of those relationships appear to correlate with CHD risk. The individual's perception of the extent to which the social network fulfills his or her needs is important (Fridlund, Stener-Bengtsson, & Wannman, 1993).

The type of social support that appears to be related to CHD mortality is not clear, although evidence for a relationship exists between perceived availability of support (support that can be called on when needed) and the development and severity of CHD (Cohen, 1988).

Ruberman and colleagues (1984) found social isolation was an independent predictor of all-cause mortality and sudden cardiac death in the Beta Blocker Heart Attack Trial. In a 1990 study by Orth-Gomer and Unden, the combined effects of lack of social ties and the CHD-prone behavior pattern was a better predictor for CHD than social isolation alone. Similarly, patients without a confidante (spouse or other) have a threefold increase of 6-month mortality after an acute myocardial infarction (Berkman, Leo-Summers, & Horowitz, 1992).

A study by Blumenthal and colleagues (1987) also found social support to be inversely related with the degree of CHD with Type A patients, but not with Type B patients. These findings could provide a possible explanation for some of the conflicting results involving TABP research. Increased availability of social support is a component of TABP modification programs. This increase in social support may contribute to the positive outcomes of the TABP interventions (Orth-Gomer, & Unden, 1990). Improved quality of relationships has been reported as a "side effect" of TABP modification (Friedman, Thoresen, & Gill, 1986).

Results from the Ischemic Heart Disease Life Stress Monitoring Program, as previously discussed, identified significantly reduced stress symptoms and a 50% reduction in cardiac-related mortality at 1 year (Frasure-Smith, & Prince, 1989). The primary focus of the intervention in this program was providing emotional support. The provision of emotional support during periods of high vulnerability to stress appears to be therapeutic (Frasure-Smith, & Prince, 1989).

Many studies speculate that social support may be a moderator of cardiovascular reactivity (Gerin, Milner, Chawla, et al., 1995). For example, Kamarck (1990) has shown that for certain types of laboratory tests, the presence of a friend reduces blood pressure and heart rate response. Other researchers have reported similar results in that the presence of a socially supportive individual attenuates cardiovascular reactivity to laboratory stresses (Lepore, Mata Allen, & Evans, 1993; Edens, Larken, & Abel, 1992).

Spiegel, Bloom, Kraemer, and Gottheil (1989) compared cancer patients who attended support group sessions with those who received only standard care. They reported that group members were less anxious and depressed and were coping more effectively with their breast cancer than the other patients. Although this study did not involve patients with CHD, it supported the premise of the positive effect of social support on patients with chronic illness.

Incorporating a measurement of social support in the nursing assessment will help the nurse identify patient needs in this area. Interventions aimed at increasing social support and decreasing social isolation will be addressed later in the chapter.

In addition to stress, the three psychosocial factors of hostility, depression, and low levels of social support have been identified as risk factors for CHD. The way stress affects each of us is as unique as the manner in which we respond to it. Some people feel anxious and overwhelmed, others get angry, still others feel depressed. Although many clinicians are able to address these psychosocial factors, the advanced-practice nurse (APN) is uniquely positioned in the current health-care environment to do so. APNs have the theoretical background and clinical expertise to properly assess, screen, and treat stress-related symptoms. The following section will identify implications for nursing care with particular emphasis upon the APN role.

Nursing Assessment

The first step in nursing assessment is to identify patients at risk. A biopsychosocial assessment of the individual should be done during an initial interview, in either an inpatient or outpatient setting. Chapter 4 addresses issues related to global assessment of the patient and evaluation of stress and other psychosocial factors. In general, during psychosocial assessment it is important to ascertain what patients perceive their needs to be. The assessment should include patients' sources of stress (family, health, work, relationships, etc.), existing coping strategies, interest in learning to manage stress, and perception of the level of social support available. For example, can they count on someone to provide them with emotional support? Do they believe that stress may be adversely affecting their health? How do they commonly react to stress (anxiety, anger, withdrawal, etc.)?

Although it is important for APNs and other clinicians to be able to identify a patient's potential psychosocial risk factors, as indicated in Chapter 4, a definitive diagnosis of the subcomponents of Type A behavior or depression requires special training and reliable, valid, and sensitive screening instruments.

PRINCIPLES AND TECHNIQUES OF STRESS MANAGEMENT

The previously described intervention studies suggest that stress management that includes the relaxation response and cognitive therapy may decrease cardiovascular reactivity, thereby decreasing CHD risk. Given their amount of patient contact, nurses are in an ideal position to identify psychosocial factors that may increase a patient's risk for CHD and to provide interventions to reduce that risk. Interventions to improve psychological distress may improve adherence to other medical regimens (Pasternak, 1996).

Stress management is a general treatment approach to a broad category of psychosocial problems. The theoretical basis for this treatment approach lies both in stress and cognitive behavioral theory (Roskies, 1987). Referring to Lazarus and Folkman's work previously discussed in the chapter, coping strategies aimed at altering a person's cognitive appraisal, and consequently interfering with the cardiovascular psychophysiologic reactivity, should reduce

CHD risk. We will now present a brief overview of stress management techniques.

The principles that guide the relaxation and stress management techniques pertain to all psychosocial risk-factor modification, so the decision on which of the techniques to use is based on the individual's values, beliefs, and individual preference. An outpatient behaviorally focused *cardiac rehabilitation program* (CRP) is strongly recommended for patients with CHD. Behaviorally oriented CRPs can screen patients who are distressed and institute appropriate stress management interventions. In addition, because CRPs occur in a group setting, they enhance social support.

The goals of a comprehensive stress management program are to increase awareness of the psychosocial factors placing the patient at risk and to help the patient develop skills to reduce that risk. Stress management includes a variety of interventions designed to induce psychophysiologic relaxation and decrease cardiovascular reactivity. Although numerous intervention strategies are used in clinical practice, we have deliberately focused on strategies that are (1) widespread, (2) have strong empirical support, or (3) are applicable to general use.

In the following section, a brief overview of stress management techniques is provided. The two main types of techniques are (1) those focused on stress management through inducement of the relaxation response and (2) cognitive behavioral techniques that target specific patient behaviors.

Relaxation Training

Relaxation training is composed of techniques that can counter the stress response. Benson (1976) characterizes the *relaxation response* (a state of deep relaxation) as the antithesis of the *stress response* and suggests that the relaxation response leads to decreased sympathetic nervous system arousal (Benson, 1975; Bulechek & McCloskey, 1992). Table 10–1 compares the physiologic stress response and the relaxation response.

The two basic elements of the relaxation response are a mental focus and a nonjudgmental attitude. The focus can be a repetition of a word, sound, phrase or muscular activity (Ben-

TABLE 10–1 Stress Response versus Relaxation Response

	Stress Response	Relaxation Response
Metabolism	Increases	Decreases
Heart rate	Increases	Decreases
Blood pressure	Increases	Decreases
Breathing rate	Increases	Decreases
Muscle tension	Increases	Decreases
Negative mood states	Increases	Decreases
Health risk	Increases	Decreases

son, 1995). Common relaxation techniques include breath focus, meditation (focus word, mantra, repetitive prayer), imagery/visualization, progressive muscle relaxation, body scan, mindfulness, yoga, and tai chi.

Box 10–1 contains a sample script the nurse can use to teach the relaxation response. Generally patients are asked to practice a technique for 10–20 minutes daily in a quiet environment. Whenever a thought or emotion enters their awareness, they should merely accept its presence without judgment. This takes regular practice. Many audiotapes are available to guide patients in their practice; at the end of this chapter a resource list is provided.

Guided imagery, or *visualization,* is a process of forming mental pictures with the involvement of all the senses (Dossey, Guzzetta, & Kenner, 1990). It can be used alone or in conjunction with other forms of relaxation. This technique can be used in a variety of settings, with many types of patients, and requires no costly equipment. The pathophysiology is the same as for other relaxation techniques. Patients are instructed to close their eyes and choose a pleasant image they can visualize, to imagine a calm, tranquil setting that evokes positive feelings and attitudes, and try to recall familiar sensations that make it seem as real as possible. The goal is for these positive images and feelings to elicit a state of calmness and contentment.

Biofeedback techniques can also be effective in reducing the physiologic symptoms of stress. *Biofeedback* has been defined as "the use of instrumentation to mirror psychophysiologic

BOX 10–1 PATIENT EDUCATION TIPS: BODY SCAN

Start by doing a breath focus/awareness. Consciously take a few deep, slow breaths. Feel your abdomen rise as you breathe in and fall as you breathe out. Slowly bring your awareness to your right great toe. Think of your toe as being made of atoms, with spaces between the atoms, so the toes feel open and spacious. Now bring your awareness to your second toe, third, fourth, and fifth toes, the ball of the foot, the arch, the top of the foot, the ankle, the calf, the knee, the space behind the knee, the thigh, and the hip. Allow the whole right leg to relax into the support of the floor, feeling spacious and light. (Slowly repeat with the left lower extremity.)

Now bring your awareness to your back, and notice each vertebra one at a time, seeing the space between the vertebrae as open and spacious, relaxing all the muscles in your back. Bring your awareness to your abdomen and to your chest, seeing the spaces between all your organs, relieving any restrictions that might be there, allowing your abdomen and chest to feel spacious and light.

Bring your awareness to your right thumb; second, third, fourth, and fifth fingers; palm of your hand; wrist, forearm, elbow, upper arm, and shoulder. Feel your whole right arm as spacious and light. (Repeat with left arm.)

Now bring your awareness to your neck and your jaw. Allow your jaw to relax. Become aware of your cheeks, your eyes, allowing the eyes to rest in their sockets, your forehead, softening the muscles, the top of your head, the back of your head.

Let your whole body rest softly into the support of the floor. Bring your awareness to your breath. With each breath in, feel the cool air; and as you breathe out, release any tension you may still be holding in your body. If you notice any part of your body still holding tension, focus your breath in the area, releasing the tension with each outward breath. Continue to focus on your breath; if your mind wanders, gently acknowledge the thoughts present and gently return to your focus. If it helps you to focus, count to yourself.

While you are breathing slowly, bring your awareness back to the room. Take a few minutes to notice the experience of yourself when your mind is quiet and body relaxed. Slowly open your eyes, take deep breaths, then stretch and yawn.

processes of which the individual is not normally aware and which may be brought under voluntary control" (Fuller, p. 3, 1977). Feedback information most commonly used in the clinical setting includes measures of muscle tension, heart rate, blood pressure, and temperature. Patients interested in learning biofeedback techniques should be referred to a center or program specializing in these techniques.

Music is another method of relaxation that nurses and other clinicians can use with their patients. Music has been shown to be as beneficial as muscle relaxation for short-term anxiety reduction (Heide & Borkovec, 1984). The effect of the music depends on the patient's responsiveness to music and personal preference. Music can be used to enhance other relaxation techniques such as imagery.

In summary, regular, daily practice of whatever relaxation technique is being practiced is encouraged. The effectiveness of a specific relaxation technique should be evaluated by the individual patient by asking questions such as, "Do I feel more relaxed and calm after practicing the technique?" and "Are my symptoms reduced?" To increase adherence, relaxation training should be prescribed in the same manner as a medical prescription. Personal instruction with multiple training sessions is best.

Reinforcement of the relaxation training with a tape for home practice is helpful. Encourage patients to keep a diary of their practice. The relaxation response helps to increase self-awareness and is important in developing other stress management skills.

Cognitive Behavioral Therapy

Everyone can function optimally at a certain level of stress, but when stress increases beyond this level, performance and efficiency decrease (Everly & Sobelman, 1987). Cognitive approaches to stress modification rely on the premise that the stress response is affected by a cognitive appraisal of the stimulus, including whether the stimulus is deemed stressful, and the extent and magnitude of the stress. Physiologic reactivity can be modified by altering the cognitive appraisal through a variety of behavioral techniques (Jacob & Chesney, 1986).

Cognitive behavioral therapy (CBT) is based on the work of Albert Ellis (1973), Aaron Beck (1976), David Burns (1989), and Donald Meichenbaum (1977). Its aim is to enable patients to understand that stress does not occur as a result of a situation or outside event but rather as a result of how they perceive or think about a situation. Although unable to change a situation, patients can learn to alter their perceptions of it; that is, they can change their thoughts and attitudes about the stressor.

According to Medich, Stuart, Deckro, and Friedman (1991), the goals of CBT are to teach patients to

1 Identify negative thoughts ("This always happens to me; I'll never get there; I'm such a jerk") that are based on assumptions or beliefs ("I must be perfect and competent at everything I undertake; I must have love and approval all the time").
2 Identify and challenge distortions in thinking (jumping to conclusions, magnification, fortune-telling).
3 Accomplish cognitive restructuring; that is, learn to substitute more realistic and self-enhancing thoughts ("It's no big deal—I'll probably be just a few minutes late; I *can* do this").
4 Develop effective coping skills (assertive communication, empathy, humor).

A four-step paradigm (stop, breathe, reflect, and choose) (Table 10–2) is often used to help patients understand the relationships among their thoughts, feelings, and behaviors (Benson & Stuart, 1992). The first two steps (*stop* and *breathe*) of the cognitive model help the patient to break the stress cycle and identify *stress warning signs*. Common warning signs

TABLE 10–2 Four-Step Stress Management Paradigm

1. *Stop* (interrupt negative stress response).
2. *Breathe* (release physical tension, and stop automatic thoughts).
3. *Reflect* (appraise situation, and identify automatic thoughts and distorted beliefs: "Is this situation really a problem? Am I overreacting? Does it serve me to be angry, depressed, etc.?").
4. *Choose* (identify coping techniques that would work here).

include muscle tension, headaches, irritability, anger, compulsive eating, smoking, and social withdrawal.

The third step in this paradigm is to teach the patient to *reflect*. Patients are instructed to write down their automatic thoughts or their immediate, negative reactions ("I'm a failure; this always happens to me; I should have known better; it's all my fault").

Once patients are able to identify their automatic thoughts, they can begin to challenge their old way of thinking using *cognitive restructuring*. For example, patients are taught to ask themselves, "Is the situation true? Am I jumping to conclusions, fortune-telling, or generalizing? What is the evidence? How do I know it will happen? Is there another way to look at the situation, and what is the worst thing that can happen? Is my anger justified? Is my anger serving me?"

The fourth step in this process involves *coping*, that is, actively choosing how to respond. The essence of coping is making conscious choices instead of reacting automatically. Patients are taught a number of coping strategies, including relaxation, journal writing, distraction, reframing (looking at a situation from a different point of view), assertive communication, social support, spirituality, and humor. As with relaxation strategies, patients choose which coping strategies work most effectively for them.

Nurses and other clinicians facilitate the effects of CBT through (1) appropriate feedback that acknowledges the patient's perceptions and feelings and (2) provision of an atmosphere of acceptance and caring (Medich, Stuart, Deckro, et al., 1991). Table 10–3 contains an example of CBT for the common scenario of waiting in a physician's office.

As part of effective coping and problem solving, patients need to learn to be assertive. *Assertive communication* involves expressing oneself directly while respecting the rights and opinions of others (Antoni, 1993). Role playing is a good method to teach and practice assertive communication skills.

Social Support

Nurses and other clinicians should help patients assess the kind and amount of social support available. Patients should be encouraged to improve the quality of their relationships as well as the number of social support networks. These networks may include (1) finding new groups to become active in, such as a club, a social support group, a church, or volunteer work; (2) cultivating new friendships; and (3) improving the quality of existing relationships. People may also consider getting a pet.

Groups can provide tremendous support to patients. Support groups can counter isolation and also allow people to feel they are helping

TABLE 10–3 Example of Cognitive Behavioral Therapy

Situation	Emotion	Thoughts	Cognitive Distortions	Rational Responses
Waiting in a doctor's office	Angry, hurt	This always happens to me.	Overgeneralization	I can wait.
		He is so rude, making me wait.	Labeling; magnification	I have a book I can read.
		He doesn't care about me.	Jumping to conclusions	The doctor probably has an emergency.
		No wonder I have HTN; This is a waste of my time.	Awfulizing	I'll do the best I can.
		I'll never get to work.	Fortune-telling	I'll probably only be a few minutes late for work.

themselves and one another (Spiegel, Bloom, Kraemer, et al., 1989).

Groups are available for every kind of chronic illness, including heart disease. Nurses and other clinicians should be aware of these resources so that they can refer patients to them. The American Heart Association is a valuable resource. Cardiac rehabilitation programs can also offer tremendous support to patients.

In summary, evaluation of the patient's response to a treatment is essential. Reports of symptom reduction, favorable improvement in psychological scores, and lifestyle are all desired outcomes of therapy. These changes will take time—weeks, months, or even years. Habits are established over extended periods of time, and it is unrealistic to expect to be able to change thoughts, feelings, and behaviors overnight. However, the APN can initiate and facilitate this process.

Being cognizant of the psychophysiologic relationship between the mind and body is essential to incorporating stress management into nursing practice. Identifying patients at risk, teaching them relaxation techniques and effective coping strategies, and referring them to appropriate resources, are all important nursing responsibilities.

CONCLUSION

In conclusion, although stress management is a vital aspect of prevention and treatment of CHD, it is only one component of a comprehensive rehabilitation process. Patients must understand the importance of modifying many aspects of their lifestyle in order to achieve maximal health benefits. Relaxation training and stress management skills will enhance the patient's ability to make optimal lifestyle changes.

Studies demonstrate that stress and associated psychosocial factors (hostility, depression, and lack of social support) increase the likelihood of morbidity and mortality in CHD patients. However, further research is needed to identify the exact mechanism by which these factors increase risk for cardiac events. Although several studies have demonstrated a positive effect for psychosocial interventions on

cardiac morbidity and mortality, additional research is warranted before definitive recommendations for practice can be made.

RESOURCES

The following relaxation audiotapes are available through the Division of Behavioral Medicine, Deaconess Hospital, Attn: One Deaconess Road, Boston, MA 10015, 617–632–9530. Each tape is $10; please make checks payable to the Deaconess Hospital. Tapes are nonrefundable.

- Basic Relaxation Exercise/Mindfulness Meditation (female voice)
  - Side 1 (20 minutes) This side introduces a basic relaxation sequence to help elicit the relaxation response, including some of the key elements, such as a breath awareness, body scan relaxation, and the use of a focus word.
  - Side 2 (20 minutes) This side offers instruction on awareness, or "mindfulness" of sensations, thoughts, and sounds. It also introduces breath and awareness as tools that enable you to integrate the relaxation response into daily activities.
- Basic Relaxation Response Exercise (male voice)
  - Side 1 (20 minutes) This tape is very similar to the other Basic Relaxation tape, except that it features a male voice.
  - Side 2 (45 minutes) Side 2 offers frequent pauses to allow you to practice techniques that elicit the relaxation response.
- Advanced Relaxation Response (female voice)
  - Side 1 (30 minutes) This side guides you through a body scan and relaxation, leading you into a relaxation response through awareness of your heart and repetition of your focus word. This tape has frequent pauses to encourage you to practice and develop ways of bringing forth the relaxation response on your own.
  - Side 2 (50 minutes) Side 2 reinforces basic skills and also guides you through a stretching routine and a series of images for healing.
- Guided Visualization with Ocean sounds/Breath and Body Awareness (female voice)
  - Side 1 (24 minutes) Side 1 is a guided body scan relaxation. It incorporates guided visualization of a sandy ocean beach, enhanced by the ocean sounds in the background.
  - Side 2 (30 minutes) Side 2 leads you through

a series of stretching exercises that will encourage a peaceful state of relaxation, awareness, and the elicitation of the relaxation response.

The following mindfulness audio tapes with Jon Kabat-Zinn, founder and director of the Stress Reduction Clinic at the University of Massachusetts Medical Center, are available by sending $10.00 per tape to Stress Reduction Tapes, P.O. Box 547, Lexington, MA 02173.

- Guided Body Scan Meditation/Guided Yoga 1 (45 minutes per side)

  □ This tape includes a body scan exercise and encourages deep states ofrelaxation. Side 2 has a sequence of mindful hatha yoga postures.

- Guided Sitting Meditation/Guided Yoga 2 (45 minutes per side)

  □ This sitting meditation has longer stretches of silence between the instruction than the body scan, to allow more time to practice mindfulness. Side 2 is a different sequence of mindful hatha yoga postures.

References

Ahern, D., Gorkin, L., Anderson, J., Tierney, C., Hallstrom, A., Ewart, C., Capone, R., Schron, E., Kornfeld, D., Herd, A., Richardson, D., & Follick, M. (1990). Biobehavioral variables and mortality or cardiac arrest in the Cardia Arrhythmia Pilot Study (CAPS). *American Journal of Cardiology, 66,* 59–62.

Allison, T., Williams, D., Miller, T., Patten, C., Bailey, K., Squires, R., & Gau, G. (1995). Medical and economic costs of psychologic distress in patients with coronary artery disease. *Mayo Clinic Proceedings 70,* 734–742.

American Psychiatric Association. (1994). *Diagnostic and Statistical Manual of Mental Disorders,* Rev. 4th ed. Washington, DC: American Psychiatric Association.

Antoni, M. (1993). Stress management strategies that work. In D. Goleman & J. Gurin (Eds.), *Mind Body Medicine.* New York: Consumer Reports Books.

Barefoot, J., Dahlstrom, W., & Williams, R. (1983). Hostility, coronary heart disease incidence and total mortality: A 25-year follow-up study of 255 physicians. *Psychosomatic Medicine, 45,* 59–63.

Barefoot, J., Dodge, K., Peterson, B., Dahlstrom, G., & Williams, R. (1989). The Cook-Medley hostility scale: Item content and ability to predict survival. *Psychosomatic Medicine, 51,* 46–57.

Beck, A. (1976). *Cognitive Therapy and the Emotional Disorders.* New York: International Universities Press.

Benson, H. (1975). *The Relaxation Response.* New York: William Morrow and Company.

Benson, H. (1995). *Timeless Healing: The Power and Biology of Belief.* New York: Scribner.

Benson, H., & Stuart, E. (1992). *The Wellness Book.* New York: Simon and Schuster.

Berkman, L., Leo-Summers, L., & Horowitz, R. (1992). Emotional support and survival after MI: A prospective population-based study of the elderly. *Annals of Internal Medicine, 117.* 1003–1009.

Blumenthal, J., Burg, M., Barefoot, J., Williams, R., Haney, T., & Zimet, G. (1987). Social support, Type A behavior, and CAD. *Psychosomatic Medicine, 49,* 331–340.

Bowling, A. (1991). Social support and social networks: Their relationship to successful and unsuccessful survival of elderly people in the community. An analysis of concepts and a review of evidence. *Family Practice, 8,* 68–83.

Bulechek, G., & McCloskey, J. (1992). *Nursing Interventions—Essential Nursing Treatments.* Philadelphia: W. B. Saunders Co.

Burns, D. (1989). *The Feeling Good Handbook: Using the New Mood Therapy in Everyday Life.* New York: William Morrow & Co.

Carney, R., Rich, M., Freeland, K., Saini, J., TeVelde, A., Simeone, C., & Clark, K. (1988). Major depressive disorder predicts cardiac events in patients with coronary artery disease. *Psychosomatic Medicine, 50,* 627–633.

Carney, R., Rich, M., TeVelde, A., Saini, J., Clark, K., & Freedland, K. (1988). The relationship between heart rate, heart rate variability, and depression in patients with coronary artery disease. *Journal of Psychosomatic Research, 32,* (2), 159–164.

Cohen, S. (1988). Psychosocial models of the role of social support in the etiology of physical disease. *Health Psychology, 7*(3), 269.

Cook, W., & Medley, D. (1954). Proposed hostility and pharisaic-virtue scales for the MMPI. *Journal of Applied Psychology, 238,* 414–418.

Dembroski, T., & Costa, P. (1987). Coronary-prone behavior: Components of the Type A pattern and hostility. *Journal of Personality, 55,* 211–235.

Dembroski, T., MacDougall, J., Costa, P., & Grandits, G. (1989). Components of hostility as predictors of sudden death and myocardial infarction in the MRFIT. *Psychosomatic Medicine, 51,* 514–522.

Dembroski, T., MacDougall, J., Williams, R., Haney, T., & Blumenthal, J. (1985). Components of Type A, hostility and anger-in: Relationship to angiographic findings. *Psychosomatic Medicine, 47,* 219–233.

Dossey, B., Guzzetta, C., & Kenner, C. (1990). *Essentials of Critical Care Nursing—Body, Mind, Spirit.* Philadelphia: J. B. Lippincott Co.

Edens, J., Larkin, K., & Abel, J. (1992). The effect of social support and physical touch on cardiovascular reactions to mental stress. *Journal of Psychosomatic Research, 36,* 371–382.

Eliot, R. (1988). *Stress and the Heart: Mechanisms, Measurements, and Management.* Mount Kisco, NY: Futura.

Ellis, A. (1973). *Humanistic Psychotherapy.* New York: McGraw Hill.

Everly, G., & Sobelman, S. (1987). *Assessment of the Human Stress Response.* New York: AMS Press, Inc.

Everly, G. (1989). *A Clinical Guide to the Treatment of the Human Stress Response.* New York: Plenum Press.

Forrester, A. W., Lipsey, J. R., Teitelbaum, M. L., Depaulo, J. R., Andrzejewski, P. L., & Robinson, R. G. (1992). Depression following myocardial infarction. *International Journal of Psychiatry in Medicine, 22,* 33–46.

Frasure-Smith, N. (1991). In-hospital symptoms of psychiatric stress as predictors of long-term outcome after myocardial infarction in men. *American Journal of Cardiology, 66,* 59–62.

Frasure-Smith, N., Lesperance, F., & Talajic, M. (1993). Depression following myocardial infarction. *Journal of American Medical Association, 270*(15), 1819–1825.

Frasure-Smith, N., Lesperance, F. & Talajic, M. (1995).

The impact of negative emotions on prognosis following myocardial infarction: Is it more than depression? *Health Psychology, 14*(5), 388–398.

Frasure-Smith, N., & Prince, R. H. (1985). The Ischemic Heart Disease Life Stress Monitoring Program: Impact on mortality. *Psychosomatic Medicine, 47,* 431–445.

Frasure-Smith, N., & Prince, R. (1989). Long-term follow-up of the Ischemic Heart Disease Life Stress Monitoring Program. *Psychosomatic Medicine, 51*(5), 485–513.

Freedland, K., Lustman, P., Carney, R., & Hong, B. (1992). Underdiagnosis of depression in patients with coronary artery disease: The role of nonspecific symptoms. *International Journal of Psychiatry in Medicine, 22*(3), 221–229.

Fridlund, B., Stener-Bengtsson, A., & Wannman, A. (1993). Social support and social network after acute myocardial infarction: The critically ill male patient's needs, choice, and motives. *Intensive and Critical Care Nursing, 9,* 88–94.

Friedman, H., & Booth-Kewley, S. (1987). The disease-prone personality: A meta-analytical view of the construct. *American Psychologist, 42,* 539–555.

Friedman, M., Thoresen, C., & Gill, J. (1986). Alteration in Type A behavior and its effect on cardiac recurrences in post myocardial infarction patients: Summary of the Recurrent Coronary Prevention Program. *American Heart Journal, 112,* 653–665.

Fuller, G. (1977). *Biofeedback: Methods and Procedures in Clinical Practice.* San Francisco: Biofeedback Press.

Gerin, W., Milner, D., Chawla, S., & Pickering, T. (1995). Social support as a moderator of cardiovascular reactivity in women: A test of the direct effects and buffering hypotheses. *Psychosomatic Medicine, 57*(1), 16–22.

Girdano, D., & Everly, G. (1986). *Controlling Stress and Tension,* 2nd ed. Englewood Cliffs, NJ: Prentice-Hall.

Glass, D. C. (1977). *Behavior Patterns, Stress, and Coronary Disease.* Hillsdale, NJ: Erlbaum.

Goldband, S., Katkin, E., & Morell, M. (1979). Personality and cardiovascular disorder: Steps toward demystification. In I. G. Sarason and C. D. Spielberger (Eds.), *Stress and Anxiety,* vol. 6. Washington, DC: Hemisphere.

Gould, K. L., Ornish, D., Kirkeeide, R., Brown, S., Stuart, Y., Buchi, M., Billings, J., Armstrong, W., Ports, T. & Scherwitz, L. (1992). Improved stenosis geometry by quantitative coronary arteriography after vigorous risk factor modification. *American Journal of Cardiology, 69*(9), 845–853.

Heide, F., & Borkovec, T. (1984). Relaxation-induced anxiety: Mechanisms and theoretical implications. *Behavioral Residents Therapeutics, 22,* 1–12.

Holahan, C. J., Moos, R. H., Holahan, C. K., & Brennan, P. L. (1997). Social context, coping strategies, and depressive symptoms: An expanded model with cardiac patients. *Journal of Personality & Social Psychology, 72*(4), 918–928.

House, J., Landis, K., & Umberson, D. (1988). Social relationships and health. *Science, 241,* 540–545.

Jacob, R., & Chesney, M. (1986). Psychological and behavioral methods to reduce cardiovascular reactivity. In K. Matthews, S. Weiss, T. Detre, T. Dembroski, B. Falkner, S. Manuck & R. Williams, Jr. (Eds.), *Handbook of Stress, Reactivity, and Cardiovascular Disease.* New York: John Wiley & Sons.

Kamarck, T. W. (1995). Affiliation moderates the effects of social threat on stress related cardiovascular responses: Boundary conditions for a laboratory model of social support. *Psychosomatic Medicine, 57,* 183–194.

Krantz, D. S., & Manuck, S. B. (1984). Acute psychophysiologic reactivity and risk of cardiovascular disease: A review and methodologic critique. *Psychologic Bulletin, 96,* 435–464.

Lazarus, R. (1966). *Psychological Stress and the Coping Process.* New York: McGraw-Hill.

Lazarus, R., & Folkman, S. (1984). *Stress, Appraisal, and Coping.* New York: Springer.

Lepore, S., Mata Allen, K., & Evans, G. (1993). Social support lowers cardiovascular reactivity to an acute stressor. *Psychosomatic Medicine, 55,* 518–524.

Lesperance, F, Frasure-Smith, N. Talajic, M. (1996). Major depression before and after myocardial infarction: Its nature and consequences. *Psychosomatic Medicine, 58,* 99–110.

Matthews, K., & Haynes, S. (1986). Type A behavior pattern and coronary disease risk. *American Journal of Epidemiology, 123,* 923–960.

Medich, C., Stuart, E., Deckro, J., & Friedman, R. (1991). Psychophysiologic control mechanisms in ischemic heart disease. *The Journal of Cardiovascular Nursing, 5*(4), 10–26.

Meichenbaum, D. (1977). *Cognitive Behavior Modification: An Integrative Approach.* New York: Plenum Press.

Mendes de Leon, C., Powell, L., & Kaplan, B. (1991). Change in coronary-prone behaviors in the Recurrent Coronary Prevention Project. *Psychosomatic Medicine, 53,* 407–419.

Mittleman, M., Maclure, M., Sherwood, J., Mulry, R., Tofler, G., Jacobs, S., Friedman, R., Benson, H., & Muller, J. (1995). Triggering of acute myocardial infarction onset by episodes of anger. *Circulation, 92*(7), 1720–1725.

Muller, J. E., Tofler, G. H., Stone, P. H. (1989). Circadian variation and triggers of onset of acute cardiovascular disease. *Circulation, 79,* 733–743.

Norbeck, J. S. (1981). Social support: A model for clinical research and application. *Advances in Nursing Science, 31,* 43–59.

Nunes, E., Frank, K., & Kornfeld, D. (1987). Psychologic treatment for the Type A behavior pattern and for CHD: A meta-analysis of the literature. *Psychosomatic Medicine, 48*(2), 159–173.

Ornish, D., Brown, S., Schewitz, L., Billings, J., Armstrong, W., Ports, T., McIanahan, S., Kireeide, R., Brand, R., & Gould, K. (1990). Can lifestyle changes reverse CHD? *Lancet, 336,* 129–133.

Orth-Gomer, K., Rosengren, A., & Wilhelmsen, L. (1993). Lack of social support and incidence of coronary heart disease in middle-aged Swedish men. *Psychosomatic Medicine, 55,* 37–43.

Orth-Gomer, K., & Unden, A. (1990). Type A behavior, social support and coronary risk. Interaction and significance for mortality in cardiac patients. *Psychosomatic Medicine, 52,* 59–72.

Pasternak, R. (1996). Spectrum of risk factors for coronary heart disease. *Journal of American College of Cardiology, 27,* 964–1047.

Post, R. M. (1992). Transduction of psychosocial stress into the neurobiology of recurrent affective disorder. *American Journal of Psychiatry, 149,* 999–1010.

Roseman, I. (1984). Cognitive determinants of emotion. In P. Shaver (Ed.), *Review of Personality and Social Psychology.* Beverly Hills, CA: Sage.

Rosenman, R., Brand, R., Jenkins, C., Friedman, M., Straus, R., and Wurm, M. (1975). Coronary heart disease is the WCGS final follow-up experience of eight and one-half years. *Journal of American Medical Association, 233,* 872–877.

Roskies, E. (1987). *Stress Management for the Healthy Type A.* New York: The Guild Press.

Ruberman, W., Weinblatt, E., Goldberg, J, & Chaudhary, B. (1984). Psychosocial influences on mortality after myocardial infarction. *New England Journal of Medicine, 311,* 552–559.

Schleifer, S., Macari-Hinson, M., Coyle, D., Slater, W., Kahn, M., Gorlin, R., & Zucker, M. (1989). The nature and course of depression following myocardial infarction. *Archives of Internal Medicine, 149,* 1785–1789.

Selye, H. (1974). *Stress Without Distress.* Philadelphia: J. B. Lippincott.

Shekelle, R., Gale, M., Ostfeld, A., & Oglesby, P. (1983). Hostility, risk of coronary heart disease, and mortality. *Psychosomatic Medicine, 45,* 109–114.

Spiegel, D., Bloom, J., Kraemer, H., & Gottheil, E. (1989). Effects of psychosocial treatment on survival of patients with metastatic breast cancer. *Lancet, 2,* 888–891.

Teplitz, L. & Siwik, D. (1994). Cellular signals in atherosclerosis. *The Journal of Cardiovascular Nursing, 8*(3), 28–48.

Toldsdorf, C. (1976). Social networks, support, and coping: An exploratory study. *Family Practice, 15,* 407–417.

Vitaliano, P., Russo, J., Bailey, S., Young, H., & McCann, B. (1993). Psychosocial factors associated with cardiovascular reactivity in older adults. *Psychosomatic Medicine, 55,* 164–177.

Wells-Federman, C., Stuart, E., Deckro, J., Mandle, C., Baim, M., & Medich, C. (1995). The mind-body connection: The psychophysiology of many traditional nursing interventions. *Clinical Nurse Specialist, 9,*(1), 59–66.

Zumoff, B., Rosenfels, R., Friedman, M., Byers, S., Rosenman, R., & Hellman, L. (1984). Elevated daytime excretion of urinary testosterone glucuronide in men with Type A behavior pattern. *Psychosomatic Medicine, 46,* 223–225.

SECTION III

SPECIAL TOPICS

CHAPTER 11

Diabetes

James A. Fain

Diabetes mellitus is a chronic disease that affects 16 million people in the United States, nearly half of whom do not yet know they have the disease (Harris, 1995). A large portion, some 3.2 million, of those diagnosed with diabetes are age 65 or older. Worldwide, 100 to 120 million people have this chronic disease. The risk for coronary heart disease (CHD) is two to four times higher in people with diabetes. CHD and other vascular diseases account for nearly 1 million hospital admissions each year among patients with diabetes, and nearly 600,000 Medicare patients with diabetes are hospitalized annually for atherosclerotic heart disease. The financial and medical burden of diabetes among the Medicare population alone is substantial, with close to $30 billion spent annually, or 27% of the entire Medicare budget (Levetan & Ratner, 1995).

Morbidity and mortality from CHD contributed to 75–80% of all deaths in people with diabetes (Vinicor, 1996), along with an increased prevalence of hypertension and lipid abnormalities. Multiple risk factors for CHD are frequently found in people with diabetes. In contrast to people without diabetes, CHD in people with diabetes appears earlier in life, affects women almost as often as men, and is more often fatal. The literature is replete with epidemiologic data suggesting that people with diabetes are more likely to have hypertension, low levels of high-density lipoprotein (HDL) (dyslipidemia), and high levels of triglycerides. Other factors associated with diabetes include obesity, smoking, hyperglycemia, and hyperinsulinemia.

The purpose of this chapter is to (1) discuss diabetes as an independent risk factor for CHD, (2) discuss the interaction between diabetes and other CHD risk factors, and (3) identify CHD risk-reduction strategies for people with diabetes.

CORONARY HEART DISEASE AND DIABETES

CHD is the most common cause of morbidity and mortality in people with diabetes. A consensus panel with expertise in clinical diabetes, epidemiology, nutrition, and cardiovascular disease was convened by the American Diabetes Association (1989) to examine a variety of issues concerned with macrovascular disease such as CHD in patients with diabetes. Commonly identified risk factors for macrovascular disease included hypertension, smoking, and lipid abnormality. The increased risk of CHD associated with diabetes has been demonstrated in several epidemiologic studies (Barrett-Connor, Cohn, Wingard, et al., 1991; Kannel, D'Agostino, Wilson, et al., 1990; Mitchell, Hazuda, Haffner, et al., 1991; Nichaman, Wear, Goff, et al., 1993).

People with type 2 diabetes mellitus are particularly at risk for CHD. This type of diabetes accounts for approximately 90% of individuals with diabetes in the United States. Typically, type 2 diabetes occurs after the age of 40, with 60–90% of individuals being obese or having a history of obesity at the time of diagnosis (D'Eramo, 1993).

In addition, CHD is of great concern in people with type 1 diabetes mellitus. Although CHD is less common in people with type 1 diabetes than in older adults with type 2 diabetes, mortality rates are still 10 times greater among individuals with diabetes when compared with those without diabetes (Harris, 1995).

CHD accounts for approximately 25% of deaths among individuals with onset of diabetes before 20 years of age. Microvascular disease is characteristic of people with type 1 diabetes, with its occurrence and progression directly related to elevated concentrations of glucose in the blood. In the Diabetes Control and Complications Trial, intensively treated subjects had a 41% reduction in cardiovascular events compared with conventionally treated patients (Diabetes Control & Complications Trial Research Group, 1993). The question of applicability of these findings to patients with type 2 diabetes has sparked considerable debate in the diabetes community. Microvascular and macrovascular complications associated with type 2 diabetes are the product of chronic hyperglycemia. Many clinicians believe that a reduction in CHD risk factors will come only with a comprehensive approach to the reduction of hyperglycemia in people with type 2 diabetes. Research has established that intensive treatment of type 2 diabetes is associated with lower cardiac-related mortality (Hellman, Regan, & Rosen, 1997).

PATHOGENESIS OF TYPE 1 AND TYPE 2 DIABETES. Type 1 diabetes has an autoimmune etiology in the majority of cases, so the general consensus is that type 1 diabetes includes a genetic component. The *major histocompatibility complex* (MHC) on chromosome 6 is the primary gene cluster associated with susceptibility to type 1 diabetes. This region codes for several molecules referred to as *human leukocyte antigens* (HLA). Increased levels of HLA-DR3 and HLA-DR4 are strongly associated with an increased risk of developing type 1 diabetes, whereas HLA-DR11 and HLA-DR15 correlate with a decreased risk of developing type 1 diabetes (Lott, 1997).

There also appear to be ethnic differences for HLA antigens. HLA typing in African-American and Latin American populations suggests similar associations with diabetes as found in the white population, but the frequency of the diabetes-associated genes is lower (Lott, 1997).

An obvious outcome of genetic analysis is the prediction of risk to family members of patients with diabetes. In order for genetic counseling to be most effective, an accurate and precise diagnosis must be made. Epidemiologic research has reported that the risk of diabetes for first-degree relatives is low, particularly for individuals with type 1 diabetes. The sibling of a child with type 1 diabetes has only a 5–10% risk of the same disease, and the risk to the offspring of a single diabetic parent is thought to be even less, i.e., 1–2% (Dorman, McCarthy, O'Leary, et al., 1995).

The pathogenesis of type 1 diabetes is characterized by an absolute insulin deficiency; thus, glucose is unable to enter muscle and adipose tissue. In most individuals, strong evidence implicates an autoimmune process in beta cell destruction. Because insulin secretory reserves are considerable, individuals with type 1 diabetes go through a period of months with no detectable abnormalities in insulin secretion or glucose metabolism. Glucose intolerance emerges when insulin secretory reserves are reduced to less than 20% of normal (Greenspan & Baxter, 1994). Continued insulin deficiency and other hormonal influences (increased levels of catecholamines, cortisol, glucagon, and growth hormone) lead to lipolysis in body tissues. As fats stored in adipose tissue are metabolized, fatty acids are produced.

The pathogenesis of type 2 diabetes involves impaired insulin secretion, insulin resistance, and abnormally elevated glucose production by the liver (DeFronzo, 1988; DeFronzo & Ferrannini, 1991). In some patients with type 2 diabetes, the primary defect starts at the level of the beta cell and manifests itself as an impairment in insulin secretion. This type of defect is more commonly seen in nonobese individuals with type 2 diabetes. In other people with type 2 diabetes, the primary defect is a sensitivity to insulin. This type of defect is more commonly seen in obese individuals with type 2 diabetes.

Insulin resistance is defined as a subnormal biologic response to a given concentration of insulin (Moller & Flier, 1991). Insulin resistance is present not only in people with type 2 diabetes, but also, to a lesser degree, in a majority of overweight individuals with normal glucose tolerance (Moller & Flier, 1991). It is even present in approximately 25% of nonobese individuals with normal glucose tolerance. In addition, research findings have provided evidence that a component of insulin resistance is inherited and may predispose family members to the development of type 2 diabetes.

Normal beta cells are able to recognize the presence of insulin resistance and augment their secretion of insulin. In the obese nondiabetic person, the compensatory response is nearly perfect, and no alteration in glucose tolerance ensues. In the person with diabetes, the beta cell response is less than perfect, and glucose intolerance ensues. Hyperinsulinemia develops not only from increased secretion of insulin by beta cells but also from impairment of insulin receptors. The additional effect of hyperglycemia causes a generalized desensitization of all cells in the body and becomes a pathogenic factor in its own right (Greenspan & Baxter, 1994).

The role of elevated blood glucose (hyperglycemia) in affecting the development and progression of CHD has long been debated. Findings from several studies suggest strongly that in both type 1 and type 2 diabetes, hyperglycemia is a major contributing factor (Diabetes Control & Complications Trial Research Group, 1993; Pyorala, Laaskso, & Uusitupa, 1987; Stern, 1995).

CHD Complications Associated with Diabetes Mellitus

CHD is the leading cause of death in people with type 2 diabetes (Pyorala, Laaskso, & Uusi-

tupa, 1987). Increases in morbidity and mortality among individuals with CHD are related to complications associated with diabetes. Diabetes-specific complications involve the vascular system for the most part. Diabetic vascular disease is classified into the two main categories of microvascular disease and macrovascular disease (Table 11–1).

Microvascular disease is a disease of small blood vessels, capillaries, and precapillary arterioles. Changes in capillaries and small vessels are manifested by thickening of the capillary basement membrane and loss of membrane function. Data from several major studies have identified hyperglycemia as the mechanism underlying the development of specific diabetic complications (Herman & Greene, 1996).

Macrovascular disease is a large vessel disease. Pathologically, macrovascular disease reflects atherosclerosis, which refers to the deposit of material (i.e., lipids) within the inner layer of vessel walls (intima). Macrovascular disease underlies abnormalities in coronary, cerebral, and larger peripheral arterial vessels. Clinically these abnormalities manifest themselves as heart disease and vascular symptoms such as intermittent claudication.

Whereas at a cellular level there may be important pathophysiologic commonalities between microvascular and macrovascular disease, symptoms are different. Patients with diabetic macrovascular disease may exhibit exertion-associated chest pain, episodic symptoms of dizziness and slurred speech caused by transient ischemic attacks, or exercise-related calf cramps (i.e., claudication) (Vinicor, 1996).

TABLE 11–1 Complications Associated with Diabetes Mellitus

Microvascular complications
  Diabetic retinopathy
  Diabetic nephropathy
  Diabetic neuropathy
  Periodontal disease
Macrovascular complications
  Coronary artery disease
  Cerebrovascular disease
  Peripheral vascular disease
  Infections

Risk Factors for Development of CHD in People with Diabetes

HYPERTENSION. Hypertension is a known CHD risk factor for people with diabetes. The prevalence of hypertension in people with diabetes is approximately twice that of hypertension in people without diabetes. In people with type 1 diabetes, hypertension might be present at the time of diagnosis, subsequently become normalized, and then return during the first 5–10 years after onset of having diabetes. In people with type 2 diabetes, hypertension is sometimes associated with what is called *syndrome X,* a constellation of findings that includes abdominal obesity, hypertriglyceridemia, and low levels of *high-density lipoprotein* (HDL) cholesterol. By the time most individuals are diagnosed with type 2 diabetes, they may have had the syndrome for several years. Syndrome X causes insulin resistance, in which glucose cannot be used efficiently and the beta cells must increase their production of insulin to compensate. The result is hyperinsulinemia. Blood glucose levels gradually rise as insulin production by the pancreas can no longer keep up with the insulin resistance, until diabetes develops.

Taken together, these abnormalities raise the incidence of angina, heart attacks, strokes, and peripheral vascular disease (Kaplan, 1989). Hyperinsulinemia increases sodium retention in the renal tubules, thereby contributing to or causing hypertension. An increased *very-low-density lipoprotein* (VLDL) production in the liver is attributed to hyperinsulinemia, leading to hypertriglyceridemia (and consequently a low HDL cholesterol level). Moreover, it is postulated that high insulin levels stimulate endothelial and vascular smooth muscle cell proliferation, by virtue of the hormone's action on growth-factor receptors, to initiate atherosclerosis (Greenspan & Baxter, 1994).

HYPERINSULINEMIA. Hyperinsulinemia is an important factor in the atherosclerotic process along with hypertension and hyperlipidemia. Epidemiologic studies have shown circulating insulin to be an important independent risk factor for atherosclerosis and have demonstrated that insulin can produce changes in vascular tissue consistent with the atherosclerotic process (Haffner, Stern, Hazuda, et al., 1990;

McPhillips, Barrett-Connor, & Wingard, 1990; Taylor, Accili, & Imai, 1994).

Type 2 diabetes is an insulin-resistant state associated with increased levels of endogenous insulin in its early stages and with increased levels of insulin needed to control glucose during therapy. If hyperinsulinemia is indeed a risk factor for atherosclerosis, it is conceivable that insulin therapy might reduce the risk of complications arising from hyperglycemia while increasing the risk of complications generated by the insulin itself. An "atherosclerotic environment" may exist for years before the onset of hyperglycemia. This possibility would help explain the lack of a time relationship between the onset of hyperglycemia and hypertension in people with type 2 diabetes (Haffner, Stern, Hazuda, et al., 1990).

HEART DISEASE. In the Multiple Risk Factor Intervention Trial, predictors of cardiovascular disease mortality were assessed among men with and without diabetes to determine the risk from cardiovascular disease. The risk in men with diabetes increased more steeply over a 12-year period than it did in men without diabetes, even after accounting for the presence of other risk factors for cardiovascular disease (i.e., high blood pressure, hypercholesterolemia, and smoking) (Fig. 11–1) (Stamler, Vaccaro, Neaton, et al., 1993).

MINORITY POPULATIONS. Type 1 diabetes mellitus is more prevalent in Native Americans, African Americans, and Mexican Americans. Compared with non-Hispanic whites, diabetes rates are 60% higher in African Americans and 110–120% higher in Mexican Americans and Puerto Ricans. The Corpus Christi Heart Project was initiated as a prospective, population-based study designed to examine the history of CHD among Mexican Americans and non-Hispanic whites. A large proportion of those individuals who had an acute myocardial infarction had diabetes. Mexican-American women were especially affected. Patients with diabetes were slightly older than those without diabetes and were more likely to have a history of a myocardial infarction, angina, or bypass surgery at the time of hospital admission (Fig. 11–2). In addition, more patients with diabetes had hypertension (more than 60%), although fewer were current smokers, than those without diabetes

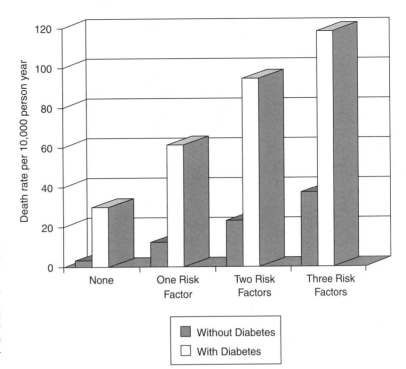

FIGURE 11–1 Age-adjusted cardiovascular disease (CVD) death rate by number of risk factors present in men screened for multiple risk factors, with and without diabetes. (Adapted with permission from Stamler, J., Vaccaro, O., Neaton, J. D., & Wentworth, D. (1993). Diabetes, other risk factors, and 12-year cardiovascular mortality for men screened in the Multiple Risk Factor Intervention Trial. *Diabetes Care, 16*(2), 434–444).

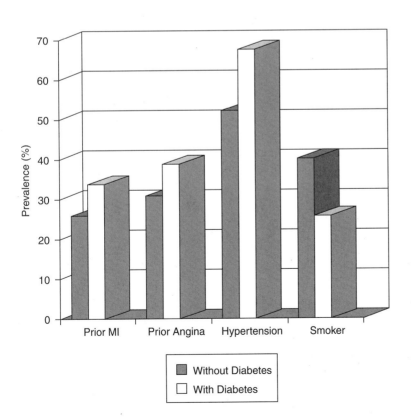

FIGURE 11–2 CHD risk factors in patients with acute MI by diabetes status (Corpus Christi Heart Project). (Based on data from Nichaman, M. Z., Wear, M. L., Goff, D. C., et al. (1993). Hospitalization rates for myocardial infarction among Mexican-Americans and non-Hispanic whites: The Corpus Christi Heart Project. *Annals of Epidemiology 3*(1), 42–48).

who had sustained a myocardial infarction. The two groups of patients had similar mean total cholesterol values (202 mg/dl versus 200 mg/dl) regardless of diabetes status.

GENDER. Although the overall cardiovascular mortality is greater among men, diabetes is the *only* disease that causes women to have cardiovascular mortality similar to that of men. In the Rancho Bernardo Study, men and women who had diabetes were compared with those who were euglycemic and had no family history of diabetes. Women with diabetes had ischemic heart disease mortality rates similar to those in men with and without diabetes (Barrett-Connor, Cohn, Wingard, et al., 1991).

A longer duration of type 2 diabetes in women was found to be associated with an increased risk of CHD. In the Nurses' Health Survey, women who were between the ages of 30 and 55 and free of CHD, stroke, and cancer were studied for an 8-year period. A strong positive association between type 2 diabetes and CHD, ischemic stroke, and cardiovascular mortality was found in middle-aged women. Both fatal and nonfatal cardiovascular events were substantially increased among women with diabetes. Diabetes was a major independent determinant of CHD. The impact of diabetes was also amplified in the presence of other risk factors such as hypertension, obesity, and cigarette smoking (Manson, Colditz, Stampfer, et al., 1991).

Reducing CHD Risk Factors in People with Diabetes

With few exceptions, preventive measures and treatment of microvascular disease are similar for people with and without diabetes (Lorber, 1994). High blood pressure and high levels of blood cholesterol are initially treated with diet and lifestyle modifications to see if these conditions can be brought under control without medication. If elevated blood cholesterol levels and blood pressure persist despite strict adherence to these measures, medication is generally needed. The emphasis on drug therapy for hypertension and dyslipidemia is greater for patients who have diabetes, because these patients have a higher risk of cardiovascular

disease. The following guidelines from the Centers for Disease Control (CDC) (1991) are helpful for health-care professionals in the detection and treatment of cardiovascular disease in people with diabetes.

AT EVERY OFFICE VISIT

- Measure the patient's blood pressure with a cuff appropriate for the patient's size.
- Ask patients whether they have had the symptoms listed in Table 11–2.

AT LEAST ONCE A YEAR

- Ask patients about their use of tobacco.
- Auscultate for bruits over large arteries, and palpate all peripheral pulses.

ONCE A YEAR

- Measure triglycerides (TG), total cholesterol (TC), and HDL cholesterol levels in the fasting state, and calculate the level of LDL cholesterol. For TG under 400 mg/dl,

$$LDL = TC - [TG \div 5] + HDL$$

- Obtain a baseline electrocardiogram in all patients with diabetes, and repeat the procedure yearly for those with clinically apparent cardiovascular disease.

Interventions aimed at reducing CHD risk factors among people with diabetes should involve all members of the health-care team. Specific strategies for decreasing CHD risk can be divided into two categories: nonpharmacologic versus pharmacologic therapies.

TABLE 11–2 Diabetes-Related Conditions and Symptoms to Ask About at Every Office Visit

Condition	Symptoms
Cerebral vascular disease	Transient blindness, dysarthria, or unilateral weakness
Coronary artery disease and congestive heart failure	Chest pain or pressure, dyspnea, orthopnea, paroxysmal nocturnal dyspnea, or edema
Peripheral vascular disease	Intermittent claudication or foot ulcers that do not heal

NONPHARMACOLOGIC THERAPIES

EXERCISE. Epidemiologic evidence suggest that regular exercise and physical fitness are associated with decreased incidence of cardiovascular disease in the general population, as well as a decreased occurrence of type 2 diabetes (Helmrich, Ragland, Leung, et al., 1991). Because persons with diabetes have an increased risk of cardiovascular disease, the role of exercise in reducing modifiable risks has primary importance. The benefits of exercise for persons with diabetes include improved functioning of the cardiovascular system; increased insulin sensitivity; and reduction in plasma cholesterol, triglycerides, and LDL, particularly in the presence of weight loss, and increase in HDL (Horton, 1988; Pollock, Wilmore, & Fox, 1984).

Moderate but regular exercise, 30 minutes a day, improves glycemic and lipid control. Exercise as easy as walking or gardening provides this control. The activity need not even be done in one 30-minute session. Exercise also has the added benefits of helping with weight loss, retarding osteoporosis, enhancing self-esteem, and improving one's sense of well-being. However, patients with diabetes should be screened for diabetic complications before beginning an exercise program. There are increased risks associated with exercise if the patient has proliferative retinopathy, CHD, nephropathy, or neuropathy (American Diabetes Association, 1989).

Epidemiologic studies suggest that exercise diminishes the mortality and morbidity from macrovascular disease in nondiabetic populations (Leon, 1987). Likewise, exercise enhances the diabetic patient's sensitivity to insulin, with a decrease in plasma insulin levels. If hyperinsulinemia is indeed a risk factor for macrovascular disease, lower insulin levels will help prevent macrovascular complications. Individuals with type 2 diabetes who exercise also report a significant decrease in plasma triglyceride levels and LDL.

SMOKING CESSATION. Smoking is an independent risk factor for CHD. In addition, smoking contributes to microvascular complications associated with diabetes caused by atherosclerosis and arteriosclerosis. Findings from the 1988 Behavioral Risk Factor Surveillance System indicated that people with diabetes smoked with the same frequency as in the general population. A higher prevalence of smoking was noted among young people between the ages of 18 and 34 as well as among African-American men with diabetes (Ford & Newman, 1991). The impact smoking has on people with and without diabetes supports the necessity of aggressive attempts to achieve smoking cessation. A smoking-cessation program may be the single most important step in reducing the risk for cardiovascular disease.

WEIGHT REDUCTION. Nutritional strategies are critical not only to monitor blood glucose levels but to control a number of other factors associated with the risk of developing diabetic complications, such as elevated blood lipids (cholesterol and triglycerides), obesity, and high blood pressure.

The American Diabetes Association (ADA) recommends that people with diabetes eat a high-carbohydrate, low-fat diet. According to the ADA's guidelines, 55–60% of the day's calories should come from carbohydrates and 30% or less from fats. The primary goal of this diet is to keep blood lipid levels low so as to reduce the risk of microvascular disease without adversely affecting blood glucose levels. For people with diabetes, it is important to control the amount of total calories, saturated fats, and dietary cholesterol eaten each day. Weight loss not only improves control of blood glucose but may lower total cholesterol, raise HDL cholesterol, and reduce elevated triglyceride levels.

PHARMACOLOGIC THERAPIES

HYPERLIPIDEMIA. To lower blood cholesterol in patients with diabetes, HMG-CoA reductase inhibitors (e.g., lovastatin, fluvastatin) or ion exchange resins (i.e., cholestyramine, colestipol) are ideal, because these drugs effectively reduce total and LDL cholesterol levels. These are major drug classes for the treatment of lipid disorders in patients who have failed to achieve target levels in spite of dietary modifications. Niacin (nicotinic acid), a lipid-modifying drug, is not commonly used in people with diabetes. It reduces the risk of CHD, but it can raise blood glucose levels, resulting in an increased risk for liver disease. If niacin is prescribed, liver function should be monitored.

Triglyceride levels above 350 mg/dl are common in people with diabetes. To reduce hypertriglyceridemia in people with diabetes, the use of a fibric acid derivative such as gemfibrozil is ideal. Yet, although gemfibrozil improves the overall lipid profile, its propensity to increase LDL cholesterol may limit its use in people with diabetes. Modest elevations in triglycerides can be treated with HMG-CoA reductase inhibitors, which are effective in lowering both triglycerides and LDL cholesterol. See Table 11–3 for a list of lipid-modifying drugs used in people with diabetes.

HYPERTENSION. To treat high blood pressure, four classes of antihypertensive drugs can be used: diuretics, beta blockers, *angiotensin-converting enzyme* (ACE) inhibitors, and *calcium channel blockers* (CCBs). Drugs that have natural or favorable effects on cholesterol levels and are considered safe for people with diabetes are ACE inhibitors such as captopril (Capoten) and enalapril (Vasotec) and CCBs such as diltiazem (Cardizem) and verapamil (Isoptin).

ACE inhibitors are the best antihypertensives for people with diabetes. They retard the progression of glomerular sclerosis and offer renal protection. They can improve glucose tolerance and are lipid-neutral. However, high doses may be detrimental to renal function in late stages of diabetes with renal insufficiency.

ACE inhibitors are particularly effective in controlling hypertension as well as reducing proteinuria when used in combination with verapamil or diltiazem. CCBs retard the progression of renal disease by decreasing accumulation of calcium in renal tissue. CCBs have no effect on glucose or lipid metabolism (Kochar & Kalluru, 1994).

Diuretic antihypertensives such as chlorothiazide (Diuril) and hydrochlorothiazide (Lopressor) and beta blockers such as propranolol (Inderal), hydrochorothiazide (Lopressor), and atenolol (Tenormin) are not as appropriate to use with patients who have elevated cholesterol levels and arteriosclerosis. Beta blockers block the warning signs of hypoglycemia. They work by impeding the action of epinephrine, the hormone responsible for producing the sweating, nervousness, and hunger that are warning symptoms of hypoglycemia. In addition, beta blockers alter lipid metabolism by increasing triglyceride and total cholesterol levels and decreasing HDL cholesterol (Kochar & Kalluru, 1994).

Diuretic antihypertensives have potential disadvantages for people with diabetes. Commonly encountered adverse effects are deterioration of glycemic control, sexual dysfunction, electrolyte imbalance, and hyperlipidemia. Hypokalemia, induced by thiazides and loop di-

TABLE 11–3 Heart Disease Drugs for People with Diabetes

| Antihypertensives (Reduce High Blood Pressure) | Lipid-Modifying Drugs | |
	Cholesterol-Reducing	*Triglyceride-Reducing*
• Angiotensin-converting enzyme inhibitors: captopril (Capoten), lisinopril (Prinivil, Zestril), enalapril maleate (Vasotec), quinapril HCl (Accupril), fosinopril sodium (Monopril)	• HMG-CoA reductase inhibitors: fluvastatin sodium (Lescol), lovastatin (Mevacor), pravastatin sodium (Pravachol), simvastatin (Zocor)	• Fibric acid derivatives: gemfibrozil (Lopid), clofibrate (Atromid S)
• Calcium channel blockers: diltiazem (Cardizem), verapamil HCl (Calan and Isoptin), isradipine (DynaCirc)	• Resins: cholestyramine resin (Questran), colestipol HCl (Colestid)	• HMG-CoA reductase inhibitors: flurastatin sodium (Lescol), simvastatin (Zocor), pravastatin sodium (Pravachol), lovastatin (Mevacor)
• Alpha blockers: doxazosin mesylate (Cardura), ? (Hydrin), clonidine HCl (Catapres)	• Fibric acid derivatives: gemfibrozil (Lopid), clofibrate (Atromid S)	

uretics, is associated with reduced insulin release and increased insulin resistance, causing further deterioration of glucose tolerance in patients with type 2 diabetes. Diuretics may also cause hyperglycemia independent of hypokalemia (Kochar & Kalluru, 1994). See Table 11–3 for a list of antihypertensive drugs used in people with diabetes.

ACE inhibitors and CCBs are recommended as drugs of first choice for hypertensive patients with diabetes. These drugs provide excellent blood pressure control, promote a better metabolic profile, and offer renoprotection (Kochar & Kalluru, 1994).

CONCLUSION

Heart disease is a major health concern for everyone, but it should especially concern people with diabetes. CHD results from multiple interacting factors, including high blood pressure, dyslipidemia, obesity, smoking, and hyperglycemia. Microvascular and macrovascular complications are responsible for a large percentage of morbidity and mortality associated with diabetes. In type 2 diabetes, multiple risk factors are present, including insulin resistance, hyperinsulinemia, glucose intolerance, dyslipidemia, hypertension, obesity, and smoking. All play a role in the development and progression of CHD, even before significant and persistent hyperglycemia is present. The benefits of glucose control, ACE inhibitors, and lipid-lowering drugs in reducing the risk for diabetes-related complications have been clearly demonstrated. The challenge is to apply the results of population-based studies to the individual with diabetes who needs assistance.

As health-care providers, we need to invest in preventive strategies and interventions so as to improve the health and reduce the risk of CHD in people with diabetes. Emphasis on education, counseling, and medical treatment is essential. Each component of care is equally important and needs the expertise and skill of various team members. Comprehensive care necessitates such a broad spectrum of knowledge that no one professional can easily provide the array of services needed. Goals can be met and comprehensive care provided only with the collaborative efforts of the individual and the members of the interdisciplinary team. Furthermore, a major reduction in the morbidity and mortality associated with diabetes will come with a comprehensive approach to the reduction of CHD risk factors.

References

American Diabetes Association. (1989). Role of cardiovascular risk factors in prevention and treatment of microvascular disease in diabetes. *Diabetes Care, 12*(8), 573–579.

Barrett-Connor E., Cohn, B. A., Wingard, D. L., et al. (1991). Why is diabetes mellitus a stronger risk factor for fatal ischemic heart disease in women than in men? *Journal of the American Medical Association, 265*(5), 627–631.

Centers for Disease Control and Prevention. (1991). *Prevention and Treatment of Complications of Diabetes: A Guide for Primary Care Practitioners,* Atlanta, GA: U.S. Department of Health and Human Services, Public Health Services, Division of Diabetes Translation.

DeFronzo, R. A., & Ferrannini, E. (1991). Insulin resistance: A multifaceted syndrome responsible for type 2 diabetes, obesity, hypertension, dyslipidemia, and atherosclerotic cardiovascular disease. *Diabetes Care, 14*(3), 173.

DeFronzo, R. A. (1988). The triumvirate: Beta-cell, muscle, liver: A collusion responsible for type 2 diabetes. *Diabetes, 37*(6), 667.

D'Eramo-Melkus, G. (1993). Type II non-insulin-dependent diabetes mellitus. *Nursing Clinics of North America, 28*(1), 25.

Diabetes Control and Complications Trial Research Group. (1993). The effect of intensive treatment of diabetes on the development and progression of long-term complications in insulin-dependent diabetes mellitus. *New England Journal of Medicine, 329,* 977–986.

Dorman, J. S., McCarthy, B. J., O'Leary, L. A., & Koehler, A. N. (1995). Risk factors for insulin-dependent diabetes. *Diabetes in America,* 2nd ed. U.S. Department of Health and Human Services, Public Health Service, Division of Diabetes Translation. (NIH Publication no. 95–1468.)

Ford, E., & Newman, J. (1991). Smoking and diabetes mellitus: Findings from the 1988 behavioral risk factor surveillance system. *Diabetes Care, 14*(10), 871.

Greenspan, F. S., & Baxter, J. D. (1994). *Basic and Clinical Endocrinology.* Norwalk, CT: Appleton & Lange, pp. 571–634.

Haffner, S. M., Stern, M. P., Hazuda, H. P., et al. (1990). Cardiovascular risk factors in confirmed prediabetic individuals: Does the clock for coronary heart disease start ticking before the onset of clinical diabetes? *Journal of the American Medical Association, 263*(21), 2893–2898.

Harris, M. I. (1995). Summary. *Diabetes in America,* 2nd ed. U.S. Department of Health and Human Services, Public Health Service, Division of Diabetes Translation. (NIH Publication no. 95–1468.)

Hellman, R., Regan, J., & Rosen, H. (1997). Effect of intensive treatment of diabetes on the risk of death or renal failure in NIDDM and IDDM. *Diabetes Care, 20*(3), 258–264.

Helmrich, S. P., Ragland, D. R., Leung, R. W., & Paffenbarger, R. S. (1991). Physical activity and reduced occurrence of non-insulin dependent diabetes mellitus. *New England Journal of Medicine, 353*(3), 147–152.

Herman, W. H., & Greene, D. A. (1996). Microvascular complications of diabetes. In D. Haire-Joshu (Ed.), *Management of Diabetes Mellitus: Perspectives of Care Across the Life Span,* 2nd ed. St. Louis, MO: Mosby–Year Book, pp. 234–280.

Horton, E. S. (1988). Role and management of exercise in diabetes mellitus. *Diabetes Care, 11,* 201–211.

Kannel, W. B., D'Agostino, R. B., Wilson, P. W., et al. (1990). Diabetes, fibrinogen, and risk of cardiovascular disease: The Framingham experience. *American Heart Journal, 115,* 672–676.

Kaplan, N. (1989). The deadly quartet: Upper body obesity, glucose intolerance, hypertriglycerides, and hypertension. *Archives of Internal Medicine, 149,* 14.

Kochar, M. S., & Kalluru, V. B. (1994). Hypertension in the diabetic patient: Controlling its harmful effects. *Postgraduate Medicine, 96*(6), 101–110.

Leon, A. S. (1987). Leisure-time physical activity levels and risk of coronary heart disease and death: The Multiple Risk Factor Intervention Trial. *Journal of the American Medical Association, 258,* 2388–2395.

Lott, J. A. (1997). *Clinical Pathology of Pancreatic Disease.* Totowa, NJ: Humana Press Inc., pp. 1–5.

Levetan, C., & Ratner, R. (1995). The economic bottom line on preventive diabetes care. *Practical Diabetology, 14*(4), 10–19.

Lorber, D. L. (1994). Complications of diabetes: Cardiovascular disease. *Practical Diabetology, 13*(2), 15.

Manson, J. E., Colditz, G. A., Stampfer, M. J., et al. (1991). A prospective study of maturity-onset diabetes mellitus and risk of coronary heart disease and stroke in women. *Archives of Internal Medicine, 151*(6), 1141–1147.

McPhillips, J. B., Barrett-Connor, E., & Wingard, D. L. (1990). Cardiovascular disease risk factors prior to the diagnosis of impaired glucose tolerance and non-insulin dependent diabetes mellitus in a community of older adults. *American Journal of Epidemiology, 131*(3), 443–453.

Mitchell, B. D., Hazuda, H. P., Haffner, S. M., et al. (1991). Myocardial infarction in Mexican-Americans and non-Hispanic whites: The San Antonio Heart Study. *Circulation, 83*(1), 45–51.

Moller, D. E., & Flier, J. S. (1991). Insulin resistance: Mechanisms, syndromes, and implications. *New England Journal of Medicine, 325*(13), 938–948.

Nichaman, M. Z., Wear, M. L., Goff, D. C., et al. (1993). Hospitalization rates for myocardial infarction among Mexican-Americans and non-Hispanic whites: The Corpus Christi Heart Project. *Annals of Epidemiology, 3*(1), 42–48.

Pollock, M., Wilmore, J., & Fox, S. (1984). *Exercise in Health and Disease.* Philadelphia: W. B. Saunders Co.

Pyorala, K., Laaskso, M., & Uusitupa, M. (1987). Diabetes and atherosclerosis: An epidemiological view. *Diabetes/ Metabolism Reviews, 3,* 463.

Stamler, J., Vaccaro, O., Neaton, J. D., & Wentworth, D. (1993). Diabetes, other risk factors, and 12-year cardiovascular mortality for men screened in the Multiple Risk Factor Intervention Trial. *Diabetes Care, 16*(2), 434–444.

Stern, M. P. (1995). Diabetes and cardiovascular disease: The common soil hypothesis. *Diabetes, 44,* 369.

Taylor, S. I., Accili, D., & Imai, Y. (1994). Perspectives in diabetes: Insulin resistance or insulin deficiency. Which is the primary cause of type 2 diabetes? *Diabetes, 43,* 735.

Vinicor, F. (1996). Features of microvascular disease of diabetes. In D. Haire-Joshu (Ed.), *Management of Diabetes Mellitus: Perspectives of Care Across the Life Span,* 2nd ed. St. Louis: Mosby–Year Book, pp. 281–308.

CHAPTER 12

—
—
—
—
—
—
—
—
—
—
—

Cardioprotective Agents: Antioxidants and Alcohol

Donna D'Agostino
Judy Costello

Despite a decrease in mortality from coronary heart disease (CHD) over the last two decades, CHD remains the number one health problem in westernized countries (Gaziano & Manson, 1996). The decline in CHD rates is partially attributable to the modification of cardiovascular risk factors such as hypertension, smoking, and elevated blood cholesterol; however, a substantial amount of variation in CHD risk remains after these cardiovascular risk factors have been taken into account (Gaziano, 1994; Todd, Woodward, Bolton-Smith, & Tunstall-Pedoe, 1995). As a result, the role of cardioprotective agents, or of other factors that may help prevent CHD, has taken on increasing importance. In particular, speculation has increased regarding the function of antioxidant vitamins (beta-carotene; alpha-tocopherol, or vitamin E; and ascorbic acid, or vitamin C;) and alcohol as possible cardioprotective agents.

Efforts aimed at the reduction of modifiable risk factors are areas in which nurses and other clinicians can have a considerable impact. It is essential that nurses and other clinicians understand the evidence supporting antioxidant use. Therefore, this chapter will explore current research examining antioxidant vitamins and al-

cohol as agents that may reduce the risk of CHD. The chapter is divided into three sections: (1) antioxidants, (2) alcohol, and (3) practice implications for cardioprotective agents. The first two sections present proposed mechanisms of actions, cardioprotective effects, and epidemiologic observations. The last section will present practice implications based on current knowledge.

ANTIOXIDANTS

Contributions from basic research, animal studies, and clinical trials have provided evidence for the possible role of antioxidants in the prevention of CHD. An appreciation of the cardioprotective role of antioxidant vitamins requires a basic understanding of *reactive oxygen species* (ROS) and oxidized *low-density lipoprotein* (LDL). The mechanisms by which oxidation causes injury are complex (Crystal, 1991); therefore, a detailed discussion of oxidation concepts is beyond the scope of this chapter. Our focus will be on general principles and behavior of ROS as these species relate to CHD. For a more in-depth discussion of the role of ROS in health and disease, the reader is referred to Kerr, Bender, and Monti (1996) and Rice-Evans and Bruckdorfer (1992).

Reactive Oxygen Species

Reactive oxygen species is a term used in the literature to describe free radicals and nonradicals that are capable of causing oxidative damage to body tissues. A *free radical* is an atom, ion, or molecule with one or more unpaired electrons (Diplock, 1991; Halliwell, 1991; Machlin & Bendich, 1987). This configuration leads to increased reactivity with other molecules, because electrons like to pair up to form stable two-electron bonds. The electron configuration allows the radical to accept electrons *(reduction)* or donate them *(oxidation)* (Burrell & Blake, 1989).

Examples of free radicals include the superoxide radical ($O_2^{\bullet}$), the hydroxyl radical ($OH^{\bullet}$), and the peroxyl radical ($LOO^{\bullet}$). Other ROS, technically not free radicals because they lack the unpaired electron, remain capable of reactivity and can therefore produce oxidative damage (Rice-Evans & Bruckdorfer, 1992). Examples of nonradicals include hydrogen peroxide (H_2O_2) and singlet oxygen ($^1O_2$).

The occurrence of ROS is a normal consequence of many biologic processes (Machlin & Bendich, 1987; Rice-Evans & Bruckdorfer, 1992). ROS can originate from endogenous and exogenous sources. *Endogenous sources* include aerobic metabolism via electron transport chains, activated leukocytes, and enzymes (Frei, 1994). *Exogenous sources* include tobacco smoke, pollutants and organic solvents, anesthetics, hyperoxic environments, pesticides, radiation, and certain medications (Machlin & Bendich, 1987).

The steady formation of ROS is balanced by the body's antioxidant defense system. Oxidative damage occurs from an imbalance in this equilibrium in favor of the ROS (Sies, 1991). ROS can cause cell damage in many ways, ranging from causing specific mutations of deoxyribonucleic acid (DNA) to changes in enzyme activity, membrane function, and lipid peroxidation (Slater, 1991). Consequences of this biologic process include aging, autoimmune diseases, acquired immunodeficiency syndrome

(AIDS), cancer, and atherosclerosis, among others (Frei, 1994). Lipid peroxidation results in the oxidation of LDL, which has been implicated in the development of atherosclerosis (Abbey, Nestel, & Baghurst, 1993). The following section will illustrate the process of endogenous radical production that leads to lipid peroxidation.

During aerobic metabolism, the oxygen molecule (O_2) undergoes a stepwise reduction to water (H_2O). In the following equation, O_2 is an electron acceptor.

$$H + O_2 \rightarrow H_2O$$

During this chain reaction, a leakage of single electrons farther up in the chain leads to the partial reduction of O_2 to the superoxide radical ($O_2^{\bullet-}$) (Frei, 1994).

$$O_2 + e^{\bullet-} \rightarrow O_2^{\bullet-}$$

The superoxide radical is relatively unreactive. However, because of its electron configuration it may act as either a reducing or an oxidizing agent. Further univalent reduction of the superoxide radical yields a nonradical species, hydrogen peroxide (H_2O_2):

$$2O_2^{\bullet-} + 2H^+ \rightarrow H_2O_2 + O_2$$

Hydrogen peroxide can diffuse considerable distances from its site of generation and is able to cross cell membranes. Therefore, damage can occur at distant sites via the reduction of hydrogen peroxide to the hydroxyl radical ($OH^{\bullet}$) (Burrell & Blake, 1989). This reduction reaction, called the *Fenton reaction,* requires a transition metal such as the ferrous (Fe^{2+}) or cuprous (Cu^+) ion as catalyst (Burrell & Blake, 1989). For example,

$$H_2O_2 + Fe^{2+} \rightarrow OH^{\bullet} + OH^- + Fe^{3+}$$

The hydroxyl radical is the most reactive and aggressive oxidizing agent (Frei, 1994). If generated in vivo, it rapidly combines with molecules in its immediate vicinity. It is capable of attacking and damaging almost every molecule found in living cells. Reactions involving the hydroxyl radical have the ability to set off chain reactions. Lipid peroxidation, one chain reaction caused by the stimulation of the hydroxyl radical (Halliwell, 1991), is the auto-oxidation of *polyunsaturated fatty acid* (PUFA) side chains. This auto-oxidation occurs when a hydrogen atom (H$^{\cdot}$) is abstracted from a PUFA (shown as PH), leading to the formation of a carbon-centered lipid radical (L$^{\cdot}$):

$$PH \rightarrow L^{\cdot} + H^{\cdot}$$

The carbon-centered lipid radical (L$^{\cdot}$) combines with oxygen (O$_2$), creating the peroxyl radical (LOO$^{\cdot}$).

$$L^{\cdot} + O_2 \rightarrow LOO^{\cdot}$$

The lipid peroxyl radical can then react with adjacent PUFA side chains to form another carbon-centered lipid radical, thereby propagating the chain reaction of lipid peroxidation (Frei, 1994). The breakdown products of this process are responsible for modifying the LDL molecule (Frei, 1994; Halliwell, 1991). Therefore, a single reaction beginning with the formation of the superoxide radical initiates the process of lipid peroxidation, which has been implicated in the development of oxidized LDL and atherosclerosis.

Oxidation of LDL and Atherosclerosis

Elevation of LDL is thought to be a significant risk factor for coronary heart disease (CHD). Yet, up to two thirds of myocardial infarction survivors have no evidence of hyperlipidemia (Luc & Fruchart, 1991). One mechanism that may predispose a person to atherosclerosis is oxidation of the LDL particle (Maxwell, 1993). As discussed previously, oxidation of LDL is induced by ROS, and this oxidation leads to lipid peroxidation. Lipid peroxidation affects the chemical and physical properties of LDL (Niki, Yamamoto, Komuro, & Sato, 1991) by modifying apolipoprotein B (Frei, 1994). The new molecules formed from this modification are no longer recognized by the classic LDL receptor but are recognized only by the "scavenger" receptors found on macrophages (Hoffman & Garewal, 1995). The macrophages are unable to remove the intracellular cholesterol

content, causing an accumulation of oxidized LDL and the production of lipid-laden foam cells (Abbey, Nestel, & Baghurst, 1993; Frei, 1994; Hoffman & Garewal, 1995). The fatty streak, composed of lipid-laden foam cells, is believed to be the earliest lesion of atherosclerosis (Hoffman & Garewal, 1995). In order to fully understand these concepts related to atherogenesis, the reader is referred to Chapter 2.

Oxidized LDL has other biologic effects important to the development of atherosclerosis. These effects include chemotactic attraction of phagocytic cells, inhibition of macrophage migration, cytotoxicity toward endothelial cells, and stimulation of platelet aggregation (Hoffman & Garewal, 1995; Maxwell, 1993). Significant animal and human in vivo evidence supports the role of oxidized LDL in atherogenesis. Antibodies against oxidized LDL have been detected in atherosclerotic lesions of rabbit aortas (Hoffman & Garewal, 1995). Autoantibodies that reacted with several forms of oxidized LDL were found in both rabbit and human plasma (Yla-Herttuala, Palinske, & Rosenreid, 1989). In human subjects, oxidized LDL has been recovered from atherosclerotic plaque (Shaik, Martini, & Quincy, 1988) as well as from human plasma (Hoffman & Garewal, 1995).

The implication that oxidized LDL promotes atherosclerosis has stimulated interest in factors that may offer protection from oxidative damage. Current theoretical approaches hypothesize that antioxidants can inhibit the oxidation of LDL and therefore prevent or slow the progression of atherosclerosis (Frei, 1994).

ROS, Oxidized LDL, and Antioxidants

The potentially deleterious reactions of ROS are controlled by antioxidant defense systems (Frei, 1994). An *antioxidant* is defined as any substance that significantly delays or prevents oxidation of a substrate and that has a low concentration relative to the oxidizable substrate (Halliwell, 1991). Thus, antioxidants act by (1) scavenging biologically important radicals, (2) preventing their formation, or (3) repairing resultant damage. In terms of ROS and human disease, experts conceptualize a balance, with ROS on one side and antioxidants on the other (Crystal, 1991). When an imbalance occurs in the equilibrium between ROS and antioxidants favoring the ROS side, oxidative stress occurs (Sies, 1991). In this situation, radical production can be damaging (Rice-Evans & Bruckdorfer, 1992), because the production of ROS overwhelms the antioxidant defense system and results in cell damage (Machlin & Bendich, 1987).

In the human body, the antioxidant defense system is extensive, consisting of both enzymatic and nonenzymatic systems (Frei, 1994). Enzymatic antioxidant defense systems include superoxide dismutases and hydroperoxidases such as glutathione peroxidase, catalase, and other hemoprotein peroxidases (Sies, 1991; Halliwell, 1991) Glutathione is the most important cellular thiol, acting as a substrate for several transferases, peroxidases, and other enzymes that prevent or mitigate the harmful effects of oxygen free radicals (DiMascio, et al., 1991). These antioxidant enzymes are primarily intracellular, so extracellular ROS must be inactivated by nonenzymatic antioxidants (Machlin & Bendich, 1987; Rice-Evans & Bruckdorfer, 1992).

Nonenzymatic antioxidants that can inactivate ROS include alpha-tocopherol (vitamin E), ascorbic acid (vitamin C), and beta-carotene (DiMascio, Murphy, & Sies, 1991; Frei, 1994). These antioxidants can be separated into lipid-soluble and water-soluble antioxidants. Vitamin E and beta-carotene are lipid-soluble and are localized to membranes and lipoproteins, whereas vitamin C is water-soluble and is present in extracellular and intracellular fluids (Frei, 1994; Maxwell, 1993). As the daily intake of these antioxidant vitamins affects the circulating blood level, low intake theoretically reduces the body's extracellular defense system against free radical damage (Machlin & Bendich, 1987) (Fig. 12–1).

Antioxidant Protection of LDL

In vitro, LDL oxidation can be prevented by naturally occurring antioxidants such as vitamin E, vitamin C, and beta-carotene (Hoffman & Garewal, 1995; Jialal & Grundy, 1993). The LDL particle contains the lipid-soluble antioxidants vitamin E and beta-carotene, which func-

tion to protect it from lipid peroxidation (Maxwell, 1993). Vitamin E, the most abundant antioxidant in LDL, is a chain-breaking antioxidant (Frei, 1994). It scavenges peroxyl radicals, thus interrupting the chain reaction of lipid peroxidation (Esterbauer, Dieber-Rotheneder, Striegl, & Waeg, 1991; Frei, 1994). The content of vitamin E in circulating LDL determines the degree of resistance to oxidation (Halliwell, 1991).

Research indicates that (1) oxidation of PUFAs in LDL is preceded by a loss of endogenous antioxidants and that (2) supplementation of the culture medium with vitamin E prevents oxidation of LDL by cells (Esterbauer, Dieber-Rotheneder, Striegl, & Waeg, 1991). Similarly, when the supply of vitamin E is depleted, the oxidation rate of LDL increases (Niki, Yamamoto, Komuro, & Sato, 1991). But the antioxidant function of vitamin E should not be viewed in isolation, because vitamin C promotes its antioxidant function.

Vitamin C functions as a first defense when ROS are generated in plasma (Hoffman & Garewal, 1995; Niki, Yamamoto, Komuro, & Sato, 1991). It reacts directly with superoxide, hydroxyl radicals, and singlet oxygen (Hoffman & Garewal, 1995), to protect LDL against oxidation, by effectively intercepting peroxyl radicals in the aqueous phase before they can attack and damage lipids (Sies & Stahl, 1995; Frei, 1991). Furthermore, vitamin C facilitates the regeneration of oxidized vitamin E, thereby maintaining the antioxidant pool within the LDL particle (Frei, 1994; Machlin & Bendich, 1987). When vitamin C and vitamin E were compared regarding the oxidative modification of LDL, vitamin C was found to be a more potent antioxidant owing to its ability to regenerate oxidized vitamin E (Jialal, Vega, & Grundy, 1990).

Beta-carotene is also present in the LDL particle but in lower concentration than vitamin E. It is the last antioxidant to be consumed under oxidizing conditions, and it functions as an anti oxidant only after vitamin E is depleted. Beta-carotene primarily quenches singlet oxygen, but it can scavenge peroxyl radicals at low physiologic oxygen tensions (Frei, 1994). The mechanism of action of beta-carotene in LDL oxidation and its relative importance as an antioxidant are unclear. Study findings on the influence of beta-carotene on LDL oxidation

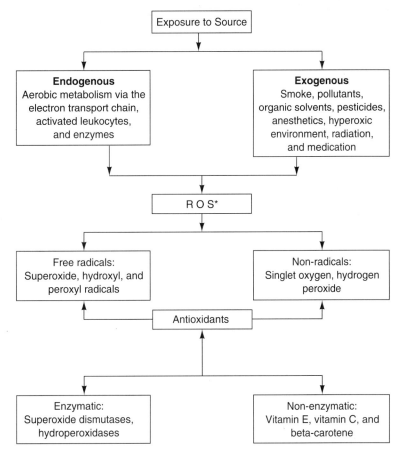

FIGURE 12–1 Proposed mechanisms for free radical formation and antioxidant action.

*ROS = reactive oxygen species composed of free radicals and non-radicals, produced by endogenous and exogenous sources, and kept in check by the function of antioxidants. An imbalance results in oxidative stress.

have been inconsistent. On one hand, beta-carotene has been shown to inhibit LDL oxidation in both cellular and cell-free systems (Jialal & Grundy, 1993). On the other hand, a 20-fold enrichment of beta-carotene levels in plasma and LDL did not enhance protection of LDL against oxidative stress (Witztum, Reaven, & Parthasarathy, 1993). Alternatively, beta-carotene may not inhibit LDL oxidation, but it may preserve endothelial function, reduce platelet aggregability, or even alter the lipoprotein profile (Gaziano & Hennekens, 1993).

In conclusion, antioxidant vitamins presumably offer protection against CHD by preventing the oxidation of LDL; however, studies have shown that the vitamins may also preserve endothelial function, affect hemostasis (Gaziano & Hennekens, 1993), and lower both LDL cholesterol and blood pressure (Trout, 1991).

Translating this theoretical research into evaluating the impact of antioxidant levels and intake on human health depends largely on evidence from epidemiologic observations and ongoing randomized trials.

Epidemiologic Observations and Ongoing Randomized Trials

Observational epidemiologic data have suggested that individuals with the highest antioxidant levels have a reduced risk of developing CHD regardless of whether antioxidants are consumed through diet or supplementation (Manson, Gaziano, Jonas, & Hennekens, 1993). Several studies have focused on antioxidant vitamin intake in female subjects. The Iowa Women's Health Study examined the relationship between antioxidant vitamins and death from CHD in 34,486 postmenopausal women (Kushi, Folsom, Prineae, et al., 1996). Data were gathered through questionnaires that assessed antioxidant vitamin intake from food and supplements. Results of the study revealed an inverse relationship between vitamin E consumption and death from CHD: The higher the intake of vitamin E, the lower the risk of death. This relationship was sustained even when the analysis was adjusted for confounding variables. However, the effect of high-dose supplementation and duration of supplementation were not well addressed. Thus, the influence of vitamin supplements was difficult to ascertain. The risk of death from CHD was not associated with intake of vitamins A and C.

The Nurses' Health Study of 87,245 female nurses examined the effects of antioxidant intake upon the primary prevention of CHD. Antioxidant intake (food and supplements) was determined from a diet questionnaire. A total antioxidant score was obtained by summing the scores for intake of vitamin E, vitamin C, and beta-carotene. Subjects who consumed the most antioxidants (highest total scores) were compared with those who consumed the least (lowest total scores). An 8-year follow-up revealed a total of 552 cases of CHD, including 115 CHD-related deaths and 437 nonfatal myocardial infarctions. After adjustment for age, smoking, and other risk factors, a decreased *relative risk* (RR) of CHD was observed for those with the highest total antioxidant vitamin score (RR = 0.54).

Of the individual antioxidants, vitamin E afforded the greatest cardioprotective benefit against CHD (RR = 0.66 for vitamin E, 0.78 for beta-carotene, and 0.80 for vitamin C). This study suggests that women taking antioxidants, particularly vitamin E, had a reduced risk of CHD (Manson, Gaziano, Jonas, & Hennekens, 1993; Stampfer, Hennekens, Manson, et al., 1993).

Similar findings with respect to the influence of antioxidant vitamins on the risk of CHD were found in a large study with male subjects. The Health Professional Follow-up Study enrolled 51,529 male health professionals aged 40–75 years. Results confirmed the association between higher vitamin E intake (at least 100 IU for a minimum of 2 years) and lower risk of CHD (RR = 0.68). Beta-carotene intake was inversely associated with risk only for current and former smokers, whereas vitamin C was not associated with a lower risk of CHD (Gaziano & Manson, 1996; Rimm, Stampfer, Ascherio, et al., 1993). An inverse correlation between plasma vitamin E and mortality from CHD was also observed in cross-cultural epidemiologic studies (Gey, Puska, Jordan, & Moser, 1991).

Other studies examined the effect of beta-carotene on CHD. The Basel Prospective Study measured baseline serum beta-carotene in 2,974 middle-aged men. Results of the study revealed an increased risk (RR = 1.53, 95% confidence interval) of death from CHD among those with the lowest plasma beta-carotene levels as compared with those who had higher levels (Gaziano, 1996). Similarly, serum beta-carotene levels of patients with CHD were found to be lower than those of control groups (Torun, Yardim, Sargin, & Simsek, 1994).

Unfortunately, results from two studies have shown that beta-carotene increases the risk of lung cancer in smokers and other high-risk groups (exposure to asbestos) (Erdman, Russell, Rock, et al., 1996; DeLuca & Ross, 1996). The Finnish Alpha-Tocopherol, Beta Carotene Cancer Prevention Study investigated the influence of vitamin E and beta-carotene on CHD in 29,133 Finnish male smokers. Subjects received 20 mg of beta-carotene and/or 50 mg of vitamin E daily. After 6 years follow-up, neither vitamin E nor beta-carotene had produced statistically significant differences in CHD mortality. In fact, subjects in the beta-carotene group had a statistically significant 18% higher risk of lung cancer and a small but significant 11% increase in mortality from ischemic heart disease. The vitamin E group had a statistically significant 50% higher rate of cerebral hemorrhage (Hennekens, Gaziano, Manson, & Buring, 1995; Hennekens & Buring, 1994).

The Beta-Carotene and Retinol Efficacy Study (CARET), a randomized, double-blind, placebo-controlled trial studying primary prevention of lung cancer and cardiovascular disease, enrolled 18,314 smokers, former smokers, and workers exposed to asbestos. Subjects received daily supplementation of 30 mg of beta-carotene and 25,000 IU of retinol (vitamin A). Results of the study revealed that after 4 years of follow-up, the active treatment group had a 28% higher incidence of lung cancer, a 17% increase in overall mortality, and a 26% increase in rate of death from cardiovascular causes (Omenn, Goodman, Thornquist, et al., 1996). The CARET study was stopped based on these findings (Greenberg & Spore, 1996).

Although the data from these blood-based and dietary-intake studies may indicate a correlation between CHD and antioxidant vitamins, criteria for identifying a causal relationship between antioxidant vitamins and CHD have not yet been met. Vitamin users may be more health-conscious than nonusers and may have other characteristics or behaviors that put them at a lower risk for CHD. Furthermore, methods used to store samples and questions regarding the stability of vitamins at the temperature used for storage may influence results (Gaziano & Hennekens, 1993). Many inconsistencies exist, necessitating the need for large numbers of participants in randomized clinical trials before conclusions can be drawn about the effect of antioxidant vitamins. Several such large, randomized trials are under way (Gaziano, 1996).

The Physicians' Health Study ($n = 22,071$), ongoing at the time of this writing, uses a double-blind, placebo-controlled design to test the effect of beta-carotene (50 mg), taken on alternate days, on the primary and secondary prevention of cardiovascular disease. A subset of the sample ($n = 333$) with a history of cardiac disease (stable angina or previous coronary revascularization) was analyzed separately to examine secondary prevention. Preliminary findings in this group revealed that subjects with a cardiac history had a 51% reduction in risk of major coronary events and a 54% reduction in risk of major vascular events. This benefit, not noted until the second year of follow-up, suggests that the benefits of antioxidant therapy may require relatively prolonged periods of administration (Manson, Gaziano, Jonas, & Hennekens, 1993). With respect to primary prevention, a subsequent analysis of data from the Physicians' Health Study revealed that after 12 years of beta-carotene supplementation, there were no differences between the treatment and placebo groups in the incidence of cardiovascular disease (Hennekens, Buring, Manson, et al., 1996).

The Women's Health Study (WHS), also on-going at the time of this writing, uses a double-blind, placebo-controlled design to examine the influence of beta-carotene (50 mg), vitamin E (600 IU), and low-dose aspirin (100 mg), taken on alternate days, in the primary prevention of cardiovascular disease and cancer in 40,000 female health professionals aged 45 years or older. The Women's Antioxidant Cardiovascular Disease Study, which evolved from the WHS, examines antioxidant use and secondary prevention of cardiovascular disease in 8,000 nurses with a documented history of cardiovascular disease. Subjects receive antioxidant supplementation of 50 mg of beta-carotene, 600 IU of vitamin E, and 500 mg of vitamin C, taken on alternate days (Hennekens, Gaziano, Manson, & Buring, 1995). The findings of these two studies are expected to further clarify the relationship between antioxidant vitamins and cardiovascular risk in women with cardiac disease.

In summary, the results of studies examining the relationship between antioxidant vitamins and CHD are promising but not conclusive. Evidence does not yet support the routine use of antioxidant vitamins as cardioprotective agents. Further results from ongoing trials are required to delineate and confirm the role of antioxidant vitamins in the prevention of CHD.

ALCOHOL

As with antioxidant vitamins, interest in the role of alcohol as a cardioprotective agent has been increasing. The cardioprotective effects of moderate alcohol consumption have been a source of debate for over a century, ever since Cabot first reported that atherosclerosis was uncommon in alcoholics (Srivastava, Vasisht, Agarwal, & Goedde, 1994). A moderate alcohol intake is considered to be one to two standard-size drinks per day (1–2 oz, or 30–50 g) (Brown, 1990).

Cardioprotective Effects of Alcohol

A number of studies have examined the influence of alcohol consumption on CHD events. The results of these studies are difficult to compare owing to differing methods of measuring

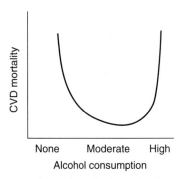

FIGURE 12–2   The U-shaped relationship between alcohol consumption and mortality from cardiovascular disease.

alcohol consumption and multiple outcome measures, including lipid levels, incidence of myocardial infarction, fatal and nonfatal CHD events, and evidence of atherosclerosis on angiography. Despite these methodologic issues, results from epidemiologic studies consistently demonstrate an inverse trend between low-to-moderate alcohol consumption and CHD. A U-shaped relationship between alcohol consumption and mortality from cardiovascular disease has been described, with heavy drinkers experiencing a higher risk of death than moderate drinkers, but moderate drinkers experiencing a lower risk of death than abstainers (Ahlawat & Siwach, 1994) (Fig. 12–2). With respect to total mortality and alcohol consumption, a J-shaped curve has been identified in which mortality increases significantly with increasing amount of daily intake (Pearson, 1996) (Fig. 12–3).

In the Framingham study, moderate alcohol consumption produced a beneficial effect in men with respect to mortality from CHD, but the findings for women were inconclusive. The

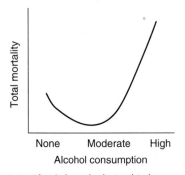

FIGURE 12–3   The J-shaped relationship between alcohol consumption and total mortality.

results also revealed that different types of alcoholic beverages have differing cardioprotective effects. For nonsmokers, consumption of beer or wine provided a greater reduction in CHD risk than spirits (Friedman & Kimball, 1986).

In a case-control study, Gaziano and co-workers (1993) investigated the relationship between alcohol consumption, lipoprotein levels, and risk of myocardial infarction (MI) in 340 subjects who had MIs and an equal number of age- and sex-matched controls. Logistic regression analyses estimated risks, revealing a significant inverse association between alcohol consumption and risk of MI ($p < .001$) after controlling for known coronary risk factors. In addition, total *high-density lipoprotein* (HDL) and its HDL_2 and HDL_3 subfractions were strongly associated with alcohol consumption ($p < .001$ for each).

Two studies investigated the relationship between alcohol consumption and angiographically documented *coronary artery disease* (CAD) (Ducimetiere, Marciniak, Milon, et al., 1993; Handa, Sasaki, Saku, et al., 1990). Both studies found that a moderate consumption of alcohol was associated with a lower incidence of CAD after controlling for other risk factors.

The influence of moderate beer consumption on blood coagulation was examined in 28 patients with CAD (Gorinstein, Zemser, Lichman, et al., 1997). Twenty-two subjects were assigned to the experimental group, while six represented the control group. Subjects in the experimental group consumed 330 ml of beer per day for 30 days. Results showed a statistically significant decrease in thrombogenic activity (specifically the activity of Factor VII and Factor VII antigens) in the experimental group.

In a cohort study involving male subjects ($n = 11,688$) enrolled in the Multiple Risk Factor Intervention Trial, the relationship between alcohol use, mortality from CHD, and HDL cholesterol levels was investigated (Suh, Shaten, Cutler, & Kuller, 1992). Subjects were assessed over a 6-year period and mortality assessed during a 3.8-year follow-up period. Study results revealed an inverse relationship between alcohol consumption and death from CHD. As alcohol intake increased by an average of seven drinks per week, the relative risk of death from CHD was .89 ($p = 0.043$). The investigators also noted that the inverse relationship could be partially explained by an increase in HDL levels.

The few studies investigating the cardioprotective effects of alcohol in female subjects demonstrate similar findings to those for male subjects. A cross-sectional study of 1,048 British women in two large centers revealed that moderate alcohol consumption was associated with lower levels of cardiovascular risk (as measured by increased HDL levels and lower triglyceride levels) (Razay, Heaton, Bolton, & Hughes, 1992). In the Nurses' Health Study, middle-aged women who consumed one alcoholic drink per day had approximately 50% lower risk of nonfatal myocardial infarction or death resulting from CHD than nondrinkers did, after other coronary risk factors were adjusted for. Although moderate alcohol intake was shown to decrease the risk of CHD and ischemic stroke, there was a small increased risk of subarachnoid hemorrhage (Stampfer, Colditz, Willett, et al., 1988). Longer-term follow-up in the Nurses' Health Study (12 years) validates the decreased risk of death from CHD for women with light to moderate alcohol intake (Fuchs, Stampfer, Colditz, et al., 1995). This benefit was greater for older women (50–70 years of age) and for those who had a greater risk of CHD (as measured by the presence of one or more coronary risk factors). Heavier drinking (more than 30 g of alcohol intake per day) was associated with increased mortality, largely owing to noncardiovascular causes, including breast cancer and cirrhosis (Fuchs, Stampfer, Colditz, et al., 1995).

Studies regarding the cardioprotective effect of alcohol have focused predominantly on the amount of alcohol consumed. Few studies have investigated the effect of frequency, type, and past history of alcohol consumption. One study investigated the influence of beer, wine, and spirits on the rate of CHD in 21 countries. Intake of all three types of alcohol (analyzed separately) revealed a significant negative correlation with CHD, although the relationship was stronger for wine ethanol ($r = -0.66$) (Criqui & Ringel, 1994).

A number of methodologic issues affect the body of research examining the influence of alcohol consumption on CHD. Two of these issues are (1) the accuracy of reporting of alcohol consumption and (2) the influence of subjects who have quit drinking because of ill health and thus are now reporting as abstainers or moderate drinkers (Marmot & Brunner, 1991). Despite issues such as these, the cardioprotective effects of moderate alcohol consumption on CHD have been well supported by large studies across diverse populations (Kannel & Ellison, 1996). In addition, all three types of alcohol—wine, beer, and spirits—have been found to reduce CHD risk (Gaziano & Manson, 1996).

The negative effects of heavy drinking have also been well documented. Excess alcohol intake has been associated with a variety of problems, including hypertension, arrhythmias, cardiomyopathy, cirrhosis, stroke, pancreatitis, accidents, fetal alcohol syndrome, and some types of cancer, including breast, upper gastrointestinal, and large bowel (Pearson, 1996; Berlin, 1996; Kannel & Ellison, 1996; Ahlawat & Siwach, 1994; Friedman & Klatsky, 1993; Srivastava, Vasisht, Agarwal, & Goedde, 1994).

Mechanism of Alcohol as a Cardioprotective Agent

The effects of alcohol consumption on CHD are complex, and the cardioprotective effects of alcohol are not well understood (Gaziano, Buring, Breslow, et al., 1993; Srivastava, Vasisht, Agarwal, & Goedde, 1994). To date, several mechanisms have been identified that may account for the cardioprotective effects of alcohol. One mechanism relates to the finding that alcohol intake increases levels of HDL cholesterol and its subfractions HDL_2 and HDL_3 (Gaziano, Buring, Breslow, et al., 1993). In fact, it has been shown that the increase in HDL levels accounts for approximately 50% of the protective effect of alcohol (Pearson, 1996). Alcohol intake has also been found to raise apolipoprotein A-I and A-4I levels (Kannel & Ellison, 1996).

A second mechanism by which alcohol may influence the development of CHD relates to the coagulation system. This effect is twofold: (1) alcohol consumption had been shown to decrease platelet aggregability and fibrinogen levels, thus reducing the likelihood of thrombosis, and (2) alcohol may enhance the breakdown

TABLE 12–1 Cardioprotective Effects of Alcohol and Proposed Mechanisms

Lipid levels	Increased HDL
	Increased HDL_2
	Increased HDL_3
	Increased apolipoprotein A
	Increased apolipoprotein A-II
Coagulation	Decreased platelet aggregability
	Increased clot breakdown
Nonalcoholic phenols and flavonoids	(Mechanisms being delineated)
Other effects	Promotion of relaxation
	Decreased stress

of clot through the increase in release of plasminogen activator (Gorinstein, Zemser, Lichman, et al., 1997; Pearson, 1996; Kannel & Ellison, 1996; Preedy & Richardson, 1994; Friedman & Klatsky, 1993; Stampfer, Colditz, Willett, et al., 1988). Others have suggested that the cardioprotective effect of alcohol could be exerted by nonalcoholic substances in particular beverages such as wine. These substances, called *phenols* and *flavonoids,* have been found to exert antioxidant properties (Pearson, 1996; Goldberg, Hahn, & Parkes, 1995). Finally, it has been suggested that alcohol may induce relaxation and thus reduce psychological stress; the decreased risk of CHD in moderate drinkers persisted after studies controlled for elevated HDL and decreased blood pressure (Handa, Sasaki, Saku, et al., 1990) (Table 12–1).

Although an inverse relationship between alcohol consumption and CHD has been established, it is clear that further research is required regarding extraneous variables and mechanism of action. Reliable measures of confounding variables in the alcohol-CHD relationship are necessary, as strong associations exist between (1) alcohol consumption and cigarette smoking and (2) alcohol consumption and high blood pressure (Suh, Shaten, Cutler, & Kuller, 1992). Other variables that may influence the association between alcohol and CHD include age, social class, and body mass index (Shaper, Wannamethee, & Walker, 1994). In addition, the frequency of consumption, type of alcohol consumed, and past history of consumption are a few of the important aspects that need to be elucidated in further study.

PRACTICE IMPLICATIONS FOR CARDIOPROTECTIVE AGENTS

In the practice setting, patients may have great difficulty interpreting the ambiguous and often confusing information regarding cardioprotective agents. Therefore, an important component of the clinician's role is to facilitate the patient's decision making by providing knowledge. The nature of informational support depends on the type of cardioprotective agent and the specific patient characteristics, such as educational level and decision-making style. Guiding principles used by the clinician should address the patient's (1) characteristics as well as current use and knowledge of cardioprotective agents, (2) intentions and interest in using cardioprotective agents, and (3) individual risk-benefit ratio regarding the use of these agents (Table 12–2). In the following sections, we have attempted to use these guiding principles to clarify practice implications for various cardioprotective agents.

TABLE 12–2 Guiding Principles for Use of Cardioprotective Agents

- Assess patient educational level and decision-making style.
- Assess current use of cardioprotective agents and other drugs.
    Alcohol: Assess type, frequency, and amount of current intake.
    Antioxidants: Note that vitamin E is contraindicated for patients on warfarin sodium (Coumadin).
- Assess intention and interest regarding use of cardioprotective agents.
    Alcohol: Note that alcohol is not recommended to prevent CHD.
    Antioxidants: Provide patient with knowledge of dietary sources; provide RDA of antioxidants; reinforce modification of classic risk factors.
- Assess patient's individual risk-benefit ratio for cardioprotective agents.
    Alcohol: Assess tendency toward excess intake of alcohol; presence of cancer, hypertension, or obesity; and family history. Note that moderate intake of alcohol may decrease risk of CAD.
    Antioxidants: Long-term supplement use has not been studied, but antioxidants have no side effects and may have protective benefits.

Antioxidants

The existing data on the beneficial effect of antioxidant vitamins are encouraging; however, much controversy exists as to the recommendation and use of supplements. Most of the evidence in favor of the use of antioxidants is based on epidemiologic studies. Unfortunately, the designs of these studies frequently prevent identification of cause-and-effect relationships. In addition, information available to date from several randomized clinical trials has shown no effect of antioxidant intake on CHD risk, and some have even revealed potential adverse effects. Although nutritional research has consistently shown lower rates of heart disease and stroke in those who consume a diet consisting of higher amounts of fruits and vegetables (Gaziano, 1996), there are a number of controversies in this area to consider.

Currently the *recommended dietary allowance* (RDA) is 15 IU of vitamin E for adult males and 12 IU of vitamin E for adult females, 60 mg of vitamin C for both adult males and females, and 5,000 IU of beta-carotene for adult males and 4,000 IU of beta-carotene for adult females. It is unclear whether the RDA should be based on levels needed for normal nutrient function or levels associated with optimal health and prevention of chronic disease (Reynolds, 1994). In many of the studies of the relationship between cardiovascular disease and antioxidant consumption, the amount of the antioxidant vitamin consumed exceeded the RDA and exceeded the amount that would be obtained by consumption of a varied diet (Abbey, Nestel, & Baghurst, 1993; Jialal & Grundy, 1993; Stampfer, Hennekens, Manson, et al., 1993; Rimm, Stampfer, Ascherio, et al., 1993).

The amount of antioxidant vitamins necessary for the prevention of CHD remains unknown. The use of antioxidants, even at one order of magnitude higher than the RDA, is not associated with toxic side effects (Pryor, 1991). Yet, fat-soluble vitamins are stored in the body and may cause adverse effects when taken in excess. And water-soluble vitamins, although readily excreted, can have adverse effects when large doses are taken for prolonged periods (Wilson, 1994).

Questions about whether or not to supplement antioxidant vitamin intake remain largely unanswered. Those in favor of supplementation feel that antioxidants may offer protection from chronic disease (Kendler, 1995). Whereas these "pro-supplementers" agree that the best source of antioxidants is in the foods consumed—namely, at least five servings of fruits and vegetables daily—they note that only 1 in 11 Americans eats five servings of fruits and vegetables daily (Anonymous, 1994). Moreover, in any recommendation, the cost to individuals should be considered in regard to particular types of food, fortified foods, or nutritional supplements, and of these, nutritional supplements are the least expensive (Blumberg, 1995). Nevertheless, vitamins cannot replace a well-balanced diet, nor can they make up for a lack of exercise or counteract the effects of smoking (Anonymous, 1994).

The Alliance for Aging is the first public health organization to recommend vitamin supplements for disease prevention. This organization has advised Americans to take large doses of vitamin C, vitamin E, and beta-carotene in addition to their diet. The daily recommendations from the Alliance for Aging include 250–1,000 mg of vitamin C, 100–400 IU of vitamin E, and 17,000–50,000 IU of beta-carotene. However, the very wide dosing ranges leave the public and clinicians with many unanswered questions.

As no consensus exists regarding the use of antioxidants, the clinician may choose to use the guiding principles mentioned previously (see Table 12–2). The first guiding principle, which advocates assessing the patient's characteristics and current use of antioxidants, gives the clinician an opportunity to review the specific antioxidants and amount being consumed as well as other drugs taken by the patient. The clinician should be aware that high levels of vitamin E should not be recommended for persons on anticoagulant therapy (Pryor, 1991). In large amounts, vitamin E can antagonize vitamin K and prolong the prothrombin time, thus potentiating the effect of oral anticoagulants (Wilson, 1994). Excess vitamin E should also not be recommended in the presence of deficiency of vitamin K (a fat-soluble vitamin critical to hemostasis). This vitamin deficiency can occur as a result of inadequate dietary intake, intestinal malabsorption syndromes, or hepato-cellular disease (Handin, 1994).

The second guiding principle advocates assessing the patient's intentions and interest regarding the use of antioxidants for disease prevention. Once the patient expresses interest in the use of antioxidants, the clinician should first recommend a diet that includes at least five servings of fruits and vegetables per day. The patient should understand that antioxidants are not a replacement for a low-fat diet, exercise, smoking cessation, and stress management. At the present time, there is far more evidence to support the benefits of modification of the classic risk factors than the use of antioxidants.

Interested patients may be provided with the recommendations from the Alliance for Aging on antioxidant vitamins, as well as a list of food sources high in antioxidants (Table 12–3). Highly motivated patients may require further informational support and ongoing monitoring for adverse responses to cardioprotective agents.

The third guiding principle advocates assessing the risk-benefit ratio for each individual patient. Although there are no known side effects from the use of antioxidants, and they may offer some protection against CHD, study findings regarding the adverse effects of antioxidant vitamins should be considered based on individual assessments. The long-term use of antioxidants has not been studied and may be associated with other health risks. It is important that patients understand the lack of scientific data verifying the amount and effectiveness of antioxidants as cardioprotective agents. In the final analysis, patients regulate their own use of antioxidants; therefore, the clinician's role is to facilitate decision making,

provide knowledge and information, and monitor for adverse effects.

Alcohol

Substantial evidence of an inverse relationship between moderate alcohol consumption and CHD risk exists. Despite this apparent benefit of moderate alcohol consumption, there is strong consensus among clinicians and researchers that a general public health recommendation to drink in order to prevent CHD is not recommended because of an adverse risk-benefit ratio (Ahlawat & Siwach, 1994; Criqui & Ringel, 1994; Gaziano, Buring, Breslow, et al., 1993; Marmot & Brunner, 1991; Shaper, Wannamethee, & Walker, 1994; Srivastava, Vasisht, Agarwal, & Goedde, 1994). Any recommendation to individuals regarding the cardioprotective effects of moderate alcohol consumption should take into account the physiologic, psychological, and metabolic effects of alcohol (Gaziano, Buring, Breslow, et al., 1993).

Several sources have outlined recommendations regarding alcohol consumption (Pearson, 1996; Gaziano & Hennekens, 1995; Ashley, Ferrence, Rankin, et al., 1994; Pearson & Terry, 1994). The same guiding principles delineated for antioxidant use can also be applied (see Table 12–2). The clinician must conduct a thorough health history that addresses the current use of alcohol, including the type, frequency, and amount consumed. In addition, individual lifestyle, potential to consume alcohol in excess, health practices, and family history of hypertension, alcoholism, liver disease, and breast cancer should be explored.

The use of standardized screening questionaires such as CAGE or MAST has been recommended for cardiac patients (Pearson & Terry, 1994; Preedy & Richardson, 1994). For patients who consume alcohol, published recommendations regarding alcohol consumption indicate that moderation consists of a daily limit of two drinks per day for men and one to one and a half drinks per day for women. These differences reflect concern for the increased incidence of breast cancer in women with alcohol consumption (Gaziano & Hennekens, 1995). Patients who consume more than the defined

TABLE 12–3 Antioxidant Food Sources

Vitamin E	Vitamin C	Beta-Carotene
Nuts and seeds	Citrus fruits	Carrots
Whole grains	Green peppers	Spinach
Legumes	Broccoli	Broccoli
Corn	Cauliflower	Squash
Seafood	Brussels	Sweet potatoes
Soy and	sprouts	Apricots
safflower oil		Cantaloupe

level for moderation should be advised to reduce their intake.

Those who do not consume alcohol should not be encouraged to start, as the risks associated with alcohol consumption should not be ignored. Moderate alcohol consumption may contribute to problems in maintaining ideal weight and an increase in triglyceride levels (particularly in women). Alcohol consumption may also have an indirect effect on the development of CHD, given that intake levels of two to three drinks per day may contribute to an increased risk of hypertension (Srivastava, Vasisht, Agarwal, & Goedde, 1994). In addition, excess consumption of alcohol on a routine and long-term basis may increase the risk of developing cardiomyopathy. For some, moderate intake may lead to heavier consumption and associated social problems. Furthermore, possible benefits must be balanced with increases in the incidence of subarachnoid hemorrhage, cancer, and other health problems. Pregnant women and patients on medications that may interact with alcohol should be advised to refrain from alcohol consumption.

CONCLUSION

The cardioprotective effects of antioxidant vitamins and moderate alcohol consumption have been the focus of much research, and findings are promising. However, the issues associated with both of these areas are complex; further research is required. Nurses should continue to provide education to patients and family members regarding classic risk-factor modification for CHD. In addition, the current status of research regarding cardioprotective agents such as antioxidant vitamins and moderate alcohol consumption should also be provided to enhance public awareness of the debate and controversies in these areas of research and allow individuals to make informed decisions regarding their health.

References

Abbey, M., Nestel, P., & Baghurst, A. (1993). Antioxidant vitamins and low-density lipoprotein oxidation. *American Journal of Clinical Nutrition, 58,* 525–532.

Ahlawat, S. K., & Siwach, S. B. (1994). Alcohol and coronary artery disease. *International Journal of Cardiology, 44,* 157–162.

Anonymous (1994). To take antioxidant pills or not? The debate heats up. *Tufts University Diet 8: Nutrition Letter* (May), 34.

Ashley, M., Ferrence, R., Rankin, J., Room, R., & Single, E. (1994). Moderate drinking & health: Best advice on low-risk drinking for individuals. *Canadian Medical Association Journal, 151(6),* 823–824.

Berlin, L. (1996). Alcohol, hypertension and cardiovascular disease. *Journal of Hypertension, 13,* 939–942.

Blumberg, J. (1995). Considerations of the scientific substantiation for antioxidant vitamins and beta-carotene in disease prevention. *American Journal of Clinical Nutrition, 62* (Suppl.), 1521s–1526s.

Brown, J. (1990). *The Science of Human Nutrition.* New York: Harcourt Brace Jovanovich.

Buring, J., & Hennekens, C. (1994). Randomized trials of primary prevention of cardiovascular disease in women: An investigator's view. *Annals of Epidemiology, 4(2),* 111–114.

Burrell, C., & Blake, D. (1989). Reactive oxygen metabolites and the human myocardium. *British Heart Journal, 61,* 4–8.

Camargo, C., Gaziano, M., Hennekens, C., Manson, J., & Stampfer, M. (1994). Prospective study of moderate alcohol consumption and mortality in male physicians. Paper presented at the American Heart Association Meeting, October, Dallas.

Crystal, R. G. (1991). Oxidants & antioxidants: Pathophysiologic determinants & therapeutic agents. *American Journal of Medicine, 91(3C),* 1S.

Criqui, M. H., & Ringel, B. L. (1994). Does diet or alcohol explain the French paradox? *Lancet, 344,* 1719–1723.

DeLuca, L., & Ross, S. (1996). Beta-carotene increases lung cancer incidence in cigarette smokers. *Nutrition Reviews, 54(6),* 178–180.

DiMascio, P., Murphy, M., & Sies, H. (1991). Antioxidant defense systems: The role of carotenoids, tocopherols, and thiols. *American Journal of Clinical Nutrition, 53,* 194s–200s.

Diplock, A. (1991). Antioxidant nutrients and disease prevention: An overview. *American Journal of Clinical Nutrition, 53,* 189s–193s.

Ducimetiere, P., Marciniak, A., Milon, H., Richard, J., & Rufat, P. (1993). Arteriographically documented coronary artery disease and alcohol consumption in French men. The Corali Study. *European Heart Journal, 14(6),* 727–733.

Erdman, J., Russell, R., Rock, C., Baura, A., Bowen, P., Burri, J., Curran-Celentano, J., Furr, H., Mayne, S., & Stacewicz-Sapuntzakis, M. (1996). Beta-carotene and the carotenoids: Beyond the intervention trials. *Nutrition Reviews, 54(6),* 185–188.

Esterbauer, H., Dieber-Rotheneder, M., Striegl, G., & Waeg, G. (1991). Role of vitamin E in preventing the oxidation of low-density lipoprotein. *American Journal of Clinical Nutrition, 53,* 314s–321s.

Frei, B. (1991). Ascorbic acid protects lipids in human plasma and low-density lipoprotein against oxidative damage. *American Journal of Clinical Nutrition, 54,* 1113s–1118s.

Frei, B. (1994). Reactive oxygen species and antioxidant vitamins: Mechanisms of action. *American Journal of Medicine, 97* (Suppl. 3A), 5s–13s.

Friedman, G. D., & Klatsky, A. L. (1993). Is alcohol good for your health? *New England Journal of Medicine, 329(25),* 1882–1883.

Friedman, L., & Kimball, A. W. (1986). Coronary heart disease mortality and alcohol consumption in Framingham. *American Journal of Epidemiology, 124(3),* 481–489.

Fuchs, C., Stampfer, M., Colditz, G., Giovannucci, E., Manson, J., Kawachi, I., Hunter, D., Hankinson, S., Hennekens, C., Rosner, B., Speizer, F., & Willett, W. (1995). Alcohol consumption and mortality among women. *New England Journal of Medicine, 332*(19), 1245–1250.

Gaziano, J. M. (1994). Antioxidant vitamins and coronary artery disease risk. *American Journal of Medicine, 97*(Suppl. 3A), 18s–21s.

Gaziano, J. M. (1996). Antioxidants in cardiovascular disease: Randomized trials. *Nutrition, 12*(9), 583–588.

Gaziano, J. M. (1996). Antioxidants in cardiovascular disease: Randomized trials. *Nutrition Reviews, 54*(6), 175–184.

Gaziano, J. M., Buring, J. E., Breslow, J. L., Goldhaber, S. Z., Rosner, B., Van Denburgh, W. W., & Hennekens, C. H. (1993). Moderate alcohol intake, increased levels of high-density lipoprotein and its subfractions, and decreased risk of myocardial infarction. *New England Journal of Medicine, 329,* 1829–1834.

Gaziano, J. & Hennekens, C. (1993). The role of beta-carotene in the prevention of cardiovascular disease. *Annals of the New York Academy of Sciences, 691,* 148–155.

Gaziano, J., & Hennekens, C. (1995). Royal College's advice on alcohol consumption. *British Medical Journal, 33,* 3–4.

Gaziano, J., & Manson, J. (1996). Diet and heart disease: The role of fat, alcohol and antioxidants. *Cardiology Clinics, 14*(1), 69–83.

Gey, K. F., Puska, P., Jordan, P., & Moser, U. (1991). Inverse correlation between plasma vitamin E and mortality from ischemic heart disease in cross-cultural epidemiology. *American Journal of Clinical Nutrition, 53,* 326s–334s.

Gey, K., Stahelin, H., & Eicholzer, M. (1993). Poor plasma status of carotene and vitamin C is associated with higher mortality from ischemic heart disease and stroke: Prospective Basel Study. *Clinical Investigation, 71,* 3–6.

Goldberg, D., Hahn, S., & Parkes, J. (1995). Alcohol and coronary heart disease: The evidence for a protective effect. *Clinica Chimica Acta, 237,* 155–187.

Gorinstein, S., Zemser, M., Lichman, I., Berebi, A., Kleipfish, A., Libman, I., Trakhtenberg, S., & Caspi, A. (1997). Moderate beer consumption and the blood coagulation in patients with coronary artery disease. *Journal of Internal Medicine, 241,* 47–51.

Greenberg, E. R., & Spore, M. B. (1996). Antioxidant vitamins, cancer, and cardiovascular disease. *New England Journal of Medicine, 334*(18), 1189–1190.

Halliwell, B. (1991). Reactive oxygen species in living systems: Source, biochemistry, and role in human disease. *American Journal of Medicine, 91*(3c), 14S–22S.

Handa, K., Sasaki, J., Saku, K., Kono, S., & Arakawa, K. (1990). Alcohol consumption, serum lipids and severity of angiographically determined coronary artery disease. *American Journal of Cardiology, 65,* 287–289.

Handin, R. (1994). Disorders of coagulation and thrombosis. In K. Isselbacher, E. Braunwald, J. Wilson, J. Martin, A. Fauci, & D. Kasper (Eds.), *Harrison's Principles of Internal Medicine.* New York: McGraw-Hill, pp. 1804–1810.

Hennekens, C., & Buring, J. (1994). Antioxidant vitamins—benefit not yet proved. *New England Journal of Medicine, 330*(15), 1080–1081.

Hennekens, C., Buring, J., Manson, J., Stampfer, M., Rosner, B., Cook, N., LaMotte, F., Gaziano, J., Ridker, P., Willett, W., & Peto, R. (1996). Lack of effect of long-term supplementation with beta-carotene on the incidence of malignant neoplasms and cardiovascular disease. *New England Journal of Medicine, 334*(18), 1146–1149.

Hennekens, C., Gaziano, J., Manson, J., & Buring, J. (1995). Antioxidant vitamin—cardiovascular disease hypothesis is still promising but unproven: The need for randomized trials. *American Journal of Clinical Nutrition, 62*(Suppl.), 1377S–1380S.

Hoffman, R. M., & Garewal, H. S. (1995). Antioxidants and the prevention of coronary heart disease. *Archives of Internal Medicine, 155*(3), 241–246.

Jackson, R., & Beaglehole, R. (1995). Alcohol consumption guidelines: Relative safety vs. absolute risks and benefits. *Lancet, 346*(8977), 716.

Jha, P., Flather, M., Lonn, E., Farkouh, M., & Yusur, S. (1995). The antioxidant vitamins and cardiovascular disease: A critical review of epidemiologic and clinical trial data. *Annals of Internal Medicine, 123*(11), 869–872.

Jialal, I., & Grundy, S. (1993). Effect of combined supplementation with alpha-tocopherol, ascorbate, and beta-carotene on low-density lipoprotein oxidation. *Circulation, 88*(6), 2780–2786.

Jialal, I., Vega, G., & Grundy, S. (1990). Physiologic levels of ascorbate inhibit the oxidative modification of low density lipoprotein. *Atherosclerosis, 82,* 185–191.

Kannel, W., & Ellison, R. (1996). Alcohol and coronary heart disease: The evidence for a protective effect. *Clinica Chimica Acta, 246,* 59–76.

Kendler, B. (1995). Free radicals in health and disease: Implications for primary health care providers. *Nurse Practitioner, 20*(7), 29–36, 43.

Kerr, M. E., Bender, C. M., & Monti, E. (1996). An introduction to free radicals. *Heart & Lung, 25*(3), 200–209.

Kok, F. J. (1993). Antioxidants and risk of myocardial infarction. *Acta Cardiologia, 48*(5), 456–457.

Kushi, L., Folsom, A., Prineae, R., Mink, P., Wu, Y., & Bostick, R. (1996). Dietary antioxidants and death from coronary heart disease in post-menopausal women. *New England Journal of Medicine, 334*(18), 115–116.

Luc, G., & Fruchart, J. (1991). Oxidation of lipoproteins and atherosclerosis. *American Journal of Clinical Nutrition, 53,* 206S–209S.

Machlin, L., & Bendich, A. (1987). Free radical tissue damage: Protective role of antioxidant nutrients. *FASEB Journal, 1*(6), 441–445.

Manson, J., Stampfer, M., Willett, W., Colditz, G., Rosner, B., Speizer, F., & Hennekens, C. (1991). A prospective study of antioxidant vitamins and incidence of coronary heart disease in women. *Circulation, 84*(Suppl. II), 546s.

Manson, J., Stamplet, M., Willett, W., Colditz, G., Speizer, F., & Hennekens, C. (1992). Antioxidant vitamin score and incidence of coronary heart disease in women. *Circulation, 86*(4) (Suppl. 1), 675s.

Manson, J. E., Gaziano, J. M., Jonas, M. A., & Hennekens, C. (1993). Antioxidants and cardiovascular disease: A review. *Journal of the American College of Nutrition, 12*(4), 426–432.

Marmot, M., & Brunner, E. (1991). Alcohol and cardiovascular disease: The status of the U-shaped curve. *British Medical Journal, 303,* 565–568.

Maxwell, S. (1993). Can anti-oxidants prevent ischaemic heart disease? *Journal of Clinical Pharmacy and Therapeutics, 18,* 85–95.

Niki, E., Yamamoto, Y., Komuro, E., & Sato, K. (1991). Membrane damage due to lipid oxidation. *American Journal of Clinical Nutrition, 53,* 201S–205S.

Omenn, G., Goodman, G., Thornquist, M., Balmes, J., Cullen, M., Glass, A., Keogh, J., Meyskens, F., Valanis, B., Williams, J., Barnhart, S., & Hammar, S. (1996).

Effects of a combination of beta-carotene and vitamin A on lung cancer and cardiovascular disease. *New England Journal of Medicine, 334*(18), 1150–1155.

Pearson, T. (1996). Alcohol and heart disease. *Circulation, 94*(11), 3023–3025.

Pearson, T., & Terry, P. (1994). What to advise patients about drinking alcohol: The clinician's conundrum. *Journal of the American Medical Association, 272,* 967–968.

Preedy, V. R., & Richardson, P. J. (1994). Ethanol-induced cardiovascular disease. *British Medical Journal, 50*(1), 152–163.

Pryor, W. (1991). The antioxidant nutrients and disease prevention—What do we need to find out? *American Journal of Clinical Nutrition, 53,* 391S–393S.

Razay, G., Heaton, K. W., Bolton, C. H., & Hughes, A. O. (1992). Alcohol consumption and its relation to cardiovascular risk factors in British women. *British Medical Journal, 304,* 80–83.

Regnstrom, J., Nilsson, J., Tornvail, P., Landou, C., & Hansten, A. (1992). Susceptibility to low-density lipoprotein oxidation and coronary atherosclerosis in man. *Lancet, 339,* 1183–1186.

Reynolds, R. (1994). Vitamin supplements: Current controversies. *Journal of the American College of Nutrition, 13*(2), 118–126.

Rice-Evans, C., & Bruckdorfer, K. (1992). Free radicals, lipoproteins and cardiovascular dysfunction. In H. Baum (Ed.), *Molecular Aspects of Medicine.* New York: Pergamon Press, pp. 5–110.

Rimm, E., Stampfer, M., Ascherio, A., Giovannucci, E., Colditz, G., & Willett, W. (1993). Vitamin E consumption and the risk of coronary heart disease in men. *New England Journal of Medicine, 328*(20), 1450–1456.

Royal College of Physicians. (1995). Alcohol and the heart in perspective. *Journal of the Royal College of Physicians of London, 29*(4), 266–271.

Salonen, J. T. (1993). The role of lipid peroxidation, antioxidants and pro-oxidants in atherosclerosis. *Acta Cardiologica, 48*(5), 457–459.

Seppa, K., Sillanaukee, P., Pitkajarvi, T., Nikkila, M., & Koivula, T. (1992). Moderate and heavy alcohol consumption have no favorable effects on lipid values. *Archives of Internal Medicine, 152,* 297–300.

Shaik, M., Martini, S., & Quincy, J. (1988). Modified plasma-derived lipoproteins in human atherosclerotic plaques. *Atherosclerosis, 69,* 165–172.

Shaper, A. G., Wannamethee, G., & Walker, M. (1994). Alcohol and coronary heart disease: A perspective from the British regional heart study. *International Journal of Epidemiology, 23*(3), 482–494.

Sies, H. (1991). Oxidative stress: From basic research to clinical application. *American Journal of Medicine, 91* (3C), 31S–38S.

Sies, H., & Stahl, W. (1995). Vitamins E and C, beta-carotene, and other carotenoids as antioxidants. *American Journal of Clinical Nutrition, 62*(Suppl.), 1315S–1321S.

Slater, T. (1991). Concluding remarks. *American Journal of Clinical Nutrition, 53,* 394S–396S.

Srivastava, L. M., Vasisht, S., Agarwal, D. P., & Goedde, H. W. (1994). Relation between alcohol intake, lipoproteins and coronary heart disease: The interest continues. *Alcohol & Alcoholism, 29*(1), 11–24.

Stampfer, M. J., Colditz, G. A., Willett, W., Speizer, F. E., & Hennekens, C. H. (1988). A prospective study of moderate alcohol consumption and the risk of coronary disease and stroke in women. *New England Journal of Medicine, 319*(5), 267–273.

Stampfer, M., Hennekens, C., Manson, J., Colditz, G., Rosner, B., & Willett, W. (1993). Vitamin E consumption and the risk of coronary heart disease in women. *New England Journal of Medicine, 328*(20), 1444–1449.

Stampfer, M., Sacks, F., Salvini, S., Willett, W., & Hennekens, C. (1991). A prospective study of cholesterol, apolipoproteins, and the risk of myocardial infarction. *New England Journal of Medicine, 325*(6), 373–381.

Suh, I., Shaten, J., Cutler, J. A., & Kuller, L. H. (1992). Alcohol use and mortality from coronary heart disease: The role of high-density lipoprotein cholesterol. *Annals of Internal Medicine, 116*(11), 881–887.

Surgeon General's Report on Nutrition and Health. (1988). Washington, DC: U.S. Government Printing Office.

Todd, S., Woodward, M., Bolton-Smith, C., & Tunstall-Pedoe, H. (1995). An investigation of the relationship between antioxidant vitamin intake and coronary heart disease in men and women using discriminant analysis. *Journal of Clinical Epidemiology, 48*(2), 297–305.

Torun, M., Yardim, S., Sargin, H., & Simsek, B. (1994). Evaluation of serum beta carotene levels in patients with cardiovascular diseases. *Journal of Clinical Pharmacy and Therapeutics, 19,* 61–63.

Trout, D. (1991). Vitamin C and cardiovascular risk factors. *American Journal of Clinical Nutrition, 53,* 322S–325S.

Wilson, J. (1994). Vitamin deficiency and excess. In K. Isselbacher, E. Braunwald, J. Wilson, I. Martin, A. Fauci, & D. Kasper (Eds.), *Harrison's Principles of Internal Medicine.* New York: McGraw-Hill, pp. 472–480.

Witztum, J. L., Reaven, P. D., & Parthasarathy, S. (1993). Studies on the ability of dietary supplementation with beta carotene to protect low-density lipoprotein from oxidative modification. *Annals of the New York Academy of Sciences, 691,* 200–206.

Wojcicki, J., Rozewicka, L., Barcew-Wizsnewska, B., Samochoweic, L., Juzwiak, S., Kadubowska, D., Tustanowski, A., Juzyszyn, Z. (1991). Effect of selenium and vitamin E on the development of experimental atherosclerosis in rabbits. *Atherosclerosis, 86,* 6–16.

Yla-Herttuala, S., Palinske, W., & Rosenreid, M. (1989). Evidence for the presence of oxidatively modified low density lipoprotein in atherosclerotic lesions of rabbit and man. *Journal of Clinical Investigation, 84,* 1086.

CHAPTER 13

Children and Coronary Heart Disease

Ellen Rukholm

This chapter will address current knowledge about children and coronary heart disease risk. *Coronary heart disease* (CHD) is caused by atherosclerosis, a slowly progressive disease of the large arteries that begins early in life but rarely produces symptoms until middle age or later. The aim of this chapter is to provide nurses and other clinicians with a better understanding of CHD risk in children and an array of tactics to deal with it. Accordingly, the onset and progression of atherosclerosis are discussed, along with the mounting epidemiologic data on the subject. Then the assessment and management of CHD risk in children are considered for both individuals and populations.

ONSET AND PROGRESSION OF ATHEROSCLEROSIS

Early Lesions

The view that atherosclerosis begins early in childhood has long been held. In fact, early aortic lesions were identified in children as young as 3 years of age in a New Orleans study carried out by Holman, McGill, Strong, and Geer (1958). Since that time evidence of the early and progressive nature of atherosclerosis has steadily mounted. Atherosclerotic fatty streaks were found to begin in the coronary arteries of children at about 13 years of age and to continue to escalate progressively throughout the teenage years and into the young-adult years (Strong, & McGill, 1962).

One study of a broad population derived from pathology laboratories in nine centers in the United States has confirmed these earlier findings (Pathobiological Determinants of Atherosclerosis in Youth, (1993). This research group studied the arteries of 1,532 individuals (black and white, male and female), 15–34 years of age, who died of causes unrelated to heart disease—that is, primarily of murder, accident, and suicide. All individuals in the age group of 15–19 years were found to have aortic lesions, and approximately one half of these also had lesions in the right coronary artery. Raised lesions in the aorta and the right coronary artery increased with age in extent and prevalence. African Americans had more extensive fatty streaks than whites. Young women had more extensive fatty streaks in the abdominal aorta, whereas young men had more in the thoracic aorta. In the right coronary artery, young men had greater extent and amount of lesions than did young women. There were no significant differences between white and black subjects in the degree of raised lesions.

The results of various studies (Holman, McGill, Strong, et al., 1958; Strong & McGill, 1962; Pathobiological Determinants of Atherosclerosis in Youth, 1993) confirm that atherosclerosis begins in childhood. These studies show that fatty streaks and fibrous plaques increase in prevalence and extent rapidly during the 15–34 years age span. Although there can be no doubt that atherosclerosis begins early in childhood and progresses steadily thereafter, nor that gender and ethnic differences exist, the link between "the natural history of atherosclerosis" (Berenson, Srinivasan, Webber, et al., p. 6, 1991) and the prevalence of CHD risk factors in children has not yet been adequately examined.

DISTRIBUTION OF CHD RISK FACTORS AMONG PEDIATRIC POPULATIONS

Risk factors may be described as the determinants that increase the likelihood of the development of CHD. In adults, major independent risk factors include cigarette smoking, hypertension, hyperlipidemia—especially *low-density lipoprotein* (LDL) cholesterol—sedentary lifestyle, stress (hostility), and being overweight. Although to date no longitudinal evidence connects these risk factors in childhood to CHD in adulthood, data exist, as already mentioned, that support the onset of atherosclerosis early in childhood.

Table 13–1 summarizes the findings of four key studies concerning CHD risk in children and adolescents. Evidence of the early and progressive nature of atherosclerotic disease led to longitudinal studies such as the Bogalusa Heart Study and the Muscatine Study. Based on these and two other well-known studies, several inferences regarding CHD risk in childhood may be drawn.

First, risk factors aggregate in families (Morrison, Namboodiri, Green, et al., 1983; Berenson, Srinivasan, Webber, et al., 1991; Lauer, Lee, & Clarke, 1988). Second, risk factors persist, or "track," from childhood into young adulthood (Webber, Cresanta, Voors, & Berenson, 1983; Lauer, Lee, & Clarke, 1988), and cluster in children (Berenson, Srinivasan, Web-

ber, et al., 1991). Berenson and co-workers (1991) reported that after the age of 13 years, the hostility subscale of Type A personality tracked into adulthood, with white male adolescents having the highest subscores. Type A personality measures have also been shown by other researchers to be stable in children through to young adulthood (Bergman & Magnusson, 1986; Steinberg, 1986; Matthews & Woodall, 1988).

Third, risk factors cluster. The relationship of obesity and body fat distribution to both hypertension and hyperlipoprotein levels is an example of clustering that has implications for clinical practice. As well, total serum cholesterol and lipoprotein cholesterol values vary by age, gender, and race (Berenson, Srinivasan, Webber, et al., 1991; Lipid Research Clinics Program, 1984; Resnicow, Morley-Kotchen, & Wynder, 1989).

The longitudinal studies carried out in Muscatine, Iowa, and Bogalusa, Louisiana, have given us normative data for key CHD risk factors (elevated blood lipids, elevated blood pressure, and obesity). Sufficient evidence to support action exists, despite gaps in our knowledge about the persistence and progression of fatty streaks in the walls of arteries of children with high lipid levels and their relationship to the development of CHD in adulthood.

Nurses and other clinicians have a role to play in assessing children who are at high risk for CHD and in managing their care. As well, nurses can participate in a population-based approach to promoting cardiovascular health in children (Harlan, 1989; Hayman & Ryan, 1994). The research evidence overwhelmingly supports the need to intervene with children and youth to encourage and support lifestyles that promote cardiovascular health and prevent cardiovascular illness later in life. In particular, hyperlipidemia, hypertension, obesity, stress (hostility), and cigarette smoking are CHD risk factors that can be altered through management of diet, physical activity, and stress and elimination of tobacco use.

A SELECTIVE REVIEW OF CHD RISK ASSESSMENT AND INTERVENTION STUDIES IN CHILDREN

It is beyond the scope of this chapter to exhaustively address the literature pertaining to CHD

TABLE 13–1 Distribution of CHD Risk Factors in Children and Adolescents

Investigator(s)	Study Design	Sample	Variables	Comments
Bogalusa Heart Study (Berenson, Srinivasan, Webber, et al., 1991)	Longitudinal and cross-sectional surveys were done. Cross-sectional surveys of the entire pediatric population took place on six different occasions over 18 years.	Sample sizes varied. The first survey, in 1973–1974, included 3,524 children 5–14 years of age. Cross-sectional surveys were repeated six times on 3,000–4,000 children at 3-year intervals.	Dietary habits, skinfold thickness, height, weight, serum cholesterol, LDL and HDL cholesterol, smoking, BP, family history, alcohol intake, use of oral contraception, Type A or B personality, gender, age, and race or ethnicity were noted.	Risk factors were "tracked" and "clustered." Clustering escalated as children moved into adolescence and was gender- and race-specific. Total serum cholesterol and lipoprotein cholesterol values were found to vary by age, gender, and race. Incidence of Type A personality increased with age for all age and both gender groups. White males had higher average scores throughout and significantly higher scores on the hostility subscale. Reliability of Type A personality findings for children under 13 years of age was questioned. Children identified with high total cholesterol levels on screening should have a complete lipoprotein profile done.
Muscatine Study (Lauer, Lee, & Clark, 1988)	Surveys took place in alternate years from 1971 until 1985.	The first sample, in 1971, consisted of 3,891 children 8–18 years of age. Then, in 1981, 2,446 eligible subjects, 67% of the first sample (some of whom had been surveyed more than once during the previous 10 years), were again surveyed at ages 20–30 years.	In the first sample, risk factors for heart disease that were measured included levels of height, weight, Quetelet Index (weight divided by height squared), triceps skinfold thickness, BP, fasting plasma cholesterol, and triglycerides. The following variables were added to the 1981 survey: use of thyroid, lipid-reducing, or oral contraceptive medications; use of tobacco and alcohol; self-reported physical activity at home and work; socioeconomic status; family history (parents or siblings) of high cholesterol, hypertension, myocardial infarction, stroke, or diabetes.	Cholesterol levels and the Quetelet Index tracked (i.e., persisted) from childhood into adulthood. Childhood total cholesterol levels were predictive of adult LDL cholesterol levels and LDL/HDL ratios. Obesity, consumption of tobacco and alcohol, and use of oral contraceptives affected LDL and HDL cholesterol levels and their ratio in subjects 20–30 years of age. Smoking more than one package of cigarettes per day was related to lower HDL cholesterol levels and higher LDL/HDL ratios, as was the adult use of oral contraceptives. Combined smoking and oral contraceptive use pushed lipid levels even higher. A family history of high cholesterol or myocardial infarction was related to high total and LDL cholesterol levels among young adults. Children with high cholesterol levels should be particularly counseled regarding diet, obesity, and smoking.

Study	Description	Sample	Measure	Findings
Lipid Research Clinics Study: multicenter prevalence trial carried out from 1972 until 1976 in seven sites in North America (Christensen, Glueck, Kwiterovich, et al., 1989; Lipid Research Clinics Program, 1984)	Study described values specific to age, sex, and race or ethnicity for total cholesterol.	Sample consisted of 13,600 (11,000 white and 2,600 black) children and adolescents 1–19 years of age.	Total plasma cholesterol levels were noted.	The Lipid Research Clinics mean for all subjects was 160.9 mg/dL, whereas the Bogalusa mean was 165.0 mg/dL. However, it should be noted that the Lipids Research Clinics study used plasma samples, whereas the Bogalusa study used serum samples. This difference is important because plasma cholesterol levels are around 3% lower than serum cholesterol levels.
Know Your Body (KYB) School Health Program started in 1975 in New York City (Resnicow, Morley-Kotchen, & Wynder, 1989)	Study measured total cholesterol levels of school-age children between 1984 and 1988.	Sample consisted of 6,585 children from 22 schools in five sites: New York City; Clarksburg, WV; Atlanta, GA; Houston, TX; and Washington, DC. Children represented a variety of racial backgrounds, including African-American, Hispanic, Asian-American, and white, so that racial/ethnic comparisons could be made. Subjects were 5–18 years of age.	Total plasma cholesterol levels, age, gender, and race or ethnicity were noted.	Mean total plasma cholesterol* for the whole population was 166.4 mg/dL ± 0.357. Gender differences were found in the total population, with girls having higher cholesterol levels (168 mg/dL ± 0.734) than boys (165 mg/dL ± 2.120). Gender differences varied among racial/ethnic groups. Mean cholesterol levels varied by race/ethnicity: 173 mg/dL ± 0.830 for African Americans, 168 mg/dL ± 0.734 for Hispanics, 165 mg/dL ± 2.120 for Asian Americans, and 163 mg/dL ± 0.537 for whites. Peak cholesterol levels for the whole population occurred at 8–10 years of age for girls and at 10 years of age for boys. These values are higher than those reported by both the Bogalusa and Lipid Research Clinics studies. HDL cholesterol levels may contribute considerably to high total cholesterol values for African American males and therefore increase the likelihood for false positives. Flexible guidelines are suggested for determining risk status in children to take into account age, race/ethnicity, and gender differences.

*Mean mg/dL ± SEM; 95% confidence interval ± 1.96 (SEM).
BP = blood pressure.

risk assessment and management in children and adolescents. Instead, an overview of selected studies, predominantly those involving multiple risk-factor assessment and intervention conducted in school settings, is presented. Table 13–2 summarizes the findings of 17 selected school studies. The majority were interventional, although a few assessed the prevalence of risk factors in school-age children.

Subjects ranged in age from kindergarten to high school age. Samples included the school, student, or family as the unit of analysis. When children and adolescents were the unit of analysis, sample sizes varied from 72 to 5,458. Many of the studies examined the combined effects of three key CHD lifestyle factors (nutrition, physical activity, and smoking). A few focused on single risk factors such as blood pressure or smoking. In those studies that identified a theoretical basis, Bandura's social learning theory predominated (Bandura, 1977, 1986). Community organization theory (Charter & Jones, 1973) and diffusion-of-innovations theory (Rogers, 1983) were employed in some studies. One study used a combination of social learning theory, the PRECEDE health-promotion model (Green, Kreuter, Deeds, et al., 1980) and the health-belief model (Becker, 1974) as its theoretical underpinning.

Some of these studies were part of larger community-based projects, such as the North Karelia project (Puska, Vartianen, Pallonen, et al., 1982) or the Stanford Five-City Project (Killen, Robinson, Telch, et al., 1989). The majority of the interventions were of short duration and curriculum-based. A few were longitudinal. Some addressed environmental changes to support children in choosing heart-healthy foods. Some involved parents, teachers, and children, using the school as an entry point to the family or using a combined family-school approach to support the child in making healthy lifestyle choices. Peer leaders were used in some studies to create an environment that enabled children and adolescents to make healthy lifestyle choices.

LEARNING DERIVED FROM SCHOOL CHD RISK-REDUCTION INITIATIVES

In general, the majority of studies reviewed showed evidence of positive behavior change in the realms of nutrition, smoking, and physical activity. The long-term impact of these changes on adult CHD mortality and morbidity remains unknown. Results from the studies confirm the need to consider the sustainability of behavior change after an intervention has ceased. In other words, are "booster" sessions necessary to sustain behavior change past kindergarten and through high school? The powerful impact of peer support and family involvement in child/adolescent heart-health programs is clearly evident. The widespread effective use of social learning theory, community organization theory, comprehensive school health theory, and health-promotion theory to guide interventions is also apparent. The incorporation of skills training, not just knowledge, into curriculum and the linkages forged between home-based and family-based and school health education programs affirm the use of these theories.

INDIVIDUAL AND POPULATION ASSESSMENT AND MANAGEMENT OF CHD RISK

The nurse, in conjunction with other clinicians, can manage cardiovascular disease prevention and health-promotion endeavors in a variety of locations such as, offices, clinics, and schools, as well as inpatient hospital settings (Hayman & Ryan, 1994). A number of settings can be used to influence the lifestyle choices and behaviors of children, including social, church, and civic groups. The approaches used in these settings can be on an individual basis, a population basis, or a combination of the two.

At the *individual level,* the nurse can contribute by assessing diet, physical activity, stress, and smoking behaviors and then providing relevant information and counseling that is age-, culture-, and gender-specific. In a school setting, nurses can assist teachers and principals by providing them with information about CHD for children and for their parents.

At the *population level,* the nurse can work with school boards to bring about system changes through the development of policies and programs for smoking prevention or cessation, healthy eating, and regular physical activity. Some resources to assist nurses in these endeavors are listed at the end of this chapter.

Text continued on page 263

TABLE 13–2 Review of Selected Cardiovascular Risk Studies Conducted in School Settings

Investigator	Sample	Design and Theory	Risk-Factor and Population Targets	Outcome Variables and Interventions	Findings
Cowell, Montgomery, & Talashek, 1992	Sample consisted of 195 high school students who participated in a cardiovascular risk-reduction program in the sixth grade.	In this longitudinal design, three cohorts retested 3–6 years after a risk-reduction program carried out in sixth grade.	Targets included stability of cardiovascular risk factors in children from sixth grade to high school, differences in risk according to gender, and curriculum.	Total cholesterol, heart rate, and BP were noted. Risk-reduction program was begun on children in sixth grade.	Risk for being overweight and having high cholesterol levels remained stable, but there were significant differences in heart rate recovery and BP. Gender differences were noted in the risk for higher cholesterol levels in girls.
Brandon & Fillingim, 1990	Sample consisted of 386 fourth-grade students, 305 with lower BP and 81 with higher BP.	Normotensive students (BP below 108/76) and elevated normotensive students (BP above 108/76) were compared before and after a physical activity program	Targets included blood pressure of fourth-grade students and curriculum.	Flexibility, muscular endurance, cardiovascular endurance, and body fat levels were noted. A physical activity program was conducted.	Fourth-graders who were fatter and had higher BP had lower cardiovascular fitness levels before and after a physical fitness program. However, their rate of fitness improvement was like that obtained by children with normal blood pressure.

Table continued on following page

TABLE 13–2 Review of Selected Cardiovascular Risk Studies Conducted in School Settings *Continued*

Investigator	Sample	Design and Theory	Risk-Factor and Population Targets	Outcome Variables and Interventions	Findings
Bernstein, Bellorado, & Bruvold, 1986	Sample consisted of 600 preschoolers, 3–5 years of age.	Nonequivalent control group was used.	Targets included nutrition and exercise knowledge in preschool children after a heart-health education program, "The Lub Dub Club" by the American Heart Association in San Francisco. Also targeted were the parents, teachers, and curriculum.	Children were provided knowledge of heart health, exercise, and nutrition. Parents and teachers assessed the usefulness and impact of the program on children.	No difference in age or gender was found between intervention and comparison groups. The intervention group's knowledge of heart health, exercise, and nutrition were significantly better than the comparison group. Parent and teacher attitudes toward the program were positive.
Killen, Robinson, Telch, et al., 1989	Sample consisted of 10th-graders in four high schools.	Quasi-experimental pretest and posttest were used. Schools were randomly assigned to control or treatment group. Social learning theory provided theoretical basis.	Targets included physical activity, nutrition, and cigarette smoking in 10th-grade students and curriculum.	In 20 sessions over 7 weeks, baseline data were gathered on physical activity, nutrition, cigarette smoking, marijuana use, and alcohol use. Height, weight, skinfold thickness, resting heart rate, and BP were retested 2 months after the sessions.	At 2 months the posttest treatment group showed knowledge gains in nutrition, physical activity, and smoking. Improvements in resting heart rate, skinfold thickness, and smoking and eating choices were reported at follow-up. More teens in the treatment group who were not exercising regularly at the baseline reported doing so at posttest.
Ellison, Capper, Goldberg, et al., 1989	Sample consisted of science students at each of two high schools.	Nonrandomized, concurrently controlled longitudinal study was conducted for 4 years.	Targets included nutrition, blood pressure, food services, and environment for high school students.	Diet diaries were evaluated for the degree of change in sodium and fat intake of food served at schools, and the effect of dietary changes on BP were noted.	Lowered intake of sodium and saturated fat occurred after the changes in school food services and resulted in favorable changes in students' BP.

Reference	Sample	Design	Targets	Variables/Measures	Findings
Harrell & Frauman, 1994	Sample consisted of 2,209 students—black, white, and "other"—in 21 rural and urban public schools in North Carolina. Socioeconomic status (L, M, H)	Schools were randomly selected for survey from three regions of the state (coastal, piedmont, and mountain).	Targets included smoking, nutrition, physical activity, and environment of children aged 8–11 years. Design of specific health policy and programs are recommended based on data.	Obesity, body mass index, smoking, diet (salt, fat), and physical activity tolerance were noted.	In the total sample 26% were obese: 33.5% of rural black, 28.5% of rural white, 22.2% of urban black, and 21.7% of urban white. More black than white children reported parents who smoked and had tried smoking themselves. Physical activity tolerance was poorer in coastal rural area than in the state overall.
Madsen, Sallis, Rupp, et al., 1993	Sample consisted of 72 Anglo adults, 68 Mexican-American adults, 80 Anglo children, and 94 Mexican-American children, which constituted the families of fifth- and sixth-grade students.	Families were surveyed at baseline, 3, 12, and 24 months.	Targets were nutrition and physical activity of fifth- and sixth-grade students and their families.	Self-recorded nutrition and aerobic exercise. Body mass index, BP, total cholesterol and lipoproteins, $V_{O_{2max}}$, and HDL/LDL ratio were noted. Intervention consisted of 18-session family-based nutrition and physical activity program.	In adults, self-reported diet changes were associated with alterations in body mass index, total cholesterol, LDL cholesterol, and SBP 1 and 2 years after baseline. No relationship was found between physical activity, self-reports, and cardiovascular risk factors. In children, no relationships between dietary self-reports and nutrition-related risk factors were found. Self-reported physical activity was related to changes in $V_{O_{2max}}$ and HDL/LDL ratio at 12 and 24 months.

Table continued on following page

TABLE 13-2 Review of Selected Cardiovascular Risk Studies Conducted in School Settings *Continued*

Investigator	Sample	Design and Theory	Risk-Factor and Population Targets	Outcome Variables and Interventions	Findings
Purath, Lansinger, & Ragheb, 1995	Sample consisted of 357 6th grade students and their parents at two central Indiana elementary schools. Students were white, black, Hispanic, and American Indian.	Survey	Targets were CHD risk factors in elementary school children, grades 1 to 5, and their parents, including family history of cardiovascular disease, dietary habits, and exercise habits.	CHD risk factors in children, such as smoking, blood pressure, cholesterol, height and weight, resting pulse, skinfold thickness, and fitness were noted. For parents, family history of high cholesterol and CHD, amount of time students' mothers exercised, cholesterol elevation, and frequency of eating out in restaurants were noted.	No significant associations were found between cholesterol and parent variables. A significant relationship was found between eating out and elevated cholesterol. If recommended screening policies of NIH, AAP, and NHLBI had been used, 66% of children with cholesterol levels above 170 mg/dL would have been missed!
Fors, Owen Hall, et al., 1989	Sample consisted of 1,204 students from 21 schools and 1,446 parents. Students were randomly assigned to one of three groups. Each group had seven schools and 20 classes. Intervention occurred during seven 2-week periods.	Quasi-experimental posttest design was used. Group A students received the "3Rs" cardiovascular health curriculum and HBP school curriculum, talked with parents, and did home BP assignment. Group B students did the same except they had no home BP pressure assignment; Group C comparison group had the usual school cardiovascular health curriculum. Post-intervention surveys were taken on three different occasions.	Targets were to gather hypertension data from 71% of family units and accomplish diffusion of HBP information from teachers to students and then to parents. Diffusion strategy was the homework assignment BP measurement. Also targeted were curriculum and family.	For students, BP measurement skills were noted immediately after education program (Groups A and B only), 4 weeks after the program (according to age, sex, race) HBP knowledge, self-esteem, and home diffusion activities for HBP risk factors and complications were noted; 4 months after the program HBP knowledge was again noted. For parents, data were collected at 4, 8, and 12 months. At 4 months after the program (according to age, race, sex, education, family income, marital status),	The higher the level of parental education, the more diffusion occurred of HBP knowledge. Diffusion was greater in white families than in black. Among both parents and students, diffusion was greater for females.

Author/Year	Sample	Design	Measures/Targets	Findings
			HBP knowledge and risk behaviors, BP measurements skills, care-seeker behavior, compliance, family interaction, level of discussion with student about HBP risk and complications were noted. At 8 months after the program, family communication patterns were noted as high-diffusion or low-diffusion. At 12 months after the program (only DBP > 90) care-seeking and medication if HBP was confirmed were noted. For teachers, a seven-item questionnaire measured fidelity and attitudes toward curriculum.	
Cohen, Felix, & Brownell, 1989	Sample consisted of 1,051 households. Nutrition program involved 233 fifth-graders. BP program involved 325 sixth-graders. Smoking prevention program involved 328 seventh-graders.	Pretest and 1-year follow-up interventional study examined parents' and children's perceptions of children's health behavior and family interaction. Social learning theory provided theoretical basis.	Targets included nutrition, BP, and smoking among fifth-, sixth-, and seventh-graders and their parents. Also targeted were teachers, peers, curriculum, and family. Parent and child baseline surveys were conducted involving three experimental peer-led interventions of four 45-minute classroom sessions (parents involved through homework assignments completed with parents, discussion regarding parents as role models, and information at the 1-year level mailed to parents (parents as "enablers"). Comparison group of teacher-led intervention involved the same content, no small-group learning, and the parent focus omitted.	Significant correlations were found between parent and student reports of diet, exercise, and fast-food consumption. Parents underestimated the rate of smoking. For BP knowledge, older peer-led groups showed a greater increase in behavior skills than teacher-led groups. For smoking, there was no difference between groups. For nutrition, both groups showed improvement, but the peer-led group had significantly lower scores on pretest than the teacher-led group.

Table continued on following page

TABLE 13-2 Review of Selected Cardiovascular Risk Studies Conducted in School Settings *Continued*

Investigator	Sample	Design and Theory	Risk-Factor and Population Targets	Outcome Variables and Interventions	Findings
Perry, Luepker, Murray et al., 1989	Sample consisted of 2,250 third-grade students in 31 urban schools in Minnesota and North Dakota and 1,100 families (Home Team).	Quasi-experimental pretest posttest factorial design involved four urban school districts, with 31 schools randomly assigned to one of four groups: school-based, home-based, school-based followed by home-based, and a no-treatment control group. Social learning theory plus health-promotion theory provided theoretical basis.	Targets included dietary fat and sodium consumption in regard to specific environmental, personality, and behavioral factors that influence children's eating patterns. Third graders and their parents were targeted. Measurements included 24-hour dietary recall (15 randomly selected subsets from each school), anthropometric measures, and urinary sodium. Teacher involvement was not extensive and no training was needed. Incentives included stickers, "Salt Sleuth" magnifying glass, team hats, etc. A grand prize was donated (trip to Disneyworld).	The school-based program, "Adventures of Hearty Heart and Friends," included a 5-week correspondence course for third graders and their parents (mailed). The correspondence package included a game motif "Player's Guide." Activities started with a story to be read by child to parent. Parent and child were advised to play games to practice the skills suggested in the story. Reinforcements included refrigerator "tip" sheet giving more detailed nutrition information and points for parent and child working together. Results were recorded on score card that was returned to the classroom. University staff were "coaches" who used tally cards, etc.	Differences between Home Team and No Home Team were found for percent of calories from saturated fat and monosaturated fat and grams of complex carbohydrates per 1,000 calories. There was lower consumption of total fat, saturated fat, and monosaturated fat 1 year later, but these differences were no longer statistically significant. No difference was found for anthropometric or urinary sodium measures. Researchers suggest that because changes were not statistically significant at 1 year, a longer intervention, and booster sessions need to be considered. Other behaviors, other socioeconomic groups, other age groups should also be tested.

| Nader, Sallis, Patterson, et al., 1989 | Sample consisted of 206 volunteers of low to middle income, Mexican American and non-Hispanic white (Anglo American) families (623 individuals), each with a fifth- or sixth-grade child. At the 24-month follow-up, 89% of families were measured | In this quasi-experimental design, half of the families were randomized to a year-long intervention, measured at 3, 12, and 24 months. Social learning theory provided the theoretical basis. The family was used as the unit of analysis | Targets included nutrition (salt/fat intake) and physical activity (a $50 incentive was paid to families for each fully completed measurement after baseline). Outcome measures were 24-hour diet recall, 3-day food record, food-frequency questionnaire, 7-day physical activity recall, physiologic submax, exercise test, body mass index, BP, pulse, serum cholesterol and lipoproteins, and urinary sodium-potassium ratio. Mediating variables were demographics, socioeconomic status, family function, confounding events, social support, knowledge, and direct observation. | Intervention families got 3 months of weekly intervention. Six to seven families met as a group for 1½ hours at the local school. Led by two graduate students, groups participated in experiential learning games, discussion, and exercise with music. Children and adults had their own sessions for part of the evening. Then families got together for review, problem solving, goal setting, and support. There were 12 weekly sessions, then 6 maintenance sessions over 9 months, with incentives and a social event at the end of that period. | Both Mexican-American and Non-Hispanic white (Anglo-American) individuals in experimental group acquired significant skills and knowledge needed for diet and physical activity changes. Experimental group reported improved diet as shown by the food-frequency index. Anglo participants lowered total fat and sodium intake on 24 recall and 3-day food records. No changes were noted in physical activity or fitness of either experimental or control groups. Anglo subjects had LDL cholesterol changes. Significant SBP and DBP changes were found for all groups. Observation confirmed diet and physical activity changes. More changes occurred in diet than in physical activity levels and more change in Anglos than in Mexican Americans. |

Table continued on following page

TABLE 13–2 Review of Selected Cardiovascular Risk Studies Conducted in School Settings *Continued*

Investigator	Sample	Design and Theory	Risk-Factor and Population Targets	Outcome Variables and Interventions	Findings
Parcel, Simons-Morton, O'Hara, et al., 1989	Sample consisted of third- and fourth-grade students in two schools assigned to intervention and two assigned to control groups. Students were Anglo, Mexican American, African American, Asian-American, and American Indian.	Quasi-experimental design had nonrandom baseline; posttest school and student measurements were used as the unit of analysis. Study took place over 2 years. Social learning theory and organizational change theory based on the Charters and Jones four-phase model provided the theoretical basis. The four phases are as follows: 1. Institutional commitment. 2. Changes in policies and practices. 3. Changes in staff roles and actions. 4. Provision of student learning activities.	Targets included behavioral capability, expectations, and self-efficacy. "Go for Health Program" classroom health education, and environmental changes in school lunch and physical education were employed to promote healthy diet and physical activity among elementary school children in third and fourth grades. Curriculum and environment (food services) were targeted.	Student-measured knowledge and self-reports of diet and physical activity were evaluated. Intervention consisted of two 4-week healthful-eating modules and one 6-week physical activity module. Nutrition was taught in blocks, one in the fall and the other in the spring. Physical activity module was divided into three 2-week modules taught at different times in the school year. A 30-minute learning activity was followed by 5–10 minutes of activities for the rest of the week. Teachers, etc. (physical education teachers, food service employees, and managers) completed an interview about the program at the end of the intervention.	Statistically significant differences were found for diet behavioral capability, self-efficacy, and behavioral expectations for salt use and frequency of physical activity.

| Flynn, Worden, Secker-Walker, et al., 1992 | Sample consisted of 5,458 students in fourth, fifth, and sixth grades. | In this quasi-experimental design, students in one pair of communities received media plus school program while students in a matched pair of communities received just the school program. Surveys were taken at baseline and annually for 4 years. | Targets included smoking curriculum, and media for students in fourth, fifth, and sixth grades. | Number of cigarettes smoked per week was noted. Over a period of 4 years students in the experimental group received media interventions plus interventions of a school smoking-prevention program. | Significant decreases in smoking occurred in the media-plus-school-program group. Cigarettes per week dropped by 41%. For those smoking yesterday the drop was 34%; for those smoking during the past week the drop was 35%. Media plus school programs were effective when targeted at high-risk groups and combined with school smoking-prevention program objectives. |

Table continued on following page

TABLE 13-2 Review of Selected Cardiovascular Risk Studies Conducted in School Settings *Continued*

Investigator	Sample	Design and Theory	Risk-Factor and Population Targets	Outcome Variables and Interventions	Findings
Puska, Vartiainen, Pallonen, et al., 1982	Sample consisted of 851 children and their parents and teachers. The children were 13 to 15 years old. Three matched pairs of schools in the United States, North Korea, and Finland were studied.	In this quasi-experimental pretest, posttest design two schools in North Karelia, Finland received intensive intervention (II), two others received a county-wide general intervention (CI), and two others formed a comparison group. Pre-post 2-year educational interventions were conducted. Multiple theories were applied.	Targets included smoking, diet, and, to a lesser degree, physical activity among children in the seventh grade.	Outcome measures included number of cigarettes smoked, BP, and total cholesterol. The smoking-prevention program (with older peer leaders) involved 10 sessions of 45 minutes each, in which information, skills training, and role plays focused on harmful effects of smoking and the social and psychological pressures to smoke. Diet intervention in the schools receiving intensive intervention (II) included replacing butter with margarine and whole milk with skim milk, buttermilk or water; using vegetable oil for cooking or salads; serving low-fat meat; avoiding egg yolks; and encouraging consumption of fish, poultry, vegetables and fresh salads. The food industry supplied reduced-salt food and salt substitutes used in cooking.	Findings from the study were mixed. Although smoking among both boys and girls increased in all three groups, the greatest increase was in the comparison group (29%). Changes in dietary fat from milk and butter occurred in both girls and boys. Total cholesterol levels were decreased in both boys and girls but more so in girls. There was some decrease in salt intake, but no consequent effect on BP.

| Walter, 1989 | Sample consisted of 3,388 New York fourth-graders. Group 1 had 2,283 lower-income students from 22 elementary schools in the Bronx. Group 2 had 1,105 middle- to upper-income students from 15 elementary schools in Westchester County. | In the Bronx all 22 schools agreed to participate and were randomly assigned to an experimental group (1,590 students from 14 schools) or a nontreatment group (693 students from eight schools). In Westchester County 485 students in eight schools were randomly assigned to a treatment group and 620 students in seven schools to a nontreatment group. PRECEDE health-promotion model, health-belief model, and social learning theory provided theoretical basis. | Targets included smoking, physical activity, and nutrition in elementary school children from differing socioeconomic groups and curriculum. | Outcome variables included ponderosity index, triceps skinfold thickness, blood pressure, postexercise pulse rate, nonfasting plasma total and HDL cholesterol, serum thiocyanate, and saliva. Mediating variables included daily diet intake reported on 24-hour diet recall, reported physical activity, cigarette smoking, and knowledge relating to prevention of CHD and cancer. | After 5 years of intervention, significant positive changes in total cholesterol and intake of fat and carbohydrates were noted. After 6 years of intervention, significant decreases were noted in smoking onset. |

Table continued on following page

TABLE 13–2 Review of Selected Cardiovascular Risk Studies Conducted in School Settings *Continued*

Investigator	Sample	Design and Theory	Risk-Factor and Population Targets	Outcome Variables and Interventions	Findings
Kelder, Perry, Klepp, et al., 1994	Sample consisted of 900 sixth-graders in a reference group and 1,198 in an intervention group, plus 363 twelfth-graders in a reference group and 1,055 in an intervention group.	Quasi-experimental intervention and comparison groups were invited to participate.	Targets included smoking, physical activity, and nutrition for all sixth graders attending public schools in 1983; they were tested annually thereafter until high school graduation.	Outcome variables included tracking of smoking, physical activity, and food choices over 6 years. Students were categorized as never smoker, experimental smoker, quitter, or weekly smoker. For physical activity, students self-reported hours of exercise per week and a physical activity score. For dietary intake, they self-reported food selections.	Results supported the early establishment and persistence of smoking, physical activity, and food-choice behaviors. Recommendations were as follows: 1. Interventions should start before sixth grade. 2. Adolescents who smoke should be considered addicted and will require smoking-cessation interventions. 3. Minnesota Heart Health Program should be implemented in schools and in communities.

BP = blood pressure.
HBP = high blood pressure.
DBP = diastolic blood pressure.
SBP = systolic blood pressure.

A discussion of the assessment and management of cholesterol, nutrition, hypertension, obesity, physical activity, cigarette smoking, and stress follows.

Cholesterol

Knowledge of all the factors that influence lipid levels is necessary in order to effectively assess and manage care. The National Cholesterol Education Program (NCEP) (1991) proposes guidelines and protocols for the identification and treatment of high cholesterol levels in children and adolescents. A total cholesterol greater than 170 mg/dL and an LDL cholesterol of 110 mg/dL are recommended cutoff points, keeping in mind that no longitudinal data have linked childhood data with adult CHD. It is also important to know HDL cholesterol and triglyceride levels, because these have been shown to be related to obesity, a modifiable risk factor. Furthermore, when the HDL/LDL ratio is higher than 3, the risk for coronary heart disease increases dramatically (Weidman, 1986). Knowledge of other factors known to affect lipid levels, such as diabetes mellitus, nephrotic syndrome, anabolic steroids, and beta blockers, is needed as well.

Views regarding cholesterol screening vary among researchers and practitioners. Researchers from the Bogalusa study suggest that all preschool children should be screened for high cholesterol. In contrast, the National Institutes of Health, the American Academy of Pediatrics, and the National Heart, Lung, and Blood Institute all advise that only children with a family history of CHD should be screened.

NCEP (1991) recommends screening of children with a family history of the premature onset of CHD (that is, less than 50 years for men and less than 60 years for women) as well as a history of any of the following: hyperlipidemia, hypertension, stroke, or diabetes mellitus in parents, aunts, uncles, grandparents, and siblings. Further, NCEP suggests that particular attention be paid to assessing and managing total cholesterol and LDL cholesterol.

Arguments against universal screening include (1) high cost, (2) potential variations in laboratory results from center to center that can result in false positive findings, (3) current

dietary recommendations for children over 2 years of age, and (4) lack of evidence of direct linkages between elevated lipid levels in childhood and CHD and death in adulthood.

Ultimately, the question needs to be asked whether in fact universal cholesterol screening in children is worth the complexity and cost to promote cardiovascular health (Walter, 1989; Walter & Wynder, 1989). Those who oppose selective screening believe that it will miss significant numbers of children with high cholesterol levels (Purath, Lansinger, & Ragheb, 1995; Resnicow, Morley-Kotchen, & Wynder, 1989). There is no doubt that screening of all preschool children would most likely identify more children at risk. However, whether high cholesterol levels in childhood are consistently linked to elevated cholesterol in adulthood is questionable and requires further research. Furthermore, it is not known whether lowering childhood levels of cholesterol will lead to lower incidence of CHD in adulthood.

At this point in time, within the context of screening, nurses have a role to play in CHD prevention through the identification of children or adolescents who have a family history of heart disease. Assessment of family history needs to take into account not only genetic predisposition but also lifestyle factors (diet, physical activity, and cigarette smoking habits) known to contribute to CHD risk. Combined high-risk screening and population-based health-promotion interventions may be one answer to the screening dilemma. Population-based health promotion is discussed later in this chapter. First, a more detailed look at genetic predisposition and current dietary recommendations for normal and hyperlipidemic children is in order.

A population-based approach has been undertaken in Canada because "no large-scale comprehensive risk-factor or nutrition surveys have been conducted" (Working Group on the Prevention and Control of Cardiovascular Disease, p. 15, 1992). Instead of screening, general healthy-lifestyle programs that promote appropriate nutrition choices, regular physical activity, and the avoidance of smoking are supported for children and adolescents within the context of their families and schools. The goal proposed by the Working Group on the Prevention and Control of Cardiovascular Disease

(1992) is "to have Canadian children adopt healthy eating and physical activity habits, maintain a healthy body weight, and avoid smoking" (p. 16). The strategy is population-based, with the long-term aim being to lower the average blood cholesterol of the population over time.

HYPERCHOLESTEROLEMIA. When high-risk screening identifies a child with hypercholesterolemia, the cause of the elevation—genetic or lifestyle factors—needs to be clarified (Mistretta & Stroud, 1990). Children identified with high cholesterol levels should have two confirming elevated fasting blood lipid tests done (Glueck, 1986). The most common form of genetic hypercholesterolemia is *heterozygous familial hypercholesterolemia,* which may be found at birth. It is an inherited autosomal dominant condition characterized by high levels of LDL cholesterol (Grundy, 1986). According to the American Heart Association, one in 200 to 500 individuals inherits this genetic disorder, which is typified by a total cholesterol of 250–500 mg/dL and the appearance of symptoms in the second decade of life, when xanthomas develop in 10–15% of cases. A more rare form, *homozygous hypercholesterolemia,* is characterized by a total cholesterol of 500–1,000 mg/dL and development of xanthomas by the age of 5 years and angina by the age of 20 years (Weidman, Kwiterovich, Arky, et al., 1986). The reader is referred to Chapter 6 for additional information on the genetic basis of hypercholesterolemia.

When elevated cholesterol levels are detected, the first considerations for children and families are lifestyle factors and possible secondary causes of hyperlipidemia. Therefore, the nurse should assess the child or adolescent for the following:

- *Use of alcohol, corticosteroids, hypothyroidism, renal disease, liver disease, and medication history.* Estrogen-containing oral contraceptives, beta blockers, and alcohol can all cause hypertriglyceridemia (Glueck, McGill, Shank, et al., 1978).
- *Diet and physical activity.* Parents or the child or adolescent can keep a daily record of dietary intake and physical activity (time in minutes for child and family members) for a week.

- *Cigarette smoking habits.* Questions to be asked include, "Do parents smoke? Does the child or adolescent smoke? How much and how often"?

To avoid the misconception that dietary cholesterol is bad, the nurse can clarify with parents that cholesterol is necessary for cellular metabolism as well as explain the significance of the HDL/LDL ratio. That is, when the ratio is higher than 3, the risk for CHD increases dramatically (Weidman, 1986). Recommendations for healthful living relevant to hypercholesterolemia are also relevant to hypertension and obesity. Dietary and physical activity recommendations can be used by the nurse in counseling individual children and their families.

Nutrition

Dietary recommendations can be applied to high-risk children or adolescents as well as to the general population. The approach taken with high-risk individuals versus the general population differs only in that very high cholesterol levels of genetic origin are likely to require medication. If dietary changes in combination with other lifestyle modifications do not significantly reduce lipid levels, then medication prescribed by a physician or advanced-practice nurse (APN) will be needed.

NCEP has a two-step dietary recommendation for hypercholesterolemic children and adolescents (Table 13–3). The Step-One dietary recommendation is the same as for healthy children. In children with hyperlipidemia, if LDL cholesterol levels are not brought below 110 mg/dL within 3 months of following the Step-One diet, then the Step-Two diet is instituted.

It is important for the nurse and all clinicians to emphasize that the recommendations are meant to foster the selection of a variety of foods and caloric intake to meet the demands of growing bodies at ideal weight levels. Overzealous parents may need to be cautioned that excessive restriction of fat content in a young child's diet may be harmful to myelination of the central nervous system (Glueck, McGill, Shank, et al., 1978). Furthermore, the NCEP low-fat dietary recommendations should be used only for children over 2 years of age. NCEP supports high-risk screening combined

TABLE 13–3 NCEP Dietary Recommendations for Healthy and Hyperlipidemic Children 2 Years of Age and Older

LDL Cholesterol Level	Saturated Fatty Acids (SFA)	Percent of Total Calories to Fats	Dietary Cholesterol
Healthy children	SFA should contribute less than 10% of total daily caloric intake.	Fats should contribute less than 30% of total daily caloric intake.	Less than 300 mg of cholesterol should be consumed daily.
Step-One diet (If LDL-C is not lowered below 110 mg/dL within 3 months, then proceed to Step-Two diet.)	SFA should contribute 8–10% of total daily caloric intake.	Same as in diet for healthy children, fats should contribute less than 30% of total daily intake.	Same as in diet for healthy children, less than 300 mg of cholesterol should be consumed daily.
Step-Two diet	SFA should contribute less than 7% of total calories.		Less than 200 mg of cholesterol should be consumed daily.

with dietary recommendations that are geared toward shifting the dietary habits of the general population so that the mean cholesterol levels of all children and adolescents in the United States are lowered. Table 13–4 provides a list of ideas that the nurse can use when counseling children and families about heart-healthy food choices.

High Blood Pressure and Obesity

Blood pressure and obesity are also critical determinants of cardiovascular health. Both systolic and diastolic pressure need to be assessed. Unlike screening procedures for cholesterol levels, less controversy exists about assessing

blood pressure. Blood pressure screening is noninvasive and less costly. The National Heart, Lung, and Blood Institute (1987) provides age and sex-specific grids that can be used to plot and track blood pressure. These grids should be used to assess children and adolescents for high blood pressure. Measurement protocols and treatment are detailed in this report, but cutoff values for high blood pressure in children and adolescents are not identified; instead, the American Academy of Pediatrics has outlined age-specific recommendations for significant and severe hypertension.

Significant hypertension is defined as a blood pressure consistently (i.e., on at least three measurements) at the 95th to 99th percentile for age and sex. *Severe hypertension* is

TABLE 13–4 Practical Tips for Heart-Healthy Eating

- Select fish, chicken and lean cuts of beef, turkey, and pork; dried beans and peas. Trim all excess fat and remove skin from poultry.
- Choose skim or low-fat (1%) milk and dairy products (i.e., milk, cheese, cottage cheese, yogurt).
- Intake of fiber and complex carbohydrates can be increased with raw fruits and vegetables (apples, carrots, celery sticks, pears, cucumbers, tomatoes, lentils, dried beans, pasta, etc.). Avoid avocados. Whole-grain breads and oatmeal cereals also increase fiber intake.
- Choose desserts like ice milk, sherbet, frozen yogurt, and homemade oatmeal cookies.
- Sprinkle oat bran onto cereals and include in cookies. Oat bran lowers total cholesterol.
- Choose canola, olive, sunflower, and corn oils, and decrease intake of shortening and hard margarines.

Data from O'Brien, L. T., Barnard, J. R., Hall, J. A., & Pritikin, N. (1985). Effects of a high complex carbohydrate low-cholesterol diet plus bran supplement on serum lipids. *Journal of Applied Nutrition, 37*(1), 31; and The ILIB Lipid Handbook for Clinical Practice.

defined as blood pressure consistently equal to or greater than the 99th percentile for age and sex.

For the nurse, the most important considerations in measuring blood pressure are correct application and the use of the appropriate cuff size. Cuffs that are too narrow or improperly applied yield falsely elevated blood pressures. As well, information concerning height and weight should be considered when assessing hypertension. It may be normal for a child who is big for his or her age to have a blood pressure higher than a child of average size.

Obesity is associated with two key risk factors for CHD, hypertension and hyperlipidemia, and persists from childhood into adulthood (Berenson, Srinivasan, Webber, et al., 1991). Both lipid levels and blood pressure have been positively influenced by interventions designed to reduce weight in overweight children and adolescents (Epstein, Kuller, Wing, et al., 1989). Hayman and Ryan (1994) recommend ongoing assessment of weight and adiposity from early childhood through adolescence.

Physical Activity

Physical activity has implications for cholesterol levels, weight control, and high blood pressure. Evidence suggests that vigorous, regular physical activity has a positive impact on lipids by decreasing total cholesterol, LDL cholesterol, and triglycerides while increasing HDL cholesterol, as well as decreasing weight and blood pressure (Hofman & Walter, 1989; Durant, Baranowski, Rhodes, et al., 1993). Weight loss and decreased anxiety and depression have also been reported (Cantwell, 1984).

Physical activity and fitness levels of children and adolescents were assessed in a Youth Risk Behavior Survey conducted by the Centers for Disease Control and Prevention in 1990. Results supported other national surveys that have found a failure of U.S. children and adolescents to participate in regular, moderate to vigorous physical activity. A cited example of such activity was playing basketball for at least 20 minutes at a level of exertion characterized by heavy breathing and a rapid heart rate (Centers for Disease Control, 1992). Studies carried out in Canada reflect similar results (Canadian De-

partment of National Health and Welfare, 1986).

Nurses can encourage children and adolescents to become more physically active. Cardiorespiratory exercise at 75% of maximal heart rate for 20–25 minutes has been demonstrated to improve cardiorespiratory fitness status (Dyment, Goldberg, Haefelc, et al., 1987), and the nurse has a role to play in promoting this kind of aerobic physical activity. One of the principles to keep in mind is that the behavior of children and adolescents is influenced by those around them. For younger children, the family is the primary environment in which patterns of healthy living are learned. For adolescents, although family remains important, peers and the school setting take on greater influence in all spheres of their lives. Hence both family and school are critical environments that can support or hinder healthy lifestyle choices.

Another consideration for the nurse making suggestions for physical activity for children and adolescents centers on growth and development. Preschoolers have limited fine motor control, so active games and play that promote feelings of fun and mastery should be encouraged. Bone growth patterns need to be considered in choosing physical activity for middle school and high school children. The epiphyses in the middle school child are not yet fused, whereas in the high school student the epiphyses are fusing and bones are calcifying while at the same time the overall growth rate is starting to slow (Riopel, Boerth, Coates et al., 1986b). Therefore, competitive long-distance running, for example, is not recommended for prepubertal children because epiphyseal growth damage may occur. Rather, physical activities that can be enjoyed and pursued throughout life, such as swimming, cycling, and tennis, should be encouraged. Physical activity should be considered neither as an expendable add-on nor as a punishment, but rather as a desirable, normal part of day-to-day living.

Cigarette Smoking

Cigarette smoking is an independent risk factor for cardiovascular disease and deserves attention here because most smokers begin this highly addictive habit during adolescence (Riopel, Boerth, Coates, et al., 1986a; Manske, Taylor, d'Avernas, et al., 1993). Furthermore, smoking has been shown to have a negative impact on serum lipids and lipoproteins (Freedman, Srinavasan, Foster, et al., 1986). These researchers state that "the start of even modest cigarette smoking during adolescence and early adulthood is independently associated with atherogenic changes in serum triglycerides, LDL, HDL, and VLDL levels" (Freedman, Srinavasan, Foster, et al., p. 207, 1986). The reader is referred to Chapter 7 for additional information about cigarette smoking and CHD risk.

In Canada, the Ontario Tobacco Research Unit combined data from national, provincial and special research studies and described the following results: "From 1983 to 1993, the percentages of Ontario male students in grades 7, 9, 11, and 13 who smoked remained steady at 23%. This increased to 28% in 1995. A similar increase was seen for young females, from 25% in 1993 to 28% in 1995. This dramatic increase is in part thought to be due to sociopolitical changes—specifically, the Canadian federal government tobacco tax rollbacks, which reduced the cost of cigarettes by approximately 50%" (Ontario Tobacco Research Unit, 1996).

In a telephone survey of adolescents in a Northern Ontario community, Blackford, Bailey, and Coutu-Wakulczyk (1994) found that peer pressure and cost were two key factors that influenced whether teenagers smoked. Young women seem to smoke for different reasons than young men, and traditional preventive programs are less successful with them. In particular, Gilchrist and co-workers (1989) recommend an emphasis on self-esteem and tension reduction in smoking intervention programs for young women. Most programs are not designed to account for gender differences, but one that was, called Fly Higher, from the Heart and Stroke Foundation of Ontario, aimed to empower girls and young women (aged 14–19) to resist the pressure to smoke (Heart and Stroke Foundation of Ontario, 1995). This study, among others, showed that interventions to prevent the onset of smoking by children and teenagers are needed.

A number of studies have shown short-term successes of programs begun at the elementary school level. However, these same studies have also demonstrated that the effects diminish during high school years (Flay, Koepke, Thomson, et al., 1989; Murray Davis-Hearn, Goldman, et al., 1988; Abernathy & Bertrand, 1992). These results suggest a need for continuing preventive programming on into the high school years. In Ontario, the largest increase in the onset of tobacco use seems to appear between grades 7 and 9 (Smart & Adlaf, 1989). This early-onset pattern is congruent with findings in the United States (Chassin, Presson, Sherman, et al., 1990) and in Great Britain (Goddard, 1989).

Manske, Taylor, d'Avernas, and Moase (1993) provide a comprehensive literature review of the need for preventive programming and guiding principles for high school smoking intervention. These authors offer a set of principles that can be used by public health nurses to create and deliver a high school smoking-prevention program. The first principle is to employ a variety of strategies, including

- Cross-curriculum learning
- Extracurricular activities
- Multi-factor health-promotion tactics
- Student participation in planning and carrying out activities incongruent with smoking

The second principle is to coordinate actions by

- Assessing needs
- Linking activities across grades
- Keeping a prevention focus
- Keeping activities balanced
- Considering the school "culture"
- Creating activities with and for high school students
- Making connections between school, home, and the community

The third principle is to incorporate subgroups in planning and implementing programs by addressing

- Gender
- Culture

Stress Management

Type A behavior, and hostility in particular, has been identified as a CHD risk factor that tracks from early adolescence into adulthood. Learning to relate effectively with others, including recognizing and managing stress, begins in childhood. Patterns of healthy lifestyles are established in childhood and learned not only within the family but also at school. The public health nurse can teach parenting skills to parents that in turn enable parents to teach their children to deal appropriately with emotional stress.

Learning (1) to recognize stress, (2) to use social supports, (3) to use personal coping tactics such as "self-talk" and relaxation, and (4) to develop a sense of self as an individual have all been shown to be adaptive ways of dealing with stress (DeV. Peters, 1990). Ability to deal with stress is closely linked to the developmental stage of the child. The preschooler and school-age child learn through play. Promoting cooperative play, respect for others, sensitivity to the needs of others, and an ability to recognize and respond appropriately to emotions in oneself and others are all skills that a child can acquire.

The period of transition from childhood to adolescence is a time of many social, emotional, and physical changes. At this time children can be particularly vulnerable to peer pressure and to other influences outside their families. Their self-esteem is easily threatened. The public health nurse or school nurse can help young adolescents who are feeling overwhelmed to recognize and deal effectively with stress.

The nurse can function as a facilitator through either direct or indirect contact with vulnerable adolescents. Providing teachers with programs that are designed to help young adolescents make decisions, communicate effectively, feel self-confident, learn to set realistic goals, and take on appropriate responsibilities is an *indirect* way that the public health nurse can act as a facilitator. Some simple stress avoidance and management techniques that the nurse can *directly* teach to young adolescents include

- Separating what cannot be changed from what can
- Breaking down problems into little parts
- Using a planner to map out school work
- Making time for fun with friends
- Eating healthy food, getting daily physical activity, and getting enough sleep

- Talking about feelings with a trusted adult

A number of excellent programs are available to help children and adolescents deal with stress effectively. The Skills for Adolescence program fosters responsibility, decision making, communication, self-confidence, and goal setting. This program is based partly on Bandura's (1977) social learning theory and emphasizes self-perceptions of competence and control, motivation, decision making, and social skills (Quest International, 1988). Another program, called Comprehensive School Health Education: Totally Awesome Strategies for Teaching Health, features numerous strategies for teaching children and adolescents how to express feelings, manage stress, and so forth. A third resource, *Too Much to Handle: Living with Stress,* is a video produced by Rainbow Educational Video that addresses the problems of students feeling overwhelmed by too many responsibilities. This video is accompanied by learning objectives, previewing questions, post video debriefing discussion questions, and suggestions for classroom activities. The video features a young adolescent male struggling with overwhelming stress and being helped by his peers.

The powerful influence of peers on child and adolescent attitudes and behavior cannot be overstated. In particular, peer support (peer counselors, peer leaders) can be instrumental in helping adolescents acquire the knowledge, skills, and confidence to make heart-healthy lifestyle choices related to eating habits, stress management, tobacco use, and physical activity. Social learning theory has been effectively applied in school-based heart-health programs. However, these applications are designed for changing individual behavior whereas the research clearly speaks to the need to move beyond the level of the individual and attempt to change the health-related actions of populations or communities.

POPULATION MANAGEMENT OF CHD RISK IN CHILDREN AND ADOLESCENTS

In the past, as mentioned, cardiac lifestyle behavioral change strategies have concentrated on the individual. However, the specter of "victim blaming" is raised when lifestyle-related cardiovascular health problems are addressed on an individual basis rather than a societal environmental one. Victim blaming can occur, for example, when a child is held responsible for eating unhealthy food even though that is the only type of food available in the school cafeteria. In this instance, an environmental, or system, change is needed so that healthy food choices are available. A population approach to managing cardiovascular health takes into account social, political, economic, and physical environmental factors (Epp, 1986).

Health promotion combines concepts of well-being and avoidance of health risks. Health-promotion and disease-prevention activities are derived from the values of individuals and society (Epp, 1986). Health promotion from a World Health Organization (1986) perspective is viewed as "a mediating strategy between people and their environments, synthesizing personal choice and social responsibility in health to create a healthier future." This perspective does not abandon medical and sociobehavioral approaches. These latter two are aimed at individuals and groups and deal with risks of illness as opposed to whole populations and socioenvironmental risk conditions (Labonte & Thompson, 1993). Hence it can be seen that health-promotion and disease-prevention activities are not incompatible. Health-promotion activities can be undertaken at the individual, group, and community levels to promote, maintain, and restore health, as well as to prevent illness (Epp, 1986). The ultimate goal of health-promotion endeavors is to improve the quality of life of children and adolescents (Raphael, Brown, Rukholm, et al., 1996).

A population approach to promoting heart health and preventing CHD in children and adolescents aims interventions at the social, political, economic, and physical environments. Such an approach does not mean that the health of the individual is ignored. Indeed, the goal is to create an environment that supports individuals in making and maintaining healthy lifestyles. The school setting offers a tremendous capacity for sustained action and far-reaching impact using a population approach. Children and the majority of adolescents attend schools. Furthermore, parents and families can be reached directly and indirectly through school newsletters and parent advisory groups (Walter, 1989; Cameron, Mutter, & Hamilton, 1991). Patterns of healthy living are established in childhood (Walter, 1989; Purath, Lansinger, & Ragheb, 1995), and there is evidence to support the effectiveness of early intervention during elementary school years (Harrell & Frauman, 1994). There is equal evidence to suggest that sustained intervention from kindergarten through to graduation from high-school is needed.

The environment in which children and adolescents live often needs to be changed to support the opportunity to make healthy lifestyle choices. Within the context of a school setting, teachers, parents, and children can together create a total healthy environment that supports healthy lifestyle choices. Creating a healthy environment might involve participation in the formation of school policies regarding smoking, food services, and physical activity. Research supports the value of health instruction (Connell, Turner, & Mason, et al., 1985; Harris, 1988) and augmented health services (Waszak & Neidell, 1991) as ways of promoting heart health in children and reducing CHD risk factors known to track from childhood into adulthood (Walter, 1989).

Comprehensive School Health Framework

A *comprehensive school health* (CSH) framework can be useful for the public health nurse interested in using a population approach because it takes into account the social, economic, and physical environment of the school. This framework can be used to address the cardiovascular health of children and adolescents in general as well as that of children from lower socioeconomic groups. Risk for CHD is greatest among lower socioeconomic groups (Epp, 1986). The potential stigma attached to singling out an already marginalized group for special attention is avoided when a CSH approach is used.

It has long been recognized that learning and health are connected (Cameron, Mutter, & Hamilton, 1991). Traditionally, the approach to improving health and thereby enhancing learning within the school setting has been to focus on health education alone. Unfortunately, this approach has proved inadequate in bringing about lifestyle changes. Many of the interventions described in the literature review were curriculum-based. Those programs that also made connections to the family and to the community, plus alterations to the school environment, tended to be more effective. It is not enough just to teach children about diseases and threats to safety. Health instruction alone cannot change health attitudes and behavior. Integration of instruction, services, and physical environment in schools in interaction with their communities is required to create an overall atmosphere conducive to and supportive of behavioral change.

A CSH framework integrates the four basic elements of instruction, services, social support, and environment (Comprehensive School Health, 1993). CSH incorporates a variety of actions and services within schools and their communities to optimize the health of children and youth, encourage and support their full development, and set them on the road to productive current and future lives. The major goals of such a framework include promotion of health and wellness; prevention of specific diseases, disorders, and injuries; intervention to aid children and youth in need or at risk; and, finally, provision of support to children already experiencing illness or disability.

Some examples of instruction, services, social support, and physical environment actions within the context of cardiovascular health that could be initiated or facilitated by the public health nurse include

- Developing school food policies that support the sale of heart-healthy foods in cafeterias
- Promoting the establishment of a school board policy for daily quality physical activity
- Developing a school board policy that prohibits cigarette smoking on or around school property
- Establishing peer support groups for cigarette smokers
- Establishing programs that help children and adolescents manage stress and resolve conflict

Essentially, a CSH approach underscores the fundamental belief that to accomplish lifestyle changes at the individual level, a supportive total atmosphere is necessary that integrates instruction, services, social support, and physical environment. In other words, change at the individual level must be supported by systemwide integration of services, support, and environment. The CSH approach aims to change the environments in which young people learn, grow, and develop as human beings. Creating supportive environments allows young people to view healthy lifestyle choices as normal, expected possibilities. Partners in creating such an environment include teachers, students, parents, families, nurses and other professionals, school boards, public health agencies, and other agencies and organizations that pertain to children and youth, to education, to health, and to social services, involving governments at all levels.

The public health nurse's roles could include those of facilitator, coordinator, and information broker. For example, as a *facilitator*, the public health nurse could bring partners together to examine existing smoking, food, and physical activity policies and programs and decide on appropriate action for a systemwide impact. In the role of *coordinator*, the public health nurse could apprise the school system of a variety of services and supports available in the community such as stress management or peer counseling programs. As *information broker*, the nurse could provide CHD risk-factor and lifestyle information to school boards, teachers, principals, children, and parents.

Diffusion Models

Best (1989) suggests that heart-health school programs have been shown to be successful and that now research is needed to learn more about how to spread, or "diffuse," heart-health promotion interventions throughout systems, institutions, and communities. According to Shea and Basch (1990), diffusion of healthy behaviors refers to the spread of healthy innovative behaviors throughout the "social networks of a community" (p. 206).

At least five large-scale studies of risk-factor intervention have been carried out in the world that have involved the community in the planning and implementation of programs and policies designed to reduce the risk of cardiovascular disease and promote heart health. These studies were The North Karelia Project (Puska et al., 1985), Heartbeat Wales (Nutbeam & Catford, 1987; Tudor-Smith, Nutbeam, Moore, & Catford, 1998), The Minnesota Heart Health Program (Carlaw et al., 1984), the Pawtucket Heart Health Project (Lefebvre et al., 1987), and the Stanford Five-City Project (Farquhar et al., 1984). All incorporated a focus on children and youth. Although a detailed examination of these studies is beyond the scope of this chapter, some relevant information is summarized in Table 13–2. The important consideration here is that all of these projects have demonstrated success in effecting lifestyle behavioral change, yet, despite the successes reported from these and other similar projects, there has been little spread, or diffusion, beyond the demonstration communities.

The use of diffusion for CHD risk communication and intervention has also been discussed in detail in Chapter 5. Diffusion occurs through two main mechanisms of communication, mass media and interpersonal relationships. The *mass media* is useful for spreading new knowledge, and *interpersonal relationships* are useful for changing attitudes and behaviors. Innovations are more likely to be adopted if they are harmonious with existing values, versatile, reversible, easy to do, easy to understand, perceived to have gains that outweigh losses, and minimally risky (Rogers, 1983). For successful spread of innovations, these characteristics need to be considered in combination with the five phases outlined by Rogers: knowledge, persuasion, decision, implementation, and confirmation.

A project called Healthy Schools Healthy Kids, outlined in Table 13–5, illustrates the diffusion-of-innovations process and may serve as a prototype for other projects. The Healthy Schools Healthy Kids project used an integrated CSH program and the diffusion-of-innovations model as part of a larger heart-health community mobilization strategy. The project started with the development of a school team composed of public health nurses, university nursing professors, staff from the local heart-health demonstration project, the director of parks and recreation for the city, a nurse from the

administrative staff of the local cardiovascular hospital, the president of the local chapter of the Heart and Stroke Foundation, and school board members, teachers, parents, and administrators. The project's goal was to use an integrated CSH and diffusion-of-innovations theory framework to effect changes across school systems to reduce the risk for CHD and promote heart health in children and adolescents. With this aim, programs and policies were developed to improve the nutrition and physical activity habits of children and discourage cigarette smoking.

Initial steps included the identification of *early adopters,* who then became members of the school team. According to the diffusion-of-innovations theory, early adopters are people who have key social positions in a community or institution that enable them to have a major impact on the adoption of an innovation across the system, institution, or community. It must be emphasized that the critical application of this aspect of the theory is to identify "key influencers" (early adopters) and get them committed to adopt the innovation. These key people are thought to have a major impact in influencing others to take on new behaviors.

The public health nurse can be crucial in identifying early adopters at the school board level as well as at the school level. The nurse can identify these individuals by looking for the characteristics of early adopters, such as a commitment to improving the heart health of children and reducing the risk of CHD and a willingness and the positional power to implement programs and policies. Often such key influencers have been personally touched by heart disease. Strategies that the public health nurse can use to find early adopters include (1) using activities such as CHD risk-factor assessments of board administrators and school teaching staff and (2) holding CHD risk-factor information-sharing sessions. These two strategies can also be used to raise awareness about the incidence and impact of heart disease and to personalize the issue so as to persuade administrators and teachers that action is needed.

After a team of key influencers has been established, they can be brought together by the public health nurse to create a vision of a heart-healthy school system. Once key influencers at the school board level have decided

TABLE 13–5   Diffusion-of-Innovations Theory Explained
and Applied by Healthy Schools Healthy Kids

Description	Central Concepts	Strategies	Application
This theory explains how innovative ideas are adopted and spread. An *innovation* is an idea that is perceived by people as original. *Diffusion* refers to how something innovative is adopted by people.	Innovations are most likely to be embraced if they are • Harmonious (with existing values) • Versatile • Alterable • Easy to do • Easy to comprehend • Perceived to have greater gains then losses Process involves five stages: • Knowledge • Persuasion • Decision • Implementation • Confirmation People can be categorized as innovators, early adopters, early majority, late majority, or late laggards. *Early adopters* are key people whose position gives them great impact on the acceptance of an innovation across the system, institution, or community.	• *Knowledge*—increasing knowledge and awareness by personalizing cardiovascular risk • *Persuasion*—using teachers as role models for students; convincing students that they will learn better if they are healthy • *Decision*—having school boards adopt Comprehensive School Health intervention for heart health and begin planning how to involve schools in heart-health program	• Heart-health risk appraisals (HRA) done for teachers and staff • Post-HRA counseling • CHD risk-factor slide presentation • Identification of key leaders in the school board system • Provision of videotape and print materials to explain comprehensive school health • School team created with school board representatives, heart-health staff, public health nurse, heart-health volunteer, Heart and Stroke Foundation staff expanded to include teachers and parents from the first eight schools. • Mission statement created regarding a vision of a heart-healthy school system • Eight schools identified by school board representatives chosen on basis of likelihood of success, enthusiasm, existing healthy activities, diverse socioeconomic status, broad geographic location, and representation from both French- and English-language areas • Logo contest • Newsletter (interschool publication by heart-health team)

Based on Rogers, E.M. (1983). *Diffusion of Innovations,* 3rd ed. New York: Free Press.

to adopt a CSH intervention, then the public health nurse can facilitate their involvement in identifying early adopters at the school level. Administrators know best who the innovators in their school system are. They can be invited to identify schools already known to be early adopters in other situations. Administrators can use criteria such as likelihood of success, enthusiasm, and existing involvement in healthy activities to identify "pilot schools." As well, diversity of socioeconomic status, geographic location, language, and culture should also be taken into account.

In the Healthy Schools Healthy Kids Project, once schools had been identified, project teams composed of a parent, teacher, and principal from each school met together in a workshop format and were invited to envision what they thought a heart-healthy school should be like. Although the project is ongoing, it is predicted that the public health nurse's role at this point will revolve around coordinating and facilitating the session as well as functioning as a CHD information broker for media activities. A logo contest across schools is planned for the future to create a heart-healthy school identity that can then be projected to the larger community. School boards will be encouraged to incorporate heart-health messages into existing school newsletters.

In the implementation phase of diffusion, it is anticipated that the nurse can provide individual schools with suggestions on how to set up a parent-teacher student committee to decide on and carry out heart-healthy activities. Furthermore, the nurse can provide a menu of activities and ideas for reducing CHD risk and promoting heart health. Finally, during the confirmation phase, the nurse can help school teams identify ways of spreading recognition of the project through incentives such as lunch bags emblazoned with the heart-health logo.

One of the lessons learned in the Healthy Schools Healthy Kids experience to date is that system change takes considerable time. Furthermore, good interpersonal relationships and a coordinated media campaign are critical for success. The most cost-effective, system wide, responsive, interactive ways of helping children and adolescents to make and maintain healthy lifestyles need to be identified. Teachers, parents, children, nurses, and school administra-

tors all need to be involved in creating and implementing their collective vision of a heart-healthy school. The nurse has a pivotal role as coordinator, facilitator, and information broker in this example of a population approach to reduce CHD risk and promote heart health.

CONCLUSIONS

Evidence of early aortic atherosclerotic changes has been documented in the aortas of children as young as 3 years of age. Several longitudinal studies have confirmed that risk factors such as hyperlipidemia, hypertension, Type A personality (hostility), and obesity track or persist from early childhood on into adulthood. Numerous school intervention studies have been conducted, either alone or as part of broad community-based heart-health intervention trials in North America and Europe. These studies confirm that lifestyle behaviors can be altered and that a school setting can offer access not only to children but also to parents and teachers.

Social learning theory is the dominant theoretical perspective used in most multiple risk-factor school programs studied to date. CSH provides a global framework for children's heart health that considers instruction, services, social support, and environment. An integrated model of CSH and diffusion of innovations not only creates connections among people (parents, children, teachers), resources (health services in the community), and environmental structures (healthy policies and programs) that support healthy lifestyle choices, but also spreads, or diffuses, changes across the entire school system.

The school serves both as a setting to support and facilitate healthy lifestyle choices for children and as an entry point the nurse can use to reach teachers and families. Nurses can participate in the identification and care of children and adolescents at high risk for the development of CHD. In addition, nurses can be involved in planning and implementing strategies to reduce the risk for CHD development and promote heart health on an individual and a population basis. The next steps to improving the cardiovascular health status of children and adolescents are to develop and test population-based diffusion strategies to create healthy social, political, economic, and physical environments.

RESOURCES

Heart and Stroke Foundation of Ontario. (1995). *Heart Smart All Stars*. A resource kit for schools produced by the Children's Heart Health Task Force, Health Promotion Branch.

Canadian Association for School Health (1991). *Comprehensive School Health: A Framework for Cooperative Action: Understanding the Framework*. White Rock, B.C. Available for $10.00 + Goods & Services Tax (Canada) from 1133-160A Street, White Rock, B.C., Canada, V4A 7G9).

Council of Chief State School Officers (1991). *Beyond the Health Room*. Washington, DC: Council of Chief State School Officers. Available for $10.00 (U.S.) from CCSSO, One Massachusetts Avenue NW., Suite 700, Washington, DC 20001-1431.

Heart and Stroke Foundation of Ontario (1995). *Fly Higher*. For information, contact Heart and Stroke Foundation of Ontario, 477 Mount Pleasant Road, Toronto, Ontario, Canada, M4S 2L9. Tel: 416-489-7111; Fax: 416-481-3439.

National Health/Education Consortium (1990). *Crossing the Boundaries Between Health and Education*. National Commission to Prevent Infant Mortality (NCIPM) and Institute for Educational Leadership. Contact NCPIM, Switzer Building Room 2014, 330 C Street S.W., Washington, DC 20201. Tel: 202-205-8364.

National School Boards Association (1991). *School Health: Helping Children Learn*. Available for $15.00 (U.S.) from NBSA, 1680 Duke Street, Alexandria, VA 22314.

Pine, P. (1987). *Promoting Health Education in Schools*. Arlington, VA: American Association of School Administrators. Available for $14.00 (U.S.) plus handling from AASA. 1901 N. Moore Street, Arlington, VA, 22209-9988.

References

Abernathy, T., & Bertrand, L. (1992). Prevention of cigarette smoking among children: Results of a four-year evaluation of the PAL program. *Canadian Journal of Public Health, 83*(3), 226–229.

Allensworth, D. (1993). Health education: State of the art. *Journal of School Health, 63*(1).

Bandura, A. (1977). *Social Learning Theory*. Englewood Cliffs, NJ: Prentice-Hall.

Bandura, A. (1986). *Social Foundations of Thought and Action*. Englewood Cliffs, NJ: Prentice-Hall.

Becker, M.H. (1974) (Ed.) *The Health Belief Model and Personal Health Behavior*. Thorofare, NJ: Slack.

Berenson, G., Srinivasan, S., Webber, L., Nicklas, T.,
Hunter, S., Harsha, D., Johnson, C., Arbeit, M., Dalferes, E., Wattigney, W., & Lawrence, M. (1991). *Cardiovascular Risk in Early Life: The Bogalusa Heart Study*. Kalamazoo, MI: Upjohn.

Bergman, L.R., & Magnusson, D. (1986). Type A behaviour: A longitudinal study from childhood to adulthood. *Psychosomatic Medicine, 48,* 134–142.

Bernstein, L.R., Bellorado, D., & Bruvold, W. (1986). Evaluation of a heart health education curriculum for preschoolers, parents, and teachers. *Health Education, 17*(3), 14–17.

Best, A. (1989). Intervention perspectives on school health promotion research. *Health Education Quarterly, 16*(2), 299–306.

Blackford, K., Bailey, P., & Coutu-Wakulczyk, G. (1994). Tobacco use in northeastern Ontario teenagers: Prevalence of use and associated factors. *Canadian Journal of Public Health, 85,* 89–92.

Brandon, L.J., & Fillingim, J. (1990). Health fitness training responses of normotensive and elevated normotensive children. *American Journal of Health Promotion, 5*(1), 30–35.

Cameron, H., Mutter, G., & Hamilton, N. (1991). Comprehensive school health: Back to the basics in the 90's. *Health Promotion, 29*(4), 2–5.

Canadian Department of National Health and Welfare (1986). *Canada Health Attitudes and Behaviours Survey: 9, 12 and 15 Year Olds, 1984–1985*. Ottawa, Canada; Ministry of Supply and Services.

Cantwell, J.D. (1984). Exercise and coronary heart disease: Role in primary prevention. *Heart and Lung, 13*(1), 6–8.

Carlaw, R., Mittelmark, M., Bracht, N., & Leupker, R. (1984). Organization for a community cardiovascular health program: Experiences from the Minnesota Heart Health Program. *Health Education Quarterly, 11,* 243–252.

Castelli, W.P., Garrison, M.S., Wilson, P.W., et al. (1986). Incidence of coronary heart disease and lipoprotein cholesterol levels: The Framingham study. *Journal of the American Medical Association, 256,* 2835–2838.

Centers for Disease Control. (1992). *Morbidity and Mortality Weekly Report, 41,* 33–35.

Charter, W., & Jones, J. (1973). On the risk of appraising nonevents in program evaluation. *Education Research, 2,* 5–7.

Chassin, L., Presson, C., Sherman, S., & Edwards, D. (1990). Four pathways to young adults' smoking status: Adolescent social psychological antecedents. Unpublished manuscript.

Christensen, B., Glueck, C., Kwiterovich, P., et al. (1980). Plasma cholesterol and triglyceride distributions in 13,665 children and adolescents: The prevalence study of lipid research clinics program. *Pediatric Research, 14,* 194–202.

Cogdon, A., & Belzer, E. (1991). Dartmouth's health promotion study: Testing the coordinated approach. *Health Promotion, 29*(4), 6–10.

Cohen, R., Felix, M., & Brownell, K. (1989). The role of parents and older peers in school-based cardiovascular prevention programs: Implications for program development. *Health Education Quarterly, 16*(2), 245–253.

Comprehensive School Health (1993). *Making Connections: A Guide for Presenters and Facilitators*. Ottawa, Canada: Ministry of Supply and Services, Canada, Canadian Association of School Health (Catalog no. H39-275/93E).

Connell, D., Turner, R., & Mason, F. (1985). Summary of findings of school health education evaluation: Health promotion effectiveness, implementation and costs. *Journal of School Health, 55*(8).

Consensus Conference: Lowering Blood Cholesterol to Prevent Heart Disease (1985). *Journal of the American Medical Association, 253*(14), 2080–2086.

Cowell, J.M., Montgomery, A.C., & Talashek, M. (1992). Cardiovascular risk stability: From grade school to high school. *Journal of Pediatric Health Care, 6*(6), 349–354.

DeV. Peters, R. (1990). Adolescent mental health promotion: Policy and practice. In R.J. McMahon, & R. DeV. Peters (Eds.), *Behaviour Disorders of Adolescence.* New York: Plenum Press, pp. 207–223.

Durant, R., Baranowski, T. Rhodes, T., Gutin, B. Thompson, W., Carroll, R., Puhl, J., & Greaves, K.A. (1993). Association among serum lipid and lipoprotein concentrations and physical activity, physical fitness, and body composition in young children. *Journal of Pediatrics, 123,* 185–192.

Ellison, R., Capper, A., Goldberg, R., Witschi, J., & Stare, F. (1989). The environmental component: Changing school food service to promote cardiovascular health. *Health Education Quarterly, 16*(2), 285–297.

Epp, J. (1986). *Achieving Health for All: A Framework for Health Promotion.* Ottawa, Ontario, Canada: Minister of Supply and Services, Canada, Health and Welfare Canada.

Epstein, L.H., Kuller, L.H., Wing, R.R., Valoski, A., & McCurley, J. (1989). The effect of weight control on lipid changes in obese children. *American Journal of Diseases of Children, 143,* 454–457.

Farquhar, J., Fortmann, S., Maccoby, N., et al. (1984). The Stanford Five City Project: An overview. In J. Matarrazzo, S. Weiss, J. Herd, N. Miller, & S. Weiss (Eds.), *Behavioral Health: A Handbook of Health Enhancement and Disease Prevention* (pp. 1154–1165). New York: John Wiley and Sons.

Flay, B.R. (1990). Youth tobacco use: Risks, patterns and control. In J. Salde & C.T. Orleans (Eds), *Nicotine Addiction: Principles and Management.* London: Oxford University Press.

Flay, B.R., d'Avernas, J., Best, J.A., Kersell, M.W., & Ryan, K.B. (1983). Cigarette smoking: Why young people do it and ways of preventing it. In P. McGrath & Firestone (Eds), *Pediatric and Adolescent Behavioral Medicine.* New York: Springer-Verlag.

Flay, B.R., Koepke, D., Thomson, S., Santi, S., Best, J.A., & Brown, K. (1989). Six-year follow-up of the first Waterloo school smoking prevention trial. *American Journal of Public Health, 79,* 1371–1376.

Flynn, B., Worden, K., Secker-Walker, R., Badger, G., Geller, B., & Costanza, M. (1992). Prevention of cigarette smoking through mass media intervention and school programs. *American Journal of Public Health, 82*(6), 827–834.

Fors, S., Owen, S., Hall, D., McLaughlin, J., & Levinson, R. (1989). Evaluation of a diffusion strategy for school-based hypertension education. *Health Education Quarterly, 16*(2), 255–261.

Freedman, D., Srinivasan, S., Foster, T., Webber, L., & Berenson, G. (1986). Cigarette smoking initiation and longitudinal changes in serum lipoproteins in early adulthood: The Bogalusa heart study. *American Journal of Epidemiology, 124*(2), 207–219.

Frerichs, R.R., Srinivasan, S.R., Webber, L.S., et al. (1976). Serum cholesterol and triglyceride levels in 3,446 children from a biracial community. *Circulation, 54,* 302–308.

Gilchrist, L., Schinke, S., & Nurius, P. (1989). Reducing

onset of habitual smoking among women. *Preventive Medicine, 18,* 235–248.

Glueck, C.J. (1986). Pediatric primary prevention of atherosclerosis. *New England Journal of Medicine, 314*(3), 175–177.

Glueck, C.J., McGill, H.C., Shank, R.E., & Lauer, R.M. (1978). Value and safety of diet modification to control hyperlipidemia in childhood and adolescence. *Circulation, 58*(2), 381a, 383a, 384a.

Goddard, E. (1989). *Smoking among Secondary School Children in England in 1988.* Office of Population Censuses and Surveys, Social Survey Division. London: Her Majesty's Stationery Office.

Green, L., W., Kreuter, M.W., Deeds, S.G., & Partridge, K.B. (1980). *Health Education Planning: A Diagnostic Approach.* Palo Alto, CA: Mayfield.

Grundy, S.M. (1986). Cholesterol and coronary heart disease: A new era. *Journal of the American Medical Association, 256*(20), 2849–2857.

Harlan, W. (1989). A perspective on school-based cardiovascular research. *Health Education Quarterly, 16*(2), 151–154.

Harrell, J., & Frauman, A. (1994). Cardiovascular health promotion in children: Program and policy implications. *Public Health Nursing, 11*(4), 236–241.

Harris, L. (1988). An Evaluation of Comprehensive Health Education in American Public Schools. New York: Metropolitan Life Foundation.

Hayman, L., & Ryan, E. (1994). The cardiovascular health profile: Implications for health promotion and disease prevention. *Paediatric Nursing, 20*(5), 509–515.

Hofman, A., & Walter, J. H. (1989). The association between physical activity and cardiovascular risk factor in children in a five-year follow-up study. *International Journal of Epidemiology, 18,* 830–835.

Holman, R. L., McGill, H. C. Jr., Strong, J. P., & Geer, J. C. (1958). The natural history of atherosclerosis: The early aortic lesions as seen in New Orleans in the middle of the 20th century. *American Journal of Pathology, 34,* 209–235.

Kannel, W.B. (1983). An overview of the risk factors for cardiovascular disease. In N.M. Kaplan, & J. Stamler (Eds.), *Prevention of Coronary Heart Disease: Practical Management of Risk Factors.* Philadelphia: W.B. Saunders, pp. 1–19.

Kelder, S., Perry, C., Klepp, K-I, & Lytle, L. (1994). Longitudinal tracking of adolescent smoking, physical activity, and food choice behaviours. *American Journal of Public Health, 84*(7), 1121–1126.

Killen, J., Robinson, T., Telch, M., Saylor, K., Maron, D., Rich, T., & Bryson, S. (1989). The Stanford adolescent heart health program. *Health Education Quarterly, 16*(2), 263–283.

King, A. (1991). Community intervention for promotion of physical activity and fitness. *Exercise and Sport Sciences Reviews, 19,* 211–259.

Labonte, R., & Thompson, P. (1993). *Promoting Heart Health in Canada: A focus on Heart Health Inequalities.* Ontario, Canada: Minister of Supply and Services, Canada, Health and Welfare Canada (Catalog no. H39-286/1993E).

Lavin, A., Shapiro, G., & Weill, K. (1992). Creating an agenda for school-based health promotion: A review of 25 selected reports. *Journal of School Health, 62*(6).

Lauer, R., Lee, J., & Clarke, W. (1988). Factors affecting the relationship between childhood and adult cholesterol levels: The Muscatine study. *Paediatrics, 82*(3), 309–318.

Lefebrve, R., Lasater, T., Carleton, R., & Peterson, G.

(1987). Theory and delivery of health programming in the community: The Pawtucket Heart Health Program. *Preventive Medicine, 16,* 80–95.

Lipid Research Clinics Program. (1984). The Lipids Research Clinics coronary primary prevention trial 1 reduction in incidence of coronary heart disease. *Journal of the American Medical Association, 251,* 351–364.

Madsen, J., Sallis, J., Rupp, J., Senn, K., Patterson, T., & Atkins, C. (1993). Relationship between self-monitoring of diet and exercise change and subsequent risk factor changes in adults and children. *Patient Education and Counselling, 21*(1–2), 61–69.

Matthews, K.A., & Woodall, K.L. (1988). Childhood origins of overt Type A behaviors and cardiovascular reactivity to behavioral stressors. *Annals of Behavioural Medicine, 10,* 71–77.

Manske, S., Taylor, T., d'Avernas, J., & Moase, O. (1993). *High School Interventions for Tobacco Control: Guiding Principles and Recommended Action for Smoking Prevention and Reduction.* Comprehensive Smoking Prevention Committee Council for a Tobacco-Free Ontario. Health Promotion Branch, Ontario Ministry of Health, Canada.

MacNeil, T. (1992). Community mobilization: The road to heart health. *Health Promotion, 30*(4), 11–13.

Mistretta, E., & Stroud, S. (1990). Hypercholesterolemia in children: Risk and management. *Paediatric Nursing, 18*(2), 162–164.

Morrison, J.A., Namboodiri, K., Green, P., Martin, J., & Glueck, C.J. (1983). Familial aggregation of lipids and lipoproteins and early identification of dyslipoproteinemia. The Collaborative Lipid Research Clinics Family Study. *Journal of the American Medical Association, 250,* 1860–1868.

Murray, D., Davis-Hearn, M., Goldman, A., Pirie, P., & Leupker, R. (1988). Four and five-year follow-up results from four seventh-grade smoking prevention strategies. *Journal of Behavioral Medicine, 11*(4), 7–8.

Nader, P., Sallis, J., Patterson, T., Abramson, I., Rupp, J., Senn, K., Atkins, C., Roppe, B., Morris, J., Wallace, J., & Vega, W. (1989). A family approach to cardiovascular risk reduction: Results from the San Diego Family Health Project. *Health Education Quarterly, 16*(2), 229–244.

National Cholesterol Education Program (1991). *Report of the Expert Panel on Blood Cholesterol Levels in Children and Adolescents.* Bethesda, MD: U.S. Department of Health and Human Services, National Institute of Health and Human Services, National Institutes of Health, National Heart, Lung, and Blood Institute (NIH Publication no. 91-2732).

National Heart, Lung, and Blood Institute (1987). Report of the Second Task Force on Blood Pressure Control in Children. *Pediatrics, 79,* 1–25.

Nutbeam, D., & Catford, J. (1987). The Welsh heart programme evaluation strategy: progress, plans and possibilities. *Health Promotion, 2,* 5–18.

O'Brien, L. T., Barnard, J. R., Hall, J. A., & Pritikin, N. (1985). Effects of a high complex carbohydrate low-cholesterol diet plus bran supplement on serum lipids. *Journal of Applied Nutrition, 37*(1), 31.

Ontario Tobacco Research Unit (1996). Tax cuts undermine Ontario tobacco strategy. *Tobacco-Free Times, 2*(1), 9–10.

Pathobiological Determinants of Atherosclerosis in Youth (PDAY) Research Group (1993). Natural history of aortic and coronary atherosclerotic lesions in youth: Findings from the PDAY study group. *Arteriosclerosis and Thrombosis, 13*(9), 1291–1298.

Parcel, G., Simons-Morton, B., O'Hara, N., Baranowski, T., & Wilson, B. (1989). School promotion of healthful diet and physical activity: Impact on learning outcomes and self-reported behavior. *Health Education Quarterly, 16*(2), 181–199.

Parcel, G., Taylor, W., Brink, S., Gottlieb, N., Engquist, K., O'Hara, N., & Eriksen, M. (1989). Translating theory into practice: Intervention strategies for the diffusion of a health promotion innovation. *Family Community Health, 12*(3), 1–13.

Perry, C., Luepker, R., Murray, D., et al. (1988). Parent involvement with children's health promotion: The Minnesota Home Team. *American Journal of Public Health, 78,* 1156–1160.

Purath, J., Lansinger, T., & Ragheb, C. (1995). Cardiac risk evaluation for elementary school children. *Public Health Nursing, 12*(3), 189–195.

Puska, P., Nissinen, A., Tuomilehto, J., et al. (1985). The community based strategy to prevent coronary heart disease: Conclusions from the ten years of the North Karelia Project. *Annual Review of Public Health, 6,* 147–193.

Puska, P., Vartiainen, E., Pallonen, U., Salonen, J., Poyhia, P., Koskela, K., & McAlister, A. (1982). The North Karelia Youth Project: Evaluation of two years of intervention on health behaviour and CVD risk factors among 13- to 15-year-old children. *Preventive Medicine, 11,* 550–570.

Quest, International. (1988). *Skills for adolescence.* Granville, OH: Quest International.

Raphael, D., Brown, I., Rukholm, E., & Hill-Bailey, P. (1996). Adolescent health: Moving from prevention to promotion through a Quality of Life approach. *Canadian Journal of Public Health, 87*(2), 81–83.

Resnicow, K., Morley-Kotchen, J., & Wynder, E. (1989). Plasma cholesterol levels of 6,585 children in the United States: Results of the Know Your Body screening in five states. *Pediatrics, 84*(6), 969–975.

Resnicow, K., Cherry, J., & Cross, D. (1993). Ten unanswered questions regarding comprehensive school health promotion. *Journal of School Health, 73*(4).

Riopel, D., Boerth, R., Coates, T., Miller, W., & Hennekens, C. (1986a). Smoking: A statement for physicians. *Circulation, 74*(5), 1192a, 1193a.

Riopel, D., Boerth, R., Coates, T., Hennekens, C., Miller, W., & Weidman, W.H (1986b). Coronary risk factor modification in children: Exercise. *Circulation, 74*(5), 1189a–1191a.

Rogers, E.M. (1983). *Diffusion of Innovations,* 3rd ed. New York: Free Press.

Shea, S., & Basch, C. E. (1990). A review of five major community-based cardiovascular disease prevention programs. Part I: Rationale, design, and theoretical framework. *American Journal of Health Promotion, 4*(3), 203–213.

Smart, R., & Adlaf, E. (1989). *Alcohol and Other Drug Use among Ontario Students in 1989: Trends Since 1977.* Toronto, Ontario, Canada: Addiction Research Foundation.

Statistics Canada and Health and Welfare Canada (1989). Coronary Heart Disease, Males 1980–86, Ages 35 to 69. Ottawa, Canada: Health and Welfare Canada.

Steinberg, L. (1986). Stability and instability of Type A behavior from childhood to young adulthood. *Developmental Psychology, 22,* 393–402.

Stephen, T., & Graham, D.F. (1993). *Canada's Health Promotion Survey 1990: Technical Report.* Ottawa, Canada: Minister of Supply and Services, Canada, Health and Welfare Canada.

Strong, J.P., & McGill, H.C. Jr. (1962). The natural history of coronary atherosclerosis. *American Journal of Pathology, 40,* 37–49.

Tudor-Smith, C., Nutbeam, D., Moore, L., & Catford, J. (1998). Effects of the Heartbeat Wales programme over five years on behavioural risks for cardiovascular disease: quasi-experimental comparison of results from Wales and a matched reference area. *British Medical Journal, 316,* 818–822.

Walter, H.J., & Hofman, A. (1987). Socioeconomic status, ethnic origin, and risk factors for coronary heart disease in children. *American Heart Journal, 113,* 812–818.

Walter, H. (1989). Primary prevention of chronic disease among children: The school-based "Know Your Body" intervention trials. *Health Education Quarterly, 16*(2), 201–204.

Walter, H., & Wynder, E. (1989). The development, implementation, evaluation, and future directions of a chronic disease prevention, program for children: The "Know Your Body" studies. *Preventive Medicine, 16*(2), 59–71.

Waszak, C., & Neidell, S. (1991). *School-Based and School-Linked Clinics, 1991.* Washington, DC: The Center for Population Options.

Webber, L. S., Cresanta, J. L., Voors, A. W., & Berenson, G. S. (1983). Tracking of cardiovascular disease risk factor variables in school-aged children. *Journal of Chronic Disease, 36,* 647–660.

Weidman, W.H. (1986). Cardiovascular risk modification childhood: Hyperlipidemia. *Mayo Clinic Proceedings, 61,* 910–913.

Weidman, W., Kwiterovich, P., Arky, R., Bilheimer, D., Blackburn, H., Boerth, R., Brown, V., Ernst, N., Lasser, N., Miller, W., Riopel, D., Schienken, R., Schonfeld, G., Strong, J., & Weinberger, M. (1986). Diagnosis and treatment of primary hyperlipidemia in childhood. *Circulation 74*(5), 1181a–1187a.

Williams, D.P., Goring, S., Lohman, T., Harsha, D., Srinivasan, S., Webber, L., & Berenson, G. (1992). Body fatness and risk for elevated blood pressure, total cholesterol, and serum lipoprotein ratios in children and adolescents. *American Journal of Public Health, 82*(3), 358–363.

Working Group on the Prevention and Control of Cardiovascular Disease (1992). *Promoting Heart Health in Canada: A Focus on Cholesterol.* Ottawa, Canada: Minister of Supply and Services, Canada, Health and Welfare Canada (Catalog no. H39-254/1992E).

CHAPTER 14

Women and Coronary Heart Disease

Pam Doyle
Glenys Hamilton

Coronary heart disease (CHD) has long been thought of as a man's disease, but it is an equally important cause of death and disability among older women (Rich-Edwards, Manson, Hennekens et al., 1995; Romeo, 1995). Despite the impact of CHD on mortality and morbidity in women, gender differences in the pathophysiology, clinical presentation, treatment outcomes, and risk-factor management have received relatively little attention. Women are biologically different from men; they have different hormones, different patterns of disease and health, and different responses to treatments and preventive strategies (Rich-Edwards, Manson, Hennekens, et al., 1995; Buring, Hennekens, 1992). In addition, women have risk factors unique to them (Rich-Edwards, Manson, Hennekens, et al., 1995).

This chapter will present the emerging body of knowledge on women and CHD. Information presented will not be limited to pure "risk"-reduction strategies, because research is limited and gaps exist. Traditional risk factors for CHD in men are also of consequence for women, although the distribution and magnitude of their effects may be different (Rich-Edwards, Manson, Hennekens, et al., 1995). Accordingly,

risk-reduction strategies delineated in other chapters may be appropriate for women as well.

The purpose of this chapter is to first orient the reader to a woman's risk for CHD by discussing landmark studies and issues. Then the reader will be presented with current research findings on CHD in women with implications for risk management. The focus will be on gender differences with respect to (1) epidemiology (clinical treatment and outcomes), (2) clinical presentation, (3) relevance of hormones and hormone replacement therapy, and (4) risk factors.

GENDER DIFFERENCES IN EPIDEMIOLOGY OF CHD

CHD is the leading cause of death in women; between 250,000 to 500,000 American women die of CHD annually (Epstein, 1993; Cochrane, 1992; Steingart et al., 1987; Wenger, 1985.) Nevertheless, most women are unaware of their risk for CHD, nor do they realize that it is higher than the risk for other diseases. For example, one out of four women will die from CHD compared with one out of nine women who will develop breast cancer (Rich-Edwards, Manson, Hennekens, et al., 1995; Steingart, et al., 1987). In fact, the mortality rate for women with CHD exceeds that for all neoplastic diseases combined (Steingart et al., 1987).

Educating women about CHD risk factors can be problematic if they appreciate the magnitude of that risk. (Romeo, 1995). Many factors may have contributed to the misconception that CHD is a man's disease. Women have been underrepresented in nearly all randomized, controlled studies on risk factors, treatment, and outcomes of CHD (Barry, 1993). Reasons for the exclusion of women include (1) fear of teratogenicity; (2) increased variability caused by a woman's menstrual cycle, pregnancy, and menopause, which complicate both design and data analysis as well as increasing cost; and (3) the false belief that sex-specific effects are unlikely to significantly influence treatment outcomes.

Research on women with CHD is in its infancy. The scientific basis for care offered to women with CHD is largely based on data extrapolated from trials in which the majority of subjects were men (Cochrane, 1992). Extrapolation of those findings to women has resulted in misinterpretations such as the belief that angina is a benign problem among women (Barry, 1993). Many clinicians maintain that the diagnosis of CHD in women is complicated by the fact that women have more chest pain than men that is less often associated with disease. This belief was supported by the initial interpretation of data from the Framingham Heart Study and by findings from the Coronary Artery Surgery Study (Amsterdam & Legato, 1993). However, in these early studies, older women were inadequately represented. The inadequate representation of older women meant that the population of women most at risk was not included. Age is perhaps the single most important factor to consider when interpreting research findings on CHD and women.

A crossover effect of age on morbidity and mortality in regard to men versus women exists. Specifically, the greatest age-related increases in CHD observed among men occur between the ages of 35 and 45 and level off by age 55 (Lerner & Lannel, 1986). In contrast, the greatest age-related increases in CHD observed among women occur after the age of 55. Only one in 17 American women younger than 60 years of age has had a coronary event, compared with one in five American men. However, after the age of 60, one in four women, as well as one in four men, dies from CHD. In addition, the annual numbers of American women and men who have myocardial infarctions show that the rate of decline has been slower among women (Rich-Edwards, Manson, Hennekens, et al., 1995).

Findings from the Myocardial Infarction Triage and Intervention (MITI) registry establish that women are an average of 9 years older than men at the time of their first myocardial infarction (Maynard & Weaver, 1992). The mean ages of the women and men in this study were 72 versus 63 years, respectively (Maynard, 1992). Findings from both the Framingham Heart Study and the Multicenter Investigation of the Limitation of Infarct Size Study indicate that women who experience myocardial infarction have poorer survival rates (Wingate, 1991; Tofler et al., 1987.). They have a 75% greater mortality rate in the first month following infarction than men do (Wenger, 1985). The incidence of reinfarction within 1 year is more than doubled for women (45% versus 20% for men), with the 5-year recurrence rate being 38% versus 13% (Wenger, 1985; Wingate, 1993). Also, women have a larger proportion of silent, or unrecognized, myocardial infarctions than men do, 34% versus 27% (Lerner & Lannel, 1986).

GENDER DIFFERENCES IN CLINICAL TREATMENT AND OUTCOMES

The increased incidence of mortality among women who experience a myocardial infarction may reflect older age, more coexisting illness at the time of onset, and suboptimal or delayed treatment (Wenger, Speroff, & Packard, 1993). Several studies indicate that women undergo less intensive or invasive evaluations than men despite equal or more severe symptomatology (Wenger, Speroff, & Packard, 1993). A study carried out by Tobin and colleagues (1987) to evaluate gender differences in referrals for coronary bypass surgery found that women were referred less often for angiography. Only 4% of the women versus 40% of men with abnormal radionuclide exercise scans were referred for angiographic study.

MITI registry data demonstrated that 14% of women versus 26% of men ($p < 0.01$) received thrombolytic therapy after myocardial infarction, and 14% of women versus 25% of men ($p < 0.01$) had coronary angiography performed during the first 24 hours of hospitalization (Maynard, 1992.) State insurance claims from Massachusetts and Maryland also indicate that men are more likely than women to undergo coronary angiography and revascularization procedures during hospitalization for known or suspected CHD (Ayanian & Epstein, 1991.) Respective rates of coronary angiography among Massachusetts and Maryland men were 27.5% and 28.7% compared with 16.1% and 17.7% for women (Ayanian & Epstein, 1991.) Respective rates for coronary revascularization for men were 15.5% and 14.1% compared with 7.4% and 6.5% for women (Ayanian & Epstein, 1991.) As a result, the clinical outcomes in women may be compromised because they undergo procedures at a later stage of disease (Ayanian & Epstein, 1991.)

Significant differences in health care offered to women and men have been hard to address. In January 1992, an invitational conference titled Cardiovascular Health and Disease in Women was convened by the National Heart, Lung & Blood Institute to address the many pressing issues regarding health-care delivery to women with CHD (Wenger, Speroff, & Packard, 1993.) Among the issues addressed at this conference was the need to educate both health professionals and women about the misconception that angina pectoris is a benign problem in women (Wenger, Speroff, & Packard, 1993.) The need to include women in randomized trials and the need to design trials especially to identify risks that may be specific to women undergoing treatment for CHD were also discussed (Wenger, Speroff, & Packard, 1993).

In response to the evidence that health-care needs of women have been neglected by medical research, the National Institutes of Health (NIH) and the U.S. Food and Drug Administration have issued policies aimed at increasing the recruitment of women in studies (Sherwin, 1994.) In addition, the U.S. Congress passed the NIH Revitalization Act of 1993, which specifically mandates inclusion of women and racial and ethnic groups in clinical studies (Sherwin, 1994.) Empowerment of women through increased participation in research studies, will help improve the standard of care women receive.

GENDER DIFFERENCES IN CLINICAL PRESENTATION OF WOMEN WITH CHD

The clinical presentation of women with ischemic-type sensations differs from that of males. Women come to emergency departments for treatment of ischemic-type symptoms significantly later than men (4.4 hours after symptoms begin for women versus 1.8 hours for men; $p = 0.006$) (Schmidt & Borsch, 1991). As myocardial cell death with irreversible loss of cellular function begins to occur within 20–40 minutes after the onset of myocardial ischemia, early intervention and treatment can dramatically reduce the loss of irreversible tissue function caused by infarction (Maynard & Weaver, 1992; Eysman & Douglas, 1992; Ayanian & Epstein, 1991.)

Women may also have a different constellation of symptoms associated with myocardial ischemia. MITI registry data revealed that 90% of both women and men who had chest pain on admission reported differing associated symptoms (Maynard, 1992.) Women complained more often of fatigue, dyspnea, nausea, and upper abdominal pain; men more often experienced diaphoresis (Maynard, 1992.) Complaints of limb weakness, dizziness, and syncope were similar in the two groups (Maynard, 1992.)

The greater prevalence of non–Q wave infarctions among women may further confound their clinical presentation (Wenger, 1985; Johansson, Bergstrand, Schlossman, et al., 1984.) Non–Q wave myocardial infarctions are associated with nonspecific ST-T wave changes, unlike the "typical" ST elevation or depression characterized with "Q wave" myocardial injury or ischemia.

HORMONES AND HORMONE REPLACEMENT THERAPY

Postmenopausal women are at greatest risk for CHD. Research findings have demonstrated that CHD is not only more prevalent among women in later years following a natural menopause, but is also more prevalent among women who experience premature menopause (Lobo, 1993; Rosenberg, Hennekens, & Rosner, 1981). Premature menopause was shown to increase the risk of CHD two- to threefold, and surgical oophorectomy increased the risk of CHD three- to sevenfold (Lobo, 1993; Rich-Edwards, Manson, Hennekens, et al., 1995; Rosenberg, Hennekens, & Rosner, 1981). These findings have raised many questions regarding the cardioprotective mechanism of estrogen.

Early animal experiments demonstrated that estrogens administered to macaque monkeys being fed a high-fat diet prevented or reduced coronary atherosclerosis (Barrett-Connor & Bush, 1991.) The cardioprotective effect of estrogen was postulated to be mediated through lipid metabolism (Barrett-Connor & Bush, 1991.) Further research has demonstrated that estrogen increases levels of *high-density lipoproteins* (HDL) and decreases levels of *low-density lipoproteins* (LDL).

Many observational studies have examined the benefit of using exogenous estrogen as a means for reducing the risk of CHD in postmenopausal women. Meta-analyses of these studies suggest that there is a 50% reduction in risk for heart disease in postmenopausal women taking unopposed estrogen (Writing Group for PEPI Trial, 1995; Stampfer, Colditz, Willett, et al., 1991). Additionally, the use of unopposed estrogen has been associated with a statistically significant reduction in angiographically defined CHD in women with chest pain (Lobo, 1993).

The risk-benefit ratio of using *hormone replacement therapy* (HRT) has been poorly understood. For example, contradictory information exists in the literature about the effect of unopposed estrogen on blood pressure. Estrogen may affect blood pressure by increasing the production of angiotensinogen, a key component of the renin-angiotensin-aldosterone system (Frisch, 1993.) Theoretically, this increased production of angiotensinogen would cause an increase in blood pressure, but differing reports indicate increases, decreases, or no change at all (Writing Group for PEPI Trial, 1995.)

Early regimens of HRT, which involved much higher doses of unopposed estrogen than currently used, were associated with definite increases in blood pressure (Journal of the American Medical Association, 1995). These early findings, along with reports on the adverse effects of higher-dose birth control pills on blood pressure and thromboembolic events, generated concern regarding the risks of HRT (Journal of the American Medical Association, 1995). In addition, there were reports of estrogen-induced endometrial cancer based on data collected during these early studies. In fact, pooled data demonstrate a sixfold increase in the incidence of endometrial cancer in women receiving unopposed estrogen replacement (New England Journal of Medicine, 1991).

This information led to the current practice of using estrogen in combination with progestin. Progestational agents are believed to reduce the risk of uterine cancer by reducing the incidence of uterine hyperplasia associated with unopposed estrogen (Wenger, Speroff, & Packard, 1993). But the addition of progestational agents has been considered problematic, because progestins have been shown to negate the cardioprotective effects of estrogen, particularly on lipoproteins (Writing Group for PEPI Trial, 1995).

At the time of this writing, only one large-scale clinical trial has been conducted on the use of HRT, the Postmenopausal Estrogen and Progestin Interventions (PEPI) trial supported by NIH, which yielded preliminary data in January 1995. The PEPI trial was a 3-year, multicenter, randomized, double-blind, placebo-controlled trial designed to assess pairwise differences between placebo, unopposed estrogen, and each of three estrogen/progestin regimens on selected CHD risk factors in healthy postmenopausal women (Writing Group for PEPI Trial, 1995). A total of 875 women aged 45–64 were randomly assigned to five treatment groups (Table 14–1). The primary endpoints designated to represent heart disease risk factors were HDL cholesterol, systolic blood pressure, serum insulin, and fibrinogen. Fibrinogen was used as a marker for blood clotting be-

TABLE 14–1   Unadjusted Mean Changes in Outcomes Measures
with Different Protocols for Hormone Replacement Therapy

			Treatment Group			
Outcome Measure	*Placebo*	*CEE*	*CEE + MPA (cyc)*	*CEE + MPA (con)*	*CEE + MP (cyc)*	*P*
HDL cholesterol (mg/dl)	−1.2	5.6	1.6	1.2	4.1	<0.001
LDL cholesterol (mg/dl)	−4.1	−14.5	−17.7	−16.5	−14.8	<0.001
Triglycerides	−3.2	13.7	12.7	11.4	13.4	<0.001
Fibrinogen (g/L)	0.2	0.2	0.5	0.01	0.01	<0.001

CEE = conjugated equine estrogen.
MPA = medroxyprogesterone acetate.
MP = micronized progesterone.
Cyc = administered daily for 12 days per month.
Con = administered daily.
Adapted from Writing Group for PEPI Trial (1995). Effects of estrogen or estrogen/progestin regimens on heart disease risk factors in postmenopausal women: The Postmenopausal Estrogen/Progestin Interventions (PEPI) Trial. *Journal of the American Medical Association, 273* (3), 199–208.

cause, based on Framingham Heart Study data, it is considered an independent risk factor for both myocardial infarction and stroke (Journal of the American Medical Association, 1995). The risk for endometrial hyperplasia was monitored through endometrial aspiration at baseline and annually with additional biopsies when there was any incidence of noncyclic endometrial bleeding (Writing Group for PEPI Trial, 1995).

The results of the PEPI indicate that estrogen taken alone or in combination with a progestin lowers LDL cholesterol and fibrinogen levels without detectable effects on postchallenge insulin or blood pressure. Although unopposed estrogen caused a more significant elevation in HDL cholesterol, estrogen in combination with progestational agents demonstrated a significant increase in this important cardioprotective lipoprotein, CEE (conjugated equine estrogen) plus cyclic MP (micronized progesterone) having the most favorable effect on HDL cholesterol. Only unopposed estrogen was associated with a statistically significant increased risk of endometrial hyperplasia or adenomatous hyperplasia compared with the other active treatments (34% versus 1%) (Writing Group for PEPI Trial, 1995). There was no increased risk for breast cancer detected at the 3-year mark (Journal of the American Medical Association, 1995).

However, the effect on breast cancer risk of adding progestins to estrogen therapy for postmenopausal women remains controversial (Colditz, Handinson, Hunter, et al., 1995). Data from the follow-up Nurses' Health Study (1978–1992) indicate that the addition of progestins to estrogen therapy does not reduce the risk of breast cancer among postmenopausal women with 5 or more years of continued use (Colditz, Handinson, Hunter, et al., 1995). However, the small number of such cases in this study precluded detailed analysis of the risk according to the duration of use and age. Also, some of the women in this study were taking 1.25 mg of conjugated estrogen compared with the currently common dose of 0.625 mg (as in the PEPI trial), and increased concentrations of estrogens may have affected the outcome measurements of this study.

These findings do suggest that women should carefully consider the risks and benefits of HRT. The only unexpected finding from the PEPI Trial was that triglyceride levels increased comparably in all active treatment arms, a result that differed significantly from the placebo group and prompted a recommendation for further study (Writing Group for PEPI Trial, 1995).

The PEPI trial admittedly did not study all of the plausible cardioprotective mechanisms of estrogen owing to time and financial constraints. One such mechanism, receiving growing support today, is estrogen-augmented coronary blood flow. Current research indicates that estrogen has both an indirect and direct effect on the coronary vascular endothelium, vascular smooth muscle, and arterial myocytes (Herrington, Braden, Williams, et al., 1994).

Normally, acetylcholine has a potent vasodilator effect on coronary arteries because of the release of endothelial-derived relaxing factor, but in atherosclerotic arteries this mechanism is impaired, and paradoxic vasoconstriction occurs (Herrington, Braden, Williams, et al., 1994). Estrogen-induced modulation of coronary vasoreactivity in the atherosclerotic arteries of women was studied by Reis and colleagues (1994), and by Herrington and colleagues (1994).

Data from these studies indicate that exogenous estrogen attenuates the abnormal coronary vasomotor response in diseased coronary arteries as manifested by increased coronary blood flow and decreased vascular resistance (Herrington, Braden, Williams, et al., 1994; Reis, Gloth, Blumenthal, et al., 1993). The modulation of coronary vasoreactivity by exogenous estrogen may occur through increased production and release of endothelial-dependent vasoactive intermediaries such as endothelial-derived-relaxing factor (Herrington, Braden, Williams, et al., 1994). Data from both of these studies suggest that estrogen normalizes endothelial-dependent vasodilator capacity through attenuation or reversal of the vasoconstrictor response to acetylcholine (Herrington, Braden, Williams, et al., 1994; Reis, Gloth, Blumenthal, et al., 1993).

Estrogen also has a direct effect on vascular smooth muscle by acting as a calcium channel blocker. Thus, estrogen modifies the kinetics of the channels through which calcium enters the cells of the heart (Katz, 1992; Reis, Gloth, Blumenthal, et al., 1993). As a calcium antagonist, estrogen reduces the amount of calcium brought into the cell, and decreased concentrations of intracellular calcium limit myocardial and smooth muscle contraction (Katz, 1992). Estrogen antagonizes calcium and endothelium-1 induced vasoconstriction, as manifested by rightward shifts of calcium concentration. These changes in the electrical properties of vascular smooth muscle cause vasodilatation of the coronary and peripheral, arteries (Reis, Gloth, Blumenthal, et al., 1993). In addition, estrogen has a direct effect on arterial myocytes that causes an increased production of humoral

vasodilator substances such as prostacyclin (Reis, Gloth, Blumenthal, et al., 1993).

Evidence strongly favors the use of HRT as a means for reducing CHD risk in women at a time when they "become especially vulnerable to heart disease," namely, after the age of 50 (Journal of the American Medical Association, 1995). It is not clear, though, whether the benefits of HRT outweigh the risks for all women, particularly women with few CHD risk factors (Colditz, Handinson, Hunter, et al., 1995). It is important to educate women in a way that will help them make informed decisions regarding HRT that are appropriate for their specific set of circumstances and consistent with their values. As the population ages, and women continue to outlive men, these issues become more important to address.

CHD RISK-FACTOR PROFILE OF WOMEN

Reduction in the risk of CHD through modification of CHD risk factors is important for women of all ages (Wenger, Speroff, & Packard, 1993). Although CHD risk factors that predict disease in men are also predictive for women, some have specific significance for women (Barry, 1993). In addition, women have risk factors that are unique to them. Understanding a woman's risk profile is an important first step in planning strategies for risk-factor modification. In the following discussion, CHD risk factors are addressed in terms of their importance for women.

Age

A woman's risk for CHD increases significantly after the age of 55, and after the age of 60, it equals that of a man's (Rich-Edwards, Manson, Hennekens, et al., 1995). Data from the Lipid Research Clinics follow-up study indicate that women have a sevenfold increase in mortality from CHD for each 10-year increment after the age of 60 (Corrao, Becker, Ockene, et al., 1990). The fact that symptomatic CHD occurs later in life for most women at risk means that preventive strategies for risk-factor modification would be most effective if young women were targeted for education and risk-factor modification.

Postmenopausal Status

As indicated, postmenopausal status increases risk for CHD, regardless of age. Women who experience early and abrupt menopause as a result of bilateral oophorectomy and who do not receive HRT have a CHD risk 2.2 to 7 times higher than premenopausal women of the same age (Rich-Edwards, Manson, Hennekens, et al., 1995; Rosenberg, Hennekens, & Rosner, 1981). In addition, women who receive HRT after surgical menopause may have a lower risk for CHD than premenopausal women (Rich-Edwards, Manson, Hennekens, et al., 1995).

Premature and natural menopause are not associated with the same sudden increase in risk for CHD as surgical menopause. Instead, increased risk is thought to be more gradual, reflecting the gradual cessation of ovarian function during the perimenopausal state (Rich-Edwards, Manson, Hennekens, et al., 1995). As previously discussed, HRT may modify risk related to postmenopausal status.

Cigarette Smoking

Research has consistently shown that the risk of CHD is two to four times higher among women who smoke 20 or more cigarettes a day than among women who do not smoke (Rich-Edwards, Manson, Hennekens, et al., 1995). In addition, the number of cigarettes smoked per day is positively correlated with an increased risk for CHD (Corrao, Becker, Ockene, et al., 1990). The risk of CHD after cessation of smoking in both women and men begins to decline within a matter of months, and within 3–5 years the level of risk is equal to that of a nonsmoker (Rich-Edwards, Manson, Hennekens, et al., 1995). Cigarette smoking is one of the most powerful and modifiable risk factors for CHD among women, especially young women (Corrao, Becker, Ockene, et al., 1990; Rich-Edwards, Manson, Hennekens, et al., 1995; Wenger, 1985). In a study done by Rosenberg and colleagues, 65% of acute myo-

cardial infarctions among women less than 50 years of age were attributable to cigarette smoking (Corrao, Becker, Ockene, et al., 1990; Wenger, 1985). Premenopausal women experience a tenfold increase in risk if they smoke 35 or more cigarettes a day compared with premenopausal women who do not smoke (Wenger, 1985). This increased risk, above and beyond a man's risk, may be due to the antiestrogenic effect cigarette smoking has in premenopausal women (Khaw, Chir, Tazuke, et al., 1988; Barron, 1984).

Epidemiologic evidence strongly supports an association between smoking and early menopause, which supports the hypothesis that smoking exerts an antiestrogenic effect (Das & Banka, 1992; Corrao, Becker, Ockene, et al., 1990; Khaw, Chir, Tazuke, et al., 1988; Baron, 1984). Additionally, there is extensive documentation that smoking accompanied by oral contraceptive use has an associated risk for myocardial infarction and cardiac-related death (Wenger, 1985).

Despite a general trend toward decreased smoking, the proportion of female teenagers who smoke has increased markedly, to an estimated 26% in 1987 (Das & Banka, 1992). In particular, smoking has increased among young and disadvantaged women, groups often targeted by cigarette advertising (Wenger, Speroff, & Packard, 1993). Also, advertising is directed to a woman's greater use of cigarettes for weight control (Wenger, Speroff, & Packard, 1993). For example, cigarette ads that boast "You can do it!" depict young, thin women smoking and having fun. A significant reduction in risk for CHD among women can be achieved by targeting this young population for smoking-cessation programs. Refer to Chapter 7 for smoking-cessation strategies to implement, with weight gain as an important consideration for this population.

Cholesterol

Although the substantial impact of HDL cholesterol on CHD risk in both women and men was evident in the Framingham cohort, HDL cholesterol has been shown to be a more powerful predictor of CHD in women than in men (Corrao, Becker, Ockene, et al., 1990; Lerner & Lannel, 1986). HDL cholesterol was an important predictor of death from cardiovascular causes among women in the Lipid Research Clinic follow-up study (Rich-Edwards, Manson, Hennekens, et al., 1995). Hong and colleagues found a statistically significant difference in the mean ratio of total cholesterol (TC) to HDL cholesterol in women with CHD (5.5) compared to women without CHD (4.2) (Romeo, 1995; Hong, Roman, Reagan, et al., 1991). In this study, the TC/HDL ratio emerged as the best predictor of CHD in women (Romeo, 1995). In addition, the Framingham study showed an elevated triglyceride level as an independent risk factor for women alone (Corrao, Becker, Ockene, et al., 1990).

Data on the primary prevention of CHD through modification of lipid profiles in healthy women are limited. For example, only 5,800 of the more than 30,000 participants enrolled in primary prevention trials of cholesterol reduction have been women. Thus, the statistical power needed to estimate the effect of cholesterol reduction in women has been inadequate (Rich-Edwards, Manson, Hennekens, et al., 1995). Although definitive evidence that lowering cholesterol levels reduces the risk of CHD in healthy women is lacking, observational data indicates that interventions to lower LDL cholesterol levels and raise HDL cholesterol levels would benefit women as well as men (Rich-Edwards, Manson, Hennekens, et al., 1995).

Diabetes

Next to smoking, diabetes has the most adverse effect on CHD mortality in women (Das & Banka, 1992; Wenger, 1985). Diabetes is a stronger risk factor for CHD in women than in men, and diabetic women are at greater risk of cardiovascular death than are diabetic men (Das & Banka, 1992; Manson, Stampfer, Colditz, et al., 1991; Rich-Edwards, Manson, Hennekens, et al., 1995; Wenger, 1985). In fact, mortality rates for CHD are three to seven times higher among diabetic women than among nondiabetic women, versus only two to four times higher among diabetic men compared with nondiabetic men (Rich-Edwards, Manson, Hennekens, et al., 1995).

In addition, women with diabetes have lipo-

protein abnormalities that are more severe and triglyceride levels that are more predictive of risk for CHD than is the case for diabetic men (Das & Banka, 1992; Gordon, Castelli, & Hjortland, 1977). Among diabetic patients with manifest CHD, women have a poorer prognosis (Das & Banka, 1992). Furthermore, the diabetic woman loses the statistical-based "protection" that other premenopausal women have against CHD (Wenger, 1985; Gordon, Castelli, & Hjortland, 1977). Diabetes impairs estrogen binding, negating the protection against CHD that endogenous estrogen provides for pemenopausal women (Rich-Edwards, Manson, Hennekens, et al., 1995).

Although it is not clear if strict glycemic control reduces the risk for CHD, there is evidence that aggressive treatment of insulin-dependent diabetes slows the development of other diabetic complications (Rich-Edwards, Manson, Hennekens, et al., 1995). Nevertheless, current risk-reduction recommendations rely on the modification of other risk factors to reduce the risk for CHD incurred by diabetes (Rich-Edwards, Manson, Hennekens, et al., 1995). For example, cigarette smoking, hypertension, obesity, and hypercholesterolemia act in synergy with diabetes (Rich-Edwards, Manson, Hennekens, et al., 1995). Therefore, reduction of these risk factors will reduce the increased risk for CHD associated with diabetes in women.

Hypertension

Systemic hypertension is a known risk factor for CHD in both women and men (Corrao, Becker, Ockene, et al., 1990). A systolic blood pressure of 160 mm Hg or greater or a diastolic blood pressure of 85 mm Hg or greater has been shown to increase the risk of CHD two- to threefold in both women and men (Corrao, Becker, Ockene, et al., 1990). Although data support effective reduction in blood pressure among women with the use of antihypertensive medications, little data exist to indicate whether the side effects of these medications are the same for women as for the white males on whom they were tested (Rich-Edwards, Manson, Hennekens, et al., 1995).

Dietary intervention and weight loss have

proved moderately successful in reducing blood pressure among women based on trials in which 30–60% of the patients were women (Rich-Edwards, Manson, Hennekens, et al., 1995). Nonpharmocologic treatment of hypertension in women should be planned according to the protocols delineated in Chapter 9. Isolated systolic hypertension is of particular concern in older women (Rich-Edwards, Manson, Hennekens, et al., 1995). This condition is more prevalent among women than in men, and is associated with an increased risk of CHD.

Antihypertensive treatment resulted in a 25% reduction in the incidence of CHD in the Systolic Hypertension in the Elderly Program (Rich-Edwards, Manson, Hennekens, et al., 1995). Pharmacologic therapies are based on trials in which the majority of subjects are men. Consequently, choosing a medication regimen for women requires extrapolation of data from these trials to women. Another problem is that the risk of hypertension for CHD increases significantly, two- to fourfold, when it is accompanied by obesity and oral contraceptive use (Romeo, 1995).

Obesity

Obesity and risk for CHD are directly and positively related (Rich-Edwards, Manson, Hennekens, et al., 1995; Romeo, 1995). In the Nurses Health Study the risk of CHD was over three times higher among women with a body mass index of 29 or higher than among those with a body mass index of less than 21 (Rich-Edwards, Manson, Hennekens, et al., 1995). Distribution of body fat is more important than overall obesity in both women and men in regard to CHD risk (Corrao, Becker, Ockene, et al., 1990; Romeo, 1995). Risk increases with a greater percentage of body fat in the abdomen as evidenced by a higher waist-to-hip ratio (Romeo, 1995), namely a ratio of greater than 0.8 (Rich-Edwards, Manson, Hennekens, et al., 1995).

It is unclear whether obesity in and of itself is an independent risk factor, or if risk is increased in obese women because of other associated risk factors such as hypertension, hypercholesterolemia, and hyperglycemia (Corrao, Becker, Ockene, et al., 1990). Data are sparse on the

efficacy of approaches to reduce upper body obesity and on the potential benefits of weight reduction in relation to CHD risk reduction in women (Rich-Edwards, Manson, Hennekens, et al., 1995; Romeo, 1995).

Oral Contraceptives

Prior to changes in the prescribing practices in the mid 1970s, women received high-dose oral contraceptives, which were associated with an increased risk for CHD (Corrao, Becker, Ockene, et al., 1990; Rich-Edwards, Manson, Hennekens, et al., 1995). Concern still exists that these high-dose oral contraceptives are atherogenic and that past usage may contribute to an increased risk for CHD among older women (Rich-Edwards, Manson, Hennekens, et al., 1995). However, a meta-analysis of 13 studies showed that there was no increased risk of CHD among past users of oral contraceptives (Rich-Edwards, Manson, Hennekens, et al., 1995). In fact, there is a rapid return to baseline risk of CHD among women who have stopped using oral contraceptives, and the duration of their use does not affect the risk. The increased risk of CHD with smoking and the use of oral contraceptives persists, though. Studies have demonstrated a sevenfold increase in risk for CHD among women who smoke and use oral contraceptives (Corrao, Becker, Ockene, et al., 1990). Targeting this population for smoking cessation is imperative.

Physical Activity

Although women have been underrepresented in studies designed to assess the relationship of exercise and risk for CHD, data generally indicate that physically active women have a 60–75% lower risk of CHD than inactive women (Rich-Edwards, Manson, Hennekens, et al., 1995). Data from the 8-year prospective study of 3,120 healthy women from the Healthy Women Study demonstrated a strong association between physical fitness and reduced rates of mortality from CHD (Rich-Edwards, Manson, Hennekens, et al., 1995). Women participating in these studies, however, have been predominantly white, educated, and middle- to upper-middle class. These women would be expected to have lower risk for CHD in any event, so results may not be generalizable (Barrett-Connor & Bush, 1991).

Psychosocial Risk Factors

Women employed outside the home may have a reduced risk for CHD (Jacobson, 1987; Hazuda, Haffner, Stem, et al., 1986; Haynes & Feinleib, 1980. The number of women participating in the workforce has risen sharply during the past 40 years, a fact that has led some to suggest women may lose their survival advantage over men (Haynes & Feinleib, 1980. This idea is based on the unsubstantiated assumption that men live fewer years than women because they work outside the home (Haynes & Feinleib, 1980). Yet, studies have consistently demonstrated that employed women have favorable HDL cholesterol levels that are not explained by the use of exogenous estrogen or by their lifestyle (Jacobson, 1987; Hazuda, Haffner, Stem, et al., 1986; Haynes & Feinleib, 1980). Women employed outside the home have significantly higher HDL cholesterol levels and lower triglyceride levels than full-time homemakers (Jacobson, 1987; Hazuda, Haffner, Stem, et al., 1986). Moreover, movement of women out of the labor force is associated with an acute drop in HDL cholesterol levels and an acute rise in triglyceride levels (Hazuda, Haffner, Stem, et al., 1986). Although the cause of these phenomena is poorly understood, possible explanations include the presence of psychological mediators (Hazuda, Haffner, Stem, et al., 1986). Employed women may be less depressed and have higher self-esteem, a greater sense of mastery and control, and less psychological stress than full-time homemakers (Rosenfield, 1989; LaRosa, 1988; Hazuda, Haffner, Stem, et al., 1986). For example, a woman's employment is associated with greater decision-making power in the family, which increases her sense of control and reduces her level of stress (Rosenfield, 1989). Perceived control over one's environment demonstrates the strongest (positive) correlation with improved cardiovascular health in women (Rosenfield, 1989; LaRosa, 1988).

Low-Dose Aspirin

The role of aspirin in the secondary prevention of CHD has been the focus of considerable research (Manson, Stampfer, Colditz, et al., 1991). In a prospective study with 87,678 registered nurses, the use of aspirin for the primary prevention of CHD in women was examined. Data from this study demonstrated that the use of one to six aspirin tablets per week was associated with a reduced risk of myocardial infarction among women (Manson, Stampfer, Colditz, et al., 1991). The valuable information derived from the Nurses' Study prompted the initiation and design of the Women's Health Study (WHS) in 1992.

The WHS was a randomized, double-blind, placebeo-controlled trial designed to test the risks and benefits of low-dose aspirin, as well as the antioxidant vitamins beta-carotene and vitamin E in the primary prevention of cardiovascular disease and cancer in healthy women (Buring & Hennekens, 1992). The results from this trial will have far-reaching public health implications. It will provide either definitive positive results on which public policy can be based or informative null results, which could then safely permit the rechanneling of already limited resources to other research areas.

The WHS is part of the Women's Health Initiative, which is the largest community-based clinical intervention and prevention trial ever conducted (Cotton, 1992). The federal government is putting $500 million into this 10-year study of diet, dietary supplements, exercise, hormone therapy (the PEPI trial), and smoking cessation as prevention for cardiovascular disease, cancer, and osteoporosis in as many as 140,000 postmenopausal women (Cotton, 1992). The Women's Health Initiative involves five of the 12 NIH organizations in Bethesda, Maryland (Cotton, 1992). Attempts to redress inattention to women as subjects of medical research are shifting into high gear as the federal government puts money where its public statements have been (Cotton, 1992).

CONCLUSION

Modification of conventional CHD risk factors is essential for both women and men. Knowledge about gender differences will facilitate the development of individualized risk-reduction programs to help meet these goals. First, women need to believe they are at risk. Women know that men are at risk for CHD, but they may not appreciate their own risk. *Perceived susceptibility* is an individual's estimated probability that he or she will encounter a specific health problem (Pender, 1987). A number of studies clearly support the importance of perceived susceptibility as a predictor of preventative behavior (Pender, 1987). For example, Fink and co-workers (1972) demonstrated that women who perceived they were susceptible to breast cancer were more likely to participate in a cancer screening program for detection of breast abnormalities. Thus, misconceptions and underestimations of risk for CHD may influence CHD risk-reduction behaviors. For women, sensitization to CHD risk, education, and counseling may become most important initial steps in CHD risk-reduction interventions.

References

Amsterdam, E.A., & Legato, M.J. (1993). What's unique about CHD in women? *Patient Care,* November 15, 1993, 21–61.

Ayanian, J.Z., & Epstein, A.M. (1991). Differences in the use of procedures between women and men hospitalized for coronary heart disease. *New England Journal of Medicine, 325*(4), 221–225.

Baggs, J., & Karch, A.M. (1987). Sexual counseling of women with coronary heart disease. *Heart & Lung. 16*(2), 154–159.

Baron, J.A. (1984). Smoking and estrogen-related disease. *American Journal of Epidemiology 119*(1), 9–22.

Barrett-Connor, E., & Bush, T.I. (1991). Estrogen and coronary heart disease in women. *Journal of the American Medical Association, 265*(14), 1861–1867.

Barry, P. (1993). Coronary artery disease in older women. *Geriatrics, 48*(Suppl. 1), 4–8.

Becker, R.C., Corrao, J.M., & Alpert, J.S. (1988). The decision to perform coronary bypass surgery in women. What are the facts? *American Heart Journal, 116*(3), 891–893.

Boogaard, M.A.K. (1984). Rehabilitation of the female patient after myocardial infarction. *Nursing Clinics of North America, 19*(3), 433–440.

Boogaard, M.A.K., & Briody, M.E. (1985). Comparison of the rehabilitation of men and women post-myocardial infarction. *Journal of Cardiopulmonary Rehabilitation, 5,* 379–384.

Buring, J.E., & Hennekens, C.H. (1992). The Women's Health Study: Summary of the study design. *Journal of Myocardial Ischemia, 4*(3):27–40.

Case, R.B., Moss, A.J., Case, N., McDermott, M., & Eberly, S. (1992). Living alone after myocardial infarction: Impact on prognosis. *Journal of the American Medical Association, 267*(4), 515–519.

Clarke, P.I., Glasser, S.P., Lyman, G.H., Krug-fite, J., &

Root, A. (1998). Relation of Results of Exercise Stress Tests in Young Women to Phases of the Menstrual Cycle. *American Journal of Cardiology. 61,* 197–199.

Cochrane, B.L. (1992). Acute myocardial infarction in women. *Critical Care Nursing Clinics of North America, 4*(2), 279–289.

Colditz, G.A., Handinson, S.E., Hunter, D.J., Willett, W.C., Manson, J.E., Stampfer, M.J., Hennekens, C., Rosner, B., & Speizer, F.E. (1995). The use of estrogens and progestins and the risk of breast cancer in postmenopausal women. *New England Journal of Medicine, 332*(24), 1589–1639.

Corrao, J.M., Becker, R.C., Ockene, I.S., & Hamilton, G.A. (1990). Coronary heart disease risk factors in women. *Journal of Cardiology. 77*(Suppl 2), 8–24.

Cotton, P. (1992). Women's Health Initiative leads way as research begins to fill gaps. *Journal of the American Medical Association, 267*(4), 469–473.

Das, B.N., & Banka, V.S. (1992). Coronary artery disease in women; How it is—and isn't—unique. *Postgraduate Medicine, 91*(4), 197–206.

Dittrich, H., Gilpin, E., Nicod, P., Cali, G., Henning, H., & Ross, J. (1988). Acute myocardial infarction in women: Influence of gender on mortality and prognostic variables. *American Journal of Cardiology, 62,* 1–7.

Ell, K.O., & Haywood, L.J. (1985). Sociocultural factors in MI recovery: An exploratory study. *International Journal of Psychiatry in Medicine. 15*(2), 157–175.

Eysman, S.B., Douglas, P.S. (1992). Reperfusion and revascularization strategies for coronary artery disease in women. *Journal of the American Medical Association, 268*(14), 1903–1907.

Fink, R., Shapiro, S., & Roester, R. (1972). Impact of efforts to increase participation in repetitive screenings for early breast cancer detection. *American Journal of Public Health, 62,* 328–331.

Frisch, M. (1993). *Stay Cool Through Menopause; Answers to Your Most-Asked Questions.* New York: Putnam Publishing Group.

Greenberg, P.S., Berge, R.D., Johnson, K.D., Ellestad, M.H., Iijas, E., & Hayes, M. (1983). The value and limitation of radionuclide angiography with stress in women. *Clinical Cardiology 6,* 312.

Gordon, T., Castelli, W.P., & Hjortland, M.C. (1977). Diabetes, blood lipids, and the role of obesity in CHD risk for women. The Framingham study. *Annals of Internal Medicine, 87,* 393–397.

Haynes, S.G., & Feinleib, M. (1980). Women, work, and coronary heart disease: Prospective findings from the Framingham Heart Study. *American Journal of Public Health, 70*(2), 133–141.

Hazuda, H.P., Haffner, S.M., Stem, M.P., Knapp, J.A., Eifier, C.W., & Rosenthal, M. (1986). Employment status and women's protection against coronary heart disease: Findings from the San Antonio Heart Study. *American Journal of Epidemiology, 123*(4), 623–640.

Herrington, D.M., Braden, G.A., Williams, J.K., & Morgan, T.M. (1994). Endothelial-dependent coronary vasomotor responsiveness in postmenopausal women with and without estrogen replacement therapy. *American Journal of Cardiology, 73,* 951–952.

Higginbotham, M.B., Morris, K.G., Coleman, R.E., & Cobb, F.R. (1984). Sex-related differences in the normal cardiac response to upright exercise. *Circulation, 70,* 357–366.

Hong, M.K., Roman, P.K., Reagan, K., Green, L.E., & Rackley, C.E. (1991). Total cholesterol/HDL ratio is the best predictor of anatomic coronary artery disease in women. *Journal of American College of Cardiology. 17*(2), 389–399.

Jacobson, B.K. (1987). Employment status and women's protection against CHD. *American Journal of Epidemiology 26*(1), 159–160.

Johansson, S., Bergstrand, R., Schlossman, D., Selin, K., Vedin, A., & Wilhelmsson, C. (1984). Sex differences in cardioangiographic findings after myocardial infarction. *European Heart Journal 5.* 374–381.

Journal of the American Medical Association (1995). PEPI in perspective; Good answers spawn pressing questions [Editorial]. *Journal of the American Medical Association, 273*(3), 240–241.

Kantowitz, N.E., & Pfeifer, M.A. (1991). Sex differences in the management of coronary artery disease. *New England Journal of Medicine, 325*(4), 226–230.

Katz, A.M. (1992). *Physiology of the Heart.* New York: Raven Press.

Khaw, K.T., Chir, M.B.B., Tazuke, S., & Barrett-Conner, E. (1988). Cigarette smoking and levels of adrenal androgens in postmenopausal women. *New England Journal of Medicine, 318*(26), 1705–1709.

LaRosa, J.H. (1988). Women's work and health: Employment as a risk factor for CHD. *American Journal of Obstetrics and Gynecology, 158,* 6(2), 1597–1602.

Lerner, D.J., & Lannel, W.B. (1986). Patterns of coronary heart disease morbidity and mortality in the sexes: A 26-year follow-up of the Framingham population. *American Heart Journal, 111*(2), 383–390.

Lobo, R.A. (1993). Hormones, hormone replacement therapy, and heart disease. In P.S. Douglas (Ed.), *Cardiovascular Health and Disease in Women.* Philadelphia: W.B. Saunders Co., pp. 153–173.

Lynn, D. (1966). The process of learning parental and sex role orientation. *Journal of Marriage and Family, 28,* 466–470.

Manson, J.E., Colditz, G.A., & Stampfer, M.J. (1991). A prospective study on maturity-onset diabetes mellitus and risk of coronary heart disease and stroke in women. *Archives of Internal Medicine, 151,* 1141–1147.

Manson, J.E., Stampfer, M.J., Colditz, G.A., Willett, W.C., Rosner, B. Speizer, F.E., & Hennekens, C.H. (1991). A prospective study of aspirin use and primary prevention of cardiovascular disease in women. *Journal of the American Medical Association, 266*(4), 521–527.

Maynard, C., & Weaver, W.D. (1992). Treatment of women with acute MI: New findings from the MITI Registry. *Journal of Myocardial Ischemia, 4*(8), 27–37.

Mark, D.B., Shaw, L.K., DeLong, E.R., Califf, R.M., & Pryor, D.B. (1994). Absence of sex bias in the referral of patients for cardiac cathetedzation. *New England Journal of Medicine, 330*(16), 1101–1106.

New England Journal of Medicine (1991). Uncertainty about postmenopausal estrogen [Editorial]. *New England Journal of Medicine, 325*(11), 800–802.

Papadoloulos, C., Beaumont, C., Shelley, S.I., & Lardmore, P. (1983). Myocardial infarction and sexual activity of the female patient. *Archives of Internal Medicine, 143,* 1528–1530.

Pender, N.J. (1987). *Health Promotion in Nursing Practice.* 2nd ed. Norwalk, CT: Appleton & Lange, pp. 37–72.

Pickett, S. (1993). Women, thrombolytic therapy, and the gender gap: Recommendations for practice. *Journal of Emergency Nursing, 19*(6), 491–497.

Rich-Edwards, J.W., Manson, J.E., Hennekens, C.H., & Buring, J.E. (1995). The primary prevention of coronary heart disease in women. *New England Journal of Medicine, 332*(26), 1758–1766.

Reis, S.E., Gloth, S.T., Blumenthal, R.S., Resar, J.R., Zacur, H.A., Gerstenblith, G., & Brinker, J.A. (1994). *Circulation, 89*(1), 52–60.

Romeo, K.C. (1995). The female heart: Physiological aspects of cardiovascular disease in women. *Dimensions of Critical Care Nursing, 14*(4), 170–177.

Rosenberg, L., Hennekens, C.H., & Rosner, B. (1981). Early menopause and the risk of myocardial infarction. *American Journal of Obstetrics and Gynecology, 139*(47), 1012–1030.

Rosenfield, S. (1989). The effects of women's employment: Personal control and sex differences in mental health. *Journal of Health and Behavior, 30,* 77–91.

Schmidt, S.B., & Borsch, M.A. (1991). Pre-hospital delay among women with acute myocardial infarction. *Journal of the American College of Cardiology.* 17(187A).

Sherwin, S. (1994). Women in clinical studies: A feminist view. *Cambridge Quarterly of Healthcare Ethics (3),* 533–538.

Stampfer, M.J., Colditz, G.A., Willeft, W.C., Manson, J.E., Rosner, B., Speizer, F.E., & Hennekens, C.H. (1991). Postmenopausal estrogen therapy and cardiovascular disease; Ten-year follow-up from the Nurses' Health Study. *New England Journal of Medicine, 325*(11), 756–762.

Steingart, R.M., Packer, M., Hamm, P., Coglianese, M.E., Gersh, B., Geltman, E.M., Sollano, J., Katz, S., Moye, L., Basta, L.L., P., Jacobson, K., Brown, E.J., Kukin, M.L., Tofler, G.H., Stone, P.H., Muller, J.E., Willich, S.N., Davis, V.G., Poole, K., Strauss, H.W., Willerson, J.T., Jaffe, A.S., Robertson, T., Passamani, E., & Braunwald, E. (1987). Effects of gender and race on prognosis after myocardial infarction: Adverse prognosis for women, particularly black women. *Journal of the American College of Cardiology, 9*(3), 473–482.

Webb, M.S., & Riggin, O.Z. (1994). A comparison of anxiety levels of female and male patients with myocardial infarction. *Critical Care Nurse* (February), 118–124.

Wenger, N.K., Speroff, L., & Packard, B. (1993). Cardiovascular health and disease in women. *New England Journal of Medicine, 329*(4), 247–256.

Wenger, N.K. (1985). Coronary disease in women. *Annual Review of Medicine, 36,* 285–294.

Wingate, S. (1991). Woman and coronary heart disease: Implications for the critical care setting. *Focus on Critical Care/AACN, 18*(3), 212–219.

Writing Group for PEPI Trial (1995). Effects of estrogen or estrogen/progestin regimens on heart disease risk factors in postmenopausal women: The Postmenopausal Estrogen/Progestin Interventions (PEPI) Trial. *Journal of the American Medical Association, 273*(3), 199–208.

CHAPTER 15

Ethnicity and Coronary Heart Disease

Catherine Pianka
Colleen Keller

Despite a decline in mortality, coronary heart disease (CHD) remains the leading cause of death in the United States, accounting for over 480,000 deaths in 1992 (American Heart Association, 1994). These mortality declines have occurred among whites, African Americans, Hispanic Americans, Asian Americans, and Pacific Islanders in two age groups: 45–64 years and 65 years and greater. For Native Americans and Alaskan natives, however, mortality rose in both age groups (Gall & Gall, 1993).

Evidence from both epidemiologic and clinical studies documents the relationship between predisposing risk factors for CHD and subsequent coronary events (Kannel, 1990). Although CHD risk factors have been less well studied in ethnic groups, the prominent risk factors of hypertension, obesity, diabetes mellitus, elevated serum lipids, cigarette smoking, and sedentary lifestyle are evident among those groups studied (Kingston & Smith, 1997; Kannel, 1990; Semjos, Cleeman, Carrol, et al., 1993). Along with these known risk factors, cultural practices, genetic factors, stressors, differences in access to health care, health maintenance behavior, and socioeconomic status are often associated with risk-factor development

(Kingston & Smith, 1997; Howard, Welty, Fabsitz, et al., 1992; Public Health Service, 1990).

African Americans, Native Americans, Hispanics, Asian Americans, and Pacific Islanders are the most widely studied ethnic groups in the United States with respect to CHD prevalence and predominant risk factors. Considerable time has been devoted to the research supporting ethnic differences because of their importance and the limited attention they have received in previous nursing texts. Strategies for decreasing risk-factor development will be addressed as nursing implications in the last section of this chapter. Because of differences in the terminology used to address cultural issues and identify populations in different regions and at different times, we have used the exact terminology in relevant research as much as possible. Therefore, the terms *race, ethnicity,* and *cultural differences* are used, as well as ethnic terms such as *Anglo, Hispanic, Native American,* and *Asian American.*

AFRICAN AMERICANS

Despite a decline in the death rate from CHD in African Americans, this disease remains the leading cause of death for both African-American males and females of all ages. The 1991 death rates for African Americans from CHD were 144.6 for males and 88.3 for females (based on a population of 100,000). The death rate is 3.5% higher for African-American males than for white males and 33% higher for African-American females than for white females (American Heart Association, 1994). Data from the National Health and Nutrition Examination Survey (NHANES) follow-up study also indicate that both African-American men and women have a greater age-adjusted mortality than their white counterparts (Cooper & Ford, 1992).

Several risk factors contribute to the development of CHD in African Americans, including hypertension, obesity, unfavorable lipoprotein profiles, diabetes mellitus, smoking, and sedentary lifestyle, all of which are more prevalent in this racial group (Lewis, Raczynski, Oberman, et al., 1991).

Hypertension

Hypertension, a prominent risk factor, accounts for much of the high incidence of CHD among African Americans. One in three has hypertension (Dixon, 1994), and at the time of the first Health and Nutrition Examination Survey (HANES I), conducted in the early 1970s, 28.2% of African Americans had mild to moderate hypertension compared with 17% of whites (Saunders, 1987). Data from NHANES II indicated that the rate of hypertension had decreased in both African American men and women yet still remained higher than for whites (Rowland & Fulwood, 1984).

Data from the 1982 Maryland Statewide Household Survey, showed that 26.8% of African Americans over 18 years of age had hypertension versus 20.1% of whites in the same age group. Differences in the age of onset of hypertension between African Americans and whites have been documented. African Americans develop hypertension at an earlier age and have a higher prevalence in all age groups (Saunders, 1987). Data from the Bogalusa Heart Study, which measured blood pressure in African American and white children 5–11 years of age, showed that African American

children had significantly higher blood pressures than white children as early as 10 years of age (Voors, Foster, Fredricks, et al., 1976). Moreover, hypertension is one and a half to two times more common in African Americans of ages 30–69 years than in whites of that age group. African-American females over 50 years of age have a higher rate of hypertension than African-American males (Saunders, 1987).

The cardiac consequences of hypertension contribute to the high number of African Americans with CHD. Early left ventricular hypertrophy is three to four times more common in this group, regardless of age, blood pressure, or medication status (Oellet, Apostolides, Entwisle, et al., 1979) and is associated with increased cardiovascular morbidity and mortality, including CHD and sudden death (Saunders, 1987).

The causes of hypertension in African Americans have been studied extensively, and a variety of theories have been postulated to explain its higher incidence. Some theories suggest that African Americans may have a genetic predisposition for hypertension (Luft, Grim, & Weinberger, 1985). Differences in sodium handling may contribute to the hemodynamic and hormonal profiles of African-American hypertensives. The role of salt in blood pressure regulation has been studied extensively and is a critical factor in hypertension. African Americans with hypertension have demonstrated salt sensitivity, expanded plasma volume, and low renin levels (Saunders, 1991). The tendency of the kidneys of African Americans to retain sodium or excrete sodium less efficiently than whites may account for the high rates of hypertension among this population (Blaustein & Grim, 1991).

Another mechanism thought to cause hypertension in African Americans is a diminished capacity to extrude sodium from smooth muscle cells, which may promote an increase in intracellular calcium that facilitates contraction and increases vasoactivity (Blaustein & Hamlyn, 1983). Finally, nephrosclerosis may be more prominent in African Americans, resulting in a decreased glomerular filtration rate and a propensity for the development of essential hypertension (Luft, Grim, & Weinberger, 1985). In one study, African-American hypertensives with normal renal function had lower renal blood flow and more angiographically identified nephrosclerotic changes than white hypertensives (Levy, Talner, Coil, et al., 1978).

Although a genetic predisposition to the development of hypertension may exist, other factors, such as obesity, stress, socioeconomic status, and environmental factors, may also contribute to this disease process in African Americans (James, 1985).

Obesity

Obesity is a prevailing problem among African Americans, especially women. African American women of every age are more likely to be obese than any other racial or ethnic group (Willianson, Kahn, & Byers, 1991). *Obesity* is defined as being more than 20% over ideal body weight, whereas *overweight* is defined as being more than 10% over ideal weight (Verity, 1993). NHANES I data showed that African-American women not overweight at baseline were 60% more likely to become obese than comparable white women. The incidence of major weight gain for African-American women was 50% higher than for white women (Williamson, Kahn, & Byers, 1991).

Data from the Coronary Artery Risk Development in Young Adults (CARDIA) and the Atherosclerosis Risk in Communities (ARIC) studies showed that African-American women in their early twenties were significantly more obese than their white counterparts, with the race difference increasing over an age span of 18–30 years (Folsom, Burke, Byers, et al., 1991). Among African-American women in the childbearing years (20–44 years), 35% were overweight compared with 25% of white women in the same age group. Among African-American women 45–55 years old, 50% were overweight.

Among African-American men, the incidence of obesity was less prevalent. Only 10% of African-American men aged 20–44 years were obese compared with 16% of white men in the same age group (Dixon, 1994). Data from the Pitt County Study (1,784 black adults) showed that more women than men were at least 20% overweight (57% versus 36%). In addition, 20% of men and 76% of women had an increased waist-to-hip ratio (Croft, Strogatz, James, et al., 1992; Keenan, Strogatz, James, et al., 1992).

Some investigators associate obesity in African Americans with a diet high in fatty and fried foods. African-American cultural influences may play a role in cooking methods. Some African Americans use fat to cook everything from biscuits and fish to greens and fruit cobblers (Dixon, 1994). Other data show that, contrary to expectations, African Americans consume more fruits and vegetables than whites and that their intake of total saturated fat is less (Swanson, Gridley, Greenberg, et al., 1993).

Cultural self-image also influences obesity in this group. Many overweight African-American women do not see their weight as a problem (Dixon, 1994). In a study of African-American women 25–64 years old, 40% of those who were moderately and severely overweight considered their figures to be attractive or very attractive, indicating a positive body image. Overweight women were less likely to exercise, less likely to skip meals, and more likely to eat between meals than those who are not overweight. These findings suggest that although African-American women may be weight-conscious, the absence of strong negative social pressure associated with a positive body image may limit weight-loss efforts (Kumanyika, 1993).

Hypercholesterolemia

Hypercholesterolemia is a known CHD risk factor for all races. Data from the Framingham study has shown that CHD risk is directly proportional to *low-density lipoprotein* (LDL) cholesterol levels and inversely proportional to *high-density lipoprotein* (HDL) cholesterol (Keller & Fleury, 1993). A number of studies have indicated that African Americans have higher levels of HDL cholesterol and lower levels of LDL and of *very low-density lipoprotein* (VLDL) cholesterol than whites (Tyroler, Hames, Krishan, et al., 1975; Heyden, Heiss, Hames, et al., 1980; Tyroler, Glueck, Christensen, et al., 1981; Morrison, Khoury, Mellies, et al., 1981). This pattern of cholesterol distribution may exert a protective effect against CHD for this group (Curry, Oliver, & Mumtaz, 1984).

The Evans County Heart Study conducted from 1960 to 1967 in Evans County, Georgia, also revealed that African-American men had a lower incidence of CHD than white men, but there was no clear racial difference among women. In addition, the development of CHD in African-American women was unrelated to serum cholesterol (Gillum & Grant, 1982).

Diabetes Mellitus

Diabetes mellitus is associated with an increased risk of CHD and is the third leading cause of death in African Americans. One in 10 African Americans aged 45–65 years has diabetes, twice the rate for whites in the same age group. Over age 65, incidence of diabetes in African Americans is three times greater than in whites. One out of every four African-American women over 55 has diabetes (Dixon, 1994).

The Evan's County study suggests that the prevalence of diabetes among African-American and white men is about equal, but there is a higher prevalence among African-American women than among white women. The Howard University study conducted in 1980–1981 showed that 50.9% of African-American women admitted for myocardial infarction were diabetic, whereas only 21% of white women admitted with the same diagnosis had the disease. African-American men had a 25.3% incidence of diabetes, whereas white men had only a 10–20% incidence (Curry, Oliver, & Mumtaz, 1984). These studies indicate that diabetes occurs more frequently in both African-American men and women than in white men and women.

As previously discussed, obesity is prevalent among African Americans, especially women. As such, obesity may contribute to the frequent occurrence of diabetes mellitus in this group. In addition, the diet of African Americans may contribute to the development of diabetes. Although some studies show that African Americans tend to have a lower caloric and fat intake than whites, others show they may consume more cholesterol and less fiber. Fiber is thought to help control levels of glucose in the blood (Dixon, 1994).

Cigarette Smoking

Cigarette smoking also contributes to CHD development. In 1965, 40% of whites smoked cigarettes compared with 43% of African Americans. By 1987, 29% of whites smoked compared with 34% of African Americans (Goldberg, 1992). These data indicate that despite overall declines in smoking, more African Americans than whites continue to smoke. The Health Interview Surveys of 1965 and 1976 showed that although the number of African-American men aged 35–64 years who smoked had declined, the number of African-American women aged 45–64 years who smoked had increased. Despite this increase, there was a noted decline in CHD in African-American women. This finding suggests that even though smoking is a potent risk factor, changes in other risk factors such as hypertension and obesity may have a greater influence on CHD mortality (Gillum & Grant, 1982).

Physical Activity

Physical inactivity has long been associated with CHD. African Americans report that they participate in leisure activities and exercise less frequently than whites (Pearson, Jenkins, & Thomas, 1991). Data from the Physical Activity for Risk Reduction study, in which 99% of the participants were African American, indicated that 31% of the sample had not participated in any type of physical activity in the previous year (Lewis, Raczynski, Oberman, et al., 1993). The Behavioral Risk Factor Surveillance Survey Data from South Carolina demonstrated that African Americans living in the South, particularly women, had lower levels of leisure-time physical activity than their white counterparts (Washburn, Kline, Lackland, et al., 1992). In a sample of 2,658 women enrolled in the CARDIA study, African-American women had significantly lower scores of physical activity than white women (Bild, Jacobs, Sidney, et al., 1993). Data from the 1985 National Health Survey found that African-American women were less likely to exercise to maintain a favorable weight (Duelberg, 1992). Barriers to physical activity by African-American women may include low income, safety concerns, and lack of time (Ford, Merritt, Heath, et al., 1991). Despite these studies, data linking activity to the development of CHD in African Americans is sparse at this time.

Although favorable declines in CHD mortality rates for African Americans have been documented, many risk factors remain prevalent among this group. The cardiovascular risk-factor profile for African Americans is summarized in Table 15–1. Strategies for decreasing these risk factors will be discussed later in the chapter.

NATIVE AMERICANS

Mortality rates for cardiovascular diseases in Native Americans are lower than for the U.S. population as a whole, but these diseases remain the leading cause of death in this group. Regional variances in the prevalence of cardiovascular disease among Native American tribes were examined in the Strong Heart Study. The morbidity and mortality rates for cardiovascular diseases among several different tribes were estimated for three major geographic areas. Four

tribes in Arizona, seven tribes in southwest Oklahoma, and three tribes from North and South Dakota were studied. Although the Strong Heart Study is ongoing at the time of this writing, preliminary data have been able to differentiate prominent cardiac risk factors in separate tribes (Howard, 1996a; Howard, Welty, Fabsitz, et al., 1992).

Hypertension

Native Americans share many CHD risk factors with other races in the United States. Hypertension, the cause of 30% of all deaths in the United States, was once thought to be uncommon among Native Americans. Studies now indicate that the prevalence of hypertension in this population ranges from 7% to 22% for adults (Welty & Coulehan, 1993) with the southwestern Arizona Pima and Oklahoma tribes having a higher incidence of hypertension than the North and South Dakota Sioux tribes (Howard, Welty, Fabsitz, et al., 1992). Research suggests, however, that the incidence for

TABLE 15–1 African-American CHD Risk-Factor Profile

Risk Factor	Prevalence
Hypertension	• Hypertension is more prevalent in African Americans than in whites (Saunders, 1987; Rowland & Fulwood, 1984).
	• Hypertension develops earlier in African Americans than in whites (Voors, Foster, Fredricks, et al., 1976).
Obesity	• African-American women at every age are more likely to be obese than other groups (Williamson, Kahn, & Byers, 1991).
	• Fewer African-American men are obese than white men (Dixon 1994).
	• African-American women are more likely to be obese than African-American men (Duelberg, 1992).
Diabetes mellitus	• Prevalence of diabetes is comparable in African-American and white men (Curry, Oliver, & Mumtaz, 1984).
	• Prevalence of diabetes is greater in African-American women than in white women (Curry, Oliver, & Mumtaz, 1984).
Serum lipids	• African Americans have higher HDL, lower LDL, and lower LVDL cholesterol levels than whites (Tyroler, Hames, Krishan, et al., 1975; Heydan, Heiss, Hames, et al., 1980; Tyroler, Glueck, Christensen, et al., 1981; Morrison, Khoury, Mellies, et al., 1981).
Cigarette smoking	• African Americans have higher rates of cigarette smoking than whites (Goldberg, 1992).
	• African-American men and women smoke fewer cigarettes per day than whites of both sexes, despite their higher incidence of smoking (Curry, Oliver, & Mumtaz, 1984).
Sedentary lifestyle	• African Americans participate in fewer physical activities and less regular exercise than whites (Lewis, Raczynski, Heath, et al., 1993; Washburn, Kline, Lackland, et al., 1992; Pearson, Jenkins, & Thomas, 1991).

Arizona and Oklahoma tribes is comparable to that of the U.S. population in general (Howard, Lee, Yeh, et al., 1996).

Obesity

Obesity has a remarkably high prevalence in Native Americans, estimated at nearly twice the national rate (Broussard, Johnson, Himes, et al., 1991). The Strong Heart Study showed high rates of obesity among three groups of Native Americans (Welty, Lee, Cowan, et al., 1992). In Pima Indians aged 20–74 years, the age-specific prevalence of overweight ranged from 31% to 78% in men and from 60% to 87% in women (Knowler, Pettitt, Saad, et al., 1991). In Navajo adults aged 20–98 years, 30% of men and 50% of women were overweight (Hall, Hickey, & Young, 1992). Data from the 1987 National Medical Expenditure Survey indicate that the prevalence of obesity in Native American men was 13.7% compared with 9.1% of U.S. men, and 16.5% in Native American women compared with 8.2% of U.S. women. Among Native Americans from Montana (Blackfeet Reservation and Great Falls), 29–41% of the women were overweight (Goldberg et al., 1991). As with African-American women versus African-American men, Native American women showed a greater prevalence of overweight than Native American men, especially between the ages of 35 and 64 years (Broussard, Johnson, Himes, et al., 1991).

Obesity has not always been a health problem for Native Americans. At the turn of the century, obesity was rare in this group. In fact, malnourishment was common, as Native Americans were faced with periods of feast and famine. Many children died from diarrhea and respiratory problems brought on by malnourishment. After 1968 massive feeding programs were started by the U.S. government, supplying foods high in fat and calories but low in fiber. Concurrently, changes from a subsistence economy to a wage-earning economy were associated with more sedentary lifestyles. With these dietary and lifestyle changes, obesity in this group developed in less than a generation (Welty, 1991).

Metabolic differences between Native Americans and other groups may predispose them to obesity when food is abundant. A study of the Tarahumara Indians of northern Mexico, relatives of the Pima, demonstrates that a traditional diet and lifestyle may prevent obesity in these ethnic groups. The Tarahumara Indians, who maintain tradition, have virtually no obesity, low cholesterol levels, and rare or nonexistent cardiovascular disease (Welty, 1991). This fact suggests that increasing rates of obesity and overweight in Native Americans contribute to their rising rates of CHD.

Diabetes Mellitus

Diabetes mellitus is extremely prevalent among Native Americans, exceeding U.S. rates, except in Alaska. The prevalence of diabetes among Indian communities in the Strong Heart Study ranged from 33% to 72% (Howard, Lee, Fabsitz, et al., 1996). The Pima Indians of the Southwest, who have the highest rates of obesity, also have the highest rates of diabetes mellitus (Welty & Coulehan, 1993). The onset of diabetes mellitus has also been occurring at a younger age in Native Americans as the prevalence of obesity and overweight increases among them (Welty, 1991). The prevalence of diabetic retinopathy in a subsample of Sioux Indians of South Dakota who underwent eye examinations was 45.3% (Howard, 1996b).

Hypercholesterolemia

Hypercholesterolemia is less common among Native American tribes than in the U.S. population as a whole. Ten percent of cardiovascular deaths in the United States are attributed to total serum cholesterol levels of greater than 219 mg/ml. The mean serum cholesterol in southwestern Indians is generally 50–60 mg/ml lower than that of whites (Howard, Davis, Pettitt, et al., 1983). Cholesterol levels are higher in the Northern Plains Indians than in the Southwest Indians but are still lower in these groups than in most other populations (Welty, 1989).

Cigarette Smoking

Cigarette smoking is uncommon among the tribes of the Southwest, but the prevalence exceeds 50% among Northern Plains Indians and Alaskan natives (Welty, Tanaka, Leonard, et al., 1987). Among tribes in Montana, 50% of the women on the reservation and 62% of the women off the reservation smoke tobacco versus 34% of the men on the reservation and 63% of the men off the reservation (Goldberg, Warren, Oge, et al., 1991). Data on smoking behavior among adolescent Native Americans are alarming. In a survey of high school seniors from 1976 to 1989 ($n = 206,919$), the prevalence of cigarette smoking was highest among Native American youth (Bachman, Wallace, O'Malley, et al., 1991).

Physical Activity

Sedentary lifestyles were prevalent among the three geographic groups in the Strong Heart Study, but little quantitative data were available. Among tribes in Montana, 46–62% of those sampled were found to lead a sedentary lifestyle (Goldberg, Warren, Oge, et al., 1991). This

sedentary lifestyle can be attributed to lifestyle changes from patterns of manual labor, hunting, and foot travel to a more mechanized way of life (Leonard & Leonard, 1985).

Although overall CHD morbidity and mortality rates for Native Americans are lower than for all other U.S. ethnic groups, differences in the prevalence of this disease among the various Indian tribes persist. These differences reflect varying risk-factor patterns, including varying lengths of exposure to factors that disrupt traditional culture and nutrition and may be related to a genetic mixing with whites. In conjunction with genetics, the major risk factors—smoking, hypertension, increased serum cholesterol, and diabetes—may contribute to the differing patterns of CHD among Native American tribes. The CHD risk-factor profile for Native Americans is summarized in Table 15–2. Further study of the risk factors for specific tribal groups should be conducted so that appropriate interventions can occur based on individual tribal needs (Welty & Coulehan, 1993).

TABLE 15–2 Native American CHD Risk-Factor Profile

Risk Factor	Prevalence
Hypertension	• Prevalence of hypertension is 7–22% for Native American adults (Kannel, 1990). • Prevalence of hypertension varies among different geographic tribes (Howard, Welty, Fabsitz, et al., 1992).
Obesity	• Native Americans have twice the national rate of obesity (Broussard, Johnson, Himes, et al., 1991). • Prevalence of obesity is greater in Native American women than in Native American men (Boussard, Johnson, Himes, et al., 1991).
Diabetes mellitus	• Native American rates of diabetes mellitus exceeds U.S. rates (Welty & Coulehan, 1993). • Pima Indians of Arizona have higher rates of obesity and diabetes mellitus than other Indian tribes (Welty & Coulehan, 1993).
Serum lipids	• Native Americans generally have lower serum cholesterol levels than the U.S. population as a whole (Howard, Welty, Fabsitz, et al., 1983; Welty, 1989).
Cigarette smoking	• Smoking is uncommon in southwestern tribes, but the prevalence exceeds 50% among Northern Plains Indians and Alaskan natives (Welty, Tanaka, Leonard, et al., 1987). • Incidence of smoking among Montana tribes exceeds 50% for women on the reservation, 62% for women off the reservation, 34% for men on the reservation, and 63% for men off the reservation (Goldberg, Warren, Oge, et al., 1991). • Native American youth have the highest prevalence of cigarette smoking among U.S. high school seniors (Bachman, Wallace, O'Malley, et al., 1991).
Sedentary lifestyle	• In Montana tribes, 46–62% lead sedentary lifestyles (Goldberg, Warren, Oge, et al., 1991).
Physical activity	• Limited quantitative data are available on Native American physical activity patterns.

HISPANIC AMERICANS

Hispanic Americans share many of the same CHD risk factors as other ethnic groups in this country but in general have lower mortality rates from the disease. Even so, CHD remains the leading cause of death in this group. A Laredo, Texas, study conducted in the 1970s examined the distribution of CHD risk factors among Hispanic Americans of low socioeconomic class. Compared with non-Hispanic Americans, they had more than a 20% lower mortality rate from CHD (Derenowski, 1990). This same conclusion was drawn from studies of Hispanics in New Mexico and California (Friis, Nanjundappa, Prendergast, et al., 1981; Becker, Wiggins, Key, et al., 1988; Schoen & Nelson, 1981).

Serum Lipids, Obesity, and Diabetes Mellitus

The San Antonio Heart Study, begun in 1979, compared CHD risk factors in Mexican-American and Anglo men and women living in three socioeconomic neighborhoods in the San Antonio area. The risk factors compared were triglyceride levels, cholesterol levels, *body mass index* (BMI), cigarette smoking, alcohol consumption, and activity levels. The results demonstrated higher triglyceride levels in both Mexican-American men and women than in their white counterparts. Mexican-American women had lower HDL cholesterol levels than Anglo women, but levels were similar for Mexican-American and Anglo men. No male-female differences in total cholesterol and LDL cholesterol levels were found for either group (Haffner, Stern, Hazuda, et al., 1986).

An increased centrality of adipose tissue, as measured by the sum of scapular-to-triceps skinfolds was associated with increased triglyceride levels in these groups. Mexican Americans of both sexes had a higher centrality index than whites in this study, indicating a higher prevalence of obesity. An inverse relationship between obesity and the HDL/total cholesterol ratio was found in Mexican Americans of both sexes, indicating that the more obese they were, the lower the HDL cholesterol level was

and the higher the risk for CHD (Haffner, Stern, Hazuda, et al., 1986).

Diabetes mellitus is three times more prevalent in both Hispanic men and women than in non-Hispanic whites. In the men studied in San Antonio, diabetes was significantly associated with increased triglyceride levels and elevated systolic blood pressure in both groups, but only Mexican-American men had an association between diabetes and decreased HDL cholesterol. No association was found between diabetes and a change in HDL cholesterol in non-Hispanic white men.

Both Mexican-American and non-Hispanic white women also had a significant association between prevalence of diabetes and elevated triglycerides, decreased HDL cholesterol levels, and increased systolic blood pressure. Only in Mexican-American women was an increased total cholesterol level also associated with diabetes. These data suggest that there is little difference in the association between diabetes and CHD risk in either group of men, but a stronger association exists in both groups of women (Mitchell, Haffner, Hazuda, et al., 1992).

Hypertension

Hypertension in Hispanics was studied in both San Antonio and Laredo, Texas. The Laredo study found that (1) low-income Mexican Americans have a higher incidence of "actual" hypertension than U.S. whites and (2) Mexican-American women have a lower incidence than white women (Stern, Gaskill, Allen, et al., 1981). The San Antonio study found that incidence of hypertension was lower in Mexican Americans in general (Mitchell, Stern, Haffner, et al., 1990), but other studies restrict these findings to Mexican-American women (Stern, Gaskill, Allen, et al., 1981; Stern & Gaskill, 1978). The San Antonio study also found that incidence of hypertension was higher in younger Mexican-American men and in older white men. Despite these age-related differences, the prevalence of hypertension in Mexican-American versus non-Hispanic white men was not statistically significant (Mitchell, Stern, Haffner, et al., 1990). Although the role of hypertension in CHD in Hispanics is not clearly defined by these studies, lower socioeconomic status and obesity each appear to play a role in diagnosis and control of hypertension.

Cigarette Smoking

The extent and pattern of cigarette smoking among Hispanics is variable. More Hispanic men than white men smoke, but Hispanic men smoke fewer cigarettes per day (Haffner, Stern, Hazuda, et al., 1986). Hispanic women smoke 30% less often than white women and use fewer cigarettes per day (Remington, Forman, Gentry, et al., 1985; Humble, Samet, Pathak, et al., 1985).

Certain sociodemographic variables have been shown to be related to smoking behavior among Hispanics. For example, smoking patterns and smoking status have been associated with educational level. In Hispanics, smoking is increased in groups with less education (Samet, Howard, Coultas, et al., 1992). NHANES data found the degree of acculturation, especially among Hispanic women, was related to smoking behavior (Coreil, Ray, & Markides, 1991). In certain groups of Hispanic women, (i.e., Mexican Americans in their 40s and Cuban Americans in their 30s), the prevalence of smoking is higher than the national average (Pletsch, 1991). These findings suggest that, in general, Hispanics have lower rates of cigarette smoking but that those rates may rise with the adoption of Anglo values and behaviors (Marin, Perez-Stable, & Vanoss-Marin, 1989).

Physical Activity

Physical activity levels were also studied in Hispanic and non-Hispanic groups. Levels of recreational physical activity were higher for Mexican Americans in San Antonio (Haffner, Stern, Hazuda, et al., 1986) but lower for those in Orange County, with little difference noted in physical activity at work between the two groups (Friis, Nanjundappa, Prendergast, et al., 1981).

Many differences in CHD incidence have been noted between Hispanic and non-Hispanic groups, with socioeconomic status playing an important role in the prevalence of CHD among Hispanics. The San Antonio Heart Study clearly demonstrated the effect of socioeconomic status on CHD development by comparing three socioeconomic groups. The incidence of diabetes mellitus in both male and female Mexican Americans declined with increasing socioeconomic status. Men of low socioeconomic status had twice the incidence of diabetes mellitus and women four times the incidence of those in higher socioeconomic groups (Stern, Rosenthal, Haffner, et al., 1984). With progression from lower to higher socioeconomic status, the incidence of obesity among Mexican-American women declined and HDL cholesterol rose. Obesity was determined using various measures, including BMI, skinfold thickness, and triglyceride levels. No consistent trends in these indicators were noted in men, although men exhibited a rise in total and LDL cholesterol levels from lower to higher socioeconomic status (Stern, Rosenthal, Haffner, et al., 1984). These data have been interpreted to suggest that as Hispanic socioeconomic status improves, the adoption of Anglo behaviors and attitudes contributes to a decline in CHD incidence. However, caution in interpreting such findings should be exercised, because differences in socioeconomic classes within a cultural group do not inherently indicate cultural assimilation into the prevailing (i.e., Anglo) culture.

With a higher incidence of diabetes mellitus, obesity, and increased triglyceride levels, Hispanics in these studies had less favorable cardiovascular profiles than whites. The CHD risk-factor profile for Hispanic Americans is summarized in Table 15–3.

Evidence suggests that despite this less favorable profile, genetic factors may be present in Hispanics that protect them from CHD, as noted by the lower CHD mortality rates. This phenomenon may be due to a genetic admixture with American Native Americans, who are relatively resistant to CHD (Coulehan, Lerner, Helzlsouer, et al., 1986). Genetic factors, if involved, may also operate differently in men and women, because this protection has been observed only in men (Mitchell, Stern, Haffner, et al., 1990). The ethnic protection from CHD in Hispanic women may be lessened by the detrimental effects of diabetes mellitus, which has a greater effect on CHD and lipid profiles in Hispanic women (Mitchell, Haffner, Hazuda, et al., 1992). Improvement of socioeconomic

TABLE 15–3 Hispanic American CHD Risk-Factor Profile

Risk Factor	Prevalence
Hypertension	• Hispanics have a lower prevalence in general of hypertension than other ethnic groups (Mitchell, Stern, Haffner, et al., 1990). • Younger Hispanic men have a higher prevalence of hypertension than white men (Mitchell, Stern, Haffner, et al., 1990).
Obesity	• Hispanics have a higher prevalence of obesity than non-Hispanic whites (Haffner, Stern, Hazuda, et al., 1986).
Diabetes mellitus	• Diabetes is three times more prevalent in Hispanics than in non-Hispanic whites (Mitchell, Stern, Haffner, et al., 1992). • Diabetes is associated with increased triglyceride levels and systolic blood pressure in Hispanic and non-Hispanic men and with decreased HDL cholesterol in Hispanic men only (Mitchell, Stern, Haffner, et al., 1992). • Hispanics and non-Hispanic white women have an association between diabetes and elevated triglycerides, decreased HDL cholesterol, and increased systolic blood pressure. Only Hispanic women had increased total cholesterol associated with diabetes (Mitchell, Stern, Haffner, et al., 1992).
Serum lipids	• Hispanics, both men and women, have higher triglyceride levels than non-Hispanic whites (Haffner, Stern, Hazuda, et al., 1986). • Hispanic women have lower HDL cholesterol levels than non-Hispanic white women (Haffner, Stern, Hazuda, et al., 1986). • HDL levels are comparable in Hispanic and non-Hispanic white men (Haffner, Stern, Hazuda, et al., 1986). • Total cholesterol and LDL cholesterol levels are comparable in both male and female Hispanics and non-Hispanic whites (Haffner, Stern, Hazuda, et al., 1986).
Cigarette smoking	• Prevalence of smoking is comparable among Hispanics and non-Hispanic whites (Stern & Gaskill, 1978). • More Hispanic men smoke than white men, but they smoke fewer cigarettes per day (Haffner, Stern, Hazuda, et al., 1986). • Fewer Hispanic women smoke than non-Hispanic white women (Remington, Forman, Gentry, et al., 1985; Humble, Samet, Pathak, et al., 1985). • Smoking is more prevalent in Hispanic groups with less education (Samet, Howard, Coultas, et al., 1992).

status, education, and acculturation appear to reduce the incidence of CHD in Hispanics. Strategies for risk-factor reduction will be discussed later.

ASIAN AMERICANS AND PACIFIC ISLANDERS

Japanese Americans form the largest group of Asian Americans in whom CHD has been studied. The Honolulu Heart Program, an extensive study of Japanese-American men living in Hawaii determined that CHD incidence in this group fell between the high rates for U.S. whites and the lower rates for Japanese men living in Japan (Yano, Reed, & McGee, 1984).

Other Asian-American and Pacific Islander groups are less well studied; however, some data are available. CHD risk factors were exam-ined in a group of Chinese, Filipino, and Japanese Americans ($n = 13,031$). In this study, the Chinese Americans had the lowest mean BMI, indicative of low obesity. The Filipino-American men and women had the highest prevalence of hypertension, and the Japanese-American men and women had the highest total serum cholesterol levels. Asian-American women in general had substantially higher rates of smoking than whites (Klatsky & Armstrong, 1991).

A major study conducted in the early 1970s compared CHD risk in men living in Hiroshima and Nagasaki, Japan, with Japanese men living on the island of Oahu. This study found that most CHD risk factors, with the exception of blood pressure, were higher in the Hawaiian group. Men in both groups with CHD had higher weights; greater subscapular skinfold thickness; higher serum cholesterol, triglyceride, and uric acid levels; and higher systolic and diastolic blood pressures. CHD risk related to smoking was also higher in the Hawaiian group despite the fact that more men in Japan were smokers (Robertson, Kato, Gordon, et al., 1977).

At the time of this writing, the Honolulu Heart Program is following a cohort of 8,086 Japanese Americans who were 45–68 years in 1965 for the development of CHD morbidity and mortality (Rodriguez, Curb, Burchfiel, et al., 1994). This study has already examined the degree of atherosclerosis in autopsy and compared it with the degree of smoking by these men. The degree of atherosclerosis in the coronary arteries was found to increase with the number of years of cigarette smoking but was not directly related to the amount of cigarettes smoked per day (Reed, Marcus, & Hayaski, 1990).

Serum cholesterol levels were also studied and compared between the groups. Cholesterol levels positively correlated with relative weight. The Hawaiian group had a 12% greater average relative weight than the Japanese group. Diet differences were evident, with the Hawaiian men consuming 23% of their calories as saturated fat compared with only 6.6% for the Japanese men (Robertson, Kato, Gordon, et al., 1977).

A similar study compared dietary habits of Japanese living in Hiroshima and ethnic Japanese from Hiroshima living in Hawaii and Los Angeles. Total energy intake was not significantly different between males and females of both groups. Intake of animal fats, saturated fatty acids, cholesterol, and simple carbohydrates was greater, and intake of complex carbohydrates was lower in the Japanese Americans than in those of Hiroshima. Japanese-American men and women also had higher serum cholesterol and triglyceride levels. HDL cholesterol was similar for the men of both groups but higher for Japanese-American women. Types IIa and IIb hyperlipidemia were twice as high in the Japanese Americans as in those of Hiroshima (Egusa, Murakami, Matsumoto, et al., 1993).

These findings suggest that westernization of dietary habits in Japanese Americans has led to increased death rates from atherosclerosis during the past 30 years. If this trend persists,

the incidence of death from CHD could continue to increase significantly for this ethnic group. Dietary changes appear to be associated with emigration patterns. The emigration of Japanese to Hawaii began in 1868 and continued for many generations. Second- and third-generation Japanese immigrants born in the United States now account for the majority of Hawaii's Japanese population. As first-generation immigrants are 70 years of age or older, and the second and third generations are in their 50s and 60s, Japanese Americans have had many years to adopt westernized dietary habits, with a resultant increase in CHD (Egusa, Murakami, Matsumoto, et al., 1993).

The longitudinal data from the Honolulu Heart Program documented positive correlations between baseline serum cholesterol and deaths from CHD at 0–6 years, 7–12 years and greater than 13 years (Stemmerman, Chyou, Kagan, et al., 1991). Although Asians historically have had low total cholesterol levels and low incidence of CHD, the westernization of some groups has had deleterious effects. For example, Asian-born Chinese living in New York City demonstrated higher levels of total cholesterol than rural and urban Chinese living in Shanghi (Pinnelas, DeLa Torre, Pugh, et al., 1992).

With changing dietary habits, the incidence of obesity has also became more prevalent among Asian Americans and Pacific Islanders. Overweight and obesity is most pronounced in Pacific Islanders, where it is reported at rates in excess of 50% in women (McGarvey, 1991; Aluli, 1991). But obesity alone is not a significant predictor of CHD in Asian Americans and Pacific Islanders. In combination with elevated blood pressure, elevated serum cholesterol and uric acid, and glucose intolerance, obesity contributes to CHD risk in these groups (Yano, Reed, & McGee, 1984).

Diabetes Mellitus

The contribution of diabetes mellitus to CHD has also been studied extensively in all Asian groups. Those with non-insulin-dependent diabetes are two to four times more likely to develop CHD than nondiabetics (Barrett-Connor & Orchard, 1985). Nondiabetic men with glucose intolerance have also been shown to have an increased CHD risk (Fuller, Shipley, Rose, et al., 1980). This increased risk may be attributed to abnormal lipids and lipoproteins, characterized by high levels of VLDL and low levels of HDL cholesterol (Pyorola, Laakso, & Uusitupa, 1987). Data from the Honolulu Heart Program support this assumption by demonstrating that men with abnormal glucose tolerance had high total and low HDL cholesterol, both of which are associated with CHD risk (Laws, Marcus, Grove, et al., 1993). Ischemic abnormalities on electrocardiogram associated with glucose intolerance and hyperinsulinemia support the hypothesis that insulin resistance underlies the increased risk for CHD in South Asian people (McKeigue, Ferrie, Pierpont, et al., 1993).

Physical Activity

Physical inactivity also plays a role in CHD development in Asian Americans and Pacific Islanders. In the Honolulu Heart Program, the highest relative risk for CHD mortality and morbidity was in those participants with the lowest physical activity index (Rodriguez, Curb, Burchfiel, et al., 1994).

Although very little data are available on CHD risk in all Asian American and Pacific Islander groups, the extensive study of Japanese Americans in the Honolulu Heart Program provides important information about this particular ethnic group. The CHD risk-factor profile for Asian Americans and Pacific Islanders is summarized in Table 15–4. Westernization of Asian Americans appears to play a significant role in the development of CHD. Further study of these American subcultures is needed to advance our knowledge of their CHD risk.

SUMMARY OF RISK FACTORS IN VARIOUS ETHNIC GROUPS

To summarize, despite some similarities in CHD risk factors among the ethnic groups discussed, there are differences in the prevalence of these risk factors. For example, African Americans have the highest incidence of hypertension, whereas Native Americans and His-

panics have the lowest. Obesity is common among all the groups, especially among African-American women and certain Native American tribes. High rates of diabetes mellitus also occur in all groups, with the highest rates among Native Americans and Hispanics. Unfavorable lipoprotein profiles are highest among Hispanic men and women, who have higher triglyceride levels than other groups, and among Japanese-American men and women, who have higher serum cholesterol and triglyceride levels than their counterparts in Japan. Cigarette smoking varies among the groups, with high rates found for African Americans, Hispanic Americans, and some Native American tribes. Physical inactivity and sedentary lifestyle are common among all these groups, although limited data are available, particularly for Native Americans and Asian Americans and Pacific Islanders.

Clearly all these ethnic groups share many common risk factors for CHD development, despite some differences in the prevalence of particular risk factors. Reduction of these risk factors is the goal of intervention. Specific intervention strategies will now be discussed.

IMPLICATIONS FOR PRACTICE

CHD is a serious health problem for all ethnic groups in the United States. Although the incidence of CHD varies among ethnic groups, the same risk factors apply, some more particularly than others for certain groups. Awareness of prevalent risk factors in each group and an understanding of related cultural beliefs, behaviors, and health practices are important in the development of programs to reduce CHD risk. Determining specific cultural variables, such as individual and group differences in health values, dietary practices, family life patterns, and ethnic health-care practices, will help to identify acceptable interventions for reduction of CHD risk (Derenowski, 1990). Interventions can be implemented through several different strategies, incorporating family involvement, community-based and school-based involvement, and role modeling.

TABLE 15–4 Asian American and Pacific Islander CHD Risk-Factor Profile

Risk Factor	Prevalence
Obesity	• Obesity is more pronounced in Pacific Islanders than in Asian Americans, with women having a 50% incidence of overweight and obesity (McGarvey, 1991; Aluli, 1991). • Obesity in conjunction with elevated blood pressure and serum cholesterol and glucose intolerance contributes to CHD in Asian Americans and Pacific Islanders (Yano, Reed, & McGee, 1984).
Serum lipids	• Japanese-American men and women have higher serum cholesterol and triglyceride levels than their counterparts in Japan (Egusa, Murakami, Matsumoto, et al., 1993). • Japanese-Amerian men consume 23% of their calories as saturated fat compared to 6.6% for their counterparts in Japan (Robertson, Kato, Gordon, et al., 1977). • HDL cholesterol levels are similar in both Japanese-American and Japanese men but higher in Japanese-American women (Egusa, Murakami, Matsumoto, et al., 1993).
Diabetes mellitus	• Japanese-American men with glucose intolerance have elevated total and lower HDL cholesterol levels (Laws, Marcus, Grove, et al., 1993).
Sedentary lifestyle	• The highest relative risk for CHD morbidity and mortality is in those Asian Americans and Pacific Islanders with the lowest physical activity index (Rodriguez, Curb, Burchfiel, et al., 1994).

Family Involvement

Family involvement is essential to initiating and maintaining lifestyle change. In many cultures, the family provides emotional and material security in times of illness (Tamez, 1981). For example, in Hispanics of lower socioeconomic status, the function of nursing the ill is assumed by mothers, grandmothers, aunts, or fathers rather than health-care professionals (Clayton-Benavidez, 1979).

CHD risk-reduction interventions should involve all family members, as each generation can benefit differently from intervention. Specific strategies for the family may include

1 Assessing family and maternal values in regard to feeding behaviors and feeding patterns that may lead to unfavorable eating habits and subsequently inadequate nutrition.
2 Assessing physical activity patterns and encouraging physical activity (e.g., sports involvement) as a lifestyle
3 Screening all children for early indications of hypertension and diabetes mellitus, especially if these disorders are prevalent in the specific ethnic group
4 Promoting early childhood awareness of heart-healthy lifestyle, which includes regular exercise and choices of healthy foods

5 Educating older children and adolescents about the dangers of cigarette smoking
6 Educating adolescents about choosing culturally relevant but healthy fast foods and managing weight
7 Providing smoking-cessation and weight-loss programs for adults
8 Providing dietary counseling for the primary food preparer, so that cultural foods can be prepared using less fat and salt

Creating an awareness of CHD risk and implementing specific age-related interventions can help reduce the incidence of CHD. Children and adolescents who learn early about healthy lifestyles are likely to become healthy adults. They also serve as role models for parents and grandparents in promoting a healthy lifestyle that will be passed down from generation to generation.

Community-Based Interventions

Community-based intervention for CHD risk reduction must take into account a community's specific health values and behaviors. Programs must be culturally relevant and geographically accessible to attract those participants for whom they are intended (Keller, 1990). Community-based strategies may include

1 Assessing the community's cultural food behaviors, meal patterns, and food preparation, then developing culturally relevant nutritional education programs to teach self-care skills (Jackson & Broussard, 1987)

2 Working with individuals or groups to identify and reduce barriers to risk reduction (e.g., lack of safe areas to exercise, prohibitive costs of healthy foods)

3 Conducting focus groups in churches and community centers to determine patterns of exercise and diet, prevalence of risk factors, health-care seeking behaviors, and value of risk reduction

4 Enlisting the help of primary care providers in community health centers to emphasize risk-reduction behaviors with their patients

5 Developing exercise and fitness programs for all age groups, as in the Zuni Diabetic Project, which teaches weight reduction and healthy eating habits to the Zuni Indians (Leonard & Leonard, 1985)

6 Providing smoking-cessation programs

7 Conducting hypertension and cholesterol screening in churches and community centers

8 Integrating programs focused at work-site intervention (e.g., the American Heart Association's work-site risk-reduction program) into community-based work settings

9 Enlisting community leaders and spokespersons to participate in risk-reduction programs that are community-specific

Before implementing any community-based programs, it is important to obtain a thorough knowledge of the community's specific CHD risk-factor prevalence and to involve individuals or groups from the community in the development of programs. The success of most programs is enhanced when community members are personally involved in their own health maintenance. Group support may also provide incentive for change in individuals.

School-Based Intervention

As 95% of American children are enrolled in school, the school becomes a natural "laboratory" in which interventions may be implemented and evaluated. School-based interventions can start children on the road to a healthy lifestyle before they develop poor health habits. Specific school-based interventions may include

1 Assessing school breakfast and lunch menus for heart-healthy foods, and enlisting help from school-based dietary consultants to plan heart-healthy menus

2 Providing physical education programs, such as after-school sports, to promote physical activity (Keller, 1990)

3 Providing nutritional programs that teach children how to choose healthy, affordable foods

4 Providing school-based programs from the American Heart Association that promote a heart-healthy curriculum as early as kindergarten (Keller, 1990)

5 Providing programs to promote early childhood awareness and education about cigarette smoking

6 Providing smoking-cessation programs for adolescents and teens

7 Screening for blood pressure to facilitate child and parent awareness of the potential for hypertension development (Keller, 1990)

8 Working with volunteer groups (e.g., American Heart Association, American Cancer Society) to conduct heart-awareness health fairs for screening and education.

All of these interventions are aimed at early awareness and education to promote heart-healthy lifestyles that can be maintained throughout a lifetime. Schools can include health education as part of an academic education for a well-rounded learning experience.

Role Modeling

Promotion of healthy behaviors can be accomplished through the use of role modeling. Those who act as role models of healthy behavior can influence others to adopt similar behaviors. Role modeling can be demonstrated in several ways, by many different people. Some methods for role modeling include

1 Using influential role models in the community (e.g., nurses, physicians, teachers)

who maintain healthy lifestyles of diet and exercise

2 Encouraging active involvement by community leaders in the promotion of group physical activities (e.g., road races, basketball or softball tournaments, exercise classes)

3 Using community leaders as public policy leaders (e.g., community cohesion in removing billboard advertisement for cigarettes and alcohol directed toward ethnic groups in ethnic neighborhoods)

4 Providing specific instruction and encouragement by health-care providers to change behaviors (e.g., smoking cessation)

5 Lobbying by parent groups affiliated with schools advocating low-fat, nutritious school menus

6 Encouraging children to act as role models of healthy behavior for parents and grandparents

Role modeling, when performed by those who are respected or admired in the community or at home, is an effective method of changing health behaviors of individuals or a community. People of all ages can act as role models of healthy living and may exert a great influence on others' personal health behaviors.

CONCLUSION

CHD remains the leading cause of death for African Americans, Native Americans, Hispanic Americans, Asian Americans, and Pacific Islanders. Except for Native Americans and Alaskan natives, declines in CHD death rates have been noted in each group. These declines may be attributed to a greater understanding of the specific incidence of CHD risk factors in these populations and the development of programs aimed at reducing risk. Cultural beliefs, behaviors, and health practices must be understood before risk-reduction programs can be implemented. A clear understanding of an ethnic group's values will provide a basis for successful intervention. Decreasing CHD risk through smoking cessation, weight reduction, physical activity, screening and monitoring for hypertension and diabetes, and diet modification can be achieved, based on the needs of a specific group.

Educational programs for CHD risk reduction should involve each member of the family. Children and adolescents who learn healthy behavior at an early age may be less likely to develop CHD later in life. Education and intervention can reduce the incidence of new cases of CHD, as well as the current incidence. Nurses and other health-care providers can play a major role in this risk reduction through creative and culturally relevant educational and motivational programs.

References

Aluli, N.E. (1991). Prevalence of obesity in a Native Hawaiian population. *American Journal of Clinical Nutrition, 53* (Suppl. 6), 1556S–1560S.

American Heart Association (1994). *Heart and Stroke Facts: 1995 Statistical Supplement.* Dallas, AHA National Center.

Bachman, J.G., Wallace, J.M., Jr., O'Malley, P.M., Johnston, L.D., Kurth, C.L., & Neighbors, H.W. (1991). Racial/ethnic differences in smoking, drinking and illicit drug use among American high school seniors, 1976–1989. *American Journal of Public Health, 81*(3), 372–377.

Barrett-Connor, E., & Orchard, T. (1985). Diabetes and heart disease. National Diabetes Data Group. *Diabetes in America* (NIH Publication no. 85-1468), XVI, 1–41.

Becker, T.M., Wiggins, C., Key, C., & Samet, J. (1988). Ischemic heart disease mortality in Hispanics, American Indians and non-Hispanic Whites in New Mexico, 1958–1962. *Circulation, 78,* 302–309.

Berinstein, D.M., Stahn, R.M., & Welty, T.K. (1997). The prevalence of diabetic retinopathy and associated risk factors among Sioux Indians. *Diabetes Care, 20*(5), 757–759.

Bild, D.E., Jacobs, D.R. Jr., Sidney, S., Haskell, W.L., Anderssen, N., & Oberman, A. (1993). Physical activity in young Black and White women: The Cardia Study. *Annals of Epidemiology, 3*(6), 636–644.

Blaustein, M.P., & Grim, C.E. (1991). The pathogenesis of hypertension: Black-white differences. In E. Saunders (Ed.), *Cardiovascular Diseases in Blacks* Philadelphia: F.A. Davis, pp. 98, 104, 106.

Blaustein, M., & Hamlyn, J. (1983). Role of natriuretic factor in essential hypertension: An hypothesis. *Annals of Internal Medicine, 98* (Suppl.), 785–792.

Broussard B., Johnson, A., Himes, J., Story, M., Fichtner, R., et al. (1991). Prevalence of obesity in American Indians and Alaskan Natives. *American Journal of Clinical Nutrition, 53,* 1535S–1542S.

Clayton-Benavidez, C. (1979). Variations and adaptations in nursing care of the elderly Mexican American. In M. Leininger (Ed.), *Transcultural Nursing.* New York: Masson Publishing USA, Inc., pp. 274–280.

Cooper, R.S., & Ford, E. (1992). Comparability of risk factors for coronary heart disease among black and whites in the NHANES I epidemiologic follow-up study. *Annals of Epidemiology, 2*(5), 637–645.

Coreil, J., Ray, L., & Markides, K.S. (1991). Predictors of smoking among Mexican Americans: Findings from the Hispanic HANES. *Preventive Medicine, 21*(4), 508–517.

Coulehan, J.L., Lerner, G., Helzlsouer, K., et al. (1986).

Acute myocardial infarction among Navajo Indians, 1976–83. *American Journal of Public Health, 76,* 412–414.

Croft, J.B., Strogatz, D.S., James, S.A., Keenan, N.L., Ammerman, A.S., Malarcher, A.M., & Haines, P.S. (1992). Socioeconomic and behavioral correlates of body mass index in black adults: The Pitt County Study. *American Journal of Public Health, 82*(6), 821–826.

Curry, C., Oliver, J., & Mumtaz, F. (1984). Coronary artery disease in blacks: Risk factors. *American Heart Journal, 108*(3), 653–657.

Derenowski, J. (1990). Coronary artery disease in Hispanics. *Journal of Cardiovascular Nursing, 4*(4), 13–21.

Dixon, B. (Ed.) (1994). *Good Health for African Americans.* New York: Crown Publishers, Inc.

Duelberg, S.I. (1992). Preventative health behavior among black and white women in urban and rural areas. *Social Science and Medicine, 34*(2), 191–198.

Egusa, G., Murakami, F., Ito, C., Matsumoto, Y., Kato, S., Okamura, M., Mori, H., Yamani, K., Hara, H., & Yamakido, M. (1993). Westernized food habits and concentrations of serum lipids in the Japanese. *Atherosclerosis, 100,* 249–255.

Folsom, A.R., Burke, G.L., Byers, C.L., Hutchinson, R.G., Heiss, G., Flack, J.M., Jacobs, D.R., & Caan, B. (1991). Implications of obesity for cardiovascular disease in blacks: the CARDIA and ARIC studies. *American Journal of Clinical Nutrition, 53,* 1515S–1518S.

Ford, E., Merritt, R., Heath, G., Powell, K., Washburn, R., Kriska, A., & Haile, G. (1991). Physical activity behaviors in lower and higher socioeconomic status populations. *American Journal of Epidemiology, 133*(12), 1246–1256.

Friis, R., Nanjundappa, G., Prendergast, T., & Welsh, M. (1981). Coronary heart disease mortality and risk among Hispanics and non-Hispanics in Orange County, California. *Public Health Reports, 96*(5), 418–422.

Fuller, J.H., Shipley, M.J., Rose, G., Jarrett, R.J., & Keen, H. (1980). Coronary heart disease and impaired glucose tolerance. The Whitehall Study. *Lancet, 1,* 1373–1376.

Gall, S.B., & Gall, T.L. (Eds.) (1993). *Statistical Record of Asian Americans.* Detroit: Gale Research, Inc.

Gillum, R., & Grant, C. (1982). Coronary heart disease in black populations. II. Risk factors. *American Heart Journal, 104*(4), 852–861.

Goldberg, R. (1992). Temporal trends and declining mortality rates from coronary heart disease in the United States. In I. Ockene, & J. Ockene (Eds.), *Prevention of Coronary Heart Disease.* Boston: Little, Brown and Company, pp. 41–68.

Goldberg, H.I., Warren, C.W., Oge, L.L., Helgerson, S.D., Pepion, D.D., LaMere, E., & Friedman, J.S. (1991). Prevalence of behavioral risk factors in two American Indian populations in Montana. *American Journal of Preventive Medicine, 7*(3), 155–160.

Haffner, S., Stern, M., Hazuda, H., Rosenthal, M., & Knapp, J. (1986). The role of behavioral variables and fat patterning in explaining ethnic differences in serum lipids and lipoproteins. *American Journal of Epidemiology, 123*(5), 830–839.

Hall, T.R., Hickey, M.E., & Young, T.B. (1992). Evidence for recent increases in obesity and non-insulin-dependent diabetes mellitus in a Navajo community. *American Journal of Human Biology, 4,* 547–553.

Heydan, S., Heiss, G., Hames, C.G., & Bartel, A.G. (1980). Fasting triglycerides as predictors of total and CHD mortality in Evans County, Georgia. *Journal of Chronic Disease, 33,* 275–282.

Howard, B.V. (1996a). Risk factors for cardiovascular disease in individuals with diabetes. The Strong Heart Study. *Acta Diabetologica, 33*(3), 180–184.

Howard, B.V. (1996b). Blood pressure in 13 American Indian communities: The Strong Heart Study. *Public Health Reports, 111* (Suppl. 2), 47–48.

Howard, B.V., Davis, M.P., Pettitt, D.J., Knowler, W.C., & Bennett, P.H. (1983). Plasma and lipoprotein cholesterol and triglyceride concentrations in the Pima Indians: Distributions differing from those of Caucasians. *Circulation, 68,* 714–724.

Howard, B.V., Lee, E.T., Fabsitz, R.R., Robbins, D.C., Yeh, J.L., Cowan, L.D. & Welty, T.K. (1996). Diabetes and coronary heart disease in American Indians: The Strong Heart Study. *Diabetes, 45 (Suppl 3),* S6–S13.

Howard, B.V., Lee, E.T., Yeh, J.L., Go, O., Fabsitz, R.R., Devereux, R.B. & Welty, T.K. (1996). Hypertension in adult American Indians. The Strong Heart Study. *Hypertension, 28*(2), 256–264.

Howard, B.V., Lee, E.T., Cowan, L.D., Favsitz, R.R., Howard, W.J., Oopik, A.J., Robbins, D.C., Savage, P.J., Yeh, J.L., & Welty, T.K. (1995). Coronary heart disease prevalence and its relation to risk factors in American Indians. The Strong Heart Study. *American Journal of Epidemiology, 142*(3), 254–268.

Howard, B., Welty, T., Fabsitz, R., Cowan, L., Oopik, A., Le, N., Yeh, J., Savage, J., & Lee, E. (1992). Risk factors for coronary heart disease in diabetic and nondiabetic Native Americans. The Strong Heart Study. *Diabetes, 41*(Suppl. 2), 4–11.

Humble, C.G., Samet, J.M., Pathak, D.R., & Skipper, B.J. (1985). Cigarette smoking and lung cancer in New Mexico's Hispanic and Anglos. *American Journal of Public Health, 75,* 145–148.

Jackson, M.Y., & Broussard, B.A. (1987). Cultural challenges in nutrition education among American Indians. *Diabetes Educator, 13*(1), 47–50.

James, S.A. (1985). Psychosocial and environmental factors in black hypertension. In W.D. Hall, E. Saunders, & N.B. Shulman (Eds.), *Hypertension in Blacks: Epidemiology, Pathophysiology and Treatment.* Chicago: Year Book Medical Publishers, Inc., pp. 132–143.

Kannel, W.B. (1990). CHD risk factors: A Framingham update. *Hospital Practice, July,* 119–130.

Keenan, N.L., Strogatz, D.S., James, S.A., Ammerman, A.S., & Rice, B.L. (1992). Distribution and correlates of waist-to-hip ratio in Black adults: The Pitt County Study. *American Journal of Epidemiology, 135*(6), 678–684.

Keller, C. (1990). Coronary artery disease in blacks. *Journal of Cardiovascular Nursing, 4*(4), 1–12.

Keller, C., & Fleury, J. (1993). Coronary heart disease in ethnic minorities. *Family and Community Health, 16*(3), 68–83.

Kingston, R.S., & Smith, J.P. (1997). Socioeconomic status and racial and ethnic differences in functional status associated with chronic diseases. *American Journal of Public Health, 87*(5), 805–810.

Klatsky, A.L., & Armstrong, M.A. (1991). Cardiovascular risk factors among Asian Americans living in Northern California. *American Journal of Public Health, 81*(11), 1423–1428.

Knowler, W.C., Pettitt, D.J., Saad, M.F., Charles, M.A., Nelson, R.G., Howard, B.V., et al. (1991). Obesity in the Pima Indians: Its magnitude and relationship with diabetes. *American Journal of Clinical Nutrition, 53* (Suppl. 6), 1543S–1551S.

Kumanyika, S., Wilson, J.F., & Guilford-Davenport, M. (1993). Weight-related attitudes and behaviors of black women. *Journal of the American Dietetic Association, 93*(4), 416–422.

Laws, A., Marcus, B., Grove, S., & Curb, J. (1993). Lipids and lipoproteins as risk factors for coronary heart disease in men with abnormal glucose tolerance. The Honolulu Heart Program. *Journal of Internal Medicine, 234,* 471–478.

Leonard, C., & Leonard, B. (1985). Zuni Diabetic Project. *IHS Primary Care Provider, 10,* 17–20.

Levy, S.B., Talner, L.B., Coil, M.N., Hall, R., & Stone, R.A. (1978). Renal vasculature in essential hypertension. Racial differences. *Annals of Internal Medicine, 88,* 12–16.

Lewis, C.E., Raczynski, J.M., Heath, G.W., Levinson, R., Hilyer, J.C. Jr., & Cutter, G.R. (1993). Promoting physical activity in low-income African American communities: The PARR project. *Ethnicity and Disease, 3*(2), 106–118.

Lewis, C.E., Raczynski, J.M., Oberman, A., & Cutter, G.R. (1991). Risk factors and the natural history of coronary heart disease in blacks. *Cardiovascular Clinics, 21*(3), 29–48.

Luft, F.C., Grim, C.E., & Weinberger, M.H. (1985). Electrolyte and volume homeostasis in blacks. In W.D. Hall, E. Saunders, & N.B. Shulman (Eds.), *Hypertension in Blacks: Epidemiology, Pathophysiology and Treatment.* Chicago: Year Book Medical Publishers, Inc., pp. 115–131.

Marin, G.M., Perez-Stable, E.J., & Vanoss-Marin, B. (1989). Cigarette smoking among San Francisco Hispanics; The role of acculturation and gender. *American Journal of Public Health, 79,* 196–198.

McGarvey, S.T. (1991). Obesity in Samoans and a perspective on its etiology in Polynesians. *American Journal of Clinical Nutrition, 53*(Suppl. 6), 1586S–1594S.

McKeigue, P.M., Ferrie, J.E., Pierpont, T., & Marmot, M.G. (1993). Association of early onset coronary heart disease in South Asian men with glucose intolerance and hyperinsulinemia. *Circulation, 87*(1), 152–61.

Mitchell, B., Haffner, S., Hazuda, H., Patterson, J., & Stern, M. (1992). Diabetes and coronary heart disease risk in Mexican Americans. *Annals of Epidemiology, 2*(1/2), 101–106.

Mitchell, B., Stern, M., Haffner, S., Hazuda, H., & Patterson, J. (1990). Risk factors for cardiovascular mortality in Mexican American and non-Hispanic whites. The San Antonio Heart Study. *American Journal of Epidemiology, 131,* 423–433.

Morrison, J.A., Khoury, P., Mellies, M., Kelly, K., Howitz, R., & Glueck, C. (1981). Lipid and lipoprotein distribution in black adults: The Cincinnati Lipid Research Clinics Princeton School Study. *Journal of the American Medical Association, 245,* 939.

Oellet, R., Apostolides, A., Entwisle, G., et al. (1979). Estimated community impact of hypertension control in a high-risk population. *American Journal of Epidemiology, 109,* 531–538.

Pearson, T.A., Jenkins, G.M., & Thomas, J. (1991). Prevention of coronary heart disease in black adults. *Cardiovascular Clinic, 21,* 263–276.

Pinnelas, D., DeLa Torre, R., Pugh, J., Strand, C., & Horowitz, S.F. (1992). Total serum cholesterol levels in Asians living in New York City: Results of a self-referred screening. *New York State Journal of Medicine, 92*(6), 245–249.

Pletsch, P.K. (1991). Prevalence of cigarette smoking in Hispanic women of childbearing age. *Nursing Research, 40*(2), 103–106.

Public Health Service (1990). *Healthy People 2000: National Health Promotion and Disease Prevention Objectives.* Washington, DC: U.S. Government Printing Office (DHHS Publication PHS 90-50212).

Pyorala, K., Laakso, M., & Uusitupa, M. (1987). Diabetes and atherosclerosis: An epidemiologic view. *Diabetes Metabolism Reviews, 3,* 463–524.

Reed, D., Marcus, E., & Hayaski, T. (1990). Smoking as a predictor of atherosclerosis in the Honolulu Heart Program. *Advances in Experimental Medicine and Biology, 273,* 17–25.

Remington, P.L., Forman, M.R., Gentry, M., et al. (1985). Current smoking trends in the United States: The 1981–83 Behavioral Risk Surveys. *Journal of the American Medical Association, 253,* 2975–2978.

Robertson, T., Kato, H., Gordon, T., Kagan, A., Rhoades, G., Land, C., Worth, R., Belsky, J., Dock, D., Miyaniski, M., & Kawamato, S. (1977). Epidemiologic studies of coronary heart disease and stroke in Japanese men living in Japan, Hawaii and California. Coronary risk factors in Japan and Hawaii. *The American Journal of Cardiology, 39,* 244–249.

Rodriguez, B.L., Curb, J.C., Burchfiel, C.M., Abbott, R.D., Petrivitch, H., Masaki, K., & Chiu, D. (1994). Physical activity and a 23-year incidence of coronary heart disease morbidity and mortality among middle-aged men: The Honolulu Heart Program. *Circulation, 89*(6), 2540–2544.

Rowland, M.L., & Fulwood, R. (1984). Coronary heart disease risk factor trends in blacks between the first and second National Health and Nutrition Examination Surveys, United States, 1971–1980. *American Heart Journal, 108,* 771–778.

Samet, J.M., Howard, C.A., Coultas, D.B., Skipper, & B.J. (1992). Acculturation, education, and income as determinants of cigarette smoking in New Mexico Hispanics. *Cancer Epidemiology, Biomarkers and Prevention, 1*(3), 235–240.

Saunders, E. (1987). Hypertension in blacks. *Medical Clinics of North America, 71,* 1013–1029.

Saunders, E. (1991). Hypertension in blacks. *Primary Care: Clinics in Office Practice, 18*(3), 607–622.

Schoen, R., & Nelson, V.E. (1981). Mortality by cause among Spanish-surnamed Californians, 1969–1971. *Social Science Quarterly, 62,* 259–271.

Semjos, C.T., Cleeman, J.I., Carrol, M.D., Johnson, C.L., Bachorik, D.S., Gorgon, D.I., Burt, V.L., Brietal, R.R., Brown, C.D., Lippel, K., & Riffend, B.M. (1993). Prevalence of high blood cholesterol among U.S. adults. *Journal of the American Medical Association, 23,* 3009–3014.

Stemmerman, G.N., Chyou, P.H., Kagan, A., Nomura, A.M., & Yano, K. (1991). Serum cholesterol and mortality among Japanese American men. The Honolulu Heart Program. *Archives of Internal Medicine, 151*(5), 969–972.

Stern, M.P., & Gaskill, S.P. (1978). Secular trends in ischemic heart disease and stroke mortality from 1970–1976 in Spanish-surnamed and other white individuals in Bexar County, Texas. *Circulation, 58,* 537–543.

Stern, M., Gaskill, S., Allen, C., Garza, V., Gonzales, J., & Waldrop, R. (1981). Cardiovascular risk factor in Mexican Americans in Laredo, Texas. II. Prevalence and control of hypertension. *American Journal of Epidemiology, 113,* 556–562.

Stern, M., Rosenthal, M., Haffner, S., Hazuda, H., & Franco, L. (1984). Sex differences in the effects of sociocultural status on diabetes and cardiovascular risk factors in Mexican Americans. The San Antonio Heart Study. *American Journal of Epidemiology, 120*(6), 834–851.

Swanson, C.A., Gridley, G., Greenberg, R.S., Schoenberg, J.B., Swanson, G.M., Brown, L.M., Hayes, R., Silverman, D., & Pottern, L. (1993). A comparison of diets of blacks and whites in three areas of the United States. *Nutrition and Cancer, 20*(2), 153–165.

Tamez, E. (1981). Familism, machisms and childrearing practices among Mexican Americans. *Journal of Psychosocial Nursing and Mental Health Services, 19,* 21–25.

Tyroler, H.A., Glueck, C.J., Christensen, B., Kwiterovich, P.O., deGratt, I., Chase, G., Mowery, R., & Tamir, I. (1981). Black-white plasma lipoprotein differences in children. *Circulation, 58* (Suppl. II), 31.

Tyroler, H.A., Hames, C.G., Krishan, I., Heyden, S., Cooper, G., & Cassel, J.C. (1975). Black-white differences in serum lipids and lipoproteins in Evans County. *Preventive Medicine, 4,* 541.

Verity, L.S. (1993). Fitness testing and aerobic programming. In R.T. Cotton & R.L. Goldstein (Eds.), *Aerobic Instructor Manual: The Resource for Fitness Professionals.* Boston: Rebok University Press and San Diego: American Council on Exercise, pp. 157–195.

Voors, A.W., Foster, T.A., Fredricks, R.R., Webber, L.S., & Berenson, G.S. (1976). Studies of blood pressure in children ages 5–14 years, in a biracial community. The Bogalusa Heart Study. *Circulation, 54*(2), 319–327.

Washburn, R.A., Kline, G., Lackland, D.T., & Wheeler, F.C. (1992). Leisure-time physical activity: Are there black-white differences? *Preventive Medicine, 21*(1), 127–135.

Welty, T. (1989). Cholesterol levels among the Sioux. *IHS Primary Care Provider, 14,* 35–39.

Welty, T. (1991). Health implications of obesity in American Indians and Alaskan Natives. *American Journal of Clinical Nutrition, 53,* 1616S–1620S.

Welty, T., & Coulehan, J. (1993). Cardiovascular disease among American Indians and Alaskan Natives. *Diabetes Care, 16* (Suppl. 1), 277–283.

Welty, T.K., Lee, E.T., Cowan, L., Fabsitz, R., Howard, B.V., Le, N., & Oopik, A. (1992). The Strong Heart Study: A study of cardiovascular risk factors in American Indians. *The IHS Primary Care Provider, 17,* 32–33.

Welty, T.K., Tanaka, E.S., Leonard, B., Rhoades, E.F., & Fairbanks, L. (1987). Indian Health Services facilities become smoke-free. *MMWR, 36,* 348–350.

Williamson, D.F., Kahn, H.S., & Byers, T. (1991). The 10-year incidence of obesity and major weight gain in black and white U.S. women aged 30–55 years. *American Journal of Clinical Nutrition, 53*(Suppl. 6), 1515s–1518s.

Yano, K., Reed, D., & McGee, D. (1984). Ten-year incidence of coronary heart disease in the Honolulu Heart Program. Relationship to biological and lifestyle characteristics. *American Journal of Epidemiology, 119*(5), 653–666.

CHAPTER 16

Radiation-Induced Coronary Artery Disease

Margaret I. Fitch
Elizabeth Keating

Oncology is the study of neoplastic diseases generally referred to as cancer. Investigation of the wide number of malignant growths that have potentially lethal sequelae has broadened the knowledge and understanding of how to manage this complex disease. However, caring for individuals diagnosed with cancer remains a challenge for today's health-care professionals.

Advances in science and medicine have influenced the ability to control cancer and prolong the survival of those diagnosed with cancer. In the 1930s, only one in five individuals diagnosed with cancer could expect to survive for 5 years or longer; today, one in three can expect to live longer than 5 years (National Cancer Institute of Canada, 1995). Primarily, this improvement in survival has been achieved through the three major cancer treatment modalities—chemotherapy, surgery, and radiotherapy.

The trends toward (1) identifying cancers earlier than in the past and (2) administering aggressive therapies have increased the survival rates for cancer patients. Additionally, larger numbers of individuals are reaching a stage of being "disease-free." Yet, any of these individuals may experience symptoms and side effects

many years after the completion of the cancer treatment (Tamlyn-Leaman, 1995). The specific side effects with which an individual may have to cope are related to the type of cancer and the treatment protocol. How well patients deal with these symptoms and side effects is often influenced by the patient's previous experience with cancer diagnosis and treatment.

This chapter will focus on one long-term side effect, radiation-induced coronary heart disease. With a growing number of individuals becoming long-term survivors of cancer, there is a cadre of people at risk for coronary difficulties many years after completing the cancer treatment. Nurses need to be alert to this potential long-term side effect, but many cardiovascular nurses and other clinicians may have limited exposure to the unique circumstances associated with care of the cancer survivor. Therefore, this chapter describes key areas of consideration in providing nursing care to individuals who receive mediastinal radiation, either at the time of the initial treatment or in the years following that treatment. Unlike previous chapters, which primarily focused on reducing CHD risk, this chapter will address the issue of living with unavoidable CHD risk within the context of cancer survival.

FACING A DIAGNOSIS OF CANCER

The impact of a cancer diagnosis and its treatment produces a burden of suffering that spans the physical, emotional, and social realms for individuals and their family members (Frank-Stromberg & Wright, 1984; Houts, Yasko, Kahn, et al., 1986; Blank, Clark, Longman et al., 1989). A cancer diagnosis is still perceived by many individuals as a "death sentence," engendering feelings of anxiety, loss of control, and helplessness (Canadian Cancer Society, 1992). Cancer treatment, in its various forms, can add to the feelings of helplessness and loss of control (Bushkin, 1993). Depending on the nature of the treatment, an individual may experience physical changes (loss of hair, loss of weight, loss of body or limb function) and treatment side effects (nausea and vomiting, fatigue, pain) (Fitch, Vachon, & Greenberg, 1995). In turn, such alterations carry the potential to influence family roles and relationships, work responsibilities, and communication with others. Clearly, cancer and its treatment can have an impact on both quantity and quality of life.

Because cancer has both a physical and psychosocial impact upon individuals, dealing with the disease and its treatment presents a myriad of issues for the person who has the cancer as well as that person's family members. Various reactions to the illness may emerge (Goldberg & Cullen, 1985; Krause, 1993). Although some individuals manage well with their situation, others experience difficulties and distress. Cancer is experienced as a single event for some people, with a defined beginning and ending, whereas for others, the cancer experience has a chronic nature (Heim, Augstiny, Schaffner, et al., 1993). Some will face recurrent disease; others may live with ongoing side effects from their treatment (Quigley, 1989; Halstead & Fernsler, 1994). In all cases, family members are affected. They, too, must cope with uncertainty and anticipated loss (Kupst, 1992; Hilton, 1994).

CONFRONTING STRESSFUL LIFE EVENTS

As individuals experience stressful events in their lives, their routine balance is disturbed (Antonovsky, 1981). They respond with a combination of feelings (emotions), thoughts (cognitions), and actions (behaviors) in an attempt to regain that sense of balance, or control. Most individuals have rather habitual ways of handling situations and usually will try to cope by using these ways. If these familiar ways do not work, a sense of distress emerges (Lazarus & Folkman, 1984).

Different people respond differently to the same event, and the same person may respond differently to the same event if it happens at different times in the person's life (Ilfeld, 1980; Folkman & Lazarus, 1980). This variation in human reaction results from a thought process called *cognitive appraisal* (Lazarus & Folkman, 1984). This process may occur at a conscious or unconscious level. When an event occurs, the individual engages in an inner dialogue to answer two questions. The first question (primary appraisal) is, "What is at stake, or how much harm is present?" Almost simultaneously the second question (secondary appraisal) arises: "Do I have the knowledge and skill to deal with this situation?" By answering these questions, the individual concludes he or she is either vulnerable (at risk) or resilient (can cope). Emotional distress emerges if the first conclusion ("I'm at risk") is reached.

Hence, the distress, or upheaval, a person feels is not inherent in the event itself, but rather is a product of the interaction between the event and the individual (Lazarus & Folkman, 1984). The process of cognitive appraisal leads an individual to assign meaning to the event. The response to the event and the subsequent approaches selected to cope with the event are based on the assigned meaning. The individual's past experiences, attitudes, skills, ideas, and feelings about the world become the frame of reference used to judge the current situation and also to choose a role to play in reacting to the event.

Illness can be conceptualized as a stressful event (Lipowski, 1969; Kiely, 1982). When illness strikes, it makes demands on an individual in a number of ways. The physical manifestations (e.g., shortness of breath, fatigue, pain), social interactions (e.g., inability to work, separation from family), and psychological shifts (e.g., increasing dependency, loss of control, altered body image) that can accompany an illness event create numerous opportunities for the individual to feel a sense of threat, harm, or loss. To a great extent, the perceptions people hold about their illness (the meaning they assign to their illness) and about the resources they have to handle illness will play an important role in how much emotional distress is experienced (Arpin, Fitch, Browne, et al., 1989). They will form an opinion about how dangerous the illness is to them (or how much inconvenience or hardship it causes, how many plans are thwarted by it, how much they risk losing because of it) and then select (either consciously or unconsciously) particular combinations of thinking, feeling, or behaving strategies to cope with the situation.

To help individuals cope with the diagnosis and treatment of cancer, it is important to understand the underlying meaning the illness has for them. Once the underlying meaning is understood, the observed behaviors may be more understandable and the direction for intervention clear.

Coping can be defined as "the ways in which individuals manipulate their environment in service of themselves or ways in which they change themselves in order to better fit the environment" (Cobb, 1976). Coping strategies serve to change the environment, change or control the meaning of the event, and control the emotional distress that has emerged. Coping strategies can also be categorized according to their focus on solving problems or handling emotions (Lazarus & Folkman, 1984). Relatively little is known about what particular combination of coping strategies a person will select. Often a person will use the coping strategies found to be successful in previous situations.

Coping with illness requires that an individual cope with a number of tasks (Moos, 1977). These tasks include (1) dealing with pain, incapacitation, the hospital environment, and treatment procedures; (2) developing relationships with professional staff; (3) preserving a reasonable emotional balance, a satisfactory image, and relationships with family members; and (4) preparing for an uncertain future. To handle these tasks successfully, people use various coping strategies (e.g., minimizing the seriousness of the situation, searching for relevant information, requesting support and reassurance, learn-

ing specific procedures related to the illness, setting concrete limited goals, rehearsing alternative outcomes, finding a general pattern of meaning) (Moos, 1977). The process of coping with illness may include a number of substantial life adjustments. Modifying the daily routine, adjusting lifestyles, dealing with role changes, grieving for losses (of abilities, hopes, income, dreams, social relationships, roles, dignity), and maintaining hope will create many demands on a person (Miller, 1983).

Cognitive appraisal is a critical factor influencing how people manage (Lazarus & Folkman, 1984). Individuals who are motivated by a challenge, feel in control of their lives, and make a strong commitment to whatever they are doing tend to cope more successfully than those who hold more negative perspectives (Kobasa, Hilker, & Maddi, 1979). In particular, negative meanings assigned to illness are associated with poor psychosocial adjustment in illness situations (Brown, Arpin, Fitch, et al., 1988).

Faced with a new illness event, such as CHD some time after treatment for cancer, memories of the former life-threatening illness return easily (Weiner & Dodd, 1993). Psychosocial issues that existed previously may resurface. Fears and concerns experienced during the past illness episode can return with intensity, and past coping patterns may emerge (Rawnsley, 1994). Helping an individual cope with the new illness event can be enhanced by understanding the individual's response to the previous event.

SURVIVORSHIP

Over 8 million people are diagnosed with cancer in the United States annually, and 5 million survive more than 5 years (American Cancer Society, 1993). In Canada, it is estimated there are at least 500,000 cancer survivors (National Cancer Institute of Canada, 1995). During the past 10 to 15 years, as the number of survivors has grown, several organizations have emerged as advocates in regard to survivorship issues (Tamlyn-Leaman, 1995).

Various definitions for the term *survivorship* in relation to cancer exist. The traditional medical perspective of a cancer survivor is one who has remained free from disease 5 years or more after diagnosis (Hassey Dow, 1991). But many people who have cancer or have had it do not use this definition (Leigh, 1992). Rather, they embrace the notion that cancer survivorship is a process that begins at the time of diagnosis (Adams, 1991; Gambosia & Ulreich, 1990; Rose, 1989). Mullan (1990), a leader within the survivorship movement in the United States, stated, "Survival, quite simply, begins when you are told you have cancer and continues for the rest of your life" (pp. 1–4).

Mullan (1985) described three seasons of survival. The first season, *acute survival,* begins with diagnosis. During this season, individuals are dealing with acute side effects of treatment, issues related to confronting mortality and intense emotions of fear and anxiety. The second season is that of *extended survival* following the completion of the initial treatment. Individuals in this season deal with severing the treatment-based supports and resisting fear of recurrence as well as adjusting to physical and psychosocial compromise. The third season, *permanent survival,* is most often associated with cure. The individual during this season focuses on long-term and late effects of cancer treatment, problems with employment and insurance, and reproductive health (Hassey Dow, 1990; Leigh, 1992).

Because survivorship is a relatively new area of study, accurate information about long-term or late effects of treatment is limited. Much of what we know is based on the experience of pediatric cancer patients (Loescher, Welch-McCaffrey, Leigh, et al., 1989). Relatively little work has been completed regarding survival rates for adult cancer patients and long-term effects of treatment. The potential for long-term psychosocial issues, though, has received some attention. The literature suggests that areas of difficulty may include psychosocial effects of physical alterations (body image and self-esteem issues), fear of cancer recurrence and death, uncertainty about the future, effects on family relationships, alterations in customary relationships with friends, reentry into the workplace, and employment and insurance discrimination (Welch-McCaffrey, Hoffman, Leigh, et al., 1989; Dudas & Carlson, 1988; Hassey Dow, 1991; Leigh, McCaffrey Boyle, Loescher, et al., 1993).

Individuals may experience difficulty planning for the future. Preoccupation with somatic ailments may be akin to a psychological cancer. Survivors acknowledge that the occurrence of physical symptoms reminiscent of the early stage of their disease triggers fears of cancer recurrence (Quigley, 1989). Investigators report that these issues are not being addressed consistently by health-care providers (Carter, 1989; Leigh, 1992).

Many potential physical sequelae exist to the major forms of cancer treatment, ranging from those that alter activities of daily living to those that represent major complications or secondary cancers (Hassey Dow, 1991; Loescher, Clark, Atwood, et al., 1990). Examples of effects that can limit activities of daily living include fatigue, arm stiffness, dermatologic problems, dental caries, and cataracts (Carnevali & Reiner, 1990). Organic complications may include sexual and reproductive dysfunction, vascular complications (lymphedema or cardiomyopathy), pulmonary complications (fibrosis), urologic complications (chronic cystitis), and gastrointestinal complications (cirrhosis). In general, the occurrence, frequency, and severity of the late effects or complications depend on many factors, including the type of cancer; the size, location, and extent of primary tumor; the intensity and type of treatment; and the age and overall health of the individual.

BIOLOGY OF CANCER

The pathogenesis (origin and development) of cancer has been attributed to certain mutations in the previously normal cell or group of cells (Rosenthal, 1991). The neoplastic process implies that the normal cellular growth-controlling mechanisms are somehow impaired because of (1) ever changing internal and external environmental factors and (2) the susceptibility of the individual to carcinogens. The resultant neoplastic cell reproduces independently in an uncontrolled and disorganized fashion and spreads from the original site to the surrounding tissues. Cancer cells are usually larger than normal cells, have bigger nuclei, are of varying sizes, and have abnormal shapes. Unlike normal cells, which have precise, specialized functions, cancer cells do not serve any useful function.

Cancer cells may arise in any body tissue at any age in response to a variety of stimuli. Stimuli may include physical or chemical agents, viruses, radiant energy, enzymes, and hormones. The mutation of cells may also be attributed to genetic or chromosomal factors. Identification of the exact cause of cancer—that is, understanding the process of transformation of a normal cell into a neoplastic cell—remains a complex problem for medical science. Given that there are over 100 different forms of cancer (Rosenthal, 1991), there is likely no single theory of causation.

Cancer treatment focuses on modifying the biologic behavior of the abnormal cells by enhancing the immune system or by using hormone or chemoradiation therapy (Moss & Cox, 1989). If the neoplastic process is not interrupted, a mass of tissue, or tumor, forms. If unchecked, this tumor may continue to grow and invade the surrounding tissues by direct extension (infiltration) or by permeation of the blood vessels or lymph system. In some instances, neoplastic cells may break away from the original tumor site and travel (metastasize) to other parts of the body.

Whether a tumor is contained within a local area or has spread to other parts of the body influences decisions about the type and extent of treatment. Cancer is potentially lethal and a challenge to treat because cancer cells can become widely disseminated throughout the body. Overall, early diagnosis of the disease is associated with better mortality and morbidity rates. Although the primary forms of treatment for cancer include surgery, chemotherapy, and radiotherapy, radiotherapy is the predominant factor influencing the subsequent development of CHD.

RADIOTHERAPY IN TREATMENT OF CANCER

Radiotherapy is an important modality in the treatment of local disease for individuals diagnosed with cancer (Moss & Cox, 1989; Coleman & Howes, 1990). Since the discovery of x-rays by Wilhelm Roentgen in 1895 and the discovery of the radioactivity of radium by Marie Curie in 1898, radiotherapy has proved itself a mainstay in cancer management. Cur-

rently an estimated 50–60% of patients diagnosed with cancer will require radiation therapy (either curative or palliative) during their illness.

The radiations of importance in the treatment of cancer consist of electromagnetic energy (waves) and subatomic particles. These radiations have the ability to displace electrons, or knock them out of their orbits around an atomic nucleus, producing the process called *ionization*. When atoms, such as living cells, are in the path of these rays, the radiations become ionized, physical and chemical changes occur in the cells, and biologic effects result (Hendrickson & Withers, 1991).

The *electromagnetic radiations* consist of x-rays and gamma rays, part of the continuous electromagnetic spectrum that includes radiowaves and light (Hendrickson & Withers, 1991). X-rays are produced in a device that accelerates electrons to high energy and then stops them in an appropriate target of copper or tungsten. Part of the stopping energy is dissipated as heat, and the rest is converted into x-rays. Gamma rays are emitted from the nucleus of a radioactive isotope. When such an unstable nucleus decays by emitting some particle, the excess energy is emitted as a monochromatic gamma ray.

The *particulate radiations* include electrons, protons, neutrons, and alpha particles (Hendrickson & Withers, 1991). Unstable atoms give up energy in the form of rays, or particles—alpha (α), beta (β) or gamma (γ)—to become more stable. The disintegration of the atom and the giving up of energy (emission of radiation) is known as *radioactivity*. It is possible to make stable chemical elements unstable by the use of nuclear reactors and high-speed particle accelerators. The rate at which atoms emit their radiation (disintegrate, or decay) is referred to as *half-life*. Half-life is the time required for one half of the atoms of a particular radioactive material to decay, or be reduced, to half its original activity. This could be hours, days, or years.

Impact of Radiation on Living Cells

The various types of radiation act on living tissues by altering, or ionizing, the atoms in the chemical systems of the cells (Hendrickson &

Withers, 1991). Ionizing radiations have the ability to affect living cells and create biologic effects. All cells, whether normal or malignant, go through a cycle of cell growth. The cell cycle consists of gap 0 (G0 is the resting/functioning phase), gap 1 (G1 is the metabolizing phase, or the phase of the commitment to reproduce), synthesis (S is the phase during which the DNA content is doubling), gap 2 (G2 is the phase for the building of energy reserves), and mitosis (M is the phase for cell division, or mitosis).

Radiotherapy does the most damage during the synthesis (S) and mitosis (M) phases of the cell cycle, because more essential cell material (i.e., DNA) is exposed during these times. Usually, the rapidly dividing malignant cells are more susceptible than are the nondividing, highly specialized normal cells. However, the ionizing rays cannot differentiate between the normal and the malignant cells and thus will damage both. Cells that divide fairly rapidly and consequently are susceptible to radiation include lymphatic tissue, bone marrow, intestinal epithelium, the germ cells of the ovaries and testes, and epithelial tissue of the skin. When these normal tissues receive radiation, the patient experiences side effects.

The ionization of living tissues, whether normal or malignant, leads to physical and chemical changes within the cell (Coleman & Howes, 1990). The energy absorbed by the nucleus of the cell can lead to chromosomal damage (mutation), cessation or temporary suppression of cellular reproduction (mitosis), blockage of immune responses, and cell membrane damage resulting in a breakdown of oxygen and nutrient supply. If the damage is minimal, the cell may recover and return to normal functioning. If maximal damage occurs, the cell will either die outright or be unable to reproduce itself. Usually the rapidly dividing cells are killed outright when irradiated. Other cells may die in the process of trying to divide or because of premature aging of the cell in which mitosis is halted.

As explained, radiation is harmful to normal tissues as well as diseased tissues (Hendrickson & Withers, 1991). Several factors influence the potential harm. A prescribed dose of radiation will be less harmful delivered in small doses over time than a large dose. Rapidly dividing cells with no specialized function are more susceptible to radiation than are slow-growing,

highly specialized cells. For example, lymphocytes and germ cells are more sensitive to radiation than are nerve cells or muscle cells.

Also, the larger the area of exposure to radiation, the greater will be the extent of the damage to the tissues. And increased tissue oxygenation enhances the effect of the radiation. But every person has an individual susceptibility to radiation, although generally a healthy person will respond more favorably than an unhealthy one.

The acute effects of radiation are a function of the dose delivered, the volume of tissue treated, and, to some degree, the rate of delivery. Normal tissues usually involved in acute reactions are the gastrointestinal tract, bone marrow, and skin. Treatment of the acute reactions is usually symptomatic, and the reactions disappear once the daily dose is decreased or the course of radiation is finished.

The late effects of radiation, directly related to fractionization of the dose and to the total dose delivered to the surrounding tissues in the treatment field, occur as early as a few months following completion of the treatment or as late as several years after radiation treatment. These effects, including tissue necrosis, fistulas, and dense fibroses, are chronic and may not bear any relationship to the earlier side effects. Radiation-induced CHD is one such side effect.

Planning for Radiotherapy

Ionizing radiation can be delivered in two ways. In *teletherapy,* the source of the radiation is some distance from the patient. The long distance is advantageous, because the dose is relatively uniform across a given volume and allows for dose-shaping, or modifying devices to be interposed between the source and the patient. In *brachytherapy,* the alternative method, the radioactive sources are placed directly into the tumor site. Overall, improvement in the power of the radiations is now combined with a more precise delivery.

Many centers are using telecobalt and linear accelerators, which provide a compact source of x-rays or electron beams. These electron beams are characterized by a high output at their center and a compact delivery. As a result, the heart, and other structures and organs further beyond the treatment target, receive relatively less radiation while there is a rapid dose buildup to the intended target.

The total dose to be given to an individual is determined by total treatment time (*protraction*), number and dose of daily treatments (*fractionation*), cell type, tolerance of the tumor bed, and response of the tumor and the patient to treatment. Despite the improvements and refinements developed in the use of radiation, tissue injury can still result. Generally, the incidence of radiation therapy complications is related to the radiation dose and fraction size.

Treatment of a tumor with radiation requires that the ionizing ray travel through normal tissue surrounding the tumor. As well, because the cancer can invade surrounding tissues, a certain margin of the normal tissue must be irradiated. The goal in radiation treatment is to achieve the greatest probability of an uncomplicated cure. The treatment course is planned with a view of effecting the least amount of harm to the normal tissue. The type of normal tissue surrounding the tumor and the ability that tissue has for repair are considered. For example, soft tissue or bone necrosis might be acceptable to achieve cure, whereas brain stem or spinal cord necrosis would not be acceptable. Normal tissues have different "tolerances" for radiation.

Thus, discussion of treatment options needs to include an examination of the *reward-risk ratio*. What potential side effects is one willing to risk in order to achieve significant tumor control with higher doses of radiation? The overall goal of radiation therapy is to eradicate the tumor while sparing normal tissues from long-term adverse effects. Undertreating a potentially curable tumor out of the fear of a complication would not be an acceptable option to most individuals. Most will accept a higher risk of injury, at some undetermined time in the future, for an improved chance of cure. It is likely that the concern regarding the development of late complications is tempered by the knowledge that the patient will often not survive long enough to experience many of these complications if the primary cancer is undertreated.

The significance of the reward-risk ratio can be demonstrated by discussing Hodgkin's disease. Kaplan (1972) determined that a 60–80% local recurrence rate existed when Hodgkin's

disease was treated with a total of 1,000 rads as opposed to a 1.3% local recurrence rate when 4,400 rads were administered. With a potentially curable disease, inadequate therapy is the greatest hazard.

CARDIAC PATHOLOGY

The focus for this chapter is on the specific late effect of radiation on the heart. According to Arsenian (1991), heart disease resulting from therapeutic radiation is well recognized. The incidence of heart disease after radiotherapy is approximately 30% (Arsenian, 1991). The heart appears to be the dose-limiting organ for thoracic irradiation, although this limitation is considered more in relation to acute side effects than potential long-term side effects. When the effects on normal vasculoconnective tissue become unduly severe, late complications of radiation therapy occur. Some of these complications may require corrective measures. They may be debilitating or even life-threatening.

The majority of radiation-induced CHD has occurred in patients previously treated for Hodgkin's disease (Byhardt & Moss, 1989). These patients tend to be younger at the time of their diagnosis and are frequently curable. Hence, they live long enough to suffer late effects. Patients treated for thymomas, seminomas (germ cell tumors), breast cancer, and lung cancer account for the remainder of the radiation-induced CHD.

Large doses of mediastinal irradiation are often administered to patients with Hodgkin's disease and non-Hodgkin's lymphoma (Gerling, Gottdiener, & Borer, 1990). The usual dose is 4,000 to 5,000 rads to the hila of both lungs and mediastinal lymph nodes. Extensive mediastinal irradiation is also given to treat the other cancers mentioned. The exposure of the heart to this amount of irradiation may cause several pathologic conditions, namely, (1) acute or chronic pericarditis, (2) transient pericardial effusion, (3) myocardial fibrosis with signs of restrictive cardiomyopathy, (4) dysfunction of the cardiac conduction system, and (5) CHD (Byhardt & Moss, 1989; Arsenian, 1992; Om, Ellahham, & Vetrovec, 1992; Benoff & Schweitzer, 1995).

The reactions of the cardiac tissues to radiation can be divided into acute, intermediate, and chronic phases. The immediate effect of radiation is inflammation of tissues followed by complete healing, or replacement with collagen and fibrosis formation. Chronic reactions result from damage to cells that are slowly dividing.

The most common cardiac complication of radiation therapy is acute or chronic pericarditis (Arsenian, 1992). *Acute pericarditis* is manifested by fever, pleuritic chest pain, a pericardial friction rub, and transient ST-T wave changes (not specific to elevation or depression). The incidence of acute pericarditis is approximately 10–15% for patients receiving over 4,000 rads to the mediastinum, with peak incidence occurring at 5–9 months after the completion of radiation treatments. This condition usually responds to nonsteroidal anti-inflammatory agents such as aspirin, indomethacin, or ibuprofen. In rare instances, pericardiocentesis or a pericardial window is required if symptoms are severe.

Chronic constrictive pericarditis may be seen more than 15 years after irradiation (Cameron, Ostersle, Baldwin et al., 1987). These patients experience a gradual worsening of dyspnea and peripheral edema. Their physical examination reveals evidence of jugular vein distention and distant heart sounds. The QRS voltage may be diminished on an electrocardiogram. It may be necessary to perform a pericardectomy to relieve these symptoms. The results of the procedure are worse in these patients than in those suffering the same symptoms from some other cause than radiation; the mortality rate appears to be about 20% (Arsenian, 1992).

Hurst (1990) reported that echocardiographic evidence of pericardial effusion occurs in approximately 39% of patients who have had mediastinal irradiation. These effusions are generally asymptomatic and do not require a specific intervention. Intervening with pericardial drainage is recommended only for an effusion that produces cardiac tamponade (Hillis, Lange, Wells, et al., 1992). The majority of these effusions resolve spontaneously within 2 years.

Large amounts of irradiation may cause myocardial fibrosis. The risk of developing myocardial disease is increased in individuals who have received cardiotoxic chemotherapy, such as doxorubicin (Arsenian, 1992). The individuals with extensive myocardial fibrosis usually develop signs and symptoms of a restrictive cardiomyopathy, such as fatigue and dyspnea. This cardiopathy is secondary to a decreased cardiac output and peripheral venous congestion. The right ventricle will often have a thickened endocardium and fibrinous deposits. Valvular thickening is characteristically left-sided and is caused by endothelial damage. The pathogenesis of myocardial fibrosis is that of radiation-induced capillary endothelial damage resulting in myocardial ischemia and injury, leading to fibrosis.

Conduction system abnormalities may result either directly from radiation damage or indirectly from vascular insufficiency. Long-term follow-up evaluations of patients many years after radiation therapy reveal that one third to one half have abnormal electrocardiograms (Watchie, Coleman, Rafflin, et al., 1987; Strender, Lindahl, Larsson, et al., 1986). Sinus tachycardia, low voltage atrioventricular block, and right bundle branch block are commonly found. The location of the heart's conduction system places it at high risk for damage from radiation. Fibrosis of the atrioventricular node is often seen. Complete heart block has also been noted in individual case reports, requiring insertion of a permanent pacemaker.

Effects of Radiation on the Coronary Arteries

Gillette and associates (1975, 1985) found that the vasculature of the heart was diminished by all fractionation schedules (the dose delivered per treatment) and with a variety of total doses of radiation. The higher the fraction size and the higher the total dose, the greater the decrease was in vasculature. The connective tissue, which is distributed between the muscle bundles throughout the heart, increases with increasing doses up to a maximum, after which increasing doses produce only small changes. The thickness of the posterior ventricular wall, as measured during diastole, increases with dose per fraction and total dose. Because of the lack of mitotic activity in the cardiac muscle, the myocardium is one of the more radioresistant tissues. Hence it is likely that most of the changes seen in heavily irradiated myocardium are a result of the radiation-induced vascular changes (Byhardt & Moss, 1989).

Large doses of irradiation may cause a marked acceleration of the atherosclerotic process, leading to CHD (Mittal, Deutsch, Thompson, et al., 1986). Atherosclerosis begins with radiation damage to the vascular endothelium. This damage induces platelet aggregation, fibrin deposition, and plaque formation.

Normally, endothelial cells provide a selective permeable barrier and a thromboresistant lining to the arterial wall. According to Ross (1990), disruption of this barrier has been shown to result in interaction between platelets and the arterial wall at sites of endothelial injury, resulting in the formation of an intimal smooth muscle proliferative response. The interaction of products released from the platelets and plasma constituents at the site of endothelial injury initiates a sequence of events: focal smooth muscle migration and proliferation lead to the development of a fibromusculoelastic lesion. Fibroblasts, which are normally found in the adventia, have been found in the intima of these patients. As smooth muscle cells migrate from the media, they are partially replaced by fibrous tissue.

A high-cholesterol diet has been found to accelerate this process in animal studies (Arton, Lofland, Clarkson, et al., 1965). Amromin and co-workers (1964) found that radiation alone produced minimal changes in the media of larger vessels. When the animals were given a high-cholesterol diet, a synergistic effect was noted, with a marked acceleration of atherosclerosis. It was thought that the degree of change was greater than what could be explained by diet alone.

The location of these lesions is an interesting phenomenon and reflects the altered pathophysiology of radiation-induced CHD. Patients with CHD attributed to mediastinal irradiation demonstrated proximal lesions of the left main, left anterior descending, and right coronary arteries, as well as at the ostium (Gottdiener, Katin, Borer, et al., 1983; Perrault, Levy, Herman, et al., 1985; Brosius, Waller, & Roberts, 1981). No distal disease has been reported. These arteries lie anteriorly in the mediastinum, in the field of radiation, and thus receive maximum doses. It is the proximal location of these

lesions that can lead to a sudden onset of symptoms, including progressive angina or even an acute myocardial infarction.

A growing number of studies have reported long-term effects regarding CHD, although the overall incidence of postirradiation lesions varies in estimates from 6% to 10–20%. The literature contains descriptions of many individual cases of myocardial infarction, mostly of young patients without major risk factors (Simon, Ling, Mendizabal, et al., 1984; Dunsmore, Loponte, & Dunsmore, 1986; McReynolds, Gold, & Roberts, 1976; Dollinger, Levine, & Foye, 1965). The average delay before onset of symptoms after completion of radiotherapy is 4 years, but symptoms may be delayed up to 15 years. Some large-scale retrospective studies have reported myocardial infarction occurring as long as 20 years after radiation to the mediastinum in the absence of other risk factors.

These reviews indicated that the incidence of severe CHD, cardiac events, and the cardiac-related death rate exceeded the expected rates based on the epidemiologic data (Annest, Anderson, & Hafermann, 1983; Boivin & Hutchison, 1982; Tommaso, Applefield, Scholis, et al., 1984). Hancock & Hoppe (1992) found that the risk of dying from heart disease was not significantly higher in patients who received a dose of mediastinal irradiation less than or equal to 30 Gy. In the control group of patients who were given doses higher than 30 Gy, the risk of dying was 3.5% times higher. This finding is of concern given that breast-conserving surgery followed by radical postoperative radiotherapy has emerged as the realistic alternative to mastectomy for many patients with early-stage breast cancer (Fuller, Haxbittle, Smith, et al., 1992). The addition of chemotherapy, either subsequent to or concurrent with radiation therapy, is being explored as well. The combined toxicities to the heart from these protocols have been documented (Valagussa, 1994) and are expected to increase as the protocols are administered to older age groups or individuals with early-stage disease.

IMPLICATIONS FOR PRACTICE

Radiotherapy has a role in the treatment of malignancy in the chest. Lung cancer and breast cancer may be effectively palliated with radiotherapy, whereas lymphomas, germ cell tumors, and seminomas can be cured. Although protection (shielding) for the heart has improved, mediastinal radiation remains a risk factor for CHD. A dose-effect relationship is present, the exact nature of which remains elusive (Stewart, Fajardo, Gillette, et al., 1995; Wallgren, 1992). A high cardiac dose (less than 4,000 rad in 20 fractions) is associated with a high incidence of cardiac disease. The risk factors for radiation-induced CHD include the total dose administered, the dose per fraction (low alpha/beta ratio), and the volume of heart irradiated.

These observations have several implications for nursing care. Prior to treatment, oncology nurses who are caring for individuals undergoing mediastinal radiation need to be certain that patients understand the potential risk factors for cardiac disease. During treatment, precautions must be taken to shield the heart from radiation. At follow-up oncology visits, the nurse needs to be alert to symptoms of dyspnea, fatigue, chest pressure, and syncopes.

The long period of time before the appearance of any cardiac difficulties can result in the patient forgetting about the previous radiation and its potential for long-term side effects. Similarly, the young age of those who may experience difficulties, and the location of the lesions (left main, left anterior descending, and right coronary arteries), leading to sudden progressive angina or even myocardial infarction in the absence of other cardiac risk factors, may catch both patient and health professional unawares. Especially for individuals who were treated for Hodgkin's disease and have survived longer than 10 years, the cardiac events occur at an age when traditional CHD factors and clinical suspicion are low.

The advanced-practice nurse can play a large role in providing the comprehensive long-term follow-up required by patients who have completed treatment. Yearly physical examinations to determine which individuals have signs and symptoms of organ toxicity and need further evaluation can be completed by a nurse practitioner. In addition to periodic or annual chest roentgenogram, evaluation via electrocardiography, and possibly echocardiography, should be utilized if individuals experience symptoms of dyspnea, fatigue, chest pressure, or syncope. This evaluation will allow for early intervention in the case of (1) potentially lethal problems, (2) identification of any rehabilitation needs, (3) education of patients and their families regarding long-term sequelae, and (4) provision of support and counseling as required.

Specific guidelines related to health maintenance and screening for CHD risk factors in patients who have survived chest malignancies should be followed. CHD risk-factor identification and modification can be incorporated into annual follow-up. The development of atherosclerosis can be slowed by means of the well-established synergistic effect of smoking cessation, regular aerobic exercise, control of hypertension and obesity, and dietary modification to a low-fat, low-cholesterol diet.

The significance of the need for follow-up guidelines will become more apparent as breast cancer survivorship increases. The ability to identify potential cardiac morbidities as this population increases can have a major impact on the cost of treatment, sense of survivorship, and ability to cope with a newly perceived threat. This population is highlighted because of the number of women at risk (left-breast cancer patients treated with mediastinal irradiation remain vulnerable to left ventricular exposure).

The nurse caring for the individual who has CHD and is confronting life-threatening illness needs to understand the meaning of the event to the patient. The nurse ought to carefully observe the patient and assess his or her mental and emotional status, as well as engage in active listening and supporting. A key area for assessment is the patient's cognitive appraisal of the situation and his or her coping resources. It is critical to discover the patient's perception of the event and whether or not adequate coping mechanisms are present. Understanding the impact of any previous cancer experience on the current situation may be key to understanding the patient's emotional response. The current episode may be reminding the individual of the previous event and influencing his or her emotional and behavioral reactions. Understanding the meaning that the current illness has for the patient places the nurse in a better position to identify the appropriate supportive intervention.

CONCLUSIONS

Radiation does constitute a risk factor for CHD. It is still unclear (1) whether abnormalities detected on functional tests of asymptomatic patients following radiation can predict cardiac complications, (2) whether postradiation CHD is related to the left ventricular volume irradiated or (3) whether the volume of lung included in the field influences the response of the heart to irradiation (Stewart, Fajardo, Gillette, et al., 1995). The best treatment approach is one of prevention. Because tolerance doses for pericardial disease are known, prevention during treatment delivery is possible. For those individuals who have received thoracic radiation and are at risk for CHD, patient education and judicious attention to symptoms are both critical.

References

Adams, M. (1991). Information and education across the phases of cancer. *Seminars in Oncology Nursing, 7*(2), 105–111.

American Cancer Society (1993). *Cancer Facts and Figures.* Atlanta: American Cancer Society.

Amromin, G.D., Gildenborn, H.L., Solomon, R., et al. (1964). The synergism of X-irradiated and cholesterol-fat feeding on the development of coronary artery lesions. *Journal of Atherosclerosis Research, 4,* 325–334.

Annest, L.S., Anderson R.P., Wei-i, L., & Hafermann, M.D. (1983). Coronary artery disease following mediastinal radiation therapy. *Journal of Thoracic and Cardiovascular Surgery, 85,* 257–263.

Antonovsky, A. (1981). *Health, Stress and Coping.* San Francisco: Jossey-Bass.

Arpin, K., Fitch, M., Browne, G., & Corey, P. (1990). Prevalence and correlates of family dysfunction and poor adjustment to chronic illness in specialty clinics. *Journal of Clinical Epidemiology, 43*(4), 373–383.

Arsenian, M.A. (1992). Heart disease after mediastinal radiotherapy. *Postgraduate Medicine, 91*(2), 211–215.

Arsenian, M.A. (1991). Cardiovascular sequelae of therapeutic thoracic radiation. *Progress in Cardiovascular Disease, 33*(5), 299–311.

Arton, C., Lofland, H.B., Clarkson, T.B., et al. (1965). Ionizing radiation atherosclerosis and lipid metabolism in pigeons. *Radiation Research, 26,* 165–177.

Benoff, L.J., & Schweitzer, P. (1995). Radiation therapy-induced cardiac injury. *American Heart Journal, 129*(6), 1236–1238.

Blank, J.J., Clark, L., Longman, A.J., & Atwood, J.R. (1989). Perceived home care needs of cancer patients and their caregivers. *Cancer Nursing, 12*(2), 78–84.

Boivin, J., & Hutchison, G.B. (1982). Coronary heart disease mortality after irradiation for Hodgkin's disease. *Cancer, 49*(12), 2470–2475.

Brosius, F.C., Waller, B.F., & Roberts, W.C. (1981). Radiation heart disease: Analysis of 16 young (aged 15 to 33 years) necropsy patients who received over 3500 rads to the heart. *American Journal of Medicine, 70,* 519–530.

Brown, G., Arpin, K., Fitch, M., & Corey, P. (1988). The meaning of illness questionnaire: reliability and validity. *Nursing Research, 37*(6), 368–373.

Bushkin, E. (1993). Signposts of survivorship. *Oncology Nursing Forum, 20*(6), 869–875.

Byhardt, R.W., & Moss, W.T. (1989). The heart and blood vessels. In W.T. Moss & J.D. Cox (Eds.), *Radiation Oncology: Rationale, Technique and Results.* 6th ed. Toronto: Mosby, pp. 277–284.

Cameron, J., Ostersle, S.N., Baldwin, J.C., et al. (1987). The etiological spectrum of constrictive pericarditis. *American Heart Journal, 113*(2, Pt. I), 354–360.

Canadian Cancer Society (1992). *Final Report on the Needs of Persons Living With Cancer Across Canada.* Toronto: Canadian Cancer Society.

Carter, B. (1989). Cancer survivorship: A topic for nursing research. *Oncology Nursing Forum, 16*(3), 435–437.

Carnevalli, D., & Reiner, A. (1990). *The Cancer Experience: Nursing Diagnosis and Management.* Philadelphia: J.P. Lippincott.

Cobb, S. (1976). Social support as a moderator of life stress. *Psychosomatic Medicine, 38,* 300–314.

Coleman, C.N., & Howes, A.E. (1990). Overall principles of cancer management: Radiation therapy. In *Cancer Manual,* 8th ed. Boston: American Cancer Society, pp. 85–97.

Cosset, J.M., Henry-Amar, M., Noordijk, E.M., & Hoope, R. (1993). Late nonmalignant complications of the treatment of lymphomas: Emphasis on long-term cardiac toxicity (Abstract). *Fifth International Conference on Malignant Lymphoma,* June 9–12, Lugano, Switzerland.

Cuzick, J., Stewart, H., Rutqvist, L., Houghton, J., Edwards, R., Redmond, C., et al. (1994). Cause-specific mortality in long-term survivors of breast cancer who participated in trials of radiotherapy. *Journal of Clinical Oncology, 12*(3), 447–453.

Dollinger, M.R., Lavine, D.M., & Foye, L.V. (1965). Myocardial infarction following radiation. *Lancet 2,* 246.

Dudas, S., & Carlson, C. (1988). Cancer rehabilitation. *Oncology Nursing Forum, 15*(2), 183–188.

Dunsmore, L.D., Loponte, M.A., & Dunsmore, R.A. (1986). Radiation-induced coronary artery disease. *Journal of American College of Cardiology, 8,* 239–244.

Fitch, M., Vachon, M., & Greenberg, M. (1995). The needs of patients attending the comprehensive cancer program. Paper presented at the 27th Clinical Oncology Society of Australia, Annual Scientific Conference, Adelaide, Australia.

Folkman, S., & Lazarus, R.S. (1980). An analysis of coping behaviour in a middle-aged community sample. *Journal of Health and Social Behaviour, 21,* 219–239.

Frank-Stromberg, M., & Wright, P. (1984). Ambulatory cancer patients' perception of the physical and psychosocial images in their lives since the diagnosis of cancer. *Cancer Nursing, 7*(2), 117–130.

Fuller, S.A., Haybittle, J.L., Smith, R.E., & Dobbs, H.J. (1992). Cardiac doses in post-operative breast irradiation. *Radiotherapy and Oncology, 25*(1), 19–24.

Gambosi, J., & Ulreich, S. (1990). Recovering from cancer: A nursing intervention program recognizing survivorship. *Oncology Nursing Forum, 17*(2), 215–219.

Gerling, B., Gottdiener, J., & Borer, J. (1990). Cardiovascular complications of the treatment of Hodgkin's disease. In M. Kacher & J. Redman (Eds.) *Hodgkin's Disease: The Consequences of Survival.* pp 267–295. Boston: Lea and Febiger.

Gillette, E.L., McChesney, S.L., & Hoopes, P.J. (1985). Isoeffect curves for radiation-induced cardiomyopathy in the dog. *International Journal of Radiation Oncology, Biology, Physics, 11,* 2091–2097.

Gillette, E.L., Maurer, G.D., & Severin, G.A. (1975). Endothelial repair of radiation damage following beta irradiation. *Radiology, 116,* 175–177.

Goldberg, R.J., & Cullen, L.O. (1985). Factors important for psychosocial adjustment to cancer: A review of the evidence. *Social Science Medicine, 20,* 803–807.

Gottdiener, J.S., Katin, M.J., Borer, J.S., Bacharach, S.L., & Green, M.V. (1983). Late cardiac effects of therapeutic mediastinal irradiation. *New England Journal of Medicine, 308,* 569–572.

Gyenes, G., Fornander, T., Carlens, P., & Rutqvist, L.E. (1994). Morbidity of ischemic heart disease in early breast cancer 15–20 years after adjuvant radiotherapy. *International Journal of Radiation Oncology, Biology, Physics, 28*(5), 1235–1241.

Halstead, M.T., & Fernsler, J.I. (1994). Coping strategies of long-term cancer survivors. *Cancer Nursing, 17*(2), 94–100.

Hancock, S.L., & Hoppe, R.T. (1992). Heart disease mortality after treatment of Hodgkin's disease (Abstract). *Proceedings of Annual Meeting of the American Society of Clinical Oncology, 11,* A1155.

Hassey Dow, K. (1991). The growing phenomenon of cancer survivorship. *Journal of Professional Nursing, 7*(1), 54–61.

Hassey Dow, K. (1990). The enduring seasons of survival. *Oncology Nursing Forum, 17*(4), 511–516.

Heim, E., Augstiny, K.F., Schaffner, L., & Valach, L. (1993). Coping with breast cancer over time and situation. *Journal of Psychosomatic Research, 37*(5), 523–542.

Hendrickson, F.R., & Withers, H.R. (1991). Principles of radiation oncology. In A.I. Holleb, D.J. Fink, G.P. Murphy (Eds.). *American Cancer Society's Textbook of Clinical Oncology.* Atlanta: American Cancer Society, pp. 35–46.

Hillis, L.D., & Lange, R.A., Wells, P.J., & Winniford, M.D. (1992). *Manual of Clinical Problems in Cardiology,* 4th ed. Boston: Little, Brown.

Hilton, A. (1994). Family communication patterns in coping with early breast cancer. *Western Journal of Nursing Research, 16*(4), 366–391.

Houts, P.S., Yasko, J.M., Kahn, S.B., Schelzel, G.W., & Marconi, K.M. (1986). Unmet psychological, social and economic needs of persons with cancer in Pennsylvania. *Cancer, 58,* 2355–2361.

Hurst, J.W. (1990). Radiation and the heart. In J.W. Hurst & R.C. Schlant (Eds.), *The Heart,* 7th ed. New York: McGraw-Hill, pp. 1529–1532.

Ilfeld, F.W. (1980). Coping styles in Chicago adults: Description. *Human Stress, 6,* 2–10.

Kaplan, H.S. (1972). Radiotherapy. In H.S. Kaplan (Ed.), *Hodgkin's Disease.* Cambridge, MA: Harvard University, pp. 281–287.

Kiely, W.F. (1982). Coping with serious illness. *Advances in Psychosomatic Medicine, 8,* 105–118.

Kobasa, S., Hilker, R.R., & Maddi, S.R. (1979). Who stays healthy under stress? *Journal of Occupational Medicine, 21,* 594–598.

Krause, K. (1993). Coping with cancer. *Western Journal of Nursing Research, 20*(6), 869–875.

Kupst, M.J. (1992). Family coping: Supportive and obstructive factors. *Cancer, 71,* 3337–3341.

Lazarus, R.S., & Folkman, S. (1984). *Stress, Appraisal and Coping.* New York: Springer Publishing.

Leigh, S. (1992). Cancer rehabilitation: A consumer perspective. *Seminars in Oncology Nursing, 8*(3), 164–166.

Leigh, S., McCaffrey Boyle, D., Loescher, L., & Hoffman, B. (1993). Psychosocial issues of long-term survival from adult cancer. In S. Groenwald, M. Hansen Frogge, M. Goodman, & C. Henke-Yarbro (Eds.), *Cancer Nursing: Principles and Practice.* Boston: Jones and Bartlett, pp. 484–495.

Lewis, F. (1986). Patient responses to illness and hospitalization. *Radiography 52*(602), 91–93.

Lipowski, Z.J. (1969). Psychosocial aspects of disease. *Annals of Internal Medicine, 71*(6), 1197–1206.

Loescher, L., Welch-McCaffrey, D., Leigh, S., Hoffman, B., & Meyskens, F. (1989). Surviving adult cancers. Part I: Physiologic effects. *Annals of Internal Medicine, 111*(5), 411–432.

Loescher, L., Clark, L., Atwood, J.R., Leigh, S., & Lamb, G. (1990). The impact of the cancer experience on long-term survivors. *Oncology Nursing Forum, 17*(2), 223–229.

McEniery, P.T., Dorosti, K., Schiavone, W.A., Pedrick, T., & Sheldon, W.C. (1987). Clinical and angiographic features of coronary artery disease after chest irradiation. *American Journal of Cardiology, 60,* 1020–1024.

McReynolds, R.A., Gold, G.L., & Roberts W.C. (1976). Coronary heart disease after mediastinal irradiation for Hodgkin's disease. *American Journal of Medicine, 60,* 39–45.

Miller, J.F. (1983). *Coping with Chronic Illness: Overcoming Helplessness.* Philadelphia: F.A. Davis.

Mittal, B., Deutsch, M., Thompson, M., & Dameshek, H. (1986). Radiation-induced accelerated coronary arteriosclerosis. *American Journal of Medicine, 81*(1), 183–184.

Moos, R.H. (1977). *Coping with Physical Illness.* New York: Plenum Press.

Moss, W.T., & Cox, J.D. (1989). *Radiation Oncology: Rationale, Technique and Results.* Toronto: Mosby.

Mullan, F. (1985). Seasons of survival: Reflections of a physician with cancer. *New England Journal of Medicine, 313,* 270–273.

Mullan, F. (1990). Survivorship: An idea for everyone. In F. Mullan & B. Hoffman (Eds.), *Charting the Journey: An Almanac of Practical Resources for Cancer Survivors.* Mount Vernon, NY: Consumers Union, pp. 1–4.

National Cancer Institute of Canada (1995). *Canadian Cancer Statistics.* Toronto: NCIC.

Om, A., Ellahham, S. & Vetrovec, G.W. (1992). Radiation-induced coronary artery disease. *American Heart Journal, 124*(6), 1598–1602.

Perrault, D.J., Levy, M., Herman, J.D. et al. (1985). Echocardiographic abnormalities following cardiac radiation. *Journal of Clinical Oncology, 3,* 546–551.

Quigley, K.M. (1989). The adult cancer survivor: Psychological consequences of cure. *Seminars in Oncology Nursing, 5*(1), 63–69.

Rawnsley, M.M. (1994). Recurrence of cancer: A crisis of courage. *Cancer Nursing, 17*(4), 342–347.

Rose, M. (1989). Health promotion and risk prevention: Applications for cancer survivors. *Oncology Nursing Forum, 16*(3), 335–340.

Rosenthal, C. (Ed.) (1991). *Neoplastic Diseases: Fundamentals of Clinical Oncology.* Chicago: Precept Press.

Ross, R. (1990). Factors influencing atherogenesis. In J.W. Hurst & R.C. Schlant (Eds.), *The Heart,* 7th ed. New York: McGraw-Hill, pp. 877–892.

Simon, E.B., Ling, J., Mendizabal, R.C., et al. (1984). Radiation-induced coronary artery disease. *American Heart Journal, 107,* 1032–1034.

Stewart, J.R., Fajardo, L.F., Gillette, S.M., & Constine, L.S. (1995). Radiation injury to the heart. *International Journal of Radiation Oncology, Biology, Physics, 31*(5), 1205–1211.

Strender, L.E., Lindahl, J., Larsson, L.E., et al. (1986). Incidence of heart disease and functional significance of change in the electrocardiogram 10 years after radiotherapy for breast cancer. *Cancer 57,* 929–934.

Tamlyn-Leaman, K. (1995). Adult cancer survivorship: Issues and challenges. *Canadian Oncology Nursing Journal, 5*(2), 45–47.

Tommaso, C.L., Applefield, M.M., Scholis, L. et al. (1984). Incidence and etiology of isolated left main coronary artery stenosis. *Chest, 86,* 284.

Valagussa, P. (1994). Cardiac effects following adjuvant chemotherapy and breast irradiation in operable breast cancer. *Annals of Oncology, 5,* 209–216.

Wallgren, A. (1992). Late effects of radiotherapy in the treatment of breast cancer. *Acta Oncologica 31*(2):237–242.

Watchie, J., Coleman, C.N., Rafflin, T.A., et al. (1987). Minimal long-term cardiopulmonary dysfunction following treatment for Hodgkin's disease. *International Journal of Radiation Oncology, Biology, Physics, 13,* 513–524.

Weiner, C.L., & Dodd, M.J. (1993). Coping amid uncertainty: An illness trajectory perspective. *Scholarly Inquiry for Nursing Practice, 7*(1), 17–35.

Welch-McCaffrey, D., Hoffman, B., Leigh, S., Loescher, L.J., & Meyskens, F.L. (1989). Surviving adult cancers. Part 2: Psychosocial implications. *Annals of Internal Medicine, 111*(6), 517–524.

Zacharias, D.R., Gilg, C.A., & Foxhall, M.J. (1994). Quality of life and coping in patients with gynecologic cancer and their spouses. *Oncology Nursing Forum, 21*(10), 1699–1706.

INDEX

Page numbers in *italics* refer to illustrations; page numbers followed by t refer to tables.